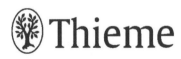

The Frontal Sinus

Surgical Approaches and Controversies

Christos Georgalas, MD, PhD, DLO, FRCS (ORL-HNS), FEBORL-HNS (Hon.)
Professor of Head and Neck Surgery
University of Nicosia Medical School
Nicosia, Cyprus;
Director of Endoscopic Skull Base Athens
Hygeia Hospital
Athens, Greece

Anshul Sama, MBBS, FRCS (Gen Surg), FRCS (ORL-HNS)
Consultant Rhinologist and Endoscopic Skull Base Surgeon
Nottingham University Hospital NHS Trust
Nottingham, UK

614 illustrations

Thieme
Stuttgart • New York • Delhi • Rio de Janeiro

Library of Congress Cataloging-in-Publication Data
is available from the publisher.

© 2022. Thieme. All rights reserved.

Georg Thieme Verlag KG
Rüdigerstraße 14, 70469 Stuttgart, Germany
www.thieme.de
+49 [0]711 8931 421, customerservice@thieme.de

Cover design: © Thieme
Cover image source: © Thieme/Martina Berge
The cover image was composed using following images
Head: © SciePro/stock.adobe.com
Drawings in circles: © Thieme/Katja Dalkowski
Typesetting by Ditech, India

Printed in Germany by Beltz Grafische Betriebe   5 4 3 2 1

ISBN 978-3-13-240052-8

Also available as an e-book:
eISBN 978-3-13-242669-6

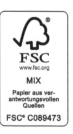

To my children, Odysseas and Fivos, born between countries, between eras, and to whom the future belongs.

To the victims and fighters of COVID-19 pandemic—those struggling to bring light in a time of darkness.

Christos Georgalas

To my wife, Sohini, for her patience and endurance.

Anshul Sama

Foreword

It is my great pleasure to write a foreword for this illuminating work which probably represents one of the most complete dissertations about the management of frontal sinus pathologies, with a special emphasis on surgical treatments. The authors have a great experience in dealing with nose and paranasal sinus pathologies, having shown a deep expertise on this argument and a clear intention to expand the limits of discovery in such a fascinating anatomical compartment; with this work they make available a huge wealth of knowledge for everyone concerned with this topic.

This book will be a valuable resource for novice surgeons approaching one of the most challenging anatomical subsites, since it provides a stepwise approach to understanding the anatomical background, the radiological aspects, and the broad spectrum of different surgical approaches to the frontal sinuses. However, it also represents a valuable tool for senior specialists, since it offers an overview of innovative advanced approaches presented by leading experts in the international surgical scene.

The essential skills to treat safely and effectively inflammatory, neoplastic, and traumatic diseases affecting the frontal sinuses are provided; in addition, the limits of different approaches and controversial topics in current practice are presented in detail.

Both external and endoscopic approaches are systematically presented, focusing on indications and contraindications, providing a step-by-step description of the surgical techniques with useful tips and tricks, as well as an overview of their complications. Additionally, the authors have included various conservative treatment strategies and minimally invasive modifications of traditional approaches which are currently employed in clinical practice.

Several photographic reproductions, crisp and clear illustrations, anatomical specimens, and representative clinical cases make the concepts easy to understand and its reading enjoyable. I could not find words to describe the stunning beauty of the images.

Finally, the authors take a look at the future, presenting the latest innovations in the field of techniques and technologies, opening new horizons toward effective and increasingly less invasive approaches which represent the frontier of contemporary surgery. The authors are to be congratulated for this masterpiece, which will become the gold standard for experts and beginners.

Highly accurate and effective works such as this are crucial to further solidify the surgical prowess of the ENT surgeons of the future.

Paolo Castelnuovo, MD, FRCSEd, FACS
Professor and Chairman
Head of Department of Otorhinolaryngology
Head of Department of Specialized Surgeries
University of Insubria
Varese, Italy

Foreword

"I wish that I knew ... when I was younger." This line from the band *Faces*, covered by Rod Stewart, captures exactly how I feel about this book on frontal sinus surgery! For me, the book captures more than 20 years of personal trial and error to find the most successful approaches to this complicated region. These approaches have been beautifully catalogued and described so that the reader can learn from the experts, who have already found success with them. Christos and Anshul have managed to compile every meaningful aspect of frontal sinus surgery and have covered it in detail. It is obvious that the descriptions and chapters have been honed by years of teaching courses, especially the "Frontal Sinus Surgery Course" in Nottingham, UK. This course has been sold out for over a decade, and I have been privileged enough to participate in it, along with my friends and colleagues. I never thought "work" could be so fun, and it is all due to my "sinus friends" (the authors and editors of this book) who

have made it so. I am sure you will like reading about and understanding the frontal sinus with this book as all the members of our group did producing it, led by Christos and Anshul!

I will leave you with another slightly silly quote—there was an advert in the States for Prego spaghetti sauce in the 1980s—and it ended with "It's in there!" The implied meaning was that everything good was in the sauce—well for *Frontal Sinus Surgery*, I can assure you "It's in there!"

James N. Palmer, MD
Professor and Director
Division of Rhinology;
Co-Director, Center for Skull Base Surgery
Department of ORL:HNS and Neurosurgery
University of Pennsylvania
Philadelphia, Pennsylvania, USA

Preface

"The most beautiful sea
hasn't been crossed yet.
The most beautiful child
hasn't grown up yet.
Our most beautiful days
we haven't seen yet."
                    –Nazim Hikmet

The last decade has brought a "democratization" of frontal sinus surgery—more and more people are interested in it, are writing about it, and are practicing it: What used to be the "final frontier" of endoscopic sinus surgery, exclusive domain of a small group of highly specialized rhinologists, is now part of the surgical armamentarium of a larger group of otolaryngologists dealing with frontal sinus pathology. This is reflected not only in practice logbooks but also in the success of dedicated frontal sinus courses (such as the Nottingham course) and the growth of publications on frontal sinus surgery over the last decade (a more than doubling in PubMed citations over the last 20 years). This book is both a result and a celebration of this trend.

There has been a proliferation of new techniques in conjunction with a better understanding of the role of surgery in the management of inflammatory disease. Although it would be elegant to present the evolution of frontal sinus surgery as a smooth transition from more traumatic (external) approaches to less invasive (intranasal) ones, reality is different: The history of frontal sinus surgery is more like a pendulum—from more extended (open) approaches to more conservative (mini functional endoscopic sinus surgery [FESS], limited FESS, balloon sinuplasty), and again back to more extended (full house FESS, Draf III, Denker), as better understanding of pathophysiology of what is primarily a medical disease makes us more humble and more open to different approaches. We understand that there is no place for "god-derived truths" in frontal sinus surgery—different approaches can be combined; different techniques, materials, and concepts have their place; and one should be careful in choosing the approach that fits the patient, the pathology, and the surgeon.

Looking back over the last 20 years makes us think how many new ideas have been introduced and subsequently abandoned. Precision medicine and the role of biologics are revolutionizing the management of inflammatory sinus disease. However, we feel that anatomy will always be key to its management as creating the space and providing local treatment to the frontal sinus will remain important. Endoscopic skull base surgery is both a product and a driving force of frontal sinus surgery techniques. Advances in reaching and operating in the frontal sinus have facilitated dealing with anterior skull base lesions and defects endoscopically, while our confidence in reaching intradural lesions has expanded the indications and applications of frontal sinus surgery.

The book is divided into five parts: Anatomy of the frontal sinus, endoscopic and open surgical techniques, management of specific frontal sinus pathologies, and controversies in managing the frontal sinus. Most parts are supplemented by video materials meant to illustrate the concepts and techniques described in the chapters.

Almost half of the book is dedicated to controversies: That is part of the book that we most cherish—we enjoyed being challenged by some of the authors, and having "crossed swords" in different settings, we consider the plurality of opinions not a weakness but a strength of the book.

Enjoy this book with an open mind, and we are looking forward to discussing the concepts, when the epidemic ends, in an open setting. Feel free to challenge us, the editors, the authors, and the publisher for anything you may disagree with. Remember:

vīta brevis,
ars longa,
occāsiō praeceps,
experīmentum perīculōsum,
iūdicium difficile.

[Life is short,
and art long,
opportunity fleeting,
experimentations perilous,
and judgment difficult.]

Christos Georgalas, MD, PhD, DLO,
FRCS (ORL-HNS), FEBORL-HNS (Hon.)
Anshul Sama, MBBS, FRCS (Gen Surg), FRCS (ORL-HNS)

Acknowledgments

We would like to thank Dr. Alexandros Poutoglidis, MD, MSc, PhD, Dr. Nikolaos Tsetsos, MD, MSc, PhD, and Dr. Amanda Oostra, MD, MSc, who very kindly reviewed and further amended the proofs.

Christos Georgalas, MD, PhD, DLO,
FRCS (ORL-HNS), FEBORL-HNS (Hon.)
Anshul Sama, MBBS, FRCS (Gen Surg), FRCS (ORL-HNS)

Contributors

Waleed M. Abuzeid, BSc (Hons), MBBS
Associate Professor;
Director of Rhinology Research
Division of Rhinology and Endoscopic Skull Base Surgery
Department of Otolaryngology
Head and Neck Surgery
University of Washington
Seattle, Washington, USA

Nithin D. Adappa, MD
Associate Professor
Department of Otorhinolaryngology
Penn Medicine
University of Pennsylvania
Pennsylvania, Philadelphia, USA

Shahzada Ahmed, MBChB, BSc (Hons), DLO, FRCS
  (ORL-HNS), PhD
Consultant Rhinologist and Skull Base & Surgeon
  Clinical Service Lead
Department of Ear, Nose and Throat (ENT) Surgery
University Hospitals Birmingham NHS Foundation Trust
Birmingham, UK

Fahad Alasousi, MBBCh, SB-ORL
ENT Senior Specialist
Endoscopic Sinus and Anterior Skull Base Surgery
Farwaniyah Hospital
Farwaniyah Governorate, Kuwait

Isam Alobid, MD
Skull Base Unit
ENT department
Hospital Clinic, Barcelona;
Professor Barcelona University
Barcelona, Spain

Abdulaziz Al-Rasheed, MD
Assistant Professor
Department of Otolaryngology
King Abdulaziz University Hospital
King Saud University
Riyadh, Saudi Arabia

Jeremiah A. Alt, MD, PhD, FACS
Associate Professor, Department of Surgery
Vice Chair, Equity, Diversity and Inclusion
Division of Otolaryngology – Head and Neck Surgery
University of Utah
Salt Lake City, Utah, USA

Klementina Avdeeva, MD
Otorhinolaryngologist
Department of Otorhinolaryngology
Clinical Diagnostic Center Medsi
Moscow, Russia

Catherine Banks, MBChB, FRACS (OHNS)
Otolaryngologist – Adult and Pediatric
Rhinology and Skull Base Surgery
Department of Otolaryngology – Head and Neck Surgery
Prince of Wales Hospital
Sydney Children's Hospital
University of New South Wales
Sydney, New South Wales, Australia

Martyn Barnes MD FRCS (ORL-HNS)
Consultant Rhinologist
Southend University Hospital NHS Foundation Trust
Essex, UK

Hazan Basak, MD
Professor
Department of Otorhinolaryngology
Head and Neck Surgery
Ankara University Medical School
Ankara University
Ankara, Turkey

Pete S. Batra, MD, FACS
Stanton A. Friedberg, MD Endowed Chair and Professor;
Clinical Leader, ENT, Dermatology, and Audiology Service
  Line;
Co-Director, Rush Center for Skull Base and Pituitary Surgery;
Medical Director, Rush Sinus, Allergy, and Asthma Center
Department of Otorhinolaryngology – Head and Neck Surgery
Rush University Medical Center
Chicago, Illinois, USA

Paolo Battaglia, MD
Professor
Department of Otorhinolaryngology
University of Insubria
Varese, Italy

Manuel Bernal-Sprekelsen, MD, PhD
Head
ENT Department
Hospital Clinic of Barcelona;
Chair of ENT Department
University of Barcelona
Barcelona, Spain

Suha Beton, MD
Department of Otorhinolaryngology, Head and
  Neck Surgery
Ankara University Medical School
Ankara University
Ankara, Turkey

Yves Brand, MD
Head of Department
Department of Otolaryngology
Cantonal Hospital Graubunden
Chur, Switzerland;
Associate Professor
University of Basel
Basel, Switzerland

Paul Breedveld, MSc, PhD
Antoni van Leeuwenhoek Distinguished Professor;
Director
3mE Graduate School;
Chair
Section of Minimally Invasive Surgery & Bio-Inspired
  Technology
Department of Bio-Mechanical Engineering;
Faculty
Mechanical, Maritime & Materials Engineering (3mE)
Delft University of Technology
Delft, the Netherlands

Hans Rudolf Briner, MD
Otorhinolaryngologist
and Head and Neck Surgeon
ORL-Zentrum Klinik Hirslanden
Zurich, Switzerland

Christian von Buchwald, MD, DMSc
Professor
Department of Otorhinolaryngology, Head & Neck Surgery
  and Audiology
Copenhagen University Hospital
Copenhagen, Denmark

Ricardo L. Carrau, MD, MBA
Professor
Department of Otolaryngology – Head & Neck Surgery;
Director of the Comprehensive Skull Base Surgery Program
The Ohio State University Medical Center
Columbus, Ohio, USA

Sean Carrie, Mb, ChB, FRCS, FRCS (ORL)
Consultant ENT Surgeon;
Honorary Senior Lecturer, Newcastle University
The Newcastle upon Tyne Hospitals NHS Foundation Trust
Newcastle upon Tyne, UK

Paolo Castelnuovo, MD, FRCSEd, FACS
Professor and Chairman
Head of Department of Otorhinolaryngology
Head of Department of Specialized Surgeries
University of Insubria
Varese, Italy

Vasileios Chatzinakis, MD, MSc
Consultant Otorhinolaryngologist – Head and Neck Surgeon
Endoscopic Sinus and Skull Base Center
Head and Neck Department
HYGEIA Hospital
Athens, Greece

Philip A. Chen, MD
ENT Specialist
Department of Otolaryngology – Head and Neck Surgery
University of Texas Health San Antonio
San Antonio, Texas, USA

Deborah Chute, MD
Associate Professor of Pathology
Department of Pathology
Cleveland Clinic
Cleveland, Ohio, USA

Caroline S. Clarke, PhD
Senior Research Associate in Health Economics
UCL Research Department of Primary Care and Population
  Health
University College London
London, UK

David B. Conley, MD
Associate Professor
Department of Otolaryngology – Head and Neck Surgery
Northwestern University
Chicago, Illinois, USA

James Constable, MD
ENT Registrar
Department of Adult Ear Nose and Throat
University Hospitals Bristol NHS Foundation Trust
Bristol, UK

John R. Craig, MD
Division Chief, Rhinology and Endoscopic Skull Base Surgery
Department of Otolaryngology – Head and Neck Surgery
Henry Ford Health System
Detroit, Michigan, USA

Anali Dadgostar, MD, MPH, FRCSC
Clinical Instructor
Department of Surgery
Faculty of Medicine
The University of British Columbia
Vancouver, Canada

Iacopo Dallan, MD
Surgeon
ENT and Phoniatric Unit
Azienda Ospedaliero-Universitaria Pisana
Pisa, Italy

John M. DelGaudio, MD, FARS
Professor and Vice Chair
Department of Otolaryngology – Head and Neck Surgery;
Chief of Rhinology;
Director
Emory Sinus, Nasal, & Allergy center
Emory University
Atlanta, Georgia, USA

**Ioannis I. Diamantopoulos, MD, DAvMed,
 Colonel HAF, FAsMA**
Consultant Otorhinolaryngologist;
Clinical Director
ENT Head & Neck Surgery Department
Hellenic Air Force General Hospital
Athens, Greece

M Reda El Badawey, MB ChB, FRCS, FRCS ORL-HNS, MD
Consultant of Otolaryngology – Head and Neck Surgery
Freeman Hospital
Newcastle upon Tyne, UK;
Associate Professor of Otolaryngology
Tanta University
Tanta, Egypt

Jean Anderson Eloy, MD, FARS
Professor and Vice Chair
Department of Otolaryngology – Head and Neck Surgery
Rutgers New Jersey Medical School
Newark, New Jersey, USA

Samer Fakhri, MD, FACS, FRCS(C)
Professor & Chair
Medical Director, ORL Specialty Clinics
Department of Otorhinolaryngology – Head & Neck Surgery
American University of Beirut Medical Center
Beirut, Lebanon;
Department of Otolaryngology
Kelsey-Seybold Clinic
Houston, Texas, USA

Judd H. Fastenberg, MD
Otolaryngologist
Department of Otorhinolaryngology – Head & Neck Surgery
Northwell Health
New York City, New York, USA

Enrico Fazio, MD
Professor
Department of Otorhinolaryngology
University of Insubria
Varese, Italy

Ulrik A. Felding, MD, PhD
ENT Specialist
Department of Otorhinolaryngology
Nordsjællands Hospital
Hillerød, Denmark

Marvin P. Fried, MD
Professor and Chair Emeritus
Department of Otorhinolaryngology – Head & Neck Surgery
Albert Einstein College of Medicine
New York City, New York, USA

**Christos Georgalas, MD, PhD, DLO, FRCS (ORL-HNS),
FEBORL-HNS (Hon.)**
Professor of Head and Neck Surgery
University of Nicosia Medical School
Nicosia, Cyprus;
Director of Endoscopic Skull Base Athens
Hygeia Hospital
Athens, Greece

Anne E. Getz, MD
Associate Professor
Otolaryngology – Head and Neck Surgery;
Associate Residency Program Director
University of Colorado School of Medicine
Aurora, Colorado, USA

Nsangou Ghogomu, MD
Otolaryngologist
Colorado Permanente Medical Group
Denver, Colorado, USA

Tomasz Gotlib, MD
Associate Professor
Department of Otorhinolaryngology – Head and Neck Surgery
Medical University of Warsaw
Warsaw, Poland

David A. Gudis, MD, FACS, FARS
Chief
Division of Rhinology and Anterior Skull Base Surgery
Department of Otolaryngology – Head and Neck Surgery;
Department of Neurologic Surgery
Columbia University Irving Medical Center
NewYork-Presbyterian Hospital
New York City, New York, USA

Edward Hadjihannas, MD
Consultant ENT Surgeon
Aretaeio Hospital
Nicosia, Cyprus

Richard J. Harvey, MD, PhD
Professor and Program Head
Rhinology and Skull Base Research Group
Macquarie University;
University of New South Wales
Sydney, Australia

Philippe Herman, MD
Head
Department of ENT, Maxillofacial and Skull Base Surgery
Skull Base Center;
Head of DMU Neurosciences Adults/Neuroscience CEO
Lariboisière Hospital, AP-HP
University of Paris
Paris, France

Roland Hettige, FRCS (ORL-HNS), MBBS, BSc, MSc
Consultant Rhinologist and ENT Surgeon
Princess Margaret Hospital,
Windsor, Berkshire, UK

Claire Hopkins, FRSC (ORLHNS), DM (Oxon)
Professor of Rhinology
King's College
London, UK

Qasim Husain, MD
Assistant Professor
Department of Otolaryngology
Hackensack Meridian School of Medicine
Seton Hall University
Coastal Ear, Nose, and Throat
Holmdel, New Jersey, USA

Dimitris Ioannidis, MD, PhD
Consultant ENT
East Suffolk and North Essex NHS Foundation Trust
Colchester, UK

Roger Jankowski, MD, PhD
Professor
ORL Department CHRU Brabois
University of Lorraine
Vandoeuvre Cedex, France

Amin Javer, MD, FRCSC, FARS
Director/Head
St. Paul's Sinus Centre
Clinical Professor of Surgery;
Research Co-Director
The University of British Columbia
Vancouver, Canada

Hari Jeyarajan, MD
Assistant Professor
School of Medicine
Department of Otolaryngology
The University of Alabama at Birmingham
Birmingham, Alabama, USA

Vivek V. Kanumuri, MD
Resident
Department of Otolaryngology–Head and Neck Surgery
Harvard Medical School
Harvard University
Cambridge, Massachusetts, USA

Apostolos Karligkiotis, MD
Professor
Division of Otorhinolaryngology – Head & Neck Surgery
Circolo Hospital and Macchi Foundation
Varese, Italy

Robert C. Kern, MD
George A. Sisson Professor of Otolaryngology;
Chair, Department of Otolaryngology
Head and Neck Surgery;
Professor, Otolaryngology – Head and Neck Surgery
Medicine-Allergy-Immunology
Feinberg School of Medicine
Northwestern University
Chicago, Illinois, USA

Nadim Khoueir, MD
Professor
Otolaryngology Head & Neck Surgery
Rhinology/Endoscopic Sinus & Skull Base Surgery
Faculty of Medicine
Saint Joseph University;
Hotel Dieu de France University Hospital;
Beirut Eye & ENT Specialist Hospital
Beirut, Lebanon

Suat Kilic, MD
Resident
Department of Otolaryngology (ENT)
Cleveland Clinic Foundation
Cleveland, Ohio, USA

Todd T. Kingdom, MD
Professor
Otolaryngology – Head & Neck Surgery and Ophthalmology;
Vice Chair, Clinical Affairs;
Director of Rhinology and Sinus Surgery
University of Colorado School of Medicine
Aurora, Colorado, USA

Claudia Kirsch, MD
Division Chief of Neuroradiology;
Professor of Neuroradiology and Otolaryngology
Department of Radiology
Northwell Health
Zucker Hofstra School of Medicine
Northwell North Shore University Hospital
Manhasset, New York, USA

Zeina Korban, MD
Assistant Professor of Clinical Specialty
Otorhinolaryngology – Head and Neck Surgery
American University of Beirut
Beirut, Lebanon

Kevin Kulendra, BSc MBBS (Hons)
   DOHNS FRCS (ORL HNS)
Consultant ENT Surgeon
Chelsea and Westminster Hospital NHS Foundation Trust
London, UK

Andreas Leunig, MD
Professor, Consultant, and Sinus Specialist
Rhinology Center Munich
Munich, Bavaria, Germany

Joshua M. Levy, MD, MPH
Associate Professor
Emory Sinus, Nasal & Allergy Center
Atlanta, Georgia, USA

Li-Xing Man, MSc, MD, MPA
Associate Professor and Residency Program Director
Rhinology and Endoscopic Skull Base Surgery
Department of Otolaryngology Head and Neck Surgery
University of Rochester Medical Center
Rochester, New York, USA

Guillermo Maza, MD
Resident Physician
Department of Otolaryngology
SIU School of Medicine
Springfield, Illinois, USA

Kelsey McHugh, MD
Assistant Professor of Pathology
Department of Pathology
Cleveland Clinic
Cleveland, Ohio, USA

Cem Meço, MD, FEBORL-HNS
President
Confederation of European Otorhinolaryngology, Head and
   Neck Surgery;
Vice President and Examiner
European Board Examination in ORL-HNS by UEMS;
Faculty
Department of Otorhinolaryngology, Head and Neck Surgery
Salzburg Paracelsus Medical University
Salzburg, Austria;
Professor and Past Chairman
Department of Otorhinolaryngology, Head and Neck Surgery
Ankara University Medical School
Ankara, Turkey

Lodovica Cristofani Mencacci, MD
Surgeon
ENT and Phoniatric Unit
Azienda Ospedaliero-Universitaria Pisana
Pisa, Italy

Stephen Morris, PhD
RAND Professor of Health Services Research
Department of Public Health and Primary Care
University of Cambridge
Cambridge, UK

David Morrissey, MBBS (HONS), FRACS (ORL)
Senior Lecturer
School of Medicine
The University of Queensland;
Otolaryngologist – Head and Neck Surgeon
Darling Downs Health Service
Toowoomba, Queensland

Salil Nair MD, FRCS ORL-HNS, FRCS Eng,
   FRCS Ed, MB ChB
Consultant ORL Surgeon
Honorary Associate Professor
University of Auckland
Auckland, New Zealand

Prepageran Narayanan, FRCS
Department of Otorhinolaryngology
Faculty of Medicine
University Malaya
Kuala Lumpur
Malaysia

Richard R. Orlandi, MD
Professor
Otolaryngology – Head and Neck Surgery;
Associate Chief Medical Officer
Ambulatory Health
University of Utah Health
Salt Lake City, Utah, USA

Charles F. Palmer, MD
Resident Physician
Department of Psychiatry and Behavioral Sciences
Department of Neurosciences
Medical University of South Carolina
Charleston, South Carolina, USA

James N. Palmer, MD
Professor and Director
Division of Rhinology;
Co-Director, Center for Skull Base Surgery
Department of ORL: HNS and Neurosurgery
University of Pennsylvania
Philadelphia, Pennsylvania, USA

Arjun K. Parasher, MD
Assistant Professor
Rhinology and Skull Base Surgery,
Department of Otolaryngology – Head and Neck Surgery
University of South Florida
Tampa, Florida, USA

Zara M. Patel, MD
Associate Professor
Director of Endoscopic Skull Base Surgery;
Rhinology – Sinus and Skull Base Surgery
Department of Otolaryngology – Head & Neck Surgery
Stanford School of Medicine
Stanford, California, USA

Michael J. Pfisterer, MD
ENT Specialist
Department of Otolaryngology – Head and Neck Surgery
Sutter Health
Fairfield, California, USA

Carl M. Philpott, MB, ChB, DLO, FRCS (ORL-HNS), MD, PGCME, SFHEA
Professor of Rhinology & Olfactology
Norwich Medical School
University of East Anglia
Norwich, UK

Giacomo Pietrobon, MD
Division of Otolaryngology and Head and Neck Surgery
IEO, European Institute of Oncology IRCCS;
Former Professor
Department of Biotechnology and Life Sciences
Division of Otorhinolaryngology
University of Insubria
Milan, Italy

Georgiy A. Polev, MD, PhD
Chief of Head and Neck Surgery Center
Ilyinskaya Hospital;
Senior Researcher
Department of Oncology and Pediatric Surgery
Dmitry Rogachev National Research Center of Pediatric Hematology, Oncology and Immunology
Moscow, Russia

Daniel M. Prevedello, MD
Professor
Department of Neurological Surgery;
Director, Minimally Invasive Cranial Surgery Program;
Co-Director, Comprehensive Skull Base Center at The James;
Director, Pituitary Surgery Program
The Wexner Medical Center
The Ohio State University
Columbus, Ohio, USA

Alkis J. Psaltis, MBBS (HONS), PhD, FRACS (ORL)
Professor of Otolaryngology – Head and Neck Surgery
University of Adelaide;
Head of Department
Otolaryngology – Head and Neck Surgery
The Queen Elizabeth Hospital
Adelaide, South Australia

Yujay Ramakrishnan, MBBChir, MA, MRCS (Ed), DOHNS, MFPM, FRCS (ORL-HNS)
Consultant Otolaryngologist
Queens Medical Centre
Nottingham, UK

Ashok Rokade, MS, DLO(RCS), FRCSI, FRCS(ORL-HNS)
Consultant ENT surgeon
Royal Hampshire County Hospital, Winchester
University Hospital Southampton, UK

Christopher Roxbury, MD
Assistant Professor of Surgery
Department of Otolaryngology – Head and Neck Surgery;
Director
Endoscopic Skull Base Surgery
UChicago Medicine
Chicago, Illinois, USA

Raymond Sacks, MBBCH, FCS (SA) ORL, FRACS
Clinical Professor and Head
Department of Otolaryngology – Head & Neck Surgery
Faculty of Medicine and Health Sciences
Macquarie University;
Clinical Professor
University of Sydney
Sydney, Australia

Anshul Sama, MBBS, FRCS (Gen Surg), FRCS (ORL-HNS)
Consultant Rhinologist and Endoscopic Skull Base Surgeon
Nottingham University Hospital NHS Trust
Nottingham, UK

E. Ritter Sansoni, MD
Assistant Professor
Department of Otolaryngology – Head and Neck Surgery
Division of Rhinology and Skull Base Surgery
Division of Head and Neck Surgery
University of Tennessee Health Science Center
Memphis, Tennessee, USA

Alfonso Santamaría-Gadea, MD, PhD
Otorhinolaryngologist and Head and Neck Surgeon
Rhinology and Skull Base Surgery Unit
Otolaryngology Service
Ramón y Cajal University Hospital
Madrid, Spain

Rodney J. Schlosser, MD
Professor and Director of Rhinology
Department of Otolaryngology – Head and Neck Surgery
Medical University of South Carolina
Charleston, South Carolina, USA

Veronica Seccia, MD, PhD
Surgeon
ENT and Phoniatric Unit
Azienda Ospedaliero-Universitaria Pisana
Pisa, Italy

Raj Sindwani, MD, FACS, FRCS(C)
Vice Chairman and Section Head
Rhinology, Sinus & Skull Base Surgery Head and Neck;
Co-Director
Minimally Invasive Cranial Base & Pituitary Surgery Program
Burkhardt Brain Tumor & Neuro-Oncology Center;
Vice Chair of Enterprise Surgical Operations
Cleveland Clinic
Cleveland, Ohio, USA

Kristine A. Smith, MD
Assistant Professor
Department of Otolaryngology – Head and Neck Surgery
Health Sciences Centre
Winnipeg, Canada

Kato Speleman, MD
Consultant
ENT & Head and Neck Surgery
AZ Sint-Jan Brugge-Oostende AV
Bruges, Belgium

Soma Subramaniam, MBBCH, MMED, FRCS (ORL)
Senior Consultant and Clinical Director;
Adjunct Assistant Professor
Department of Otolaryngology – Head & Neck Surgery
Ng Teng Fong General Hospital
National University Hospital Singapore
Singapore

Pavol Šurda, MD
Consultant Rhinologist and Skull Base Surgeon
Guy's and St Thomas' NHS Foundation Trust
London, UK

Bobby A. Tajudeen, MD
Head
Section of Rhinology and Skull Base Surgery;
Vice, Research Affairs;
Assistant Professor
Department of Otorhinolaryngology
Rush University Medical Center
Chicago, Illinois, USA

Neil Cheng-Wen Tan, FRCS(ORL-HNS), MEd, PhD
Consultant Rhinologist and Honorary Senior Lecturer
Royal Cornwall Hospital
University of Exeter Medical School
Truro, United Kingdom

Dennis Tang, MD
Assistant Professor of Surgery
Division of Otolaryngology - Head and Neck Surgery
Cedars-Sinai Medical Center
Los Angeles, California, USA

Ing Ping Tang, FRCS
Consultant ORL-HNS
ORL-HNS Department
University of Malaysia, Sarawak
Sarawak, Malaysia

Osama Tarabichi, MD
Department of Otolaryngology – Head and Neck Surgery;
Department of Genetics
Washington University School of Medicine
St. Louis, Missouri, USA

Marc A. Tewfik, MDCM, MSc, FRCSC
Associate Professor
Department of Otolaryngology – Head & Neck Surgery
McGill University Health Centre
Montreal, Quebec, Canada

Kiranya E. Tipirneni, MD
Resident Physician
Department of Otolaryngology and
  Communication Sciences
State University of New York Upstate Medical University
Syracuse, USA

Mario Turri-Zanoni, MD
Professor
Unit of Otorhinolaryngology – Head & Neck Surgery
University of Insubria;
ASST Sette Laghi
Circolo Hospital and Macchi Foundation
Varese, Italy

Benjamin K. Walters, MD
ENT Resident
San Antonio Military Medical Center
United States Air Force
San Antonio, Texas, USA

Bradford A. Woodworth, MD, FACS
James J. Hicks Endowed Professor of Otolaryngology;
Adjunct Professor of Neurosurgery;
Vice Chair of Clinical Affairs
Department of Otolaryngology
University of Alabama at Birmingham;
Senior Scientist
Gregory Fleming James Cystic Fibrosis Research Center
Birmingham, UK

**Peter John Wormald, MD, FAHMS, FRACS, FCS(SA),
  FRCS (Ed), MBChB**
Chairman (Otolaryngology)
Head and Neck Surgery
Professor of Skull Base Surgery
University of Adelaide
Adelaide, Australia

Ahmed Youssef, MD, MRCS
Fellow
Department of Otolaryngology – Head and Neck Surgery
Queen Elizabeth Hospital Birmingham
Birmingham, UK

Contents

Foreword vi
Paolo Castelnuovo

Foreword vii
James N. Palmer

Preface... viii

Acknowledgments ix

Contributors x

Videos.. xxx

Section I   Anatomy of the Frontal Sinus and Frontal Recess 1

1.   Developmental Bases of the Anatomy of the Frontal Sinus................................... 2
     Roger Jankowski

1.1   Introduction 2

1.2   Frontal Sinuses and Ethmoid Lateral Masses
      have Different Evolutionary and
      Developmental Origins 2

1.2.1   The Ethmoid Develops from the Olfactory
        Cartilaginous Capsule 2
1.2.2   The Frontal Sinuses Pneumatize after
        Erythropoietic Bone Marrow Conversion into
        Fatty Marrow 3

1.3   The Nitric Oxide "Story" of the Paranasal
      Sinuses Makes them Play a Role in Blood
      Oxygenation on Demand 3

1.4   Pneumosinus Dilatans and Arrested
      Pneumatization Could Bear Witness to
      Sinus Development 5

1.4.1   Pneumosinus Dilatans........................ 5
1.4.2   Arrested Pneumatization 6

1.5   Conclusion 7

2.   Radiological Anatomy... 9
     Claudia Kirsch

2.1   Introduction 9

2.2   Lamina Papyracea.......................... 12

2.3   Uncinate Process........................... 12

2.4   Floor of Olfactory Recess 13

2.5   Agger Nasi Air Cell 13

2.6   Accessory Air Cells 14

2.7   Anterior Ethmoidal Artery 14

2.8   Bulla Ethmoidalis 15

2.9   Middle Turbinate........................... 15

2.10 Conclusion 15

3.   Applied Surgical Anatomy 18
     Iacopo Dallan, Lodovica Cristofani Mencacci, and Veronica Seccia

3.1   General Considerations 18

3.2   Applied Anatomy for Endonasal
      Approaches 18

3.3   Applied Anatomy for External Approaches . 21

3.3.1   Coronal Approach............................ 21
3.3.2   Transpalpebral Approach 22

3.4   Blood Supply 22

3.5   Innervation 22

3.6   Anatomical Variations and Surgical
      Considerations 23

3.7   Conclusions 23

Section II   Endoscopic Surgical Approaches to Frontal Sinus Disease.......................... 25

4.   Draf Frontal Sinusotomy I and IIa 26
      Andreas Leunig and Hans Rudolf Briner

4.1   Indications 26

4.2   Surgical Steps 26

4.3   Tips and Tricks 28

4.4   Case Examples 28

4.5   Complications Management.......................... 47

4.6   Conclusion 50

5.   Draf Frontal Sinusotomy IIb 52
      Kevin Kulendra, Ahmed Youssef, and Shahzada Ahmed

5.1   Indications 52

5.2   Anatomy 52

5.3   Surgical Steps 52

5.3.1 Lateral Approach.......................... 52

5.3.2 Median Approach 52

5.4   Tips and Tricks 53

5.5   Complications.......................... 53

6.   Extended Draf IIb and Other Modifications of the Lothrop Procedure 54
      Vivek V. Kanumuri, Qasim Husain, Suat Kilic, Michael J. Pfisterer, Osama Tarabichi, and Jean Anderson Eloy

6.1   Introduction 54

6.2   Indications 54

6.3   Surgical Steps 54

6.3.1 Overview of Standard Draf IIb.......................... 54

6.4   Modifications of the Standard Draf IIb
      Procedure 55

6.4.1 Modified Hemi-Lothrop Procedure (Eloy IIC).... 55
6.4.2 Modified Mini-Lothrop Procedure (Eloy IID) 55
6.4.3 Modified Subtotal-Lothrop Procedure (Eloy IIE) . 55
6.4.4 Modified Central-Lothrop Procedure (Eloy IIF) .. 56

6.5   Tips and Tricks 57

6.6   Case Examples 57

6.6.1 Example 1.......................... 57
6.6.2 Example 2.......................... 57
6.6.3 Example 3.......................... 57

6.7   Complications.......................... 57

6.7.1 Recurrence and Chronic Scarring.......................... 57
6.7.2 Cerebrospinal Fluid Leak.......................... 57
6.7.3 Orbital Injury 58
6.7.4 Anterior Ethmoid Artery Injury 58

7.   The Frontal Sinus Rescue Procedure.......................... 59
      Fahad Alasousi, Anali Dadgostar, and Amin Javer

7.1   Indications 59

7.2   Surgical Steps 59

7.2.1 Step 1 60
7.2.2 Step 2 60
7.2.3 Step 3 60
7.2.4 Step 4 60

7.3   Reverse Frontal Rescue Procedure 60

7.4   Complications.......................... 60

7.5   Tips and Tricks 62

7.6   Conclusion 62

8. **Draf III (Endoscopic Modified Lothrop)— Inside-Out and Outside-In Approaches** 64

Christos Georgalas, Vasileios Chatzinakis, Klementina Avdeeva, Georgiy A. Polev, and Anshul Sama

8.1 **Indications** 64

8.1.1 Relative Contraindications 64

8.2 **Surgical Steps** 64

8.3 **Lateral-to-Medial/Inside-Out Technique** 64

8.4 **Outside-In/Medial-to-Lateral Technique** 66

8.5 **Tips and Tricks** 70

8.6 **Case Examples** 70

8.6.1 A Case of Allergic Fungal Rhinosinusitis with Fronto-orbital Mucocele 70

8.6.2 A Case of Chronic Frontal Sinusitis with a High Posterior Frontal (Type 3) Cell 71

8.6.3 A Case of Chronic Frontal Sinusitis—Riedel's Procedure Reversal 72

8.7 **Postoperative Management** 72

8.8 **Complications and their Management** 73

8.8.1 Skull Base Injury and Cerebrospinal Fluid Leak .. 73
8.8.2 Hemorrhage 73
8.8.3 Orbital Injury 74
8.8.4 Skin Injury 74
8.8.5 Stenosis of the Frontal Sinus Neo-ostium 74

9. **Transseptal Approach** 76

Bobby A. Tajudeen and Pete S. Batra

9.1 **Background and CT Review** 76

9.2 **Indications and Contraindications** 76

9.3 **Advantages** 77

9.4 **Disadvantages** 77

9.5 **Surgical Steps** 77

9.6 **Tips and Tricks** 78

9.6.1 Case Example 78

9.7 **Complications** 78

10. **Endoscopic Endonasal Orbital Transposition for Lateral Frontal Sinus Lesions** 81

Paolo Castelnuovo, Mario Turri-Zanoni, Enrico Fazio, Paolo Battaglia, and Apostolos Karligkiotis

10.1 **Indications** 81

10.2 **Surgical Steps** 82

10.3 **Tips and Tricks** 83

10.4 **Case Example** 83

10.5 **Complications** 84

11. **The Role of Frontal Sinus in Anterior Skull Base Surgery and the Transcribriform Approach** 87

E. Ritter Sansoni, Raymond Sacks, and Richard J. Harvey

11.1 **Indications** 87

11.2 **Surgical Steps** 89

11.3 **Tips and Tricks** 91

11.4 **Complications** 91

12. **Extended Endonasal Anterior Skull Base Approaches** 93

Soma Subramaniam, Guillermo Maza, Daniel M. Prevedello, and Ricardo L. Carrau

12.1 **Indications** 93

12.2 **Surgical Steps** 93

12.2.1 Principles 93
12.2.2 Operative Setup 94
12.2.3 Surgical Technique 94
12.2.4 Reconstruction 95
12.2.5 Postoperative Considerations 95

12.3 **Tips and Tricks** 96

12.4 **Case Examples** 96

12.4.1 Esthesioneuroblastoma (Transcribriform Approach) 96
12.4.2 Tuberculum Sellae Meningioma: Endoscopic Transtuberculum/Transplanum Approach 96

12.5   Complications and Management 96

12.5.1 Vascular Complications........................ 96
12.5.2 Cranial Nerve Injury........................... 99

12.5.3 Cerebrospinal Fluid Fistulas.................... 99
12.5.4 Postoperative Infection........................ 99
12.5.5 Other Complications 99

13.   Revision Endoscopic Frontal Sinus Surgery 101

Salil Nair and Peter John Wormald

13.1   Introduction 101

13.2   Indications 101

13.2.1 Ongoing Mucosal Disease..................... 102
13.2.2 Incomplete Dissection........................ 102
13.2.3 Lateralization of the Middle Turbinate 102
13.2.4 Scarring and Synechiae 103
13.2.5 Neo-Osteogenesis............................ 103

13.3   Patient Selection.......................... 103

13.4   Preoperative Planning 104

13.4.1 Analyzing the Computed Tomography Imaging . 104
13.4.2 Computer-Assisted Navigation during Surgery . 104
13.4.3 Endoscopes and Equipment................... 104

13.5   Choice of Procedure 104

13.6   Surgical Steps 105

13.6.1 The Axillary Flap Technique................... 105
13.6.2 Frontal Sinus Mini-Trephine 106

13.7   Specific Scenarios......................... 107

13.7.1 Retained Cells in the Frontal Recess or Extending into the Frontal Sinus (Draf I or International Classification of Extent of Endoscopic Frontal Sinus Surgery Grades 1–3)... 107
13.7.2 A Narrow Frontal Ostium and/or Extensive Supra Agger/Bulla Frontal Cells, or Ongoing Significant Burden of Disease (CRSwNP, Aspirin-Sensitive Asthma, Allergic Fungal Disease [Draf III/EFSS 6])..................... 107

13.8   Tips and Tricks 109

13.9   Case Example 109

13.10   Complications: Management 111

13.10.1 Scarring and Restenosis...................... 111
13.10.2 Anterior Ethmoid Artery..................... 111
13.10.3 Orbital Injury 112
13.10.4 Cerebrospinal Fluid Leak.................... 112

14.   Complications of Frontal Sinus Surgery 113

David Morrissey and Alkis J. Psaltis

14.1   Introduction 113

14.2   Epidemiology and Etiology 113

14.3   Specific Complications of Endoscopic Approaches to the Frontal Sinus 113

14.3.1 Failure to Accomplish the Specific Aim of the Procedure 113
14.3.2 Pain... 115
14.3.3 Bleeding..................................... 115
14.3.4 Infection 116

14.3.5 Scar/Stenosis 117
14.3.6 Mucocele Formation 117
14.3.7 Anterior Skull Base Injury/Cerebrospinal Fluid Leak 118
14.3.8 Orbital Injury............................... 119

14.4   Prevention of Complications............... 119

14.4.1 Preoperative Planning........................ 120
14.4.2 Perioperative Technique...................... 120
14.4.3 Postoperative Care 120

15.   Delivery of Topical Therapy to the Frontal Sinus 122

John R. Craig and Nithin D. Adappa

15.1   Introduction 122

15.2   Basic Science Research on Topical Distribution to the Sinuses................ 122

15.3   Clinical Research on Topical Distribution to the Sinuses............................ 124

15.3.1 Tips and Tricks............................... 125

15.4   Conclusion 125

16. Postoperative Management: Dressings and Toilet.. 126

Neil Cheng-Wen Tan and Peter John Wormald

16.1 Natural History of Sinus Ostia after Surgery 126

16.2 Intranasal Packing 126

16.2.1 Nonabsorbable Packs....................... 126
16.2.2 Absorbable Packings 127

16.3 To Pack or Not to Pack 128

16.4 Inert Stents 129

16.5 Drug-Eluting Stents 129

16.6 Postoperative Care.......................... 130

16.6.1 Saline Irrigations............................ 130
16.6.2 Endoscopic Debridement 130
16.6.3 Topical Treatments.......................... 130

16.7 Conclusion 131

17. Office-Based Frontal Sinus Procedures 133

Joshua M. Levy and John M. DelGaudio

17.1 Indications 133

17.1.1 Anatomic Considerations 133
17.1.2 Patient Selection 133
17.1.3 Frontal Sinusitis............................ 134
17.1.4 Frontal Mucoceles........................... 134
17.1.5 Nasal Polyps 134

17.2 Surgical Steps/Anesthesia.................. 135

17.3 Postoperative Management and Procedures................................ 135

17.3.1 Nasal Irrigations and Topical Therapies 136

17.4 Tips and Tricks 136

17.4.1 Case Examples.............................. 136

17.5 Controversies 138

17.5.1 Balloon Catheter Dilation 138

17.6 Emerging Technologies 139

17.7 Conclusion 139

Section III   Open Surgical Approaches to Frontal Sinus Disease 141

18. Mini- and Maxi-Trephines.. 142

David A. Gudis, Charles F. Palmer, and Rodney J. Schlosser

18.1 Indications 142

18.2 Surgical Steps.............................. 142

18.3 Tips and Tricks 144

18.4 Case Example 144

18.5 Complications.............................. 144

19. Osteoplastic Flap Approach with and without Obliteration 146

Arjun K. Parasher and James N. Palmer

19.1 Indications 146

19.2 Surgical Steps.............................. 146

19.2.1 Osteoplastic Flap without Obliteration......... 146
19.2.2 Osteoplastic Flap with Obliteration 148

19.3 Tips and Tricks 149

19.4 Complications: Management 149

19.5 Conclusion 149

20. Riedel's Procedure and Cranialization of the Frontal Sinus 150

Kato Speleman and Anshul Sama

20.1 Riedel's Procedure 150

20.1.1 Historic Perspective 150
20.1.2 Indications 151
20.1.3 Technique 151

20.2 Cranialization of the Frontal Sinus......... 151

20.2.1 Historic Perspective 151
20.2.2 Indications 152
20.2.3 Technique 153

Section IV   Management of Specific Frontal Sinus Conditions..................................... 155

21.   Frontal Sinus Barosinusitis... 156
Ioannis I. Diamantopoulos

21.1   Epidemiology and Etiology 156

21.2   Clinical Presentation and Investigations... 156

21.3   Management........................... 157

21.4   Case Example (Courtesy of Christos Georgalas) 159

22.   Frontal Sinus in Patients with Cystic Fibrosis.. 161
Kiranya E. Tipirneni, Hari Jeyarajan, and Bradford A. Woodworth

22.1   Epidemiology and Etiology 161

22.2   Clinical Presentation and Investigations... 161

22.2.1 Radiographic Abnormalities in Cystic Fibrosis and the Frontal Sinus........................ 162

22.3   Management........................... 163

22.3.1 Medical Therapy 163
22.3.2 Nasal Saline Irrigations 163

22.3.3 Corticosteroids 163
22.3.4 Topical Antibiotics 163
22.3.5 Oral Antibiotics 164
22.3.6 Dornase Alfa................................. 164
22.3.7 Cystic Fibrosis Transmembrane Conductance Regulator modulators 164
22.3.8 Surgical Therapy 164
22.3.9 Endoscopic Approaches 165

22.4   Complications: Management 169

23.   Pneumosinus Dilatans... 173
Ing Ping Tang, Yves Brand, and Prepageran Narayanan

23.1   Introduction 173

23.2   Epidemiology and Etiology 173

23.3   Clinical Presentation and Investigations... 173

23.4   Diagnosis............................... 173

23.5   Management.............................. 174

23.6   Complications............................ 174

23.7   Conclusion 174

24.   Frontal Sinusitis in Chronic Rhinosinusitis without Nasal Polyposis 176
Kristine A. Smith, Jeremiah A. Alt, and Richard R. Orlandi

24.1   Introduction 176

24.2   Epidemiology 176

24.3   Pathophysiology 177

24.3.1 Anatomic Factors........................... 177

24.3.2 Physiological Factors 178

24.4   Management.............................. 178

24.4.1 Medical Management 178
24.4.2 Surgical Management 179

24.5   Conclusion 180

25.   Frontal Sinus Surgery in CRSwNP, AFRS, and ASA Triad 182
Nsangou Ghogomu and Robert C. Kern

25.1   Epidemiology and Etiology 182

25.1.1 Chronic Rhinosinusitis with Nasal Polyps 182
25.1.2 Aspirin-Exacerbated Respiratory Disease 182
25.1.3 Allergic Fungal Sinusitis 182

25.2   Clinical Presentation and Investigations... 182

25.2.1 Chronic Rhinosinusitis with Nasal Polyps 182

25.2.2 Aspirin-Exacerbated Respiratory Disease 182
25.2.3 Allergic Fungal Sinusitis 183

25.3   Management Overview................... 183

25.3.1 Chronic Rhinosinusitis with Nasal Polyps 183
25.3.2 Aspirin-Exacerbated Respiratory Disease 183
25.3.3 Allergic Fungal Sinusitis 183

25.4 Extent of Surgery and Outcomes 183

25.4.1 Goals of Surgery 183
25.4.2 Effect of Extent of Surgery on Outcomes for Maxillary and Ethmoid Sinuses 184
25.4.3 Effect of Extent of Surgery on Outcomes for the Frontal Sinus............................... 184

25.5 Case Examples 185

25.5.1 Samter's Triad Successfully Managed with Draf IIa... 185
25.5.2 Samter's Triad Only Controlled after Draf III 185
25.5.3 Nasal Polyp Recurrence in Frontal Ostium Managed in the Office 185
25.5.4 Allergic Fungal Sinusitis Presenting with Proptosis 186

25.6 Complications............................. 186

26. Frontal Sinus Mucoceles 188

James Constable and Anshul Sama

26.1 Terminology 188

26.2 Epidemiology 188

26.3 Pathology 188

26.4 Clinical Presentation 188

26.5 Investigations............................ 189

26.6 Classification............................. 189

26.7 Management.............................. 190

26.8 Outcomes 193

26.9 Conclusion 193

27. Frontoethmoidal Osteomas 195

Christos Georgalas and Edward Hadjihannas

27.1 Epidemiology and Etiology 195

27.2 Histology................................. 196

27.3 Clinical Presentation and Investigations ... 196

27.4 Management.............................. 196

27.5 Approaches for Frontoethmoidal Osteomas 197

27.5.1 External Approaches 197
27.5.2 Endoscopic Approaches 197

27.6 Summary................................. 199

27.7 Case Examples 200

27.7.1 Case 1....................................... 200
27.7.2 Case 2....................................... 201
27.7.3 Case 3....................................... 202
27.7.4 Case 4....................................... 202

28. Frontal Inverted Papilloma 205

Paolo Battaglia, Apostolos Karligkiotis, Giacomo Pietrobon, Paolo Castelnuovo, and Mario Turri-Zanoni

28.1 Epidemiology and Etiology 205

28.2 Clinical Presentation and Investigations ... 207

28.3 Management.............................. 208

28.4 Case Examples 211

28.4.1 Case 1....................................... 211
28.4.2 Case 2....................................... 211
28.4.3 Case 3....................................... 211

28.5 Complications: Management 212

29. The Frontal Sinus: Fibro-Osseous Lesions 217

Catherine Banks and Raymond Sacks

29.1 Fibrous Dysplasia 217

29.1.1 Epidemiology and Etiology 217
29.1.2 Clinical Presentation and Investigations........ 218
29.1.3 Management 219

29.2 Ossifying Fibroma........................ 220

29.2.1 Epidemiology and Etiology 220

29.2.2 Clinical Presentation and Investigations........ 221
29.2.3 Management 222
29.2.4 Surgical Steps................................ 222
29.2.5 Consent 222

29.3 Summary................................. 223

30. Malignant Disease Involving the Frontal Sinus 226

Dennis Tang, Christopher Roxbury, Kelsey McHugh, Deborah Chute, and Raj Sindwani

30.1 Epidemiology and Etiology 226

30.2 Clinical Presentation and Investigation 229

30.3 Staging 230

30.4 Management 230

30.5 Case Example 231

30.6 Complications: Management 231

30.7 Tips and Tricks 232

31. Acute Frontal Osteomyelitis: Intracranial and Orbital Complications 233

Ashok Rokade and Dimitris Ioannidis

31.1 Epidemiology and Etiology 233

31.1.1 Epidemiology 233
31.1.2 Etiology 234

31.2 Clinical Presentation and Investigations ... 234

31.2.1 Orbital Complications 234
31.2.2 Intracranial Complications 235
31.2.3 Osseous Complications 236
31.2.4 Investigations 236

31.3 Management 238

31.3.1 Frontal Sinus Drainage Techniques 238
31.3.2 Management of Orbital Complications 240
31.3.3 Management of Intracranial Complications 240

31.3.4 Management of Osseous Complications 241

31.4 Case Examples 241

31.4.1 Case 1: Subperiosteal Abscess
(Contrast-Enhanced CT) 241
31.4.2 Case 2: Orbital Abscess (Magnetic Resonance
Imaging) 241
31.4.3 Case 3: Cerebral Abscess (Magnetic Resonance
Imaging) 241
31.4.4 Case 4: Epidural Abscess
(Contrast-Enhanced CT) 241
31.4.5 Case 5: Subdural Abscess
(Contrast-Enhanced CT) 241
31.4.6 Case 6: Pott's Puffy Tumor 241

32. Fungal Frontal Sinusitis: Allergic and Nonallergic 244

Fahad Alasousi, Anali Dadgostar, Amin Javer, and Carl M. Philpott

32.1 Introduction 244

32.2 Epidemiology and Etiology 244

32.2.1 Invasive 244
32.2.2 Noninvasive 244

32.3 Clinical Presentation and Investigations ... 245

32.3.1 Invasive 245
32.3.2 Noninvasive 245

32.3.3 Special Considerations in Frontal Sinus Fungal
Disease 246

32.4 Management 247

32.4.1 Medical Management 247
32.4.2 Surgical and Postoperative Management in the
Frontal Sinus 247
32.4.3 Complications: Management 247

32.5 Conclusion 248

33. Frontal Sinus Trauma and Its Management 250

Ulrik A. Felding and Christian von Buchwald

33.1 Epidemiology and Etiology 250

33.1.1 Anatomy 250
33.1.2 Trauma Mechanism 250

33.2 Clinical Presentation and Investigations ... 251

33.2.1 Initial Examination of the Patient 251
33.2.2 Imaging and Paraclinical Investigations 251

33.3 Management 251

33.3.1 Surgical Techniques 251
33.3.2 Surgical Decision-Making 252

33.4 Case Example 253

33.5 Complications: Management 253

34. Cerebrospinal Fluid Leak in the Frontal Sinus: Endoscopic Management 256

Hari Jeyarajan, Benjamin K. Walters, and Bradford A. Woodworth

34.1 Epidemiology and Etiology 256

34.1.1 Etiologies.................................. 256

34.2 Clinical Presentation and Investigations ... 257

34.3 Management............................. 258

34.3.1 Surgical Management 258
34.3.2 Endoscopic versus Open Repair 259

34.3.3 Postprocedural Care.......................... 259
34.3.4 Postprocedural Adjuvants 259
34.3.5 Outcomes 260

34.4 Case Examples 260

34.5 Complications: Management 260

34.6 Conclusion 263

Section V   Controversial Topics in Current Practice.. 267

35. The Use of Flaps in Frontal Sinus Surgery 268

Nadim Khoueir and Philippe Herman

35.1 Published Evidence 268

35.1.1 Background................................. 268
35.1.2 Rationale for Flaps 268
35.1.3 Literature Review and Surgical Techniques..... 269

35.2 Controversies and Opinions............... 270

35.2.1 Promising Outcome for Flaps................. 270

35.2.2 Recommendation for Future Studies........... 270
35.2.3 Flaps Feasibility............................. 271
35.2.4 Illustrative Cases........................... 271

35.3 Surgical Tips 273

35.4 Unanswered Questions 273

36. Osteitis and the Frontal Sinus 275

Christos Georgalas

36.1 Introduction 275

36.2 Epidemiology and Etiology 275

36.2.1 Definitions 275
36.2.2 Histology: Pathophysiology.................. 275
36.2.3 Allergy.................................... 276
36.2.4 Bacteriology............................... 276
36.2.5 Biofilms................................... 277
36.2.6 Incidence.................................. 277

36.3 Clinical Presentation and Investigations ... 277

36.3.1 Radiological Features......................... 277
36.3.2 Clinical Implications......................... 278
36.3.3 Prognostic Factor 278

36.4 Management.............................. 278

36.5 Case Example 279

36.6 Summary................................. 280

36.7 Key Points................................ 280

37. Extreme Lateral Lesions: What Is the Limit of Endoscopic Surgery?.......................... 282

Cem Meco, Suha Beton, and Hazan Basak

37.1 Published Evidence 282

37.1.1 Traditional External Approaches for Far Lateral
Lesions...................................... 282
37.1.2 Endonasal Endoscopic Surgery and Evolution of
Lateral Disease Management.................. 283

37.1.3 Evolution of Far Lateral Frontal Sinus Surgery:
Exploring Limits of ESS 285

37.2 Controversies and Opinions............... 287

37.3 Unanswered Questions 294

38. Use of Image Guidance Technology: Mandatory or Not.. 299

Judd H. Fastenberg, Marvin P. Fried, and Waleed M. Abuzeid

38.1 Introduction 299

38.1.1 Indications 299

38.1.2 Applications................................ 300

38.2 Published Evidence 300

38.2.1 Complications 300
38.2.2 Revision Rate 300
38.2.3 Clinical and Quality-of-Life Outcomes 301
38.2.4 Medicolegal Concerns 301
38.2.5 Cost.. 301

38.3 Controversies and Opinions................ 301

38.3.1 Indications 301
38.3.2 Surgical Training 301
38.3.3 Future Use................................. 301

38.4 Unanswered Questions 301

39. Balloon Technology in the Frontal Sinus: Useful or Gimmick 304

Claire Hopkins and Roland Hettige

39.1 Published Evidence 304

39.1.1 Level 1 Evidence 304
39.1.2 Nonrandomized Studies 307

39.2 Controversies and Opinions................ 307

39.2.1 Diffuse versus Localized CRS 308
39.2.2 Polyp Disease.............................. 309
39.2.3 Miscellaneous Uses......................... 309

39.2.4 Contraindications............................. 309
39.2.5 Preoperative Preparation 309
39.2.6 Training Requirements 310
39.2.7 Complications 310

39.3 Unanswered Questions 311

39.3.1 Cost-Effectiveness............................ 311
39.3.2 Extrapolation to Wider Patient Cohort......... 312

40. Minimum versus Maximal Surgical Sinusotomy 314

Anne E. Getz and Todd T. Kingdom

40.1 Published Evidence 314

40.1.1 Balloon Dilation............................. 314
40.1.2 Draf I..................................... 315
40.1.3 Draf IIa................................... 315
40.1.4 Draf IIb................................... 315
40.1.5 Draf III 316

40.2 Controversies and Opinions................ 316

40.3 Case Studies............................... 316

40.3.1 Case 1.................................... 316
40.3.2 Case 2.................................... 317
40.3.3 Case 3.................................... 317

40.4 Unanswered Questions 317

41. Patient-Reported Outcome Measures and Outcomes in Frontal Sinus Surgery: Do They Make a Difference? 320

Yujay Ramakrishnan, M. Reda El Badawey, and Sean Carrie

41.1 Published Evidence 320

41.1.1 Patient-Reported Outcome Measures in Rhinology 320
41.1.2 Patient-Reported Outcome Measures in Frontal Sinus Treatment 321

41.2 Controversies and Opinions................ 321

41.3 Unanswered Questions 324

42. Symptoms of Frontal Sinus Disease: Where Is the Evidence?................................. 325

Zara M. Patel

42.1 Published Evidence 325

42.2 Controversies and Opinions................ 326

42.3 Case Examples 327

42.3.1 Case 1.................................... 327

42.3.2 Case 2.................................... 328
42.3.3 Case 3.................................... 328
42.3.4 Case 4.................................... 330
42.3.5 Case 5.................................... 330

42.4 Unanswered Questions 331

43. Anatomy and Classification of Frontoethmoidal Cells.................................. 333
Tomasz Gotlib, Anshul Sama, and Christos Georgalas

43.1 Introduction 333

43.2 Published Evidence 333

43.3 Controversies and Opinions................ 336

44. To Drill or Not to Drill 340
Alfonso Santamaría-Gadea, Isam Alobid, and Manuel Bernal-Sprekelsen

44.1 Published Evidence 340

44.2 Indications for Drilling Approaches of the Frontal Sinus 340

44.3 Results of Drilling Approaches of the Frontal Sinus 341

44.4 Complications.............................. 342

44.5 Controversies and Opinions................ 342

44.6 Unanswered Questions 342

45. Indications for Operating the Frontal Sinus: Primary Surgery or Always Second Line?...... 344
Nsangou Ghogomu and David B. Conley

45.1 Introduction 344

45.2 Controversies and Opinions............... 344

45.2.1 Does OMC/Frontal Recess Obstruction Cause Frontal CRS?................................ 344
45.2.2 Is Anterior Ethmoidectomy (Draf I) Optimal as First-Line Surgery for Frontal CRS?......... 346
45.2.3 What Are the Clinical Characteristics of Patients Who Fail Draf I? 346
45.2.4 Why Is Draf I not Successful in Some Patients with Frontal CRS?.................... 347
45.2.5 Is Primary Draf IIa Effective as an Initial Surgical Intervention for Frontal CRS? 347

45.3 Case Studies.............................. 348

45.3.1 Case 1: Mild Diffuse CRSwNP Involving the Frontal Sinus................................. 348
45.3.2 Case 2: Failed Draf I Procedure Requiring at least Draf IIa—Ciliary Dysfunction? 348
45.3.3 Case 3: Severe CRSwNP Requiring EMLP as Initial Surgical Intervention................... 348
45.3.4 Case 4: Odontogenic Frontal CRS 348

45.4 Unanswered Questions 349

46. Economic and Quality-of-Life Evaluation of Surgery and Medical Treatment for Chronic Rhinosinusitis 351
Caroline S. Clarke, Carl M. Philpott, and Steve Morris

46.1 Published Evidence 351

46.1.1 What is Known about the Economic Burden of Chronic Rhinosinusitis?...................... 351
46.1.2 What Are the Wider Costs of CRS?............ 352
46.1.3 What Is the Impact of CRS on QOL?........... 352
46.1.4 Cost and Cost-Effectiveness of Treatment for CRS 353

46.2 Controversies Surrounding the Cost-Effectiveness of Treatment for CRS 354

46.3 Unanswered Questions and Future Research 355

47. Training Models and Techniques in Frontal Sinus Surgery 358
Abdulaziz Al-Rasheed, Philip A. Chen, and Marc A. Tewfik

47.1 Introduction 358

47.2 Published Evidence 358

47.3 Controversies and Opinions................ 360

47.4 Unanswered Questions 361

48. Augmented Reality in Frontal Sinus Surgery 363
Pavol Šurda and Martyn Barnes

48.1 Role of Augmented Reality in Preoperative Planning 363

48.2 Role of Augmented Reality during Surgery 363

49. Robotic Surgery: Beyond DaVinci 366
Paul Breedveld

49.1 Published Evidence 366

49.1.1 Shortcomings of DaVinci...................... 366

49.2 Steering at Greater Simplicity 366

49.3 Steering at Reduced Dimensions 367

49.4 Controversies and Opinions................ 367

49.4.1 Maneuvering beyond DaVinci................. 367

49.5 Maneuvering Like a Snake 368

49.6 Future Steps toward Clinical Practice...... 369

49.7 Unanswered Questions 369

50. Pathophysiology of the Failed Frontal Sinus and Its Implications for Medical Management 371
Li-Xing Man, Zeina Korban, and Samer Fakhri

50.1 Introduction 371

50.2 Failure due to Errors in Patient Selection .. 371

50.3 Local Causes of Recalcitrant Frontal Sinus Disease................................... 371

50.4 Systemic Causes of Recalcitrant Frontal Sinus Disease.............................. 374

50.5 Conclusion 376

Index 378

Videos

Video 4.1 CRSwNP, Draf type I (Case 1)... 29

Video 4.2 CRS, Draf type I (Case 2).. 32

Video 4.3 CRS, Draf type IIa example 2 (Case 3)... 35

Video 4.4 CRS, Draf type I, axillary flap approach (Case 4)... 38

Video 4.5 CRS, Draf type IIa example 1 (Case 5)... 40

Video 4.6 CRS, Draf type IIa, concha bullosa (Case 6).. 44

Video 4.7 CRSwNP, Draf IIa approach (Case 7).. 47

Video 6.1 Modified Hemi-Lothrop procedure for recurrent left frontal mucocele 55

Video 6.2 Modified subtotal Lothrop procedure for cholesterol granuloma of the right frontal sinus 56

Video 6.3 Modified central lothrop procedure for left frontal mucocele 57

Video 7.1 Frontal sinus rescue procedure 62

Video 8.1 Lateral fronto-orbital mucocele Draf III approach (Case 8.6.1).............................. 71

Video 8.2 Outpatient endoscopic view after Draf III for fronto-orbital mucocele (Case 8.6.1) 72

Video 8.3 Live surgery – Inside out Draf III with laterally based flap (Case 8.6.2)...................... 72

Video 8.4 Outpatient endoscopic view after Draf III for recurrent frontal sinusitis (Case 8.6.2) 72

Video 9.1 Transeptal frontal sinus approach for frontal sinus mucocele with osteogenesis (Case 9.6.1) 78

Video 13.1 Frontal drillout... 111

Video 17.1 Frontal mucocele – Intact bulla approach: example 1 137

Video 17.2 Frontal mucocele – Intact bulla approach: example 2 137

Video 17.3 Frontal sinus mucocele – Trans bulla approach... 137

Video 17.4 Outpatient endoscopic frontal polypectomy – example 1 138

Video 17.5 Outpatient endoscopic frontal polypectomy – example 2 138

Video 22.1 Frontal sinus surgery in a cystic fibrosis (CF) patient 165

Video 27.1 Case 3 – Draf III for a frontal osteoma.. 202

Video 27.2 Endoscopic removal of a giant frontal sinus osteoma...................................... 202

Video 34.1 Post traumatic cerebrospinal fluid (CSF) leak.. 260

Video 34.2 CSF/Dural repair post resection of meningioma 260

Video 36.1 Case example Osteitis – Draf IIb performed as part of Live surgery on a patient with frontal sinusitis... 280

Video 36.2 Case example: Draf III performed in the same patient following osteitis recurrence........ 280

Video 37.1 Far lateral right frontal recurrent inverted papilloma...................................... 297

Video 37.2 Frontal cholesteatoma. Extending far lateral to middle cranial fossa and temporalis muscle... 297

Section I

Anatomy of the Frontal Sinus and Frontal Recess

1 Developmental Bases of the
Anatomy of the Frontal Sinus   *2*

2 Radiological Anatomy   *9*

3 Applied Surgical Anatomy   *18*

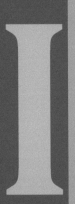

1 Developmental Bases of the Anatomy of the Frontal Sinus

Roger Jankowski

Abstract

The frontal sinus starts its development after birth. Pneumatization in the frontal bone leads multiple gas-filled cavities to coalesce and form a polylobed cavity, which finally communicates with the lateral mass of the ethmoid. Nitric oxide (NO), the gas produced throughout life by the sinus epithelium, is actively released into the nasal cavity to be mixed up with the inspiratory airflow. At the level of the alveolar capillary membrane, nitric oxide facilitates the alveolar oxygen transfer into the bloodstream and increases arterial blood oxygenation. Thus, the frontal sinus and the other paranasal sinuses, or the maxillary and sphenoid sinuses (the ethmoid is not a sinus), cannot be seen as physiologically meaningless cavities.

This modern concept of paranasal sinuses development and physiology challenges the classical concept, proposed more than a century ago by Zuckerkandl, Mouret, and others, suggests that sinuses are ethmoidal cells which expand into the frontal, maxilla, and sphenoid bones and remain ventilated and drained through small openings called ostia. Neither the osteoclastic attribute necessary to the respiratory mucosa for bony expansion, nor the ventilation function of the ostium could have ever been demonstrated.

This chapter summarizes evidence in favor of the modern concept of frontal sinus development.

Keywords: paranasal sinuses, ethmoid, nitric oxide, arrested pneumatization, pneumosinus dilatans, evo-devo

1.1 Introduction

The frontal sinus starts its development after birth. Pneumatization in the frontal bone leads multiple gasfilled cavities to coalesce and form a polylobed cavity, which finally communicates with the lateral mass of the ethmoid.[1] Nitric oxide (NO), the gas produced throughout life by the sinus epithelium, is actively released into the nasal cavity to be mixed up with the inspiratory airflow.[2] At the level of the alveolar capillary membrane, nitric oxide facilitates the alveolar oxygen transfer into the bloodstream and increases arterial blood oxygenation. Thus, the frontal sinus and the other paranasal sinuses, or the maxillary and sphenoid sinuses (the ethmoid is not a sinus),[1] cannot be seen as physiologically meaningless cavities.

This modern concept of paranasal sinuses development and physiology challenges[3] the classical concept, proposed more than a century ago by Zuckerkandl,[4] Mouret,[5,6] and others, suggests that sinuses are ethmoidal cells which expand into the frontal, maxilla, and sphenoid bones and remain ventilated and drained through small openings called ostia. Neither the osteoclastic attribute necessary to the respiratory mucosa for bony expansion,[7] nor the ventilation function of the ostium[3] could have ever been demonstrated. This chapter summarizes evidence in favor of the modern concept of frontal sinus development.

1.2 Frontal Sinuses and Ethmoid Lateral Masses have Different Evolutionary and Developmental Origins

1.2.1 The Ethmoid Develops from the Olfactory Cartilaginous Capsule

The human ethmoid bone structure seems a priori to result from a remodeling of the anterior cranial base over the last several million years of evolution, since bipedalism began in our primate ancestors.

The mammalian quadruped ethmoid is formed by two olfactory chambers. They are separated from each other by the perpendicular plate, from the respiratory nasal passages lying below by the transverse lamina and from the skull base posteriorly by the cribriform plate through which the olfactory nerves pass to the olfactory bulb. These chambers open anteriorly in a vestibule which is common to the olfactory and respiratory noses.[1] They are entirely covered with olfactory mucosa and the surface of the olfactory mucosa is increased manyfold by the development of the transverse ethmoturbinates into the chambers.[8]

Bipedalism freed the hand and so humans acquired the upright posture. This evolutionary process led to the bending of skull base, a retraction of the snout occurred and the orbits migrated anteriorly.[9] According to the evo-devo theory,[1] the complex evolutionary craniofacial remodeling led to the squeezing of the mammalian ethmoturbinals and to the loss of their olfactory mucosa. As a result the lateral masses of the ethmoid were formed. In humans, olfactory mucosa remained located at the upper recess of the olfactory clefts and at the cribriform plates. The olfactory bulb shifted from a posterior almost vertical position to a superior horizontal position, following the development of the frontal lobes of the brain. Moreover, the transverse lamina disappeared and so the anatomical partition between the olfactory and respiratory epithelium led to the formation of the nose as a single organ.

In fact, human development tells us that the olfactory and respiratory parts of the nasal cavity are of different origins. The olfactory part develops from the olfactory placodes which invaginate toward the brain into olfactory pits. On the other hand, the respiratory part develops beneath the olfactory pits at the expense of the oral cavity by a remodeling of the bones of the secondary palate.[1] The olfactory pits differentiation give rise to all the anatomical structures of the fibrocartilaginous nose (alar and septolateral cartilages, olfactory fascia, and mucosa).[10-12] The fibrocartilaginous nose is attached to the anterior skull base, thanks to the embryological spreading of the tip end mucosa of the olfactory pits into the reliefs of the olfactory cartilaginous capsule that develops in the mesenchyme between the brain and olfactory pits around the eighth week of embryological formation. This olfactory cartilaginous capsule is the forerunner of the ethmoid bone which ossifies after birth. By contrast, the bones forming the respiratory nose (inferior turbinates, palatal apophyses of the maxilla and palatal bones, pterygoids, and vomers) despite their profound remodeling and repositioning remain attached to the maxillary bones. Even the vomer that forms the septum of the respiratory part of the nose below the septum of the olfactory nose. The septum is formed by the quadrangular cartilage and the perpendicular plate.

The ethmoid cartilage or bone appears to be involved in housing the olfactory mucosa in all the vertebrates, since the most primitive ones like the agnathan fish. Fish and amphibians do not have paranasal sinuses. Bony pneumatic recesses that resemble sinuses can only be observed in terrestrial animals. Bone pneumatization actually appears associated with life in earth that form paranasal sinuses and concerns not only the paranasal bones but also the petrous bones in humans and may even extend throughout other skeletal pieces of bone in birds (vertebrae, ribs, girdles, and proximal limb elements).[7]

1.2.2 The Frontal Sinuses Pneumatize after Erythropoietic Bone Marrow Conversion into Fatty Marrow

Bone pneumatization appears in fact as a biological mechanism, which follows the same rules independently of the developing bone. Pneumatization seems to proceed by the replacement of the erythropoietic bone marrow with "empty" sac diverticula. These diverticula might not be filled with air during the initial stage of their formation but with some gas resulting from the biochemical resorption of bone marrow. This gas may finally escape when the bony diverticula communicates with the respiratory tract. Many diverticula may form one single part of bone around the initial one, into which they drain successively.

These stages of bone pneumatization have been observed both in animals[13-15] and humans.[16] In the pigeon, a large proportion of the skeleton becomes pneumatized by conversion of the erythropoietic bone marrow

into fatty marrow. This phenomenon starts at 1 month after hatching. At the age of 6 months posthatching, bone marrow has been displaced, its volume has decreased in correlation to the increasing pneumaticity and conversion to fatty marrow.[15] Bone pneumatization has also been well studied in young children using MRI of the bone marrow at the level of the sphenoid.[16,17] Until the age of 4 months, the basisphenoid contains red bone marrow. At this time, sphenoid marrow commences fatty conversion with most individuals showing significant fatty marrow conversion by the age of 2 years. After 3 years of age most children demonstrate pneumatized diverticula in association to fatty conversion images. With respect to the sphenoid, complete pneumatization occurs between the ages of 1 and 5 years. Thus, the authors conclude that fatty change before pneumatization is a normal developmental process and should not be misinterpreted as a pathological condition.[16]

Nothing is known about fatty conversion of the bone marrow before pneumatization in the frontal bones. However, images of arrested pneumatization (see next section) suggest that the mechanism of pneumatization in the frontal should be similar to the sphenoidal one.

Almost nothing is known about the process of pneumatization at the cellular and tissue levels, and even less about pneumatization processes. However, the nitric oxide "story" of the sinuses that might be the clue to understand how pneumatization occurs.

1.3 The Nitric Oxide "Story" of the Paranasal Sinuses Makes them Play a Role in Blood Oxygenation on Demand

The role and function of the paranasal sinuses, that is the frontal, maxillary and sphenoid bony cavities, have long been debated. Paranasal sinuses may have no function but could have been coopted in evolution for their beneficial effects in many domains: Head lightening, energetics, maintaining strength with minimizing materials, assistance in facial growth and architecture, skull base widening for the support of the large palate to accommodate the permanent dentition, functional pillars for dispersal of masticatory forces, protection for the brain, thermal insulation for central nervous system and sense organs, increase of the surface area for the olfactory mucosa, resonance of the voice, etc.

The true, genuine function of the paranasal sinuses may, however, have been inferred, in the context of evolution, from their ability to produce, store, and release NO (▶ Fig. 1.1). The discovery of the physiological role of NO produced by blood vessel endothelial cells as a powerful vasodilator was awarded the Nobel Prize for Medicine in 1998. Until this discovery, this gas was regarded as merely an atmospheric pollutant, with no biological role.

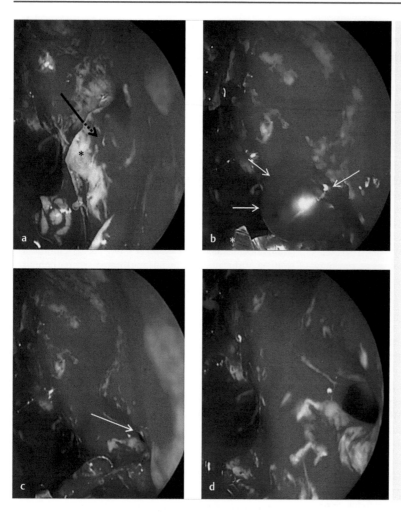

Fig. 1.1 Ostial emission of a gas bolus of maxillary origin during left ethmoidectomy **(a)**, the lower part of the unciform apophysis (*) adjacent to the presumed position of the maxillary ostium (*arrow*), **(b)** introducing the mobile bit of the retrograde forceps (*) in the infundibulum reveals a gas bolus (*arrows*), **(c)** ablating the lower part of the unciform apophysis partially reveals the maxillary ostium, **(d)** the maxillary ostium appears open.

In fact, its physiological role extends to many other cell and tissue functions, notably in the respiratory, nervous, and immune systems. The presence of NO in exhaled air was discovered in 1991.[18]

The role of the upper airway system in NO production was demonstrated by measuring exhaled NO in tracheostomized subjects at the cannula, oral and nasal cavity; levels were low in the cannula, intermediate in the oral, and high in the nasal cavity.[19] Nasal administration of NO synthetase (NOS) inhibitors showed, no significantly reduced production. Maxillary sinus catheterization revealed a much higher level of NO in the maxillary sinus than that of the exhaled air in the nose, approximating in some subjects the maximum authorized atmospheric concentration of 25 ppm.[20,21] Moreover, iterative sinus sampling revealed rapid recovery of NO levels, suggesting the continuous sinus production. Intrasinus injection of NOS inhibitors reduced NO levels by 80%, confirming the active enzymatic NO synthesis in the sinus.[21] Finally, maxillary sinus mucosa biopsy demonstrated that the enzyme responsible for this continuous NO production was iNOS (NOS-2),[22] the classically inducible calcium-independent isoform of the NO synthetase enzyme, which was located at the apical pole of the epithelium covering the inner surface of sinus cavity.[21] The surprise was that iNOS, which had never been detected in healthy tissue, was spontaneously and permanently active in the sinus epithelium.[2] In contrast, only weak NO synthetase activity was detected in the epithelium of the nasal cavity.[21]

It takes less than 3 minutes for the depleted sinus NO reserve to fully recover, and it has been shown that intermittent NO bolus release by the sinuses can be induced by humming for about 10 seconds during nasal expiration.[23] The mean nasal exhaled NO rate in humming is about five fold higher than in silent nasal expiration.[24] Humming causes the exhaled airflow to vibrate, and its impact on NO flowrate seems to be related to the vibration frequency.[24] The role of acoustic vibrations in sinus ostium patency has already been described in 1959 by Guillerm et al[25]. Regarding ultrasound, which, added the nasal aerosol therapy, and facilitated the sinus drug penetration.

Humming like ultrasonorization of inhaled air is, however, not a normal function. However, speaking, shouting, crying, laughing, snoring, etc. also cause intermittent vibrations of the nasal airflow, which could physiologically stimulate repeated, independent NO boli release by paranasal sinuses. Sinus ostia are classically passive openings of the bony cavities as no nerves, vessels, or muscles can be found in their surface. Therefore, the functional role of a sphinchter could be given in their mucosal line.[26] We have, however, recently observed during endoscopic procedures under general anesthesia that paranasal sinuses ostia could be active structures controlling the independent opening and closure of the different paranasal sinuses, thereby being able to control the release of NO boli into the nasal airflow. What we have observed is a relatively quick, edematous, reversible swelling of the circumferential mucosa bordering the ostium.[27] Our hypothesis is that this lies in the physiology of the cells bordering the ostium. Such a mechanism is present in the guard cells surrounding the leaves stomata that are controlling gas exchange (CO_2, O_2, H_2O) in plants. Stomata, located in the plant epidermidis, consist of a pair of guard cells, and their enclosing pore. Stomata open and close through turgor changes driven by massive ion fluxes. They mainly occur through the guard cell plasma membrane and tonoplast. Fine control of stomatal aperture is achieved through an exquisite sensitivity of the guard cells to multiple environmental and endogenous signals including light, humidity, temperature, CO_2, plant water status, and plant hormones. Signals like vibrations in the nasal airstream, sinus content or concentration of NO, humidity, temperature, etc. could in the same way drive the physiology of the cells surrounding the paranasal sinuses ostia.

These hypotheses would be worth testing, because NO appears as a regulator of respiratory exchange in lung physiology, modulating the respiration/perfusion ratio, reducing pulmonary vascular resistance, and facilitating alveolar oxygen transfer into the bloodstream. Adding NO to the inspiratory circuit of intubated patients reduces pulmonary vessel resistance and enhances arterial blood oxygenation.[28] Other reports confirm that adding small amounts of NO (10-100 ppb) to inhaled air has significant impact on pulmonary vessel resistance and arterial blood oxygenation in acute respiratory distress syndrome.[29,30] Compared to oral respiration, nasal respiration reduces pulmonary vessel resistance and enhances arterial blood oxygenation in healthy subjects.[28,31] Adding 100 ppb NO to ambient orally inhaled air reproduces the effect of nasal respiration.[31] Moreover, it has been shown that endogenous NO produced by paranasal sinuses is inhaled at similar concentrations in normal breathing,[32,33] and the level of exhaled NO is significantly higher in populations living under hypoxic conditions in the Tibetan highlands than in control populations living at low altitude.[34] Thus, NO produced in the upper airway system may act in an "aerocrine" fashion to enhance pulmonary oxygen uptake in humans.[28]

Finally, the genuine function of the paranasal sinuses might be to produce NO, thanks to the epithelium lying on their walls and to store NO, thanks to the closure function of their ostia. It could be achieved by turgor changes in the ostial epithelial cells, and to release NO on demand when increased oxygenation of the blood is needed. Different kinds of vibrations of the nasal airstream may not be the only signals inducing the opening of the ostium, and research needs to continue.

1.4 Pneumosinus Dilatans and Arrested Pneumatization Could Bear Witness to Sinus Development

1.4.1 Pneumosinus Dilatans

Pneumosinus dilatans is a disease that produces an abnormal expansion of a paranasal sinus cavity, which contains only gas and is lined by normal mucosa. The bony walls are displaced outwardly and cause either embossing or intracranial, orbital, and ethmoidal encroachment (▶ Fig. 1.2).

We found that pneumosinus dilatans are associated with intense remodeling of the bone surrounding the sinus cavity, showing substitution of normal lamellar trabecular bone by osteoid trabeculae, with a high

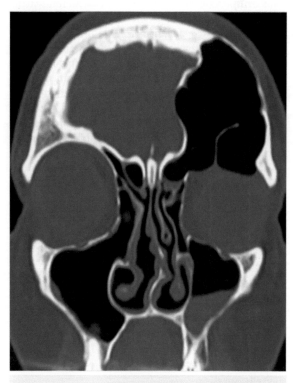

Fig. 1.2 Pneumosinus dilatans is a disease that produces an abnormal expansion of a paranasal sinus cavity. It contains only gas and is lined by normal mucosa. The bony walls are displaced outwardly aimed to cause embossing or intracranial, orbital and ethmoidal encroachment.

number of osteoclasts intermingled with the osteoblasts reflecting the simultaneous bone resorption and formation. These pathological findings show similarities to bone from active Paget's disease. Compared with normal lamellar bone, the poorly mineralized osteoid bone from pneumosinus dilatans appears to be very sensitive to mechanical forces and subsequent remodeling. 18-Labeled sodium fluoride Positron Emission Tomography–Computed Tomography (NaF PET-CT) showed significant increase in ^{18}F-NaF uptake highlighting the pneumosinus dilatans walls, in accordance with intense bone remodeling. By contrast, no abnormal uptake of fluorine-deoxyglucose was observed on FDG PET-CT, in accordance with the normal histological aspect of the sinuses mucosa.[35]

Thus, pneumosinus dilatans appears to be an osteogenic disease. Interestingly, NO is known as an important signaling molecule in bone, with its concentration used to control the balance between bone formation and resorption.[36] We were not able to measure NO during surgery, which simply consisted in reopening the sinus cavity into the ethmoid lateral mass, but this intervention was sufficient to stop evolution of disease and restore ossification of sinuses bony walls.[35] Our hypothesis is that pneumosinus dilatans could be the bony consequence of elevated concentration and/or pressure of NO inside a sinus cavity. Our experience is that pneumosinus dilatans can be controlled on the long term by apparently allowing NO to escape the sinus again.

This hypothesis about the pathogeny of pneumosinus dilatans could bear witness to the development of the sinus cavity during infancy. NO might be produced by bone marrow regression, allowing each sinus cavity to expand and find an opening into the nasal cavity. Once NO concentration inside the sinus can be controlled by a well-functioning ostium, the size and shape of the sinus cavity stabilize.

This mechanism of paranasal sinus formation may explain why the size and shape of sinuses are highly variable, showing asymmetry in most people, and that they can develop in some areas independently of biomechanical forces.

Sinus hyperpneumatization may be explained in the same way and should be distinguished from pneumosinus dilatans. Hypersinuses[37] describe those sinuses which have developed beyond the usual size. Although, the sinus is larger than usual, it does not extend beyond the normal boundaries of the frontal, maxillary or sphenoid bone. Their walls are normal and their content is gaseous. There is no facial bossing or intracranial, orbital or ethmoidal encroachment (▶ Fig. 1.3). The patient is clinically totally asymptomatic.

Hyperpneumatization may also affect the temporal bone, and even in rare cases the occipital bone and the first vertebrae (atlas and axis).[38] The signals that initiate bone marrow regression and allow its replacement by pneumatized cavities in some selected bones are not known.

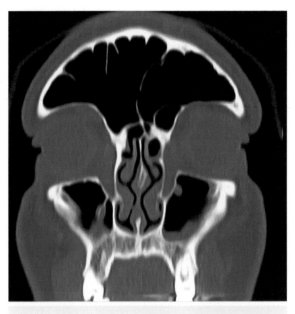

Fig. 1.3 Hyperpneumatization of the frontal bone. Although the sinus is larger than usual, it does not extend beyond the normal boundaries of the frontal bone. There is no facial bossing or intracranial, orbital or ethmoidal encroachment.

1.4.2 Arrested Pneumatization

Looking at the shape of adult paranasal sinuses, it seems as if more than one spot was pneumatized in each bone to build up their anatomy. The bony septa that usually partially divide the adult sinus cavities may be remnants among the multiple spots of bone marrow degeneration that after coalescence formed a single sinus cavity in each bone. Images of arrested pneumatization, which have been described at the level of the sphenoid bone to eliminate serious differential diagnosis like chondrosarcoma, osteomyelitis, bone metastasis, or fibrous dysplasia,[39] seem also to bear witness to the multiple-spot sinus excavation development.[1]

Arrested pneumatization is usually limited to the part of the bone in which it occurred and seems to correspond to one (sometimes two or three) spot(s) of bone marrow degeneration that (have) not fulfilled the conditions to be pneumatized and remained sequestered in the bone (▶ Fig. 1.4). It is described as a usually incidental discovery on CT imaging of a zone of abnormal ossification in a site of usual pneumatization. The zone of abnormal ossification has to present two of the four following criteria to be eligible to the diagnosis of arrested pneumatization: well-circumscribed, sclerotic margins with narrow transition zone, regions of internal fat density, regions of internal soft tissue density, and curvilinear internal calcifications.[39]

Images of arrested pneumatization have been found in the sphenoid, frontal, and maxillary, but not in the

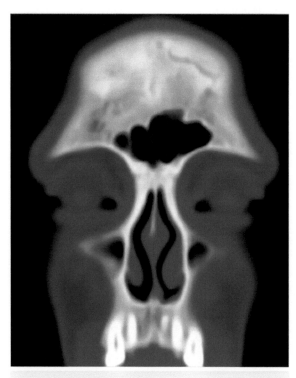

Fig. 1.4 Arrested pneumatization in the frontal bone. The zone of abnormal ossification has to present two of the four following criteria to be eligible for the diagnosis of arrested pneumatization: well-circumscribed, sclerotic margins with narrow transition zone, regions of internal fat density, regions of internal soft tissue density, curvilinear internal calcifications.

ethmoid bone. These data have been interpreted as indirect argument to support a different origin between the lateral masses of the ethmoid bones and other paranasal sinuses as arrested pneumatization can only occur in bones that pneumatize.[40]

1.5 Conclusion

The modern concept of frontal sinus development proposes new clues to improve classical surgical techniques and develop modern frontal sinus surgery.

References

[1] Jankowski R, ed. The Evo-Devo Origin of the Nose, Anterior Skull Base and Midface. Paris; 2013

[2] Lundberg JO. Nitric oxide and the paranasal sinuses. Anat Rec (Hoboken) 2008;291(11):1479–1484 PubMed

[3] Jankowski R, Nguyen DT, Poussel M, Chenuel B, Gallet P, Rumeau C. Sinusology. Eur Ann Otorhinolaryngol Head Neck Dis 2016;133 (4):263–268

[4] Zuckerkandl E. Normale und Pathologische Anatomie der Nasenhöle und ihrer pneumatischen Anhänge. 2nd ed. Vienna: W. Braumuller; 1893

[5] Mouret J. Anatomie des cellules ethmoïdales. Rev Laryngol; 1898

[6] Mouret J. Rapports du sinus frontal avec les cellules ethmoidales. Rev Laryngol; 1901

[7] Witmer L. The phylogenic history of paranasal air sinuses. In: T Koppe HN, KW Alt, eds. The paranasal sinuses of higher Primates—Development, Function, and Evolution. Chicago: Quintessence Publishing Co, Inc; 1999

[8] Moore W, ed. The mammalian skull. Cambridge: Cambridge University Press; 1981

[9] Márquez S, Tessema B, Clement PA, Schaefer SD. Development of the ethmoid sinus and extramural migration: the anatomical basis of this paranasal sinus. Anat Rec (Hoboken) 2008;291(11):1535–1553 PubMed

[10] Jankowski R. Marquez p. Embryology of the nose: the evo-devo concept. World J Otorhinolaryngol 2016;6(2):33–40

[11] Jankowski R, Rumeau C, de Saint Hilaire T, et al. The olfactory fascia: an evo-devo concept of the fibrocartilaginous nose. Surg Radiol Anat 2016;38(10):1161–1168 PubMed

[12] Jankowski R. Septoplastie et rhinoplastie par désarticulation: histoire, anatomie et architecture naturelles du nez. Paris: Elsevier Masson; 2016:370

[13] O'Connor PM. Pulmonary pneumaticity in the postcranial skeleton of extant aves: a case study examining Anseriformes. J Morphol 2004;261(2):141–161 PubMed

[14] O'Connor PM. Postcranial pneumaticity: an evaluation of soft-tissue influences on the postcranial skeleton and the reconstruction of pulmonary anatomy in archosaurs. J Morphol 2006;267(10):1199–1226 PubMed

[15] Schepelmann K. Erythropoietic bone marrow in the pigeon: development of its distribution and volume during growth and pneumatization of bones. J Morphol 1990;203(1):21–34 PubMed

[16] Aoki S, Dillon WP, Barkovich AJ, Norman D. Marrow conversion before pneumatization of the sphenoid sinus: assessment with MR imaging. Radiology 1989;172(2):373–375 PubMed

[17] Szolar D, Preidler K, Ranner G, et al. Magnetic resonance assessment of age-related development of the sphenoid sinus. Br J Radiol 1994;67(797):431–435 PubMed

[18] Gustafsson LE, Leone AM, Persson MG, Wiklund NP, Moncada S. Endogenous nitric oxide is present in the exhaled air of rabbits, guinea pigs and humans. Biochem Biophys Res Commun 1991;181 (2):852–857 PubMed

[19] Lundberg JO, Weitzberg E, Nordvall SL, Kuylenstierna R, Lundberg JM, Alving K. Primarily nasal origin of exhaled nitric oxide and absence in Kartagener's syndrome. Eur Respir J 1994;7(8):1501–1504 PubMed

[20] Lundberg JO, Rinder J, Weitzberg E, Lundberg JM, Alving K. Nasally exhaled nitric oxide in humans originates mainly in the paranasal sinuses. Acta Physiol Scand 1994;152(4):431–432 PubMed

[21] Lundberg JO, Farkas-Szallasi T, Weitzberg E, et al. High nitric oxide production in human paranasal sinuses. Nat Med 1995;1(4):370–373 PubMed

[22] Lundberg JO, Weitzberg E, Rinder J, et al. Calcium-independent and steroid-resistant nitric oxide synthase activity in human paranasal sinus mucosa. Eur Respir J 1996;9(7):1344–1347 PubMed

[23] Weitzberg E, Lundberg JO. Humming greatly increases nasal nitric oxide. Am J Respir Crit Care Med 2002;166(2):144–145 PubMed

[24] Maniscalco M, Weitzberg E, Sundberg J, Sofia M, Lundberg JO. Assessment of nasal and sinus nitric oxide output using single-breath humming exhalations. Eur Respir J 2003;22(2):323–329 PubMed

[25] Guillerm R, Badre R, Flottes L, Riu R, Rey A. [A new method of aerosol penetration into the sinuses]. Presse Med 1959;67(27):1097–1098 PubMed

[26] Flottes L, Clerc P, Riu R, Devilla F, eds. La physiologie des sinus. Paris: Librairie Arnette; 1960

[27] Jankowski R, Rumeau C. Physiology of the parnasal sinus ostium: endoscopic observations. Eur Ann Otorhinolaryngol Head Neck Dis, Submitted

[28] Lundberg JO, Lundberg JM, Settergren G, Alving K, Weitzberg E. Nitric oxide, produced in the upper airways, may act in an 'aerocrine' fashion to enhance pulmonary oxygen uptake in humans. Acta Physiol Scand 1995;155(4):467–468 PubMed

[29] Gerlach H, Rossaint R, Pappert D, Falke KJ. Time-course and dose-response of nitric oxide inhalation for systemic oxygenation and pulmonary hypertension in patients with adult respiratory distress syndrome. Eur J Clin Invest 1993;23(8):499–502 PubMed

[30] Puybasset L, Rouby JJ, Mourgeon E, et al. Inhaled nitric oxide in acute respiratory failure: dose-response curves. Intensive Care Med 1994;20(5):319–327 PubMed

[31] Lundberg JO, Settergren G, Gelinder S, Lundberg JM, Alving K, Weitzberg E. Inhalation of nasally derived nitric oxide modulates pulmonary function in humans. Acta Physiol Scand 1996;158(4):343–347 PubMed

[32] Busch T, Kuhlen R, Knorr M, et al. Nasal, pulmonary and autoinhaled nitric oxide at rest and during moderate exercise. Intensive Care Med 2000;26(4):391–399 PubMed

[33] Gerlach H, Rossaint R, Pappert D, Knorr M, Falke KJ. Autoinhalation of nitric oxide after endogenous synthesis in nasopharynx. Lancet 1994;343(8896):518–519 PubMed

[34] Beall CM, Laskowski D, Strohl KP, et al. Pulmonary nitric oxide in mountain dwellers. Nature 2001;414(6862):411–412 PubMed

[35] Jankowski R, Kuntzler S, Boulanger N, et al. Is pneumosinus dilatans an osteogenic disease that mimics the formation of a paranasal sinus? Surg Radiol Anat 2014;36(5):429–437 PubMed

[36] van't Hof RJ, Ralston SH. Nitric oxide and bone. Immunology 2001;103(3):255–261 PubMed

[37] Urken ML, Som PM, Lawson W, Edelstein D, Weber AL, Biller HF. Abnormally large frontal sinus. II. Nomenclature, pathology, and symptoms. Laryngoscope 1987;97(5):606–611 PubMed

[38] Petritsch B, Goltz JP, Hahn D, Wendel F. Extensive craniocervical bone pneumatization. Diagn Interv Radiol 2011;17(4):308–310 PubMed

[39] Welker KM, DeLone DR, Lane JI, Gilbertson JR. Arrested pneumatization of the skull base: imaging characteristics. AJR Am J Roentgenol 2008;190(6):1691–1696 PubMed

[40] Kuntzler S, Jankowski R. Arrested pneumatization: witness of paranasal sinuses development? Eur Ann Otorhinolaryngol Head Neck Dis 2014;131(3):167–170 PubMed

2 Radiological Anatomy

Claudia Kirsch

"The beginning of wisdom is the definition of terms."
— Socrates

Abstract

The complex variable frontal sinus drainage pathway anatomy on radiographic imaging appears different viewed endoscopically; however, awareness of the multiple alternate drainage pathways is vital to prevent potential surgical complications and is confounded by redundant and confusing terminology. Despite newer imaging techniques, major complications from frontal sinus surgery still occur. This chapter's goal is to improve radiographic visualization and understanding of the frontal sinus drainage pathway anatomy starting from development to the multitude of presentations found on computed axial tomography of the paranasal sinuses. The following mnemonic is a helpful reminder that "radiology of the frontal sinus drainage pathway requires you to Look Precisely UP FOR AN Accessory air cell, Ethmoidal Arteries, and BE Mentally Trained." This mnemonic is a reminder to visually check on the CT scan critical anatomy, the "Look Precisely **UP FOR AN** Accessory Air cell, Ethmoidal Arteries, and **BE** Mentally Trained" represent the "Lamina Papyracea" of the orbit, the "Uncinate Process," "Floor of the Olfactory Recess," "Agger Nasi air cell," "Accessory Air cells," "Ethmoidal Arteries," and **BE** Mentally Trained" reminds one to look at the "Bulla Ethmoidalis" and "Middle Turbinate." This chapter highlights these critical structures' development, and presents in more detail their radiographic anatomy.

Keywords: paranasal sinus computed axial tomography (CT), frontal sinus drainage pathway, agger nasi, uncinate process, floor of the olfactory recess, lateral lamella, accessory air cells, bulla ethmoidalis, middle turbinate

"Radiology of frontal sinus drainage pathways requires you to "Look Precisely UP FOR AN Accessory air cell, Ethmoidal Arteries, and BE Mentally Trained."

2.1 Introduction

Like fingerprints, the frontal sinus and frontal sinus drainage pathways are unique and mutable in each and every individual including identical twins.[1,2,3] Understanding the complex frontal sinus drainage pathways' variable anatomy with both radiographic and endoscopic imaging is important to prevent potential surgical complications and is confounded by often redundant and confusing terminology.[4] This chapter on radiographic anatomy will attempt to clarify this anatomy and utilize the standardized accepted terms outlined in the 2014 European Position Paper on the Anatomical Terminology of the Internal Nose and Paranasal Sinuses.[5]

The variegated frontal sinus drainage anatomy on computed axial tomography (CT) that clearly defines bony margins does not have the same appearance on stereotactic localization with overlying mucosa and tissue when viewed through the nostrils by an endoscope (▶ Fig. 2.1, ▶ Fig. 2.2, ▶ Fig. 2.3, ▶ Fig. 2.4, ▶ Fig. 2.5, ▶ Fig. 2.6). In addition, a surgeon maneuvering in this unique tight space with angled endoscopes and instruments must mentally recreate this anatomy.[6,7] Despite newer imaging techniques, major complications from frontal sinus surgery occur in 2.7% of patients.[8,9,10] The goal of this chapter is to define the radiographic anatomy of the frontal sinus drainage pathways from their first origins to the final variable anatomy, providing a checklist to prevent missing critical anatomical variants.

When viewing a radiographic image, search patterns with a set list of items aid clinicians in what to look for and help avoiding mistakes including "satisfaction of search." This occurs after identifying a unique finding; a clinician forgets to double check and misses a second critical finding. In the narrow complex radiographic frontal sinus drainage pathway, this mnemonic is helpful: radiology of the frontal sinus drainage pathway requires you to "Look Precisely UP FOR AN Accessory air cell, Ethmoidal Arteries, and BE Mentally Prepared." This mnemonic reminds radiologists to check each radiograph for key areas, namely "Look Precisely" is reminder to assess the LP or "Lamina Papyracea" of the orbit. UP represents the "Uncinate Process," FOR, the "Floor of the Olfactory Recess" including the delicate lateral lamella, AN represents the "Agger Nasi air cell," the "Accessory Air cells," and "Ethmoidal Arteries" are self-explanatory, BE represents the "Bulla Ethmoidalis" and Mentally trained or MT the "Middle Turbinate." This chapter briefly discusses the development of these critical structures and details their radiographic anatomy.

The frontal sinuses form at approximately the fifth week of gestation along with the branchial arches, pouches, and primitive gut. The anterior opening or stomodaeum includes the maxillary arch above, mandibular arch and frontonasal prominence anteriorly and superiorly dividing the nasal prominences and nasal aperture.[11] During the seventh and eighth weeks of gestation, the nasal capsule lateral wall develops mesenchymal ridges above the palatal shelves and eventually form the complex frontal sinus drainage pathways, including ramified ethmoturbinals, extending perpendicular to the lateral wall, with smaller exoturbinals and larger endoturbinals, extending to the medial nasal septum.

Mechanisms of ethmoid sinus formation are debatable as recent mammalian ethmoid sinus development research

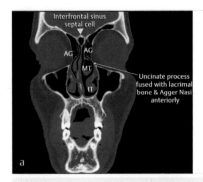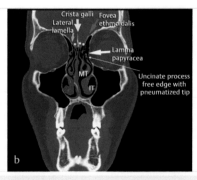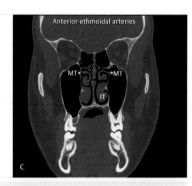

Fig. 2.1 (a) Coronal CT scan through the frontal sinus anteriorly. Small yellow arrowhead, —interfrontal sinus septal cell; AG, agger nasi air cell; IT, inferior turbinate; MT, middle turbinate. Note the concha bullosa in the left MT lateral deviation of the inferior AG and UP, and rightward nasal septal deviation abutting the right inferior turbinate restricting airflow in the right inferior meatus. (b) Coronal CT scan posterior to ▶ Fig. 2.1a of frontal sinus at the crista galli—yellow arrow. The left fovea ethmoidalis is denoted by the blue arrow. There is slight flattening of right fovea ethmoidalis, the increased obliquity of the right lateral lamella—purple arrow, is at greater risk for injury. Lamina papyracea—white arrow, and uncinate process free edge with a pneumatized tip marked (^) and long thin arrow. Note middle turbinate (MT) lamella attaches to floor of the olfactory recess at junction of lateral lamella and cribiform plate. The left MT concha bullosa has two superior attachments marked by (*) asterisks. There is rightward nasal septal deviation abutting the right inferior turbinate restricting airflow in the right inferior meatus. IT, inferior turbinate. (c) Coronal CT scan posterior to ▶ Fig. 2.1a, b. The middle turbinate (MT) lamella extends horizontally to the medial maxillary sinus, denoted by a *MT, a dividing point for ethmoid air cells anteriorly drain with the frontal recess to the infundibulum, ethmoidal air cells posteriorly drain with the sphenoethmoidal recess. IT, inferior turbinate. Note the slight indentation of the superior lamina papyracea demarcating anterior ethmoidal arteries; the presence of left accessory supra bulla air cells means the anterior ethmoidal artery may extend inferiorly.

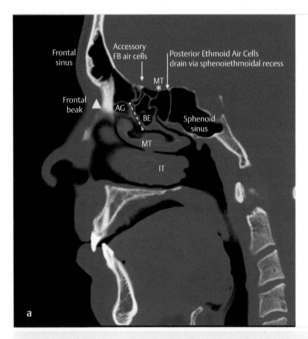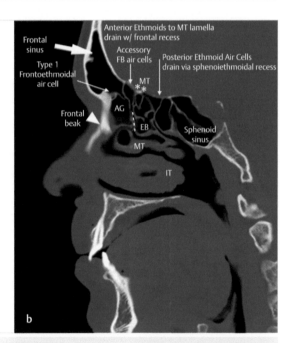

Fig. 2.2 (a) Sagittal CT scan of the same sinus as in ▶ Fig. 2.1a–c. The right frontal sinus drainage pathway (FSDP) is demarcated by the fine dotted line. Frontal beak—small arrowhead. AG, agger nasi air cell is the anterior margin of FSDP; BE, bulla ethmoidalis air cell, the posterior margin of FSDP. Note accessory frontal bulla air cells above BE, placing anterior ethmoidal artery at risk during surgery. (b) Sagittal CT scan of the left frontal sinus drainage pathway—fine dotted line, of sinus in ▶ Fig. 2.1a–c. Frontal beak—small arrowhead. AG, agger nasi air cell, the anterior margin of the FSDP; BE, bulla ethmoidalis air cell, the posterior margin of FSDP; IT, inferior turbinate; MT, middle turbinate. The left MT concha bullosa is partially visualized, with two thin lamellae attaching superiorly.

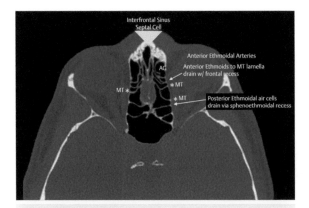

Fig. 2.3 Axial CT scan of sinus in ▶ Fig. 2.1 and ▶ Fig. 2.2. AG, agger nasi air cell; the anterior margin of frontal sinus drainage pathway; IT, inferior turbinate; MT, middle turbinate. Note the attachments of the MT laterally to the lamina papyracea.

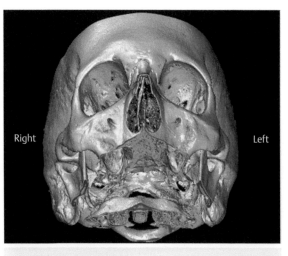

Fig. 2.4 Bony 3D reformations of sinus in ▶ Fig. 2.1, ▶ Fig. 2.2, ▶ Fig. 2.3, similar to endoscopic appearance when covered by mucosa, note rightward nasal septal deviation.

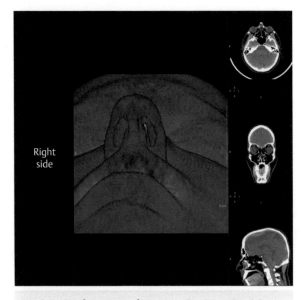

Fig. 2.5 3D reformations of sinus in ▶ Fig. 2.1, ▶ Fig. 2.2, ▶ Fig. 2.3, ▶ Fig. 2.4 with overlying mucosa, similar to endoscopic appearance, note rightward nasal septal deviation and how overlapping structures limit visualization of frontal nasal sinus drainage pathway (FSDP). Far left CT axial, coronal, and sagittal images are reference points for angulation and visualization.

notes that on all radiographic images there is a "stacking appearance" of the thin transverse bone plates or "ethmoturbinals." The infolding of the ethmoturbinals increases surface area and these eventually become the ethmoid labyrinth losing their olfactory mucosa, which remains only in the olfactory grooves. In evo-devo theories, the endoturbinals form overlapping shelves flattening and curving atop each other, like onion skin layering[12] (▶ Fig. 2.1a, b). At approximately the 25th to 28th week of

gestation, three medially directed projections arise from the lateral wall. The first ethmoturbinal's or "nasoturbinal" ascending anterior component develops into the agger nasi, the inferior projection of the maxilloturbinate becomes the maxillary sinus, and the superior projection transforms into the ethmoidoturbinate.[11] The first ethmoturbinal's descending portion forms the uncinate process while the remaining portion regresses. At the fourth fetal month, a medial outpouching above the superior uncinate process forms and after birth develops into the frontal sinus.

The second ethmoturbinal becomes the middle turbinate, later becoming an important radiographic landmark seen well on the sagittal plane because when the attachment of the middle turbinate switches from attaching superiorly to a horizontal component extending to the lamina papyracea, this becomes a dividing line for the separate drainage pathways of the anterior and posterior ethmoidal air cells (▶ Fig. 2.1c, ▶ Fig. 2.2a, b, ▶ Fig. 2.3). Therefore, in front of the second ethmoturbinal are the developing anterior ethmoid air cells and located behind it are the developing posterior ethmoid air cells. The third ethmoturbinal becomes the superior turbinate, the fourth and fifth ethmoturbinals usually regress, although occasionally form a supreme turbinate. The persistent lamellar attachments of the first and second ethmoturbinals to the lateral nasal wall remain radiographically and surgically important as identifiers for frontal sinus drainage pathways.[13] With this developmental pathway in mind, let's use the mnemonic radiographically to examine the frontal sinus drainage pathways and "Look Precisely UP FOR AN Accessory air cell, Ethmoidal Arteries, and BE Mentally Trained." In the coronal plane, the easily radiographically identifiable landmark of the "Lamina Papyracea" and upward pointing "Uncinate Process" remind us

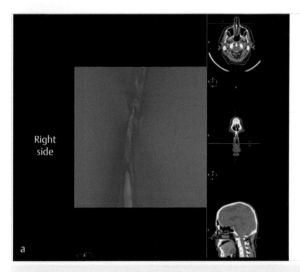 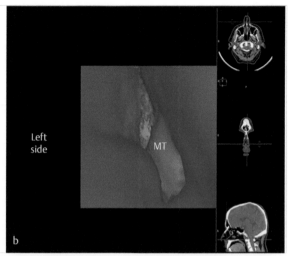

Fig. 2.6 (a) CT 3D reformations with endoscopic view through the right inferior meatus upward. The far left axial, coronal and sagittal CT scans with the thin yellow line demonstrating angle and upward visualization to the frontal sinus drainage pathway obscured by rightward nasal septal deviation. **(b)** CT 3D reformations with endoscopic view through the left inferior meatus upward. The far left axial, coronal and sagittal CT scans with thin yellow line demonstrating angle and upward visualization to the frontal sinus drainage pathway obscured by the left middle turbinate (MT) concha bullosa.

to "Look Precisely UP FOR the two thinnest bones at surgical risk, namely the "Lamina Papyracea" and " lateral lamella at the Floor of the Olfactory Recess" (▶ Fig. 2.1b).

2.2 Lamina Papyracea

"Look Precisely" at the Lamina Papyracea.

The lamina papyracea arises from the ethmoid bone and, like its name, is the paper-thin orbital plate forming the lateral ethmoid sinus border and medial orbital margin (▶ Fig. 2.1a, b, ▶ Fig. 2.3). The thin lamina papyracea may have a focal dehiscence in up to 10% of the population, and iatrogenic surgical risks may increase with anatomical sinus variations.[14,15] If the lamina is disrupted, not all is lost so long as the orbital periosteum remains intact, the disruption may be of little or no consequence.[16] Typically, the lamina papyracea and maxillary ostium are in the same plane; however, variations occur, and in some cases, the lamina papyracea may extend medial to the maxillary ostium, putting it at risk for injury.[17,18] Interestingly, post-functional endoscopic sinus surgery, the lamina papyracea may also deviate medially.[19]

There are three major structures that can insert onto the lamina papyracea including the agger nasi air cell (▶ Fig. 2.1a), the middle turbinate basal lamella demarcation point for the anterior and posterior ethmoidal air cells (▶ Fig. 2.1c, ▶ Fig. 2.3), and rarely the uncinate process.[20,21,22,23] On imaging, check for fracture deformities, dehiscence or ethmoid sinuses located medial to the maxillary ostium or lateral to the maxillary ethmoidal suture, or air cells along the superior maxillary sinus

orbital margin and inferior medial orbital margin termed "Haller's air cells."[7,18,23,24,25,26,27,28]

In the majority of patients, the agger nasi cell extends into the lamina papyracea as shown in ▶ Fig. 2.1a. The upward component of the agger nasi air cell may also give a component of bone to the bulla lamella anteriorly and posteriorly.[22] Inadvertent damage through the lamina puts the orbital medial rectus muscle at risk for injury and may form a potential route for orbital emphysema and infection resulting in an orbital cellulitis. Even more worrisome is the concern for damage to the anterior ethmoidal artery that may result in an intraorbital hematoma.[15,23,29]

2.3 Uncinate Process

"Look Precisely UP"—The Uncinate Process.

In Latin, the term uncinate means "hooked out growth."[25] The curved uncinate process (UP) is a bony leaflet pointing upward, easily noted on a coronal CT scan, as marked by an ^ and long white arrow on ▶ Fig. 2.1b. The UP is believed to be a vestige of the ethmoidal turbinal and first arises from the lateral nasal wall at approximately 11 to 12 weeks' gestation, projecting below the middle turbinate.[20] By 17 weeks' gestation, the UP is well formed between the middle turbinate and the yet to be formed ethmoidal bulla, which as noted previously will end up in parallel to the anterior ethmoid bulla running in a slight curve from anterior superior to posterior inferior.[20] The posterior free margin lies as in the evo-devo theory of development, parallel to the anterior margin of the ethmoidal bullae[5,12,20]

(▶ Fig. 2.1b). The air space above the upper edge of the UP marked by the ^ is the hiatus semilunaris opening into the ethmoidal infundibulum.[4,5,21,22]

The UP anterior ascending convex margin may rarely pneumatize ▶ Fig. 2.1b, or deviate medially fusing with the middle turbinate, or extend upward fusing with the skull base or laterally to the lamina papyracea, abutting the lamina papyracea creating a recessus terminalis and atelectatic infundibulum.[23] The UP has three components: anteriorly, the UP attaches to the lacrimal bone and at times the agger nasi air cell medially (▶ Fig. 2.1a) or the middle turbinate and posteriorly to the perpendicular process of the palatine bone and inferior turbinate ethmoidal process. The superior portion has multiple variable ways of attaching that alter the frontal sinus drainage pathway[24,25] (▶ Fig. 2.1b). Researchers have noted at least six types of attachments,[26] including a type I, with the superior attachment of the UP to the lamina papyracea; type II, the UP extends upward to the ethmoid roof or skull base; type III, the UP attaches to the middle turbinate, and may bend either medially or laterally, or become hypertrophied or pneumatized (▶ Fig. 2.1b). When the tip of the uncinate process is pneumatized, it may be referred to as an uncinate bullae[21,22,23,24,25] (▶ Fig. 2.1b). The most common variation of the UP occurring approximately 50 to 60% is attachment to the lamina papyracea with attachment to a posterior medial agger nasi air cell, about 18 to 20% to the junction of the lamina papyracea, cribriform plate, and middle turbinate, to the ethmoid roof only 3 to 6%, and to the middle turbinate rarely at only 1.4%.[25,27] In chronic rhinosinusitis, the most frequent findings is a UP bent or folded medially with increased contact along the middle turbinate.[25,26] In the frontal sinus drainage pathway, a type I attachment of the superior UP to the lamina papyracea alters the pathway and is significantly associated with frontal sinusitis.[25] One must always radiographically assess the superior UP, especially if it bends laterally or inserts onto the lamina papyracea creating a "recessus terminalis" of the ethmoidal infundibulum, with fusion of the UP to the lamina papyracea of the lateral wall.[5,7,16,18] The UP is the medial wall of the inferior hiatus semilunaris and attaches to the lateral wall anteriorly at the end of the infundibulum. The attachment of the superior UP alters the pathway of the superior infundibulum. When the uncinate extends superiorly to the skull base or middle turbinate, the infundibulum is contiguous with the frontal recess.

2.4 Floor of Olfactory Recess

"Look Precisely UP "FOR"–Floor of Olfactory Recess

In the floor of the olfactory recess, the lateral lamella of the cribriform plate is the thinnest skull bone and the bone most at risk, and if disrupted, may result in a cerebrospinal fluid (CSF) leak[16,23] (▶ Fig. 2.1b). Along the inferior lateral cribriform margin is the superior anterior attachment of the middle turbinate[18] (▶ Fig. 2.1b). The attachment of the lateral lamella of the cribriform plate and insertion of the superior aspect of the middle turbinate, as well as the horizontal lamina cribrosa, the inferior boundary and floor of the olfactory recess, are best identified on CT in the coronal plane (▶ Fig. 2.1b). The midline cribriform plate separates the anterior cranial fossa from the nasal cavity (▶ Fig. 2.1b, ▶ Fig. 2.3). Intracranially, the olfactory fossa is subdivided medially by the vertical crista galli (▶ Fig. 2.1b). The term "cribriform" means perforated like a sieve, and the perforations allow for extension of the olfactory neural filaments. The superior margin of the olfactory fossa is the horizontal fovea ethmoidalis and roof of the ethmoid sinus (▶ Fig. 2.1b). The cribriform plate lateral lamella is the medial aspect of the ethmoid roof, and this bone is thinner than the adjacent lateral orbital process of the frontal bone usually only 0.1 to 0.2 mm in thickness. The right and left lateral lamella may be variable in both length and angulation. When the lateral lamella is short and vertical, the risk of injury decreases; however, as the lateral lamella increases in length vertically and in obliquity, the risk of injury is increased[16,18,30,31] (▶ Fig. 2.1b). Keros classified three types determined by the length of the lateral lamella and how inferior the lamina cribrosa is relative to the orbital process of the frontal bone. Type I is 1 to 3 mm, type II is 4 to 7 mm, and type III is greater than 8 mm.[30] Assessing the increasing and variable length of the lateral lamella is important, as the olfactory fossa extends more inferiorly, the thin elongated lateral lamella is at greater risk for injury when manipulated or during a middle turbinectomy or ethmoidectomy. Disruption of this bony connection may result in a CSF leak.[16,18]

2.5 Agger Nasi Air Cell

"Look Precisely UP FOR "AN"–Agger Nasi Air Cell.

The first ethmoid turbinal is the origin of the agger nasi air cell and the UP, and variable attachments of the uncinate process may result in alternative radiographic presentations of agger nasi air cells (▶ Fig. 2.1a). The UP origin is intimately related to the agger nasi air cell and forms its posterior and medial wall attaching posteriorly[11,13,22] (▶ Fig. 2.1a, b). The term "agger" comes from the Latin meaning an elevation, mound, or heap and refers to the small elevation formed by the base of the maxillary ethmoidal crest, on the nasal cavity lateral wall, located between the olfactory sulcus above and middle meatus. The "agger" bone is pneumatized in up to 98.5%[22] of adults, and the pneumatized air cell, the "agger nasi," is the most anteriorly located ethmoidal air cell (▶ Fig. 2.1a, b; ▶ Fig. 2.2a, b). The anterior wall of the agger nasi air cell is the maxillary frontal process, the lateral wall is the lacrimal bone, and the variable medial margin the UP.[13,14,22] The agger nasi air cell can be found anterior to the middle turbinate.[5,22] Although the anterior agger nasi cell is separate from the UP, the posterior agger nasi is related to the superiorly extending UP.[22] The majority of the time, the medial agger nasi air cell and UP insert on the lamina papyracea with a small bony leaflet extending to the bulla lamella dividing the frontal recess anterior to posterior in a vertical orientation from the bulla ethmoidalis to the medial agger nasi cell, with the frontal sinus drainage pathway extending medially and posteriorly[22] (▶ Fig. 2.1a, b; ▶ Fig. 2.2b). If an enlarged agger nasi cell displaces the uncinate tip medially where it attaches to the middle turbinate, the frontal drainage pathway is displaced posteriorly.[22]

2.6 Accessory Air Cells

"Look Precisely UP FOR AN Accessory air cell...—The Accessory Air Cell(s)."

Adding to the complexity of the frontal sinus drainage pathway are variable accessory air cells including air cells arising from the frontal process of the maxilla or "frontoethmoidal" air cells classified by Kuhn into four types, and air cells adjacent to the bullae ethmoidalis or "suprabullar" air cells (▶ Fig. 2.1a–c; ▶ Fig. 2.2a, b; ▶ Fig. 2.3).

Accessory air cells related to the frontal process of the maxilla and ethmoid are referred to as "frontoethmoidal" air cells. Variations with multiple frontal ethmoidal air cells with the agger nasi cell are often seen and are classified by Kuhn into four types: A type 1 configuration is one frontoethmoidal air cell above the agger nasi. Type 2 is a two or more air cells above the agger nasi and below the orbital roof. Type 3 is a single frontoethmoidal air cell extending from the agger nasi into the frontal sinus, above the frontal beak. Type 4 is an isolated air cell in the frontal sinus not contiguous with the agger nasi, that may pneumatize from the frontal recess, and as recently modified from the original classification should extend greater than 50% of the vertical height of the frontal sinus[32,33] (Fig. 2.1a). The classification of air cells becomes more complex as one or more air cells may be present, located either medially, anteriorly, or posteriorly.[5,34] The 2014 European Position Paper suggests that the frontoethmoidal air cells should be classified as anterior, medial, or posterior in relation to the frontal recess and inner walls of the frontal sinus.[5] Additional methods to identify these air cells are proposed; however, the number of air spaces affecting the frontal sinus drainage pathway is really the most critical information.[34,35] Accessory air cells may displace the uncinate superiorly along the lamina papyracea with the uncinate forming the medial margin and roof of the air cells.[22] Enlarged accessory air cells may also displace the uncinate

insertion onto the middle turbinate or skull base, accessory air cells extending to the medial skull base may displace the uncinate insertion medially onto the skull base or middle turbinate, and the narrowed frontal sinus drainage pathway is displaced laterally.[22,28] When frontoethmoidal air cells are located near the skull base laterally, this narrows and displaces the frontal sinus opening medially, although previous literature may use the term, "ostium"; this is considered technically incorrect, as it implies a two-dimensional structure.[5] Enlarged frontoethmoidal air cells may extend to the skull base forming a blind recess or abutting the anterior bulla ethmoidalis (Fig. 2.2a, b). Type III cells extending into the floor of the frontal sinus may be located medial or lateral to the frontal sinus ostium; when located medially displacing the floor of the frontal sinus, they are also termed "interfrontal sinus septal cell" (ISSC)[28] (Fig 2.1a).

Additional accessory air cells not associated with the maxillary frontal process and instead associated with the bulla ethmoidalis and skull base are referred to as suprabullar cells.[5,7,27,34] A frontal bulla air cell or suprabullar air cell(s) are pneumatized air cells along the anterior skull base and frontal sinus obstructing the frontal sinus drainage pathway (Fig. 2.2a, b). On a coronal CT scan, these may appear as an isolated frontal sinus cell. A suprabullar cell or cells are by definition located above the bulla ethmoidalis[28,34] (Fig. 2.2a, b).

2.7 Anterior Ethmoidal Artery

Look Precisely UP FOR AN Accessory air cell, **Ethmoidal Arteries....**

The anterior ethmoidal artery (AEA) arises as a branch from the ophthalmic artery and is identified on a coronal CT by finding a small anterior notch along the medial orbital wall at the level of the ethmoid air cells[18,36,37] (Fig. 2.1c). Preoperative identification of the vessel is essential to avoid surgically violating it, which may result in retraction of the vessel and a retro-orbital hematoma.[38] The AEA is usually located between the second and third lamellae, at the axilla of the middle turbinate,[38,39] on average approximately 11 mm from the posterior wall of the lateral recess[40] (Fig. 2.1c; Fig. 2.2a, b; Fig. 2.3). When the notch abuts the fovea ethmoidalis or lateral lamella, the AEA is shielded during surgery.[18,36] However, when supraorbital accessory air cells are present, which is up to 26 to 35% of the time,[18,36,41] the artery can traverse in the ethmoid air cells, putting it at greater risk for injury.[18,38,41] Although the majority of AEAs are in the suprabullar or supraorbital recess, the vessel may be in the suprabullar recess or roof of the ethmoid bulla.[38,40] Importantly, the AEA may travel below the skull base and be dehiscent. A lower hanging AEA may be seen more often with a longer lateral lamella or supraorbital pneumatization.[38]

2.8 Bulla Ethmoidalis

"Look Precisely UP FOR AN Accessory air cell, Ethmoidal Arteries, and BE..."

The bulla ethmoidalis (BE) or ethmoid bulla is usually the largest anterior ethmoid air cell, although can be small and undeveloped in approximately 8% of patients[5,26] (Fig. 2.2a, b). The anterior margin of the BE is the posterior margin of the frontal recess, inferior semilunar hiatus, and ethmoidal infundibulum.[5] The BE is usually a large single air cell opening into the hiatus semilunaris or retrobullar recess. The majority of time, the BE or multiple air cells' openings extend into the superior hiatus semilunaris.[5,42,43] Occasionally, the BE may extend into the ethmoidal infundibulum, or may have multiple air cells with multiple openings with three main categories of ethmoidal development including simple, compound, and complex.[43]

2.9 Middle Turbinate

*"Look Precisely UP FOR AN Accessory air cell, Ethmoidal Arteries, and BE **Mentally Trained."***

The middle turbinate arises from the ethmoid bone. The most anterior portion of the middle turbinate fuses with the agger nasi air cell and creates a curved air space referred to as the "axilla." Superiorly and anteriorly the MT attaches in a vertical plane to the skull base at the lateral margin of the cribriform plate, in the same plane as the lateral lamella of the cribriform plate (▶ Fig. 2.1a–c). Following the middle turbinate posteriorly in the coronal plane, the attachment referred to as the "basal lamella" changes into a posterior horizontal attachment to the lamina papyracea of the medial orbital wall (▶ Fig. 2.1c; ▶ Fig. 2.2a, b; ▶ Fig. 2.3). The attachment divides the ethmoidal air cells into anterior and posterior air cells with different drainage patterns. In addition, there may be pneumatization of the middle turbinate, referred to as concha bullosa (▶ Fig. 2.1c; ▶ Fig. 2.2a, b; ▶ Fig. 2.6b). Although there is no clear association with concha bullosa and sinus disease, there is an association with a concha bullosa and contralateral deviation of the nasal septum that again may support the evo-devo theory of development and the stacked layered configuration within the paranasal sinuses[44] (▶ Fig. 2.1a, b; ▶ Fig. 2.5, ▶ Fig. 2.6a).

2.10 Conclusion

In summary, the radiographic anatomy of the frontal sinus drainage pathways requires one to "Look Precisely UP FOR AN Accessory air cell, Ethmoidal Arteries, and BE Mentally Trained." This mnemonic is a reminder to double check the thin bony lamina papyracea for medial displacement, fracture deformities or dehiscence, or inferior medial orbital wall Haller's air cells (▶ Fig. 2.1a–c; ▶ Fig. 2.2a, b; ▶ Fig. 2.3). In addition, look for the structures inserting onto it, including the agger nasi air cell, MT, and especially an UP abutting the lamina papyracea creating a "recessus terminalis."

After assessing the lamina papyracea, the UP free edge is readily found in the coronal plane on CT pointing upward and may have variable presentations including deviation medially or laterally and possible tip pneumatization (▶ Fig. 2.1b). Most commonly, the UP attaches superiorly into the lamina papyracea. The UP thin bony leaflet is the key surgically for access to the ethmoid infundibulum, and one of the most frequent pathological findings in chronic rhinosinusitis is a medially bent UP contacting the MT.

Next, the important "floor of the olfactory recess" includes the cribriform plate and the thin bony lateral lamella at risk for surgical injury on the coronal CT. The longer and more inferiorly displaced lateral lamellas and the olfactory fossa, as per the Keros classification, the greater the risk for intraoperative injury of the lateral lamellas and inadvertent CSF leaks or meningoceles allowing for direct communication into the anterior cranial fossa and concomitant infection risks (▶ Fig. 2.1b; ▶ Fig. 2.2a, b; ▶ Fig. 2.3).

Next, the important "agger nasi" air cell, usually found pneumatized in most all individuals, by definition, the most anterior component of the ethmoid sinus, just posterior to the lacrimal bone and in front of the free edge of the UP, believed to be a remnant of the first ethmoturbinal. The degree of pneumatization and attachment of the superior agger nasi air cell may alter the frontal sinus drainage pathways (▶ Fig. 2.1a, b; ▶ Fig. 2.2a, b; ▶ Fig. 2.3).

Adjacent to the agger nasi air cell, look for neighboring accessory air cells, when arising from the frontal process of the maxilla and ethmoid; these are frontoethmoidal air cells that may extend either medial, lateral, or posteriorly relative to the frontal recess and inner frontal sinus. When the air cells are located above the bulla ethmoidalis, these are "suprabullar" cells, their presence may imply variable drainage patterns of the ethmoidal arteries (▶ Fig. 2.1a, b; ▶ Fig. 2.2a, b; ▶ Fig. 2.3).

Look for the anterior ethmoidal notch on coronal CT and note if it is abutting the fovea ethmoidalis or lateral lamella, which is protective for the artery during functional endoscopic surgery; however, pneumatization of air cells above the ethmoidal notch, that may occur in up to a third of patients, may be indicative of the ethmoidal artery extending freely through the ethmoid sinus, at risk for injury during surgery, and for retraction into the orbit with a retrobulbar hematoma (▶ Fig. 2.1c).

Look for the bulla ethmoidalis forming the frontal sinus outflow pathway posterior margin and neighboring air cells, and next to it the MT (▶ Fig. 2.2a, b). Following the

MT simultaneously in the coronal and sagittal planes, note how the "basal lamella" attachment initially extending to the thin lateral margin of cribriform plate at the junction of the lateral lamella, then switches posteriorly into a lateral horizontal (▶ Fig. 2.1a–c) attachment to the lamina papyracea of the medial orbital wall. In the sagittal plane, this demarcates the anterior and posterior ethmoidal air cells and their drainage pathways. All of these key anatomical findings contribute to the formation of the unique and variable drainage patterns of the frontal sinus. Because each frontal sinus drainage pathway is unique, even varying in the same patient from side to side, each of these critical anatomical structures need to be assessed, and having a search pattern helps, so when looking at these radiographically, remember to "Look Precisely UP FOR AN Accessory air cell, Ethmoidal Arteries, and BE Mentally Trained."

References

[1] Nambiar P, Naidu MD, Subramaniam K. Anatomical variability of the frontal sinuses and their application in forensic identification. Clin Anat. 1999; 12(1):16–19

[2] Kjær I, Pallisgaard C, Brock-Jacobsen MT. Frontal sinus dimensions can differ significantly between individuals within a monozygotic twin pair, indicating environmental influence on sinus sizes. Acta Otolaryngol. 2012; 132(9):988–994

[3] Besana JL, Rogers TL. Personal identification using the frontal sinus. J Forensic Sci. 2010; 55(3):584–589

[4] Daniels DL, Mafee MF, Smith MM, et al. The frontal sinus drainage pathway and related structures. AJNR Am J Neuroradiol. 2003; 24(8):1618–1627

[5] Lund VJ, Stammberger H, Fokkens WJ, et al. European position paper on the anatomical terminology of the internal nose and paranasal sinuses. Rhinol Suppl. 2014; 24(24):1–34

[6] Bassiouni A, Wormald PJ. Role of frontal sinus surgery in nasal polyp recurrence. Laryngoscope. 2013; 123(1):36–41

[7] Farneti P, Riboldi A, Sciarretta V, Piccin O, Tarchini P, Pasquini E. Usefulness of three-dimensional computed tomographic anatomy in endoscopic frontal recess surgery. Surg Radiol Anat. 2017; 39(2):161–168

[8] Eloy JA, Svider PF, Setzen M. Preventing and managing complications in frontal sinus surgery. Otolaryngol Clin North Am. 2016; 49(4):951–964

[9] Folbe AJ, Svider PF, Eloy JA. Advances in endoscopic frontal sinus surgery. Oper Tech Otolaryngol–Head Neck Surg. 2014; 25:180–186

[10] Hoskison E, Daniel M, Daudia A, et al. Complications of endoscopic frontal sinus surgery. Otolaryngol Head Neck Surg. 2010; 143 suppl 2:272

[11] Al-Bar MH, Lieberman M, Casiano RR. Surgical Anatomy and Embryology of the Frontal Sinus. Berlin, Heidelberg: Springer; 2016:15–33

[12] Jankowski R, Perrot C, Nguyen DT, Rumeau C. Structure of the lateral mass of the ethmoid by curved stacking of endoturbinal elements. Eur Ann Otorhinolaryngol Head Neck Dis. 2016; 133(5):325–329

[13] Hwang PH, Abdolkhani A. Embryology, anatomy and physiology of the nose and paranasal sinuses. Otorhinolaryngol Head Neck Surg. 2003; 17:2009–2455

[14] Vaid S, Vaid N, Rawat S, Ahuja AT. An imaging checklist for pre-FESS CT: framing a surgically relevant report. Clin Radiol. 2011; 66(5):459–470

[15] Rene C, Rose GE, Lenthall R, Moseley I. Major orbital complications of endoscopic sinus surgery. Br J Ophthalmol. 2001; 85(5):598–603

[16] Amine MA, Anand V. Anatomy and complications: safe sinus. Otolaryngol Clin North Am. 2015; 48(5):739–748

[17] Meyers RM, Valvassori G. Interpretation of anatomic variations of computed tomography scans of the sinuses: a surgeon's perspective. Laryngoscope. 1998; 108(3):422–425

[18] O'Brien WT, Sr, Hamelin S, Weitzel EK. The preoperative sinus CT: avoiding a "close" call with surgical complications. Radiology. 2016; 281(1):10–21

[19] Cunnane ME, Platt M, Caruso PA, Metson R, Curtin HD. Medialization of the lamina papyracea after endoscopic ethmoidectomy: comparison of preprocedure and postprocedure computed tomographic scans. J Comput Assist Tomogr. 2009; 33(1):79–81

[20] Wake M, Takeno S, Hawke M. The uncinate process: a histological and morphological study. Laryngoscope. 1994; 104(3 Pt 1):364–369

[21] Zhang L, Han D, Ge W, et al. Anatomical and computed tomographic analysis of the interaction between the uncinate process and the agger nasi cell. Acta Otolaryngol. 2006; 126(8):845–852

[22] Wormald PJ. The agger nasi cell: the key to understanding the anatomy of the frontal recess. Otolaryngol Head Neck Surg. 2003; 129(5):497–507

[23] Huang BY, Lloyd KM, DelGaudio JM, Jablonowski E, Hudgins PA. Failed endoscopic sinus surgery: spectrum of CT findings in the frontal recess. Radiographics. 2009; 29(1):177–195

[24] Isobe M, Murakami G, Kataura A. Variations of the uncinate process of the lateral nasal wall with clinical implications. Clin Anat. 1998; 11(5):295–303

[25] Srivastava M, Tyagi S. Role of anatomic variations of uncinate process in frontal sinusitis. Indian J Otolaryngol Head Neck Surg. 2016; 68(4):441–444

[26] Stammberger HR, Kennedy DW, Bolger W, Anatomic Terminology Group. Paranasal sinuses: anatomic terminology and nomenclature. Ann Otol Rhinol Laryngol Suppl. 1995; 167:7–16

[27] Landsberg R, Friedman M. A computer-assisted anatomical study of the nasofrontal region. Laryngoscope. 2001; 111(12):2125–2130

[28] Wormald PJ. Three-dimensional building block approach to understanding the anatomy of the frontal recess and frontal sinus. Oper Tech Otolaryngol–Head Neck Surg. 2006; 17(1):2–5

[29] Bhatti MT, Schmalfuss IM, Mancuso AA. Orbital complications of functional endoscopic sinus surgery: MR and CT findings. Clin Radiol. 2005; 60(8):894–904

[30] Keros P. [On the practical value of differences in the level of the lamina cribrosa of the ethmoid]. Z Laryngol Rhinol Otol. 1962; 41:809–813

[31] Adeel M, Ikram M, Rajput MS, Arain A, Khattak YJ. Asymmetry of lateral lamella of the cribriform plate: a software-based analysis of coronal computed tomography and its clinical relevance in endoscopic sinus surgery. Surg Radiol Anat. 2013; 35(9):843–847

[32] Kuhn FA. Chronic frontal sinusitis: the endoscopic frontal recess approach. Oper Tech Otolaryngol–Head Neck Surg. 1996; 7(3):222–229

[33] Wormald PJ, Chan SZ. Surgical techniques for the removal of frontal recess cells obstructing the frontal ostium. Am J Rhinol. 2003; 17(4):221–226

[34] Pianta L, Ferrari M, Schreiber A, et al. Agger-bullar classification (ABC) of the frontal sinus drainage pathway: validation in a preclinical setting. Int Forum Allergy Rhinol. 2016; 6(9):981–989

[35] Wormald PJ, Bassiouni A, Callejas CA, et al. (2016, December). The International Classification of the radiological Complexity (ICC) of frontal recess and frontal sinus. In International Forum of Allergy & Rhinology

[36] Souza SA, Souza MM, Gregório LC, Ajzen S. Anterior ethmoidal artery evaluation on coronal CT scans. Rev Bras Otorrinolaringol (Engl Ed). 2009; 75(1):101–106

[37] Gotwald TF, Menzler A, Beauchamp NJ, zur Nedden D, Zinreich SJ. Paranasal and orbital anatomy revisited: identification of the ethmoid arteries on coronal CT scans. Crit Rev Computed Tomogr. 2003; 44(5):263–278

[38] Jang DW, Lachanas VA, White LC, Kountakis SE. Supraorbital ethmoid cell: a consistent landmark for endoscopic identification of the anterior ethmoidal artery. Otolaryngol Head Neck Surg. 2014; 151(6):1073–1077

[39] Lee WC, Ming Ku PK, van Hasselt CA, van Hasselt CA. New guidelines for endoscopic localization of the anterior ethmoidal artery: a cadaveric study. Laryngoscope. 2000; 110(7):1173–1178

[40] Simmen D, Raghavan U, Briner HR, et al. The surgeon's view of the anterior ethmoid artery. Clin Otolaryngol. 2006; 31(3):187–191

[41] Chung SK, Dhong HJ, Kim HY. Computed tomography anatomy of the anterior ethmoid canal. Am J Rhinol. 2001; 15(2):77–81

[42] Wright ED, Bolger WE. The bulla ethmoidalis: lamella or a true cell? J Otolaryngol. 2001; 30(3):162–166

[43] Setliff RC, III, Catalano PJ, Catalano LA, Francis C. An anatomic classification of the ethmoidal bulla. Otolaryngol Head Neck Surg. 2001; 125(6):598–602

[44] Stallman JS, Lobo JN, Som PM. The incidence of concha bullosa and its relationship to nasal septal deviation and paranasal sinus disease. AJNR Am J Neuroradiol. 2004; 25(9):1613–1618

3 Applied Surgical Anatomy

Iacopo Dallan, Lodovica Cristofani Mencacci, and Veronica Seccia

Abstract

The frontal sinus is widely considered the most challenging chamber to approach during endoscopic sinus surgery, due to its position, anatomical variability, and close relationship with critical orbital and skull base structures.

A careful knowledge of the relevant anatomy is mandatory to minimize complications and enable the surgeon to improve his/her surgical confidence, to correctly understand normal variants from pathological conditions and choose the right surgical approach for any given situation.

Last but not least, it should be emphasized the essential role of radiological evaluation as an integral part of the diagnostic path; incorrect or missed visualization of radiological images may lead to catastrophic complications.

Keywords: frontal sinus, frontal recess, applied surgical anatomy, anatomy, endonasal approach, external approach

3.1 General Considerations

The frontal sinus is usually a paired, triangular, pyramid-shaped cavity extending between the anterior and posterior tables of the ascending portion of the frontal bone. The frontal bone, in which it is contained, contributes to the formation of the floor of the anterior cranial fossa and the roof of the orbits; it articulates with the ethmoid, sphenoid, parietal, and nasal bones, as well as with the zygoma and the maxilla. The anterior wall of the frontal sinus begins at the nasofrontal suture line and ends below the frontal bone protuberance. It is covered by the pericranium, frontalis muscle, subcutaneous fat, and more superficially the skin. The posterior wall of the frontal sinus is a plate of thin, compact bone. It forms the anteroinferior limit of the anterior cranial fossa, separated from the frontal lobe only by the meningeal layers. It presents an upper vertical portion that gradually curves downward and becomes almost horizontal as it forms the part of the orbital roof. The medial wall of the frontal sinus is represented by the intersinus septum, a triangular-shaped segment of bone that separates the frontal sinuses into two independently draining sinus cavities. It may be so laterally deviated that the two sinuses may differ significantly from each other in size, shape, and height. However, the most inferior portion of this intersinus septum is always located in the same plane as the nasal septum and close to or at the midline.[1] At this level, it is continuous with the crista galli, the perpendicular plate of the ethmoid, and the nasal spine of the frontal lobe. Each sinus may be divided by intrasinus septations into further incomplete chambers and recesses,[1] and pneumatization of these additional cells

may occasionally extend into the crista galli. Their drainage generally occurs into the nasal cavity through their own outflow tract, at the level of the infundibulum, next to the normal frontal sinus outflow tract.[2]

The inferior wall of the frontal sinus is formed by the orbital roof laterally and the nasoethmoid complex medially. It is made of thin bone, specially in its lateral part, making possible the gradual erosion from chronic inflammatory diseases and subsequent orbital complications. The medial part of the inferior wall of the frontal sinus corresponds to the nasoethmoid complex. The very anterior part of the inferior wall is exactly above the roof of the nose; it is made of thick bone from the nasal spinous process of the frontal bone, the frontal process of the maxilla, and the upper part of the nasal bones.[1]

3.2 Applied Anatomy for Endonasal Approaches

The frontal sinus outflow tract has been defined in different ways over the years, from different authors.[1,3,4]

It is currently described as an hourglass which consists mainly of three structures: the frontal sinus infundibulum, ostium, and recess; its narrowest part is taken at the level of the frontal sinus infundibulum.[5]

The frontal sinus outflow tract is often considered synonymous of the term "frontal recess" even if these are two separate entities; the European Position Paper (EPOS) on the Anatomical Terminology of the Internal Nose and Paranasal Sinuses[45] defines the **frontal recess** as the most anterosuperior part of the ethmoid, inferior to the frontal sinus opening. Wormald and colleagues describe the frontal recess as the space posterior to the frontal beak, between the lamina papyracea and the vertical lamella of the middle turbinate continuing onto the lateral wall of the olfactory fossa, anterior to the basal lamella of the middle turbinate.[6] The drainage of the frontal sinus through the frontal recess is complex and is influenced by several anatomical structures, such as the presence of additional air cells and the attachments of the uncinate process,[44] as it will be described below.

The **frontal sinus infundibulum** is a funnel-shaped area formed by the most inferior aspect of the frontal sinus that leads to the frontal sinus ostium. The **ostium** is the narrowest area of the transition zone from the frontal sinus to the frontal recess with its anterior edge formed by the frontal sinus beak and the posterior edge formed by the skull base.[67] The **frontal recess** is bounded posteriorly by the anterior wall of the ethmoidal bulla (if this reaches the skull base), anteroinferiorly by the agger nasi, laterally by the lamina papyracea, and inferiorly by the terminal recess of the ethmoidal infundibulum, if present.

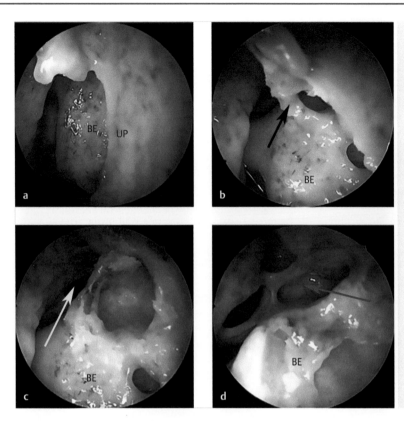

Fig. 3.1 (a–d) Sequential endoscopic views of the frontal recess. BE, bulla ethmoidalis; UP, uncinate process; *black arrow*, superior part of the uncinate process; *yellow arrow*, frontal sinus opening; *red arrow*, suprabullar cell.

Anatomically speaking, the **uncinate process** is a thin structure that runs almost in the sagittal plane from anterosuperior to posteroinferior. Posteriorly, it attaches to the perpendicular process of the palatine bone and the ethmoidal process of the inferior turbinate. Anteriorly, it is attached to the lacrimal bone and may have a common attachment to the medial surface of the agger nasi and the middle turbinate.[45] Its superior attachment is really very variable, with at least six "common" variations described.[67] Most frequently, the uncinate process attaches to the lamina papyracea or to the skull base or to the middle turbinate. If the uncinate process attaches to the skull base or turns medially, the frontal recess opens directly into the *ethmoidal infundibulum*.[45] If the uncinate process attaches laterally onto the lamina papyracea or the base of an agger nasi cell, the frontal sinus drains into the *middle meatus*. In this case, we observe the so-called "terminal recess" (recessus terminalis) that means a blind end of the ethmoidal infundibulum superiorly. In other and simple words, the superior attachment of the uncinate process determines whether the frontal sinus has a medial or lateral drainage pathway.

Additional ethmoidal cells may be present along the frontal recess and infundibulum. This extreme anatomical variability represents the main element that makes the frontal sinus surgery challenging; because of the complexity of these anatomical and spatial relationships, a surgeon not adequately skilled and trained may confuse these cells even with the frontal sinus itself and so getting disoriented.

Among ethmoidal cells, the **agger nasi cell** is described as the most anterior cell of the ethmoid and it sits above the insertion of the middle turbinate into the lateral nasal wall[6] (▸ Fig. 3.1). It has a variable degree of pneumatization, and if particularly large, it may narrow the frontal recess posteriorly and/or laterally the nasolacrimal duct or directly pneumatize the lacrimal bone.[45] As a matter of fact, the agger nasi cell represents the anterior border of the frontal recess. In cases of very large agger nasi cell, this cell can be confused with frontal sinus itself. Above the agger nasi cell other cells can be found, more or less extending into the frontal sinus. Different names have been given to these anterior cells extending superiorly, including *supra agger cell* and *supra agger frontal cell* (▸ Fig. 3.2).[90] Historically, the so-called "frontal infundibular" cells, that is, cells belonging to the anterosuperior ethmoidal cells, have been classified by Bent and colleagues[7] in four types. A *type I* frontal cell is a single anterior ethmoid cell located superior to the agger nasi. This kind of cell do not involve the sinus itself, but occlude the frontal recess. *Type II* frontal cells consist of a series of small anterior ethmoid cells located superior to the agger nasi, but below the orbital roof. *Type III* frontal cells are small cells arising superior to the agger nasi, but contiguous with it, and extending into the frontal sinus. A *type IV* cell is an isolated cell arising within the frontal sinus.

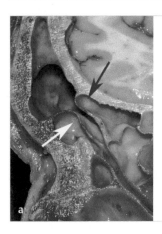
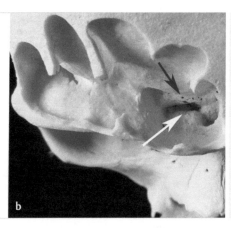

Fig. 3.2 (a,b) Frontal sinus: sagittal and frontal views (right side). White arrow, supra agger frontal cell; blue arrow, supra-orbital cell.

According to the European Position Paper on Anatomical Terminology, we also prefer to name type III and IV as *frontoethmoidal cells*. It must be stressed that regardless the names used in different papers, that unfortunately can be confusing, we would like to present a logic perspective on 3D anatomy of these spaces. So, as a matter of fact, the **agger nasi cell** and the **other anterosuperior cells** (*supra agger cell* and *supra agger frontal cell*) represent anterior structures, located in the anterior border of the frontal recess/sinus. On the other side, the **bulla ethmoidalis** and the **suprabullar cells** represent important elements in the posterior frontal recess/sinus. The bulla ethmoidalis is described as the largest anterior ethmoidal cell, but it should be noted that in 8% of cases it is poorly or not developed. If the ethmoidal bulla reaches the skull base, it forms the posterior border of the frontal recess. If the bulla does not touch the ethmoidal roof, a suprabullar recess is described.[45] Wormald and colleagues prefer to consider this recess as a *cell*, and we agree with them. In the group of the suprabullar cells, according to Wormald, we can identify the *supraorbital cell*, the *suprabullar cell*, and the *supra bulla frontal cells*. The **suprabullar cell** lies above the ethmoidal bulla but does not enter the frontal sinus, while a **supra bulla frontal cell** originates in the suprabullar region and pneumatized along the skull base into the posterior aspect of the frontal sinus. The **supraorbital (ethmoid) cell** is described as a cell that pneumatized around, anterior or posterior to the anterior ethmoidal artery over the roof of the orbit. If a **supraorbital cell** is present, it can be a challenging element during endoscopic surgery. As said, it is a well-pneumatized posterior cell in the anterior ethmoid complex that extends laterally into the frontal bone over the orbit and narrows the frontal recess by pushing it anteriorly (▶ Fig. 3.3). To be more precise, the European Position Paper on Anatomical Terminology has proposed to abandon this last term and use the term supraorbital recess,[45] but we still prefer to consider these spaces as cells. Recently, a medial group of cells, named **frontal septal cells**, have been described as medially placed cells of the anterior ethmoid or the inferior frontal sinus, in close relationship with the

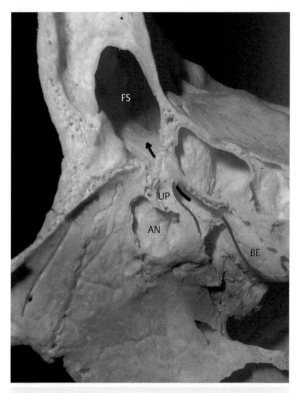

Fig. 3.3 Sagittal view of a dry skull, showing a right frontal sinus and its relationship with the ethmoidal complex. AN, agger nasi; BE, bulla ethmoidalis; FS, frontal sinus; UP, uncinate process. Black arrow indicates the drainage of the frontal sinus; the green line indicates a supraorbital cell; the blue line indicates the anterior shape of the bulla ethmoidalis; the pink line indicates the posterior aspects of the uncinate process. As clearly evident, in the upper part, the uncinate process joins the agger nasi cell.

interfrontal sinus septum. These cells push the drainage pathway laterally and often posteriorly.[6]

The *anterior ethmoidal artery (AEA)* is very often found during frontal recess surgery. AEA is a branch of the ophthalmic artery and enters the ethmoidal complex passing through the anterior ethmoidal foramen. In well-pneumatized sinuses, the artery does not run in the skull base. It usually runs along with the anterior ethmoidal nerve, with an oblique direction, from posterolateral to anteromedial. The artery is most often found in the suprabullar recess/cell (85%)[45] and enters the anterior cranial fossa usually passing through the lateral lamella of the cribriform plate. After traveling intracranially, the AEA then reenters the nasal cavity and divides into multiple branches, including the anterior septal branch and the anterior lateral nasal branch. These branches feed the anterosuperior part of the septum and the middle turbinates. The meningeal branches of AEA feed the falx cerebri surrounding brain tissue.

When dealing with more extended transnasal procedures, in which the frontal sinus floor is drilled out, other critical landmarks should be kept in mind. The position of the lacrimal sac and duct could be relevant when performing such an approach. The duct is covered anteromedially by the frontal process of the maxilla, while posteriorly this role is given by the lacrimal bone. The position of the agger nasi cell and its pneumatization can be relevant in lacrimal pathway identification.

When a Draf III is planned and performed via a medial-to-lateral technique, the position of the first olfactory fiber should be known. Conceptually, this landmark defines the anterior limit of the anterior cranial fossa, but in reality, the anteriormost part of the olfactory fossa can extend even anteriorly to the first olfactory fibers, thus making this landmark not completely safe. In this respect, a more accurate landmark seems to be the *septal branch of the AEA*. Anteriorly to this last landmark drilling should be considered safe. It must be stressed that the identification of such landmarks in the midline in vivo application cannot be easy, and whenever possible, a lateral-to-medial approach should be advised. In fact, anatomopathological conditions and even previous treatments can make identification of these medial landmarks challenging. A more reliable landmark recently described for the superior septectomy in Draf III procedure is the *nasofrontal beak* (NFB).[8] Only in 2% of the patients the NFB presents a direct contact with olfactory fossa, but this contact is limited to the midline regions.

3.3 Applied Anatomy for External Approaches

Endonasal endoscopic approach became the dominant surgical method of management of the frontal sinus, eclipsing the more aggressive external procedures. However, they still maintain a specific role in contemporary rhinological and skull base surgery. So, according to the pathology to treat, the frontal sinus can be approached, managed, or even removed through external approaches. Hereafter, we present anatomical details of the coronal and superior transpalpebral approaches to the frontal sinus, used by the first author in selected cases.

3.3.1 Coronal Approach

The coronal approach is a very versatile external approach to the frontal sinus. It requires an arc-shaped skin incision extending from one pretragal region to the other that is performed parallel and posteriorly to the hairline, connecting both the preauricular regions.

One of the anatomical keypoint of this approach is represented by the temporoparietal fascia (TPF), which comprises a fascial layer just under the subcutaneous tissue in the temporal region extending to the parietal region.[9] The TPF is the lateral extension of the galea and is continuous with the superficial muscular aponeurotic system (SMAS). The temporal branches of the facial nerve, usually in variable number,[9,10] are deep to the TPF above the zygomatic arch. Between the TPF and the superficial layer of the deep temporal fascia, the so-called *areolar tissue* can be found. In close proximity of the zygomatic arch, the superficial fat pad lies, enveloped between a duplication of the superficial layer of deep temporal fascia, that reaches the superior surface of the zygomatic arch in its medial and lateral borders. The deep temporal fat pad lies between the superficial and deep layer of the deep temporal fascia. So, dissection on the subgaleal plane, within the *areolar tissue*, is easy and safe until approaching the upper edge of the zygomatic arch. Inferior to this level, subgaleal dissection carries the risk of injury to the temporal and frontal branches of the facial nerve. Therefore, the surgeon will need to dissect in a more deep plane, usually working deep to the superficial layer of the deep temporal fascia. In this way, the upper surface of the zygomatic arch can be reached safely.

Another anatomical element to keep in mind during a coronal approach of the frontal sinus is the temporalis fascia, a strong aponeurotic layer covering the temporalis muscle. It splits into two main layers: the superficial and the deep. As said, the superficial usually splits in two layers that is attached to the lateral and the medial margins of the zygomatich arch, enveloping the superficial fat pad. Within the superficial fat pad lies the zygomatic branch of the superficial temporalis artery and a branch of the maxillary nerve. An appropriate releasing of the connection of the flap with the temporalis fascia (at the level of the anterior aspect of the superior temporal line) allows the coronal flap to be retracted anteroinferiorly in a very easy way. If the coronal flap is harvested in a subperiosteal (subpericranium) plane since the beginning, the pericranium may be dissected free at the end of the procedure, if needed for reconstructive purpose.[11]

Finally, the position of the supraorbital and supratrochlear nerves and vessels should be emphasized when dealing with the final dissection phases of flap harvesting, once in close relationship with the orbital rim (▶ Fig. 3.4). In some cases, the supraorbital neurovascular bundle passes through a complete foramen, and this canal should be opened inferiorly in order to release adequately the flap. In more fortunate cases, the bundle runs in a

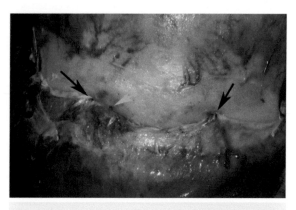

Fig. 3.4 Coronal approach—external view (final phases of flap harvesting). Black arrows indicate the supraorbital neurovascular bundles; green arrow indicates the supratrochlear artery.

groove, and makes surgery easier. The supraorbital nerve gives a branch to the frontal sinus. The supratrochlear bundle lies more medial than the supraorbital one and perforates the orbital septum to pass superiorly on the forehead. At this level, there is usually a rich anastomotic connection between branches of the supraorbital, supratrochlear, and frontal branch of the superior temporal arteries. More medially, just superior to the medial palpebral ligament, the dorsal nasal artery penetrates the orbital septum (medially to the supratrochlear artery) to join the angular artery close to the medial canthus. This artery feeds, at least partially, the lacrimal sac.

3.3.2 Transpalpebral Approach

Transpalpebral endoscopic-assisted approach to the frontal sinus can be considered as a useful, minimally invasive alternative in selected cases of frontal sinus disease. In this case, the aid of the endoscope significantly increases the range of application.

The superior eyelid is formed, from an anterior to posterior perspective, by two lamellae: the anterior lamella is formed by the skin and orbicularis oculi muscle; the posterior one is formed by the Mueller palpebral muscle and levator aponeurosis. Between these two lamellae lies the orbital septum, a membranous sheet that originates from the orbital rim at the arcus marginalis and is continuous with the periorbita and periosteum of the external surface of the cranium. It is pierced by vessels and nerves superomedially. Medially, it lies behind the medial palpebral ligament, while laterally, it is anterior to the lateral palpebral ligament. The superior orbital septum becomes thinner as it approaches the free margin of the eyelid; it is attached to the Müller muscle and superior tarsus inferiorly and ends within the pretarsal skin.[12]

The fat pads of the upper eyelid include a medial (whitish) and a central fat (more yellow) pad. Superior tarsal plate provides support for the eyelid, with its

lateral and medial canthal tendons, giving the tarsoligamentous sling. The upper eyelid retractor system is formed mainly by the levator palpebrae and its aponeurosis. The Müller's sympathetic muscle in the upper lid should be considered as an accessory tendon of the levator palpebrae. On the anterior surface of the upper tarsus, the marginal arterial arcade (mainly from the medial palpebral and lacrimal arteries) runs. So, the blood supply for the superior eyelid greatly depends on ophthalmic artery (with lesser contributions from infraorbital, temporal, transverse facial, and angular arteries).[13] The retro-orbicularis oculi fat lies above the orbital septum and expands from the mid-supraorbital rim to the lateral orbital rim. Moving laterally, dissecting in a suborbicularis plane, the orbital rim (at the level of the frontozygomatic suture) is reached. Just behind the orbital septum, in the superolateral part, the orbital (or upper) lobe of the lacrimal gland is visible, lying above the lateral extension of the levator palpebrae fascial system. As a matter of fact, the critical anatomical landmark to safely identify the orbital rim is represented by the orbicularis oculi muscle (▶ Fig. 3.5). As said, dissecting on the undersurface of this muscle allows an easy and safe identification of the bony rim, and thus allows a complete exposure of the area of interest without damaging noble structures (especially the levator palpebrae system). During the exposure of the anterior frontal sinus wall, care should be taken in the identification of the supraorbital bundle (▶ Fig. 3.6).

3.4 Blood Supply

Arterial supply of the frontal sinus is mainly provided by terminal vessels of the supraorbital artery and supratrochlear arteries that penetrate the frontal sinus. Branches of anterior falcine artery, anterior ethmoidal artery are also involved in the vascularization of the frontal sinus.[4] Minor vessels arise from the sphenopalatine system; its very terminal branches reach the frontal sinus through the nasofrontal recess and infundibulum. The venous drainage follows different pathways that include mainly the superior ophthalmic vein. In more details, it is provided by anastomotic veins in the supraorbital notch, connecting the supraorbital and superior ophthalmic vessels. Also, valveless, diploic veins draining the superior sagittal and sphenoparietal sinuses are involved.[1,14]

3.5 Innervation

Innervation comes from the ophthalmic nerve (first division of the trigeminal nerve), a purely sensory nerve. Just before entering the orbit via the superior orbital fissure, the ophthalmic nerve divides into three branches: the lacrimal, the nasociliary, and the frontal nerves. Among them, the frontal nerve provides major supply to the frontal sinus mucosa innervation. It divides into two

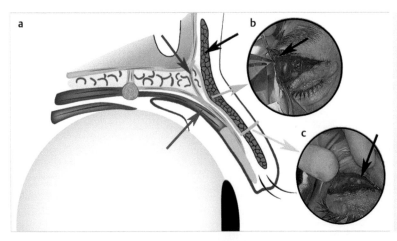

Fig. 3.5 (a–c) Schematic drawings of the superior eyelid and anterior orbital anatomy (sagittal view). Black arrow indicates the orbicularis oculi muscle; yellow line indicates the skin–muscle incision (as seen in **c**, right side); green line indicates the suborbicularis oculi muscle dissection (as seen in **b**, right side); blue arrow indicates the orbital septum; red arrow indicates the Müller's muscle.

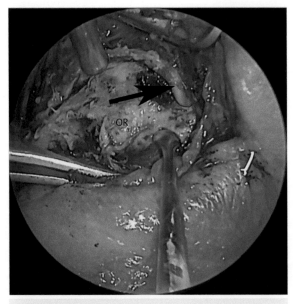

Fig. 3.6 Superior eyelid approach (endoscopic anterior view—right side). OR, orbital rim. Black arrow indicates the supraorbital bundle (passing through the supraorbital foramen).

branches: the larger supraorbital and smaller supratrochlear nerves. The supraorbital in turn gives off a smaller medial branch that brings sensory innervation to the frontalis muscle, the upper eyelid, the galea aponeurosis, and the frontal sinus mucosa. Autonomic innervation of mucosal glands accompanies the neurovascular bundle supplying the frontal sinus.[2,15]

3.6 Anatomical Variations and Surgical Considerations

Anatomical variations, as already mentioned, are well documented in literature and well experimented in clinical practice. The frontal sinus should be considered nothing but a pneumatization within the squama of the frontal bone and may present different degrees of pneumatization: hypoplasia, complete aplasia, or, conversely, hyperpneumatization of the frontal sinus are not uncommon findings.[4]

Moreover, if the frontal sinus extends largely to the dorsal region, it will reach the olfactory groove, the anterior borders of which will form a prominent ridge, the so-called "crista olfactoria."[16] It can be easily damaged during surgical procedures, resulting in opening the anterior cranial fossa.

Anyway, the real complexity of these areas, especially when dealing with an *endonasal approach*, cannot be fully described in an anatomical chapter and should be well understood in the preoperative imaging case by case. In this respect, we advise the surgeon to strictly collaborate with a dedicated radiologist in order to understand very deeply radiological imaging.

3.7 Conclusions

The endoscopic surgical approach to the frontal sinus still remains a challenge, and requires a deep anatomical knowledge and adequate surgical skills. Its risks are mainly related to the close relationship of frontal sinus contracts with critical orbital and skull base structures as well as to its anatomical features. It is therefore essential to have a thorough awareness of the anatomical relationship with close vital structures along with the most recurring anatomical variants in order to perform the safest surgery possible and to avoid complications. Moreover, the knowledge of the "surgical anatomy" for external approach is essential when dealing with this kind of patients.

References

[1] Levine HL, Clemente MP, eds. Sinus surgery: endoscopic and microscopic approaches. New York, NY: Thieme; 2005
[2] Duque CS, Casiano RR. Surgical anatomy and embryology of the frontal sinus. In: Kountakis SE, Senior BA, Draf W, eds. The Frontal sinus. Germany: Springer; 2005

[3] Friedman M, Bliznikas D, Ramakrishnan V, et al. Frontal sinus surgery 2004: update of clinical anatomy and surgical techniques. Oper Tech Otolaryngol–Head Neck Surg. 2004; 15(1):23–31

[4] Lang J, ed. Clinical Anatomy of the Nose, Nasal Cavity and Paranasal Sinuses. New York, NY: Thieme; 1989

[5] Saini AT, Govindaraj S. Evaluation and decision making in frontal sinus surgery. Otolaryngol Clin North Am. 2016; 49(4):911–925

[6] Wormald PJ, Hoseman W, Callejas C, et al. The International Frontal Sinus Anatomy Classification (IFAC) and Classification of the Extent of Endoscopic Frontal Sinus Surgery (EFSS). Int Forum Allergy Rhinol. 2016; 6(7):677–696

[7] Bent JP, Cuilty-Siller C, Kuhn FA. The frontal cell as a cause of frontal sinus obstruction. Am J Rhinol. 1994; 8:185–191

[8] Craig JR, Petrov D, Khalili S, et al. The nasofrontal beak: A consistent landmark for superior septectomy during Draf III drill out. Am J Rhinol Allergy. 2016; 30(3):230–234

[9] Babakurban ST, Cakmak O, Kendir S, Elhan A, Quatela VC. Temporal branch of the facial nerve and its relationship to fascial layers. Arch Facial Plast Surg. 2010; 12(1):16–23

[10] Gosain AK, Sewall SR, Yousif NJ. The temporal branch of the facial nerve: how reliably can we predict its path? Plast Reconstr Surg. 1997; 99(5):1224–1233, discussion 1234–1236

[11] Yaşargil MG, Reichman MV, Kubik S. Preservation of the frontotemporal branch of the facial nerve using the interfascial temporalis flap for pterional craniotomy. Technical article. J Neurosurg. 1987; 67 (3):463–466

[12] Dallan I, Castelnuovo P, Sellari-Franceschini S, eds. Endoscopic orbital and transorbital approaches. Endo: Press GmbH; 2015

[13] Rootman J, ed. Diseases of the Orbit: A Multidisciplinary Approach. Philadelphia, PA: Wolters Kluwer Health/Lippincott Williams & Wilkins; 2014

[14] Janfaza P, Nadol JB Jr, Galla RJ, et al, eds. Surgical anatomy of the head and neck. Philadelphia, PA: Lippincott Williams & Wilkins; 2001

[15] Shankland WE. The trigeminal nerve. Part II: the ophthalmic division. Cranio. 2001; 19(1):8–12

[16] Stucker FJ, de Souza C, Kenyon GS, et al, eds. Rhinology and Facial Plastic Surgery. Berlin, Heidelberg, Germany: Springer; 2009

Section II

Endoscopic Surgical Approaches to Frontal Sinus Disease

4 Draf Frontal Sinusotomy I and IIa   *26*

5 Draf Frontal Sinusotomy IIb   *52*

6 Extended Draf IIb and Other Modifications of the Lothrop Procedure   *54*

7 The Frontal Sinus Rescue Procedure   *59*

8 Draf III (Endoscopic Modified Lothrop)— Inside-Out and Outside-In Approaches   *64*

9 Transseptal Approach   *76*

10 Endoscopic Endonasal Orbital Transposition for Lateral Frontal Sinus Lesions   *81*

11 The Role of Frontal Sinus in Anterior Skull Base Surgery and the Transcribriform Approach   *87*

12 Extended Endonasal Anterior Skull Base Approaches   *93*

13 Revision Endoscopic Frontal Sinus Surgery   *101*

14 Complications of Frontal Sinus Surgery   *113*

15 Delivery of Topical Therapy to the Frontal Sinus   *122*

16 Postoperative Management: Dressings and Toilet   *126*

17 Office-Based Frontal Sinus Procedures   *133*

II

4 Draf Frontal Sinusotomy I and IIa

Andreas Leunig and Hans Rudolf Briner

Abstract

A surgeon experienced in endoscopic frontal sinus surgery will be able to apply tailored surgical techniques to a broad range of indications such as chronic inflammatory diseases (chronic rhinosinusitis with or without polyps), cysts, mucoceles, fungal infections, and even benign and malignant sinus pathologies. However, the endoscopic technique is not the solution for all problems of the sinuses. It is important for the surgeon to respect technical (e.g., equipment) limitations as well as their own, experience-related, limitations of the endoscopic endonasal techniques. This chapter describes the authors' philosophy of frontal recess and sinus surgery.

Keywords: FESS, minimally invasive, mucosa-sparing surgical technique, frontal recess, frontal sinus, uncinate process, agger nasi cell, frontoethmoidal cell, bulla intact approach, axillary flap

4.1 Indications

Functional endoscopic sinus surgery (FESS) is the surgical treatment of choice for chronic rhinosinusitis (CRS) that has not responded well to conservative treatments.[1,2,3,4,5] There are further indications such as mucoceles or mucopyoceles of the frontal sinus (FS), revision surgery,[6,7] and also benign and even malignant tumors,[5,8,9,10,11] if these are approachable endoscopically.

Although widely practiced, issues such as the timing of surgery and the extent of the surgery itself generate an ongoing discussion.[12,13,14] The extent of endoscopic procedures ranges from balloon dilation and Draf types I, IIa, and IIb to extensive procedures like Draf type III.[15] Current evidence does not clarify whether minimal or extended techniques are best for different patient populations.[5,14,16,17] However, the choice of the treatment concept and surgical approach remains based on the individual patient's disease and anatomy, as well as the surgeon's experience and skills.

4.2 Surgical Steps

The first and most important step in FESS is the "infundibulotomy," in which the medial wall of the ethmoid infundibulum (i.e., the uncinate process [UP]) is removed to get access to the anterior ethmoid. To ensure that this step is carried out correctly and to prevent postoperative synechiae and iatrogenic complications (particularly likely with an atelectatic ethmoid infundibulum), it is essential to understand the anatomy of the UP and the frontoethmoidal complex.[5,18,19]

The UP is a hook-shaped structure composed of a thin bony plate that is covered by mucosa on both sides and lies in an approximately parasagittal plane. It may attach superiorly to the lamina papyracea (LP), skull base, or middle turbinate (MT). This feature has important technical implications in FS operations. With the correct removal of the anterior and posteroinferior portions of the UP, the natural maxillary sinus opening can be seen. Furthermore, resection of the inferior portion of the UP generally exposes a domelike structure that resembles an inferiorly opened anterior ethmoid cell. This structure is the superior blind end of the ethmoidal infundibulum that is formed by the lateral bending of the UP and is called the "terminal recess (TR)." The latter is often mistaken for an agger nasi cell (ANC) or for the FS itself, when it is extending far cranially. The TR is distinguished by having anterior, medial, lateral (orbit), and posterior walls. Since the TR and ANC commonly share the same posteromedial wall (fusion), removal of the ANC leads to removal of the posterior wall of the TR, but at a higher and more anterior location. It is essential to identify and preserve the mucosa in the FR and hence to protect the natural drainage pathway of the FS.

According to the EPOS document,[20] the terms "frontal recess" and "FS drainage pathway" usually refer to two separate entities. The opening of the FS is best defined in the sagittal section on CT; here the contours of the FS and FR have been described as forming an hourglass, the narrowest part of which is taken as the frontal sinus opening (FSO). The area below the natural FSO, the FR, extends from the insertion of the MT to the anterior ethmoidal artery (AEA) and is delimited anteroinferiorly by the agger nasi (AN), laterally by the LP, posteriorly by the anterior wall of the ethmoidal bulla (EB)—if this reaches the skull base—and inferiorly by the TR of the ethmoidal infundibulum, if present. The use of the term "ostium" in relation to the opening of the FS is incorrect, as it implies a two-dimensional structure. The term "nasofrontal" or "frontonasal duct" has been abandoned as the drainage pathway of the FS is not a true duct.

If the UP attaches superiorly to the MT or to the anterior skull base (ASB), the natural FSO will be clearly visible immediately after removal of the superior portion of the UP. It may also be visible after resection of the inferior part of the UP, since its outflow tract runs lateral to the UP and the FS drains directly into the ethmoid infundibulum. Here it is dangerous to dissect medial to the superior attachment of the UP with the risk of perforating the lateral lamella of the cribriform plate resulting in a CSF leak. The natural FSO may not be visible in complex anatomical situations where multiple frontoethmoidal cells (FEC) are present.[21] In these more challenging cases, an intraoperative navigation system is helpful and strongly recommended.[22]

Table 4.1 International Frontal Sinus Anatomy Classification (IFAC) according to Wormald et al[5]

Cell type	Cell name	Definition	Abbreviation
Anterior cells (push the drainage pathway of the frontal sinus medially, posteriorly, or posteromedially)	Agger nasi cell	Cell that sits either anterior to the origin of the middle turbinate or directly above the most anterior insertion of the middle turbinate into the lateral nasal wall	ANC
	Supra agger cell	Anterolateral ethmoidal cell, located above the agger nasi cell (not pneumatizing into the frontal sinus)	SAC
	Supra agger frontal cell	Anterolateral ethmoidal cell that extends into the frontal sinus. A small SAFC will only extend into the floor of the frontal sinus, whereas a large SAFC may extend significantly into the frontal sinus and may even reach the roof of the frontal sinus	SAFC
Posterior cells (push the drainage pathway anteriorly)	Supra bulla cell	Cell above the bulla ethmoidalis that does not enter the frontal sinus	SBC
	Supra bulla frontal cell	Cell that originates in the supra bulla region and pneumatizes along the skull base into the posterior region of the frontal sinus. The skull base forms the posterior wall of the cell	SBFC
	Supraorbital ethmoid cell	An anterior ethmoid cell that pneumatizes around, anterior to, or posterior to the anterior ethmoidal artery over the roof of the orbit. It often forms part of the posterior wall of an extensively pneumatized frontal sinus and may only be separated from the frontal sinus by a bony septation	SOEC
Medial cells (push the drainage pathway laterally)	Frontal septal cell	Medially based cell of the anterior ethmoid or the inferior frontal sinus, attached to or located in the interfrontal sinus septum, associated with the medial aspect of the frontal sinus outflow tract, pushing the drainage pathway laterally and frequently posteriorly	FSC

Table 4.2 Extent of frontal sinus surgery according to Draf[15] and Wormald et al[5]

Draf classification	Wormald et al	Anatomical correlation
	Grade 0	No removal of tissue
Type I	Grade 1	Removal of ethmoidal cell below the frontal sinus outflow tract
Type IIa	Grade 2–3	Removal of frontoethmoidal cell within or above the frontal sinus outflow tract
Type IIb	Grade 4–5	Removal of internal beak unilateral partial or complete
Type III	Grade 6	Removal of internal beak bilateral

According to W. Draf, the extent of FS surgery (EFSS) is classified into types I, IIa, IIb, and III. A new international classification with grade 0 to 6 about the EFSS according to P.J. Wormald et al subclassifies Draf types IIa and IIb into grades 2–3 and 4–5, respectively.

The main difference between the various approaches lies in the extent of the FSO and/or enlargement based on the individual anatomy (see ▶ Table 4.1 and ▶ Table 4.2).

For example, in the type 2b procedure, the natural FSO is maximally enlarged from the LP to the nasal septum. The most extensive endonasal FSO is the Draf type III drainage procedure, also known as the median drainage or modified endoscopic Lothrop procedure. In both type 2b and type 3 procedures, powered instrumentation (drills, burs) are used to remove the floor of the FS between the two laminae papyracea, the interfrontal septum, and the superior nasal septum to establish sufficient drainage from the FS.

4.3 Tips and Tricks

The following points should be noted when dissecting in the area of the frontal recess and the FSO:

- **Anatomy:** It is important to assess the individual anatomical variation of the frontal recess displayed on coronal, axial, and sagittal CT scans.[5,21]
- **Bloody surgical field:** A clear surgical field (epinephrine vasoconstriction!) is important to avoid excessive tissue resection, that is, always maintain normal mucosa.
- **Instruments:** Suitably angled instruments and telescopes (e.g., 45 degrees) should be used. Generally, the instrument is positioned below the endoscope. If only anatomical structures located far in the cranium (e.g., large supra agger frontal or large supra bulla frontal cells [LSBFC]) should be removed, the instrument is positioned above the endoscope. Cutting instruments are preferred to avoid stripping mucosa.[23]
- **Middle turbinate:** The MT should not be fractured, as the lateralized turbinate often results in obstruction the frontal recess.
- **Agger nasi cell:** In the case of a large ANC, the instrument is inserted posteriorly between the skull base and bony plate (dorsal wall of the ANC), and the plate is carefully fractured forward and downward. After complete dissection, the "door" into the frontal recess and sinus is open.
- **Frontal recess:** Minimally invasive dissection and preservation of mucosa is important to promote fast healing and to avoid scarring in the frontal recess.
- **Frontal sinus opening:** If the natural FSO cannot be visualized after removal of the uncinate process, EB or ANC or other FEC, the cause is usually a thin, intact bony plate still obstructing the plane of the natural FSO, which should be removed with a suitable angled instrument.
- **Frontal sinus:** If FS dissection is done with good visibility and adequate instruments, there is no need for blind probing of the frontal recess or natural FSO. This avoids unnecessary stripping of the mucosa, and denuding bone. Injury of mucosa and denuding bone will produce fibrosis and scar tissue as well as osteitis and new bone formation, resulting in stenosis and obstruction of the FS outflow tract.
- **Anterior ethmoidal artery:** The most reliable landmark to identify the AEA is the insertion of the MT basal lamella at the ASB. This is the posterior access to the frontal recess. The AEA is usually located 10 to 15 mm dorsal to the point where the roof of the ethmoid begins to turn upward into the dorsal wall of the FS.[24]
- **Frontoethmoidal cell:** The surgical principle of dissecting FEC (e.g., large supra agger frontal or LSBFC) is the

same as dissecting an ANC; however, in very rare case, the limits may be reached dissecting this FEC by using the endonasal route due to limits of available instruments. Before using a combined endoscopic–external approach, a drill out procedure may solve this individual problem.

- **Supraorbital ethmoid cell:** This cell can be managed by using computer-assisted surgery in order to identify both the FSO and the supraorbital cell ostium; the wall between them should be identified and removed to create an open access to the FS.
- **Suprabullar cell:** This cell arises near the ethmoid bulla lamella at the level of the ASB and basically narrows the frontal recess from behind.
- **Interfrontal sinus septal cell:** The anatomy varies a lot, for example, pneumatization in the lower interfrontal sinus septum or also in the upper part or even in the crista galli. The ostium is typically located anterior and medial to the FSO.
- **Computer-assisted surgery:** It should be used to increase confidence, to have "on-site CT anatomy" when operating in the frontal recess, and to achieve a significantly higher identification rate of anatomical structures (e.g., FEC).[22]
- **Powered instrumentation:** These devices may facilitate dissection in the frontal recess by reducing polyps bulk or large amounts of crushed bone and avoiding mucosal stripping and injury.
- **Outcome:** The post-op outcome is strongly influenced by the degree of mucosal preservation, the complete (if necessary) dissection of FEC, and skillful handling of the MT.[5]
- **Postoperative care:** This should be performed with proper equipment and personalized skillful postoperative debridement with adequate visualization of the FSO and proper medication, if needed.
- **Overall outcome:** Overall outcome hinges upon three questions: why, when, and how should we treat? Have a clear diagnosis and treatment concept that defines why and when surgery is indicated, taking into account patient symptoms, imaging, and preoperative medication. Know which surgical technique and what degree of opening of the FS are needed. These factors also determine the postoperative treatment (debridement, postoperative medication).[25]

4.4 Case Examples

Case 1: Example (Video 4.1):
- Indication: CRS with nasal polyps on the left.
- International frontal sinus anatomy classification (IFAC), ANC, and supra bulla cell (SBC) on the left.
- Draf type I or EFSS grade 1 (bulla intact approach).
- (X degrees) denotes endoscope angle (see ▶ Fig. 4.1–▶ Fig. 4.16).

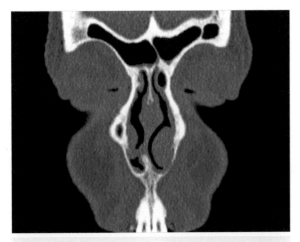

Fig. 4.1 Coronal CT scan with an agger nasi cell on the left.

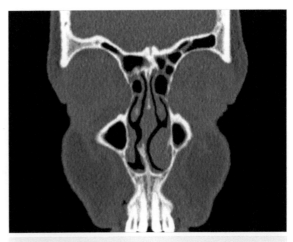

Fig. 4.2 Coronal CT scan with a supra bulla cell on the left.

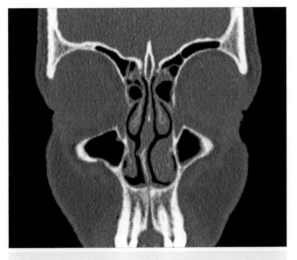

Fig. 4.3 Coronal CT scan with inflamed mucosa in the frontal recess on the left.

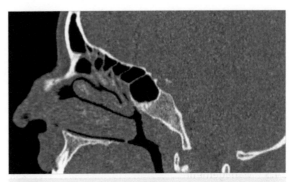

Fig. 4.4 Sagittal CT scan shows the relation between the agger nasi and the supra bulla cell on the left.

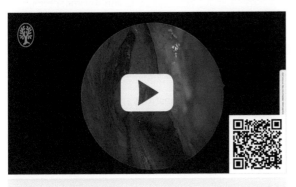

Video 4.1 CRSwNP, Draf type I (Case 1)

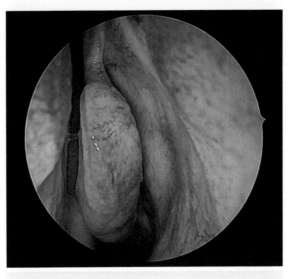

Fig. 4.5 Left nasal cavity with septum, middle turbinate, and uncinate process (0 degrees).

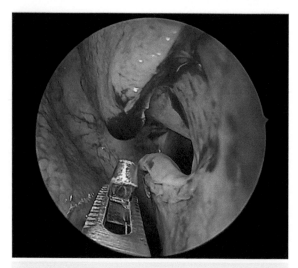

Fig. 4.6 Swinging door technique, cutting through the uncinate process and exposing the maxillary sinus opening using the small back-biting instrument (0 degrees).

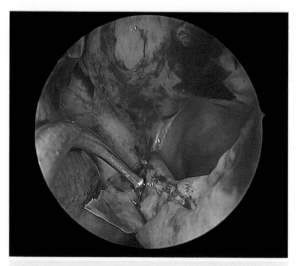

Fig. 4.7 Dissecting the inferior bony part of the uncinate process using Castelnuovo sinus probe (0 degrees).

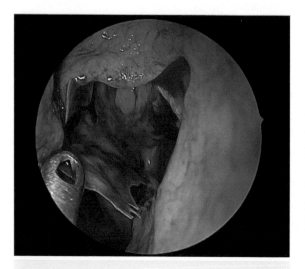

Fig. 4.8 Removing the uncinate process using a small Blakesley forceps (0 degrees).

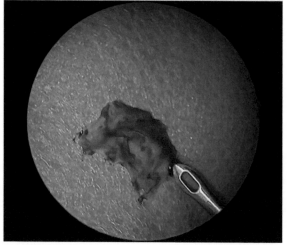

Fig. 4.9 Specimen of the uncinate process (0 degrees).

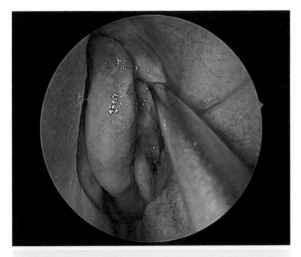

Fig. 4.10 Dissecting remnants of the uncinate process using a straight Kuhn spoon (0 degrees).

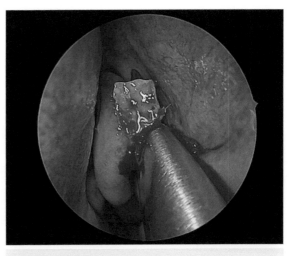

Fig. 4.11 Removing remnants of the uncinate process using a Kerrison punch (0 degrees).

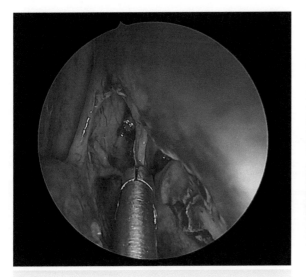

Fig. 4.12 Removing bony lamellas in the frontal recess using a Stammberger Rhinoforce II forceps (45 degrees).

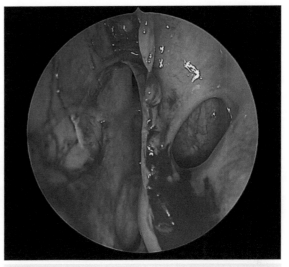

Fig. 4.13 Frontal sinus drainage pathway with intact supra bulla cell on the left (45 degrees; compare ▶ Fig. 4.16).

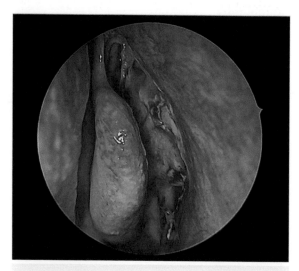

Fig. 4.14 Anterior ethmoid and frontal recess following "infundibulotomy" with intact ethmoidal bulla technique (0 degrees; compare ▶ Fig. 4.15). Note: no bleeding = no need for nasal packing.

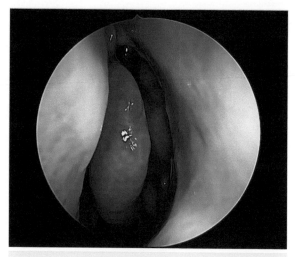

Fig. 4.15 Anterior ethmoid with intact ethmoidal bulla 3 months postsurgery (0 degrees; compare ▶ Fig. 4.14).

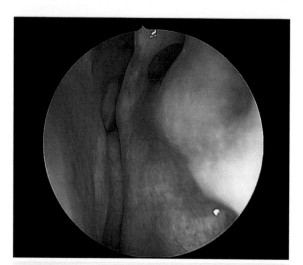

Fig. 4.16 Left frontal sinus drainage pathway with intact supra bulla cell 3 months postsurgery (45 degrees; compare ▶ Fig. 4.13).

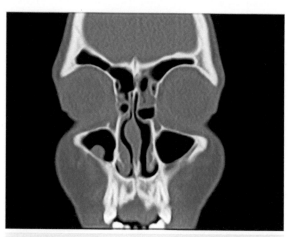

Fig. 4.17 Coronal CT scan with an agger nasi cell and frontoethmoidal cell (supra bulla cell) on the left.

Case 2: Example (Video 4.2):
- CRS on the left.
- IFAC, ANC, and SBC on the left.
- Draf type I or EFSS grade 1.
- (X degrees) denotes endoscope angle (see ▶ Fig. 4.17–▶ Fig. 4.29).

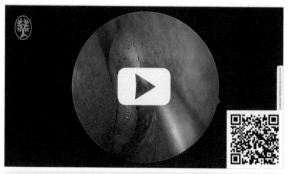

Video 4.2 CRS, Draf type I (Case 2)

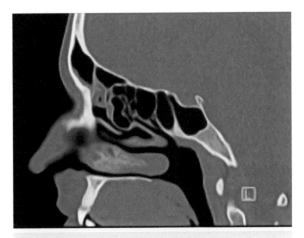

Fig. 4.18 Sagittal CT scan with an agger nasi cell and frontoethmoidal cell (supra bulla cell) on the left.

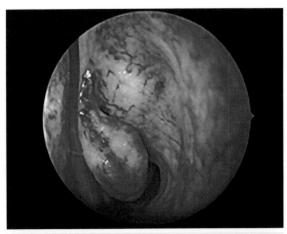

Fig. 4.19 Septum, middle turbinate, uncinate process, and prominent agger nasi on the left (0 degrees).

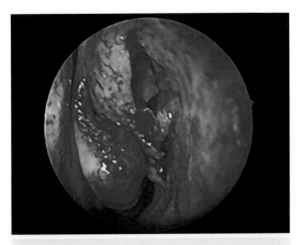

Fig. 4.20 Incised uncinate process and anterior wall of an agger nasi cell (0 degrees).

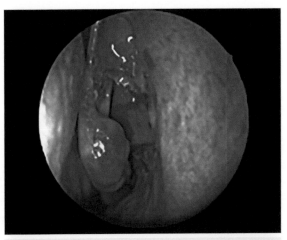

Fig. 4.21 Anterior ethmoid after removal of the uncinate process and anterior wall of an agger nasi cell (0 degrees).

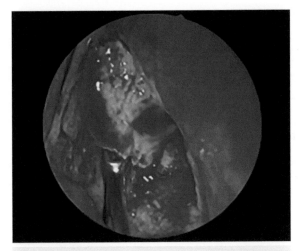

Fig. 4.22 Dissecting and elevating the medial posterior wall (fusion) of the uncinate process and an agger nasi cell (45 degrees).

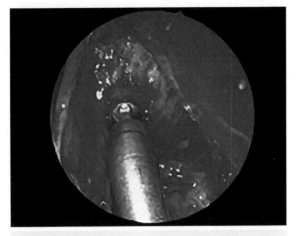

Fig. 4.23 Removing of bony lamella in the frontal recess using a Stammberger circular cutting punch (45 degrees).

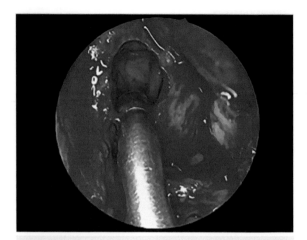

Fig. 4.24 Extending the approach from top down using a Stammberger circular cutting punch (45 degrees).

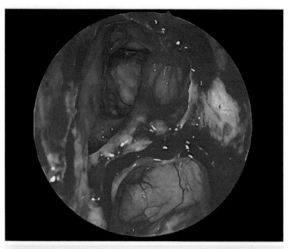

Fig. 4.25 Frontal recess with remnants of the ethmoidal bulla, frontal sinus opening, and intact supra bulla cell (45 degrees; compare ▶ Fig. 4.29).

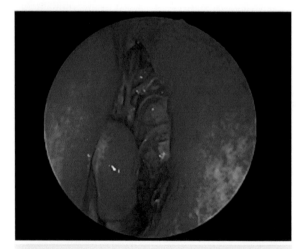

Fig. 4.26 Anterior ethmoid after removal of the uncinate process, ethmoidal bulla, and agger nasi cell (45 degrees; compare ▶ Fig. 4.28). Note: no bleeding = no need for nasal packing.

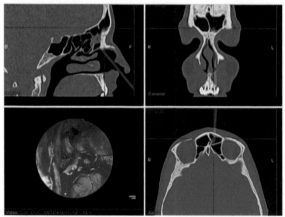

Fig. 4.27 Computer-assisted surgery located in the frontal recess on the left (45 degrees).

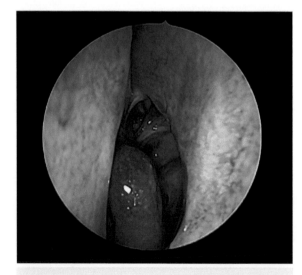

Fig. 4.28 Three months postsurgery middle meatus and anterior ethmoid (45 degrees; compare ▶ Fig. 4.26).

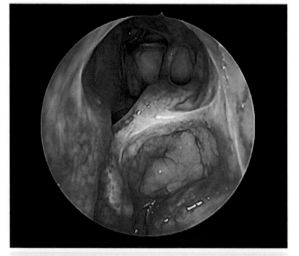

Fig. 4.29 Frontal recess 3 months postsurgery with remnants of the ethmoidal bulla, frontal sinus opening, and intact supra bulla cell (45 degrees; compare ▶ Fig. 4.25).

Case 3: Example (Video 4.3):
- CRS on the right.
- IFAC, ANC, supra agger cell (SAC), and supra agger frontal cell (SAFC) on the right.
- Draf type IIa or EFSS grade II.
- (X degrees) denotes endoscope angle (see ▸ Fig. 4.30–▸ Fig. 4.42).

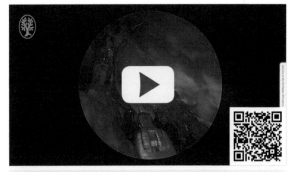

Video 4.3 CRS, Draf type IIa example 2 (Case 3)

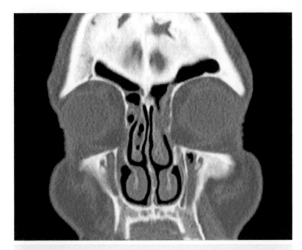

Fig. 4.30 Coronal CT scan with an agger nasi cell and supra agger frontal cell on the right.

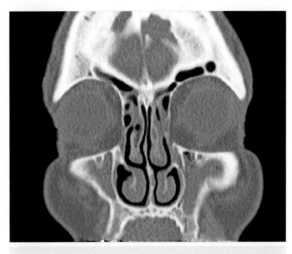

Fig. 4.31 Coronal CT scan with an agger nasi cell, supra agger, and supra agger frontal cell on the right.

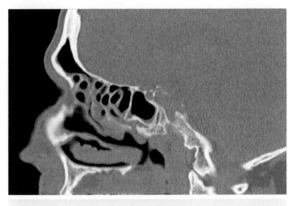

Fig. 4.32 Sagittal CT scan with an agger nasi cell, supra agger, and supra agger frontal cell on the right.

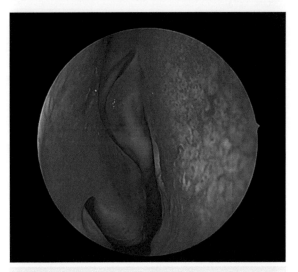

Fig. 4.33 Inferior turbinate, uncinate process, concha bullosa, and nasal septum following endoscopic septoplasty (0 degrees).

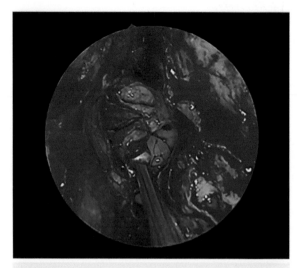

Fig. 4.34 Identifying access to the frontal sinus using a Kuhn-Bolger frontal sinus curette (45 degrees).

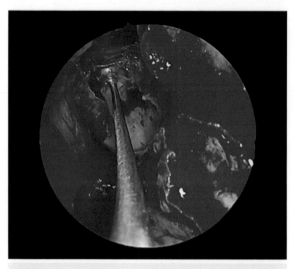

Fig. 4.35 Identifying the posterior wall of a supra agger frontal cell using a Castelnuovo frontal sinus probe (45 degrees).

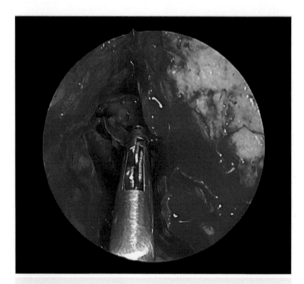

Fig. 4.36 Removing of the posterior wall of a supra agger frontal cell using a Stammberger Rhinoforce II forceps (45 degrees).

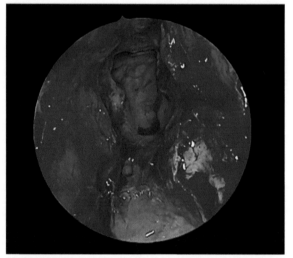

Fig. 4.37 Frontal recess after exposing the frontal sinus opening (45 degrees).

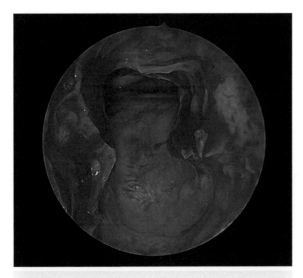

Fig. 4.38 Frontal recess and sinus with anterior ethmoidal artery following complete dissection and removal of a supra agger and supra agger frontal cell (45 degrees; compare Fig. 4.42).

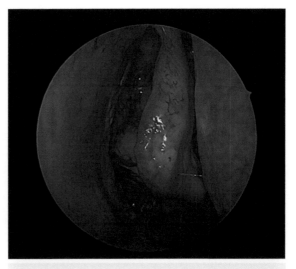

Fig. 4.39 Anterior and posterior ethmoid following removal of the uncinate process, ethmoidal bulla, basal lamella, and agger nasi cell (0 degrees; compare Fig. 4.41). Note: no bleeding = no need for nasal packing.

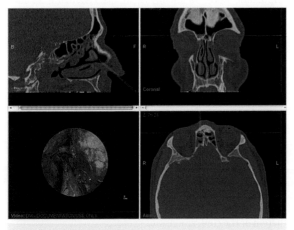

Fig. 4.40 Computer-assisted surgery with supra agger frontal cell on the right.

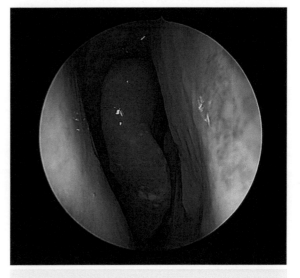

Fig. 4.41 Middle meatus 3 months postsurgery on the right (45 degrees; compare ▶ Fig. 4.39).

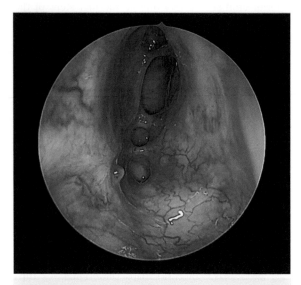

Fig. 4.42 Frontal recess 3 months postsurgery on the right (45 degrees; compare ▶ Fig. 4.38).

Case 4: Example (Video 4.4):
- CRS on the left.
- IFAC and ANC on the left.
- Draf type I or EFSS grade 1 (axillary flap approach).
- (X degrees) denotes endoscope angle (see
  ▶ Fig. 4.43–▶ Fig. 4.50).

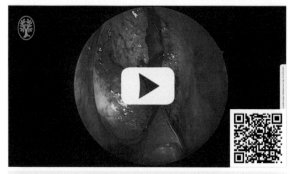

Video 4.4 CRS, Draf type I, axillary flap approach (Case 4)

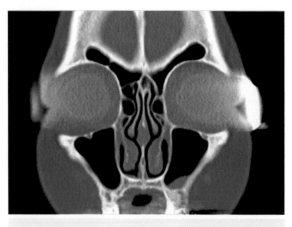

Fig. 4.43 Coronal CT scan with agger nasi cell on the left.

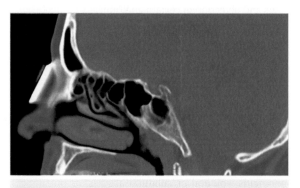

Fig. 4.44 Sagittal CT scan with agger nasi cell on the left.

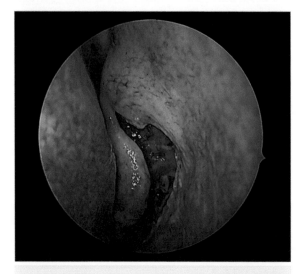

Fig. 4.45 Middle meatus and agger nasi after removal of the uncinate process (0 degrees).

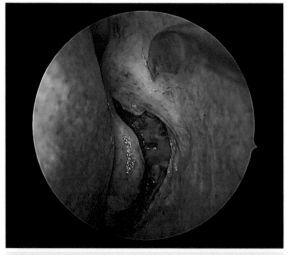

Fig. 4.46 Incision line for axillary flap approximately 1 cm above and anteriorly to the axilla of the middle turbinate (0 degrees).

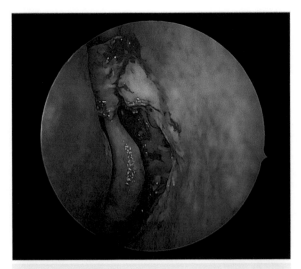

Fig. 4.47 Raised axillary mucosal flap placed over the root of the middle turbinate (0 degrees).

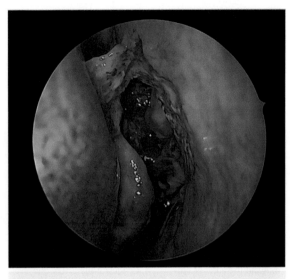

Fig. 4.48 Removed anterior wall of agger nasi cell with wide access to the frontal recess and sinus (0 degrees).

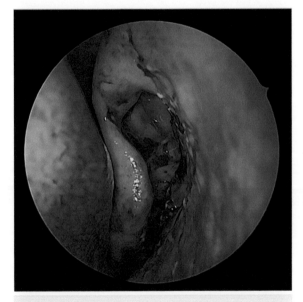

Fig. 4.49 Finally, putting back the axillary flap around the axilla of the middle turbinate to cover the denuded bone (0 degrees; compare ▶ Fig. 4.50).

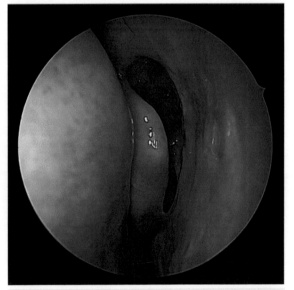

Fig. 4.50 Middle meatus 3 months postsurgery (0 degrees; compare ▶ Fig. 4.49).

Case 5: Example (Video 4.5):
- CRS with nasal polyps on the left.
- IFAC and LSBFC on the left.
- Draf type IIa or EFSS grade 3.
- (X degrees) denotes endoscope angle (see
  ▶ Fig. 4.51–▶ Fig. 4.68).

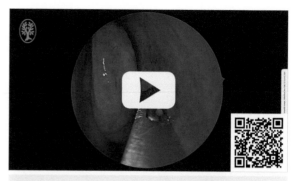

Video 4.5 CRS, Draf type IIa example 1 (Case 5)

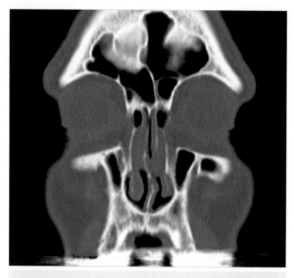

Fig. 4.51 Coronal CT scan with an agger nasi cell and large supra bulla frontal cell on the left.

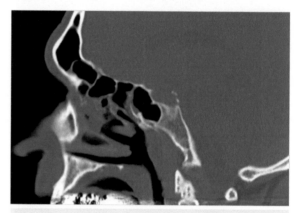

Fig. 4.52 Sagittal CT scan with an agger nasi cell and large supra bulla frontal cell on the left.

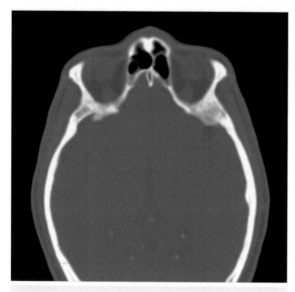

Fig. 4.53 Axial CT scan with a supra bulla frontal cell on the left.

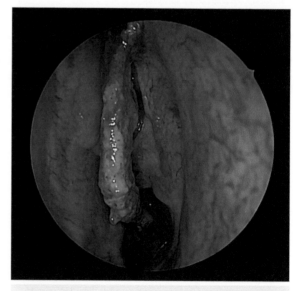

Fig. 4.54 Septum, middle turbinate, polypoid mucosa on the anterior wall of the ethmoidal bulla, and uncinate process (0 degrees).

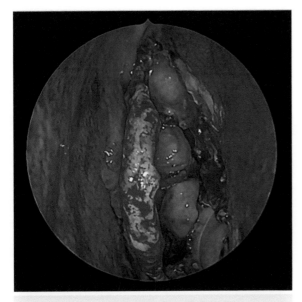

Fig. 4.55 Anterior and posterior ethmoid following removal of the uncinate process, ethmoidal bulla, and basal lamella (45 degrees).

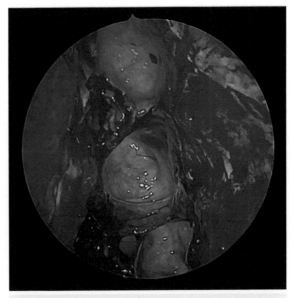

Fig. 4.56 Frontal recess, agger nasi cell, and ethmoid roof (45 degrees).

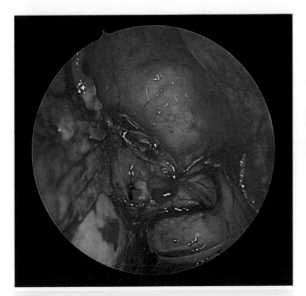

Fig. 4.57 Identifying drainage pathway medial posterior between the opposite mucosae (45 degrees).

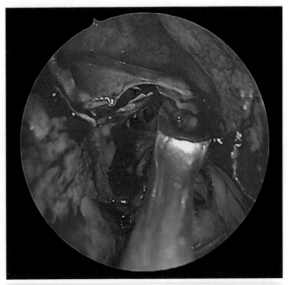

Fig. 4.58 Elevating medial posterior the wall of the uncinate process and agger nasi cell. Raised bony fragments should be removed (45 degrees).

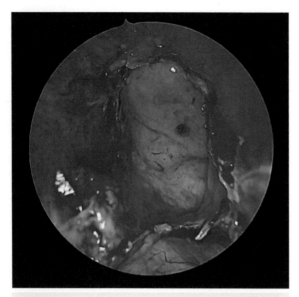

Fig. 4.59 Exposure of a large supra bulla frontal cell on the left (45 degrees).

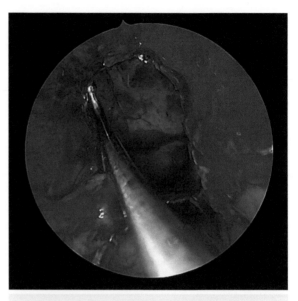

Fig. 4.60 Dissecting the medial wall and drainage pathway using a Castelnuovo frontal sinus probe (45 degrees).

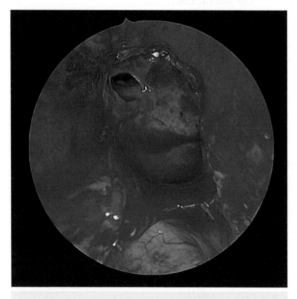

Fig. 4.61 Opened frontal sinus (45 degrees).

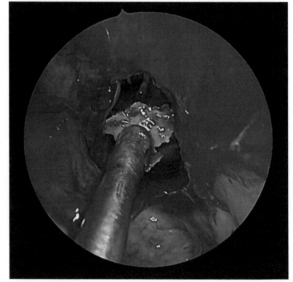

Fig. 4.62 Removing bony fragments using a Stammberger circular cutting punch (45 degrees).

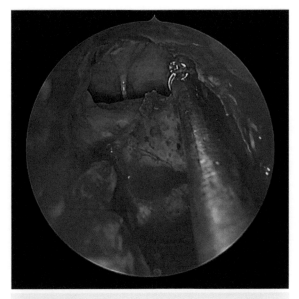

Fig. 4.63 Enlarging access to the frontal sinus laterally by removing parts of a large supra bulla frontal cell (45 degrees).

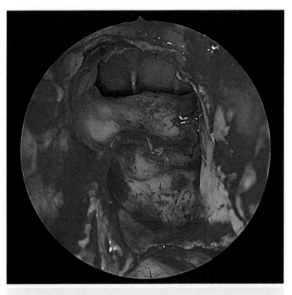

Fig. 4.64 Frontal recess and sinus after removal of a large supra bulla frontal cell (45 degrees; compare ▶ Fig. 4.68).

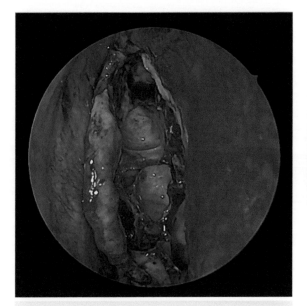

Fig. 4.65 Anterior and posterior ethmoid after removal of the uncinate process, ethmoidal bulla, basal lamella, and agger nasi cell (0 degrees; compare ▶ Fig. 4.67). Note: no bleeding = no need for nasal packing.

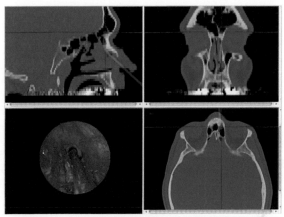

Fig. 4.66 Computer-assisted surgery located in large supra bulla frontal cell on the left (45 degrees).

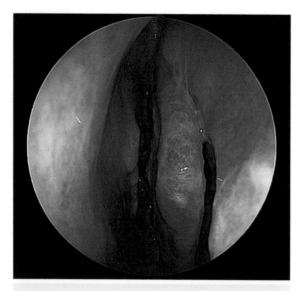

Fig. 4.67 Three months postsurgery with slight adhesion of the middle turbinate laterally and wide access to the olfactory cleft on the left (0 degrees; compare ▶ Fig. 4.65).

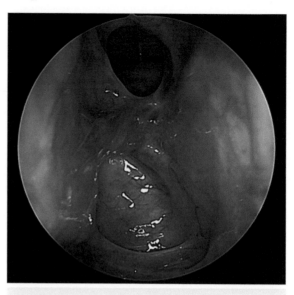

Fig. 4.68 Frontal sinus outflow tract 3 months postsurgery on the left (45 degrees; compare ▶ Fig. 4.64).

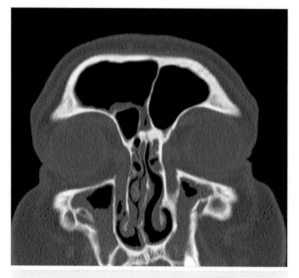

Fig. 4.69 Coronal CT scan with an agger nasi cell and large supra agger frontal cell on the right.

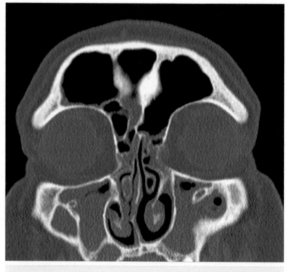

Fig. 4.70 Coronal CT scan with inflamed mucosa in the frontal recess on the right.

Case 6: Example (Video 4.6):
- CRS with concha bullosa on the right.
- IFAC, large supra agger frontal cell (LSAFC) on the right, and LSBFC.
- Draf type IIa or EFSS grade 3.
- (X degrees) denotes endoscope angle (see
  ▶ Fig. 4.69–▶ Fig. 4.82).

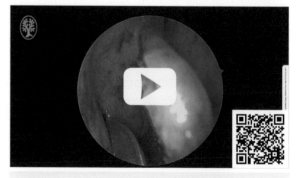

Video 4.6 CRS, Draf type IIa, concha bullosa (Case 6)

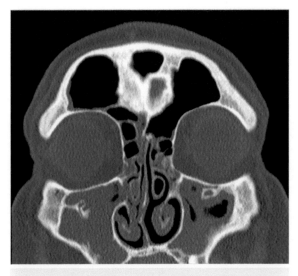

Fig. 4.71 Agger nasi cell and two frontoethmoidal cells (large supra agger frontal cell and large supra bulla frontal cell) on the right.

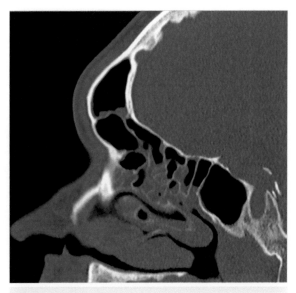

Fig. 4.72 Sagittal CT scan with an agger nasi cell and two frontoethmoidal cells (large supra agger frontal cell and large supra bulla frontal cell).

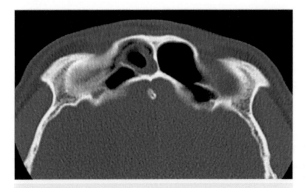

Fig. 4.73 Axial CT scan with two frontoethmoidal cells (large supra agger frontal and large supra bulla frontal cell) on the right.

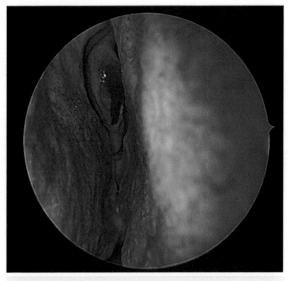

Fig. 4.74 Nasal cavity on the right (0 degrees).

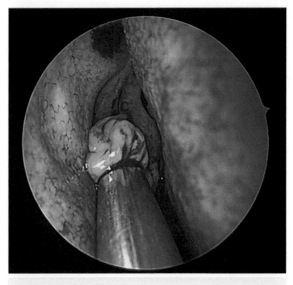

Fig. 4.75 After removed lateral lamella of a concha bullosa suctioning of mucus retention (0 degrees).

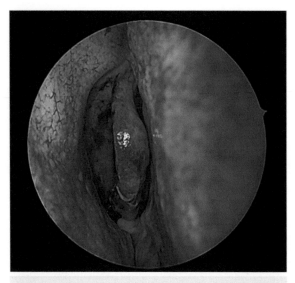

Fig. 4.76 Middle meatus after dissecting the concha bullosa (0 degrees).

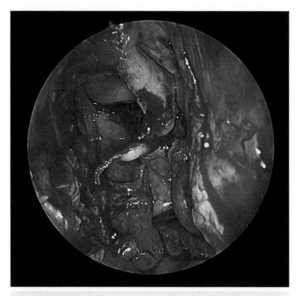

Fig. 4.77 Identification of the medial wall of a large supra agger frontal and large supra bulla frontal cell on the right (45 degrees).

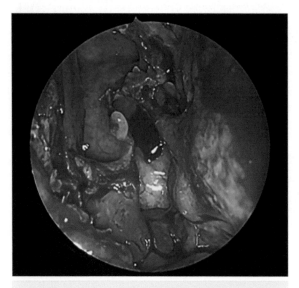

Fig. 4.78 Identification of the frontal sinus outflow tract, where mucosa of a large supra agger frontal cell is facing mucosa of a large supra bulla frontal cell (45 degrees).

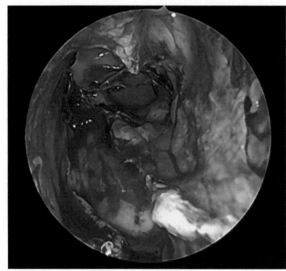

Fig. 4.79 Access in the frontal sinus is between the two frontoethmoidal cells following removal of the cranial and posterior wall of a large supra agger frontal cell (45 degrees).

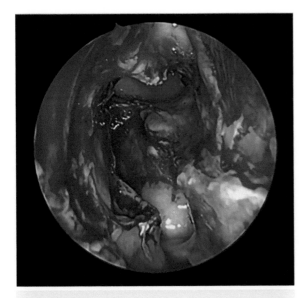

Fig. 4.80 Frontal sinus after complete dissection and removal of a large supra agger frontal and supra bulla frontal cell on the right (45 degrees; compare ▶ Fig. 4.82). Note: no bleeding = no need for nasal packing.

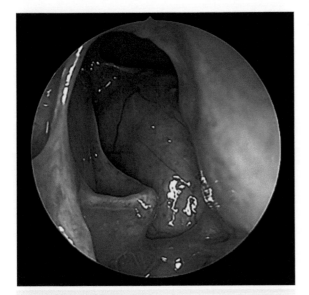

Fig. 4.82 Frontal recess and sinus 3 months postsurgery (45 degrees; compare ▶ Fig. 4.80).

Case 7: Example (Video 4.7):
- CRS with nasal polyps (white out) on the right.
- IFAC and LSAFC on the right.
- Draf type IIa or EFSS grade 3.
- (X degrees) denotes endoscope angle (see ▶ Fig. 4.83–▶ Fig. 4.94).

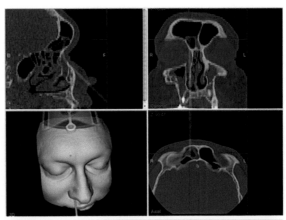

Fig. 4.81 Computer-assisted surgery with two frontoethmoidal cells (large supra agger frontal cell and large supra bulla frontal cell) on the right.

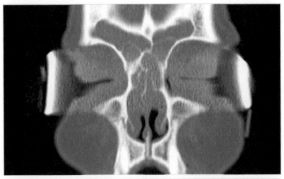

Fig. 4.83 Coronal CT scan with a "white out" on both sides and large supra agger frontal cells on both sides. Note aspirin exacerbated respiratory disease.

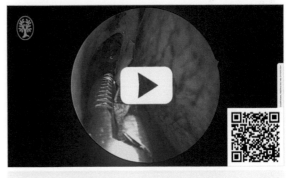

Video 4.7 CRSwNP, Draf IIa approach (Case 7)

4.5 Complications Management

- Floppy MT and middle meatal collapse:
  - *How to avoid:* Do not fracture MT and preserve mucosa and MT attachment.

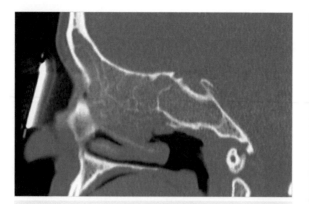

Fig. 4.84 Sagittal CT scan with an agger nasi and large supra agger frontal cell on the right.

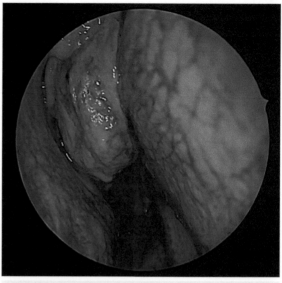

Fig. 4.85 Middle meatus with nasal polyps, middle turbinate, and septum on the right (0 degrees).

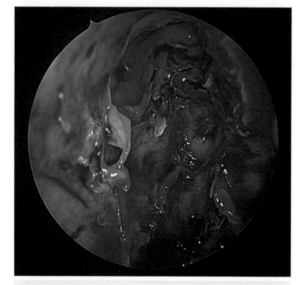

Fig. 4.86 Identification of a large supra agger frontal cell (45 degrees).

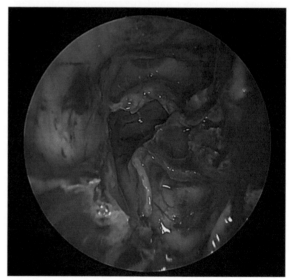

Fig. 4.87 Access in frontal sinus medial posterior of a large supra agger frontal cell on the right (45 degrees).

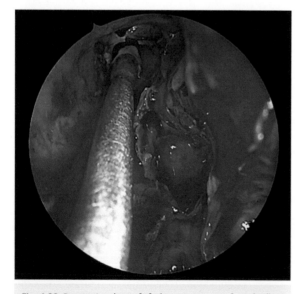

Fig. 4.88 Penetrating the roof of a large supra agger frontal cell on the right using a Stammberger circular cutting punch (45 degrees).

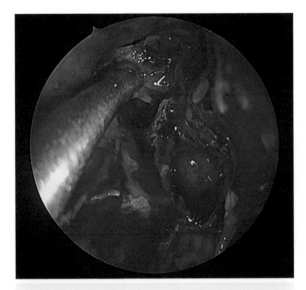

Fig. 4.89 Removing the roof of a large supra agger frontal cell ("uncapping the egg") using a Stammberger circular cutting punch (45 degrees).

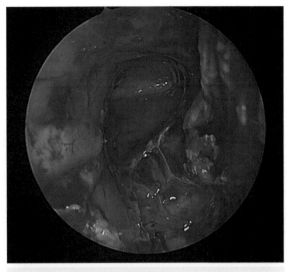

Fig. 4.90 Frontal sinus after complete dissection and removal of a large supra agger frontal cell on the right (45 degrees; compare ► Fig. 4.94).

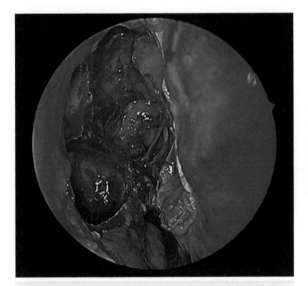

Fig. 4.91 Anterior, posterior ethmoid and sphenoid sinus on the right (0 degrees; compare ► Fig. 4.93). Note: no bleeding = no need for nasal packing.

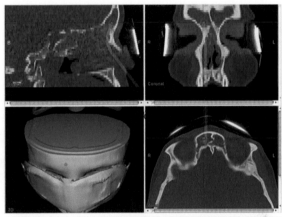

Fig. 4.92 Computer-assisted surgery with a large supra agger frontal cell on the right.

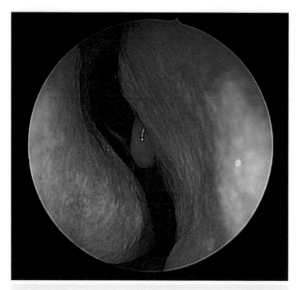

Fig. 4.93 The ethmoid cavity 6 months postsurgery on the right (0 degrees; compare ▶ Fig. 4.91).

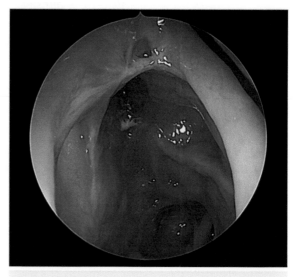

Fig. 4.94 Frontal recess and sinus following complete dissection and removal of a large supra agger frontal cell on the right 6 months postsurgery (45 degrees; compare ▶ Fig. 4.90). Note recurrent nasal polyps. Aspirin exacerbated respiratory disease.

- *What to do, if it happens:* Pack ethmoidal cavity to prevent uncontrolled lateralization. Use controlled synechiae technique (synechia provocation between the MT and the nasal septum)! If desperate, perform partial resection of parts of the MT, which may block frontoethmoidal drainage.
- ASB CSF leak:
  - *How to avoid:* Use a regular CT checklist to analyze ASB (e.g., Keros type, etc.).
  - *What to do if it happens:* Dura repair and post-op CT scans!
- AEA bleeding:
  - *How to avoid:* Clear the surgical field by using epinephrine vasoconstriction.
  - *What to do, if it happens:* Bipolar coagulation! If desperate, packing.
- Orbit/AEA intra-/retro-orbital hematoma:
  - *How to avoid:* Clear the surgical field by using epinephrine vasoconstriction.
  - *What to do if it happens:* Endoscopic endonasal decompression and/or lateral canthotomy and cantholysis!
- Orbit laceration or penetration of the medial orbital wall:
  - *How to avoid:* Use a CT checklist to analyze a "dangerous infundibulum" and using the swinging door technique to resect UP.
  - *What to do, if it happens:* Repair the LP, if appropriate. Do not resect orbital content; we recommend oral antibiotics and avoidance of blowing the nose!
- Frontal recess and sinus stenosis, headache and mucocele formation:

  - *How to avoid:* Complete dissection of obstructing air cell in the frontal recess, preserve mucosa, and avoid circular mucosa injury.
  - *What to do if it happens:* Multiplanar CT scan and, if necessary, revision FS surgery using navigation!

4.6 Conclusion

In a nutshell, endoscopic endonasal surgery of the frontal recess and sinus requires a profound understanding of the anatomy due to its inherent complexity, as variation is normal and access is usually around the corner in a narrow space. There is no simple FR and sinus. Hence, skillful surgical technique is necessary to open the FSO drainage, which can be blocked by one, two, or combinations of multiple FEC. To open the "door" to these cells, the UP and ANC are key structures, which should be removed carefully but completely by using adapted surgical techniques and proper curved instruments in a clear surgical field. The surgical approach is always tailored to individual anatomy and disease of the patient.

References

[1] Dautremont JF, Rudmik L. When are we operating for chronic rhinosinusitis? A systematic review of maximal medical therapy protocols prior to endoscopic sinus surgery. Int Forum Allergy Rhinol. 2015; 5 (12):1095–1103

[2] Kennedy DW. Functional endoscopic sinus surgery. Technique. Arch Otolaryngol. 1985; 111(10):643–649

[3] Messerklinger W. Background and evolution of endoscopic sinus surgery. Ear Nose Throat J. 1994; 73(7):449–450

[4] Stammberger H. Endoscopic endonasal surgery: concepts in treatment of recurring rhinosinusitis. Part II. Surgical technique. Otolaryngol Head Neck Surg. 1986; 94(2):147–156

[5] Wormald PJ, Hoseman W, Callejas C, et al. The International Frontal Sinus Anatomy Classification (IFAC) and classification of the extent of endoscopic frontal sinus surgery (EFSS). Int Forum Allergy Rhinol. 2016; 6(7):677–696

[6] Cohen NA, Kennedy DW. Revision endoscopic sinus surgery. Otolaryngol Clin North Am. 2006; 39(3):417–435, vii

[7] Morrissey DK, Bassiouni A, Psaltis AJ, Naidoo Y, Wormald PJ. Outcomes of revision endoscopic modified Lothrop procedure. Int Forum Allergy Rhinol. 2016; 6(5):518–522

[8] Langdon C, Herman P, Verillaud B, et al. Expanded endoscopic endonasal surgery for advanced stage juvenile angiofibromas: a retrospective multi-center study. Rhinology. 2016; 54(3):239–246

[9] Ledderose GJ, Betz CS, Stelter K, Leunig A. Surgical management of osteomas of the frontal recess and sinus: extending the limits of the endoscopic approach. Eur Arch Otorhinolaryngol. 2011; 268(4):525–532

[10] Rawal RB, Gore MR, Harvey RJ, Zanation AM. Evidence-based practice: endoscopic skull base resection for malignancy. Otolaryngol Clin North Am. 2012; 45(5):1127–1142

[11] Timperley DG, Banks C, Robinson D, Roth J, Sacks R, Harvey RJ. Lateral frontal sinus access in endoscopic skull-base surgery. Int Forum Allergy Rhinol. 2011; 1(4):290–295

[12] Bassiouni A, Naidoo Y, Wormald PJ. When FESS fails: the inflammatory load hypothesis in refractory chronic rhinosinusitis. Laryngoscope. 2012; 122(2):460–466

[13] Fokkens WJ, Lund VJ, Hopkins C, et al. European position paper on rhinosinusitis and nasal polyps 2020. Rhinol Suppl. 2020:20(58):1–464

[14] Orlandi RR, Kingdom TT, Hwang PH, et al. International consensus statement on allergy and rhinology: rhinosinusitis. Int Forum Allergy Rhinol. 2016; 6 Suppl 1:S22–S209

[15] Draf W. Endonasal microendoscopic frontal sinus surgery: the fulda concept. Oper Tech Otolaryngol Head Neck Surg. 1991; 2(4):234–240

[16] Eloy JA, Marchiano E, Vázquez A. Extended endoscopic and open sinus surgery for refractory chronic rhinosinusitis. Otolaryngol Clin North Am. 2017; 50(1):165–182

[17] Landsberg R, Segev Y, Friedman M, Fliss DM, Derowe A. A targeted endoscopic approach to chronic isolated frontal sinusitis. Otolaryngol Head Neck Surg. 2006; 134(1):28–32

[18] Simmen D, Jones N. Operative procedures: a step-by-step safe and logical approach. In: Simmen D, Jones N, eds. Manual of Endoscopic Sinus Surgery and Its Extended Applications. Stuttgart: Thieme; 2014:50–104

[19] Stammberger H. Functional Endoscopic Sinus Surgery. The Messerklinger Technique. Philadelphia, PA: B. C. Decker; 1991

[20] Lund VJ, Stammberger H, Fokkens WJ, et al. European position paper on the anatomical terminology of the internal nose and paranasal sinuses. Rhinol Suppl. 2014; 24(24):1–34

[21] Leunig A, Sommer B, Betz CS, Sommer F. Surgical anatomy of the frontal recess: is there a benefit in multiplanar CT-reconstruction? Rhinology. 2008; 46(3):188–194

[22] Oakley GM, Barham HP, Harvey RJ. Utility of image-guidance in frontal sinus surgery. Otolaryngol Clin North Am. 2016; 49(4):975–988

[23] Mus L, Hermans R, Jorissen M. Long-term effects of cutting versus non-cutting instruments in FESS. Rhinology. 2012; 50(1):56–66

[24] Simmen D, Raghavan U, Briner HR, et al. The surgeon's view of the anterior ethmoid artery. Clin Otolaryngol. 2006; 31(3):187–191

[25] Noon E, Hopkins C. Review article: outcomes in endoscopic sinus surgery. BMC Ear Nose Throat Disord. 2016; 16:9

5 Draf Frontal Sinusotomy IIb

Kevin Kulendra, Ahmed Youssef, and Shahzada Ahmed

Abstract

An endoscopic Draf IIb frontal sinusotomy is usually performed under general anesthesia. We will describe the common indications for surgery and the key surgical steps. This may be performed following a Draf IIa or be performed bilaterally and then converted to a Draf III. Anatomically this involves removal of all the cells leading up to the frontal recess including the anterolateral attachment of the middle turbinate, then removal of the floor of the frontal sinus between the lamina papyracea laterally and the nasal septum medially.

Keywords: endoscopic, Draf IIb, frontal sinus, surgical approach

5.1 Indications

- Frontal sinusitis needing drainage that might not be achieved by Draf I or IIa (▶ Fig. 5.1a).
- Frontal sinus or frontal recess tumors.
- Frontal sinus access, for example, to repair cerebrospinal fluid (CSF) fistulas or approach lateral frontal sinus mucoceles.
- Revision frontal sinus surgery.

5.2 Anatomy

The frontal sinus recess is a three-dimensional (3D) corridor that is bounded anteroinferiorly by the agger nasi cell, medially by the anterolateral attachment of middle turbinate, laterally by lamina papyracea, posteriorly by the anterior wall of the ethmoid bulla, and inferiorly by the terminal recess of the ethmoidal infundibulum (see Chapter 3). All these structures are lined by a mucous membrane, which is often intimately related to the dis-ease process that is being treated and has to be considered in the healing phase.

5.3 Surgical Steps

5.3.1 Lateral Approach

- Following on from a Draf IIa, remove the anterolateral attachment of the middle turbinate just in front its vertical attachment. This can often be undertaken with through biting forceps to avoid injury to the skull base from excessive turbinate manipulation.
- The floor of the frontal sinus (frontal beak) is then removed anteromedially up to the nasal septum to further maximize the drainage pathway. The anterior limit of bone resection is reached when the undersurface of the anterior wall of the frontal sinus is visualized through the new frontal sinus opening. The posterior limit is the posterior wall of the frontal sinus laterally and the first olfactory filament medially (▶ Fig. 5.1b).
- Care is taken to preserve as much mucosa as possible to reduce the postoperative nasal crusting and stenosis.

5.3.2 Median Approach

- An incision is marked in the mucosa of the roof of the nose with a monopolar needle diathermy starting at the axilla of the middle turbinate vertically up to the roof of the nose and back vertically down medially on the nasal septum to the same level as the lateral axillary incision.
- The mucosa is carefully dissected in a subperiosteal plane posteriorly until the first olfactory filament is clearly visualized (▶ Fig. 5.2). Drilling 7 mm anterior to the first olfactory filament allows entry into the floor of the frontal sinus in 91% of frontal sinuses.[1] Drilling posterior to the first olfactory filament will result in an iatrogenic CSF leak[2] and should be avoided.

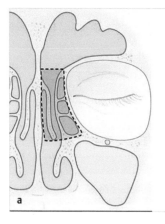 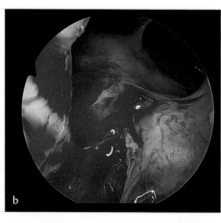

Fig. 5.1 (a) Left Draf IIb drainage showing area of bone resection. **(b)** Left Draf IIb with frontal sinus floor resected from the lamina papyracea to the nasal septum plus the anterolateral attachment of the middle turbinate also resected.

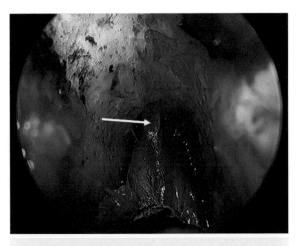

Fig. 5.2 Arrow illustrating the first olfactory filament in the roof of the left nasal cavity identified during the median approach to the frontal sinus.

- This window into the floor of the frontal sinus is then gradually widened to the same limits as the lateral approach: medially to nasal septum, laterally to lamina papyracea and skin, anteriorly to the front wall of the frontal sinus, posteromedially to the first olfactory filament, and posterolaterally to the posterior wall of the frontal sinus. This is all undertaken under direct vision.
- Care is taken to preserve as much mucosa as possible to reduce postoperative nasal crusting and stenosis.

5.4 Tips and Tricks

- Have appropriate frontal sinus instruments: as a minimum 0 degrees and angled (either 30- or 45-degree) Hopkins rod endoscopes, a frontal sinus seeker, frontal sinus bone punch, and angled frontal sinus drills.
- Utilize image guidance for all frontal sinus surgery cases.[3]
- Appreciation of key anatomical landmarks is vital such as the first olfactory filament and the posterior wall of the frontal sinus.
- Preservation of the frontal recess mucosa and periosteum can reduce the risk of stenosis. This can be enhanced with the use of septoturbinal flaps.[1]
- Gently packing the surgical cavity with 1:1,000 or 1:10,000 adrenaline on neuropatties can help decongest the mucosa as well as achieve hemostasis.

- Enhance 3D anatomical appreciation with cadaveric and simulation training.

5.5 Complications

- CSF leak.
- Orbital injury.
- Epistaxis.
- Orbital ecchymosis
- Synechiae.
- Stenosis of frontal recess.

Complications may be minimized with the use of meticulous surgical technique and careful pre-op analysis of the patient's CT scan in multiplanar views.

Recommended Readings

Chiu AG, Vaughan WC. Using the frontal intersinus septal cell to widen the narrow frontal recess. Laryngoscope. 2004; 114(7):1315–1317

Cho SH, Lee YS, Jeong JH, Kim KR. Endoscopic above and below approach with frontal septotomy in a patient with frontal mucocele: a contralateral bypass drainage procedure through the frontal septum. Am J Otolaryngol. 2010; 31(2):141–143

Upadhyay S, Buohliqah L, Vieira Junior G, Otto BA, Prevedello DM, Carrau RL. First olfactory fiber as an anatomical landmark for frontal sinus surgery. Laryngoscope. 2016; 126(5):1039–1045

Dubin MG, Kuhn FA. Endoscopic modified Lothrop (Draf III) with frontal sinus punches. Laryngoscope. 2005; 115(9):1702–1703

Draf W. Endonasal micro-endoscopic frontal sinus surgery: the Fulda concept. Oper Tech Otolaryngol Head Neck Surg. 1992; 2:234–240

May M, Schaitkin B. Frontal sinus surgery: endonasal drainage instead of an external osteoplastic approach. Oper Tech Otolaryngol Head Neck Surg. 1995; 6:184–192

Schatkin B. Endoscopic approaches to the frontal sinus. In Myers EN, ed. Operative Otolaryngology: Head and Neck Surgery. Philadelphia, PA: Saunders Elsevier; 2008:121–126

References

[1] Fiorini FR, Nogueira C, Verillaud B, Sama A, Herman P. Value of septo-turbinal flap in the frontal sinus drill-out type IIb according to draf. Laryngoscope. 2016; 126(11):2428–2432

[2] Wormald PJ. The frontal sinus. In: Jones N, ed. Practical Rhinology. London, UK: Edward Arnold Ltd; 2010:105–111

[3] American Academy of Otolaryngology – Head and Neck Surgery. Position Statement: Intra-Operative Use of Computer Aided Surgery. Available at: http://www.entnet.org/content/intra-operative-use-computer-aided-surgery. 2012. Accessed April 25, 2018

6 Extended Draf IIb and Other Modifications of the Lothrop Procedure

Vivek V. Kanumuri, Qasim Husain, Suat Kilic, Michael J. Pfisterer, Osama Tarabichi, and Jean Anderson Eloy

Abstract

This chapter further explores endoscopic surgical approaches to frontal sinus disease. Specifically, it highlights the Draf IIb approach and its extended modifications, namely, the modified hemi-Lothrop, modified mini-Lothrop, modified subtotal-Lothrop, and modified central-Lothrop approaches. These are extended approaches meant to address refractory chronic frontal sinusitis. These approaches are often used after failure of a more limited frontal sinusotomy such as a Draf I or Draf II as described in the previous chapters. As with other endoscopic sinus procedures, the end goal is to create a patent outflow pathway and to allow access for appropriate topical therapy for long-term management.

Keywords: frontal sinus, endoscopic sinus surgery, Draf IIb, Draf IIc, modified mini-Lothrop, extended frontal sinusotomy, modified hemi-Lothrop procedure, hemi-Lothrop procedure, modified mini-Lothrop procedure, modified subtotal-Lothrop procedure, Eloy modifications

6.1 Introduction

A standard Draf IIb is a unilateral wide frontal sinusotomy that opens the floor of the frontal sinus from the lamina papyracea (medial orbital wall) laterally to the nasal septum medially.[1,2,3,4] A number of modifications to this approach have been described in recent years involving combinations of ipsilateral and contralateral frontal sinus-otomies, and septectomies to allow for improved access and additional instrumentation.[5,6,7] These modifications and their indications are described in this chapter.

6.2 Indications

As described earlier, the extended endoscopic surgical approaches to the frontal sinus delineated in this chapter are indicated for patients with chronic rhinosinusitis who have failed appropriate medical management.[5,8] These patients have often also failed more limited frontal sinus approaches such as the Draf I or IIa approaches. These extended approaches are also useful in the cases of hard-to-access frontal sinus soft-tissue tumors, such as those in the lateral recesses, or in other isolated frontal sinus lesions.[5,9] A number of modifications to these approaches (▶ Table 6.1) have been described and are detailed here with their more specific indications.

6.3 Surgical Steps

6.3.1 Overview of Standard Draf IIb

The surgical steps of the standard Draf IIb (see Chapter 5 for complete description) are as follows (▶ Fig. 6.1):

1. Position the patient supine with the head extended slightly to obtain improved access to the frontal sinus.
2. Prepare the nose and nares with oxymetazoline-soaked pledgets.
3. Examine the nasal cavity bilaterally using 4-mm 0-, 30-, and 70-degree endoscopes.
4. Inject the uncinate process and the middle turbinate (axilla and head) with 1% lidocaine with 1:100,000 epinephrine.
5. Identify the frontal recess using anatomical landmarks as described in Chapter 2. A small ball probe can be used to gently identify the area of the frontal sinus recess, though this is not always feasible based on the extent of disease. Caution must be used when probing given the potential for distorted anatomy, and the proximity of the cribriform plate to the frontal sinus recess. Image guidance can often help with this step.
6. Using a combination of powered instrumentation, bone curettes, and different through-cutting instruments creates a wide frontal sinusotomy extending from the lamina papyracea laterally to the nasal septum medially.

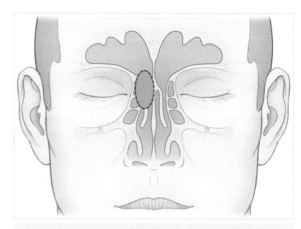

Fig. 6.1 Illustration of the Draf IIB procedure (coronal). (This image is provided courtesy of Chris Gralapp, Fairfax, CA.)

Table 6.1 Classification of endoscopic approaches to the frontal sinus

Draf	Eloy modification	Description
I	I	Anterior ethmoidectomy with drainage of the frontal sinus recess without touching the frontal sinus outflow pathway
IIA	IIA	Removal of the anterior ethmoidal cells and frontal cells protruding into the frontal sinus outflow pathway creating an opening between the middle turbinate medially and the lamina papyracea laterally
IIB	IIB	Removal of the frontal sinus floor between the nasal septum medially and the lamina papyracea laterally
	IIC	Ipsilateral removal of the frontal sinus floor between the nasal septum medially and the lamina papyracea laterally; superior septectomy for access from the contralateral side and enhanced access to the lateral supraorbital frontal sinus and supraorbital ethmoid regions. This also provides binostril, bimanual manipulation; previously described as a **modified hemi-Lothrop procedure**
	IID	Contralateral removal of the frontal sinus floor between the nasal septum medially and the lamina papyracea laterally with addition of an intersinus septectomy for drainage of the diseased frontal sinus to the contralateral recess; previously described as a **modified mini-Lothrop procedure**
	IIE	Ipsilateral removal of the frontal sinus floor between the nasal septum medially and the lamina papyracea laterally; superior septectomy for access from the contralateral side and enhanced access to the lateral supraorbital frontal sinus and supraorbital ethmoid regions; intersinus septectomy for access to the entire posterior wall of the frontal sinus; preservation of the contralateral frontal sinus recess; previously described as a **modified subtotal Lothrop procedure**
	IIF	Central resection of the frontal sinus floor bilaterally, with a superior septectomy and frontal intersinus septectomy, while preserving both frontal sinus recesses; also termed a **modified central-Lothrop procedure**
III	III	Bilateral removal of the floor of the frontal sinus anterior to the middle turbinates from one lamina papyracea to the next with superior septectomy and inter sinus septectomy; also termed a modified Lothrop procedure

Source: Reproduced with permission of Eloy JA, Vazquez A, Liu JK, Baredes S. Endoscopic approaches to the frontal sinus: modifications of the existing techniques and proposed classification. Otolaryngol Clin North Am 2016; 49:1007–1018.

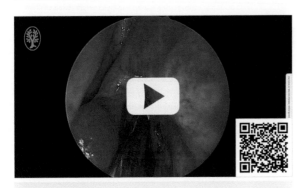

Video 6.1 Modified Hemi-Lothrop procedure for recurrent left frontal mucocele.

6.4 Modifications of the Standard Draf IIb Procedure

6.4.1 Modified Hemi-Lothrop Procedure (Eloy IIC)

This modification to the Draf IIb follows steps 1 to 6 but combines the standard Draf IIb with a superior septectomy (▶ Fig. 6.2 and ▶ Video 6.1).[10,11,12,13] This allows bimanual binostril manipulation and enhanced access to the lateral frontal sinus recess and supraorbital ethmoid cell via a cross-court angle through the contralateral nasal cavity (▶ Fig. 6.2c, d).

6.4.2 Modified Mini-Lothrop Procedure (Eloy IID)

This approach combines the standard Draf IIb on the *contralateral* side (with respect to disease pathology) with a frontal intersinus septectomy (▶ Fig. 6.3).[14,15] It is indicated when ipsilateral access to the affected frontal sinus is not feasible due to scarring or other obstructive pathology.

6.4.3 Modified Subtotal-Lothrop Procedure (Eloy IIE)

This approach combines the standard Draf IIb on the ipsilateral side with *both* a superior nasal septectomy and a frontal intersinus septectomy (▶ Fig. 6.4 and ▶ Video 6.2).[16,17] This procedure is indicated for bilateral frontal sinus disease, including large unilateral frontal sinus tumors, and large posterior frontal sinus

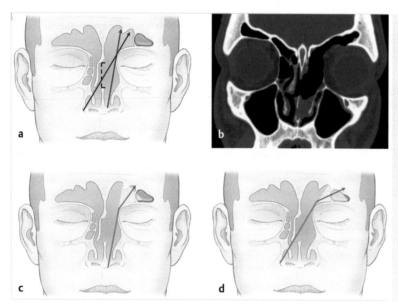

Fig. 6.2 Illustration of the modified hemi-Lothrop (Eloy IIC) procedure (coronal). **(a)** Drawing in the coronal plane showing the approach to the contralateral frontal sinus with the Eloy IIC procedure. **(b)** Postoperative coronal CT scan after a modified hemi-Lothrop. **(c,d)** Binostril bimanual instrumentation. *Bracket* in depicts superior septectomy window. *Red arrow* depicts limited lateral access via the ipsilateral nasal cavity. *Blue arrow* depicts improved lateral access. (These images are provided courtesy of Chris Gralapp, Fairfax, CA.)

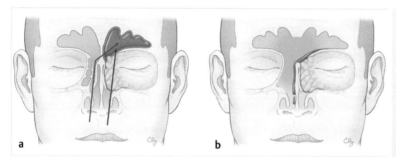

Fig. 6.3 (a) Illustration of the modified mini-Lothrop (Eloy IID, blue arrow) procedure in a patient for whom ipsilateral frontal sinusotomy (red arrow) is not feasible due to fat prolapse (coronal). **(b)** Drainage via the contralateral nasal cavity after the Eloy IID procedure. (These images are provided courtesy of Chris Gralapp, Fairfax, CA.)

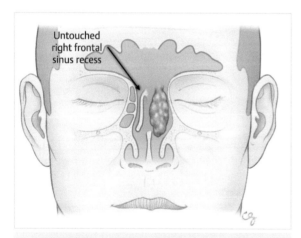

Fig. 6.4 Illustration of bilateral frontal sinus access with the Eloy IIE (modified subtotal Lothrop) procedure with preservation of the contralateral frontal sinus recess. (This image is provided courtesy of Chris Gralapp, Fairfax, CA.)

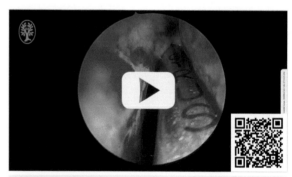

Video 6.2 Modified subtotal Lothrop procedure for cholesterol granuloma of the right frontal sinus.

encephaloceles. This approach allows for bimanual binostril instrumentation and access to both frontal sinuses while preserving the contralateral middle turbinate and frontal sinus outflow pathway.

6.4.4 Modified Central-Lothrop Procedure (Eloy IIF)

This approach combines bilateral removal of the medial aspect of the frontal sinus floor with a superior nasal septectomy and frontal intersinus septectomy (▶ Fig. 6.5).[5],[6] The bilateral frontal sinus outflow pathways are left intact. This procedure is indicated for frontal sinus

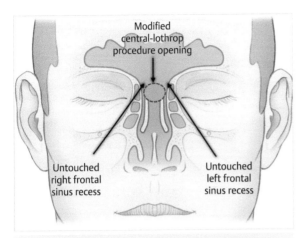

Fig. 6.5 (a) Illustration of the modified central Lothrop (Eloy IIF) procedure (coronal). (This image is provided courtesy of Chris Gralapp, Fairfax, CA.)

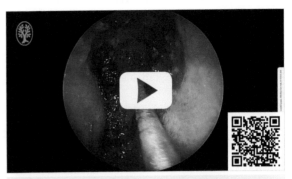

Video 6.3 Modified central lothrop procedure for left frontal mucocele.

disease largely confined to the midline, including certain frontal sinus mucoceles.

6.5 Tips and Tricks

Tips for additional difficulties that may be encountered in these procedures are outlined in ▶ Table 6.2.

6.6 Case Examples

6.6.1 Example 1

Video 6.1 demonstrates the use of the modified hemi-Lothrop (Eloy IIC) procedure in a patient with a recurrent left frontal sinus mucocele.

6.6.2 Example 2

Video 6.2 demonstrates the use of the modified subtotal-Lothrop (Eloy IIE) procedure in a patient with a cholesterol granuloma of the right frontal sinus and posterior table dehiscence.

6.6.3 Example 3

Video 6.3 demonstrates the use of the modified central-Lothrop (Eloy IIF) procedure in a patient with a left frontal sinus mucocele with medial extension and orbital dehiscence.

6.7 Complications

6.7.1 Recurrence and Chronic Scarring

The most important factor in achieving symptom resolution in frontal sinus surgery is maintenance of a patent drainage pathway. Given the additional instrumentation and dissection required in the above approaches,

Table 6.2 Tips and tricks

Difficulties/nuances	Technical solution(s)/significance
Identification of frontal sinus recess with ball probe	Aim the ball probe superiorly and medially, away from the medial orbital wall
Presence of agger nasi cells	Takedown of agger nasi and Suprabullar improves visualization of the frontal sinus infundibulum
Risk of postoperative scarring	Limit the use of power tools when feasible, and maximize mucosal preservation
Transillumination witnessed in the medial canthal region	May indicate that the supraethmoidal cell rather than frontal sinus was opened. It may also suggest that the frontal sinus is poorly pneumatized
Avoiding anterior ethmoid injury with sinus probe	When entering the frontal sinus, direct the probe medially and anteriorly to avoid injuring the anterior ethmoid artery

particular attention is needed to maintain adequate mucosal preservation, particularly in the area of the frontal sinus outflow pathway.[18] Insufficient care can lead to chronic scarring and recurrence. Rarely, this can present in the form of a mucocele, which in the frontal sinus often necessitates more aggressive management in the form of endoscopic and/or open marsupialization.

6.7.2 Cerebrospinal Fluid Leak

A cerebrospinal fluid (CSF) leak is of special concern for the large and difficult-to-access lesions for which the approaches described in this chapter are ideal. Given the significant variability in frontal sinus anatomy between patients, the most important step in avoiding this complication may be careful preoperative assessment and knowledge of anatomic landmarks.[18] If encountered intraoperatively, the CSF leak can be repaired using a number of techniques and grafts (including allogenic materials, free mucosal graft harvested from the nasal septum or hard palate, temporalis fascia, or in severe and large defect a nasoseptal pedicled flap).[18]

6.7.3 Orbital Injury

Injury to the orbit presents a particular risk in extended frontal sinus approaches given the need to extend a frontal sinusotomy all the way to the thin lamina papyracea (on both sides in some cases) for maximal freedom of movement, access with surgical instrumentation, and for providing an outflow pathway. Preoperative evaluation of any defects in the lamina papyracea is crucial.[19] Orbital fat herniation is often the first sign of disruption of the lamina. If encountered, prompt triage and evaluation is necessary.[18] Intraoperative ophthalmology consultation may be indicated.

6.7.4 Anterior Ethmoid Artery Injury

Although rare, a particularly feared complication in frontal sinus surgery is orbital hemorrhage, which can lead to permanent blindness.[18] This is often a result of damage to the anterior ethmoid artery, which can be easily encountered upon initial entry to the frontal sinus. Carefully directing the frontal sinus probe away from the medial orbital wall, anteriorly, can help prevent this injury.[18]

References

[1] Weber R, Draf W, Kratzsch B, Hosemann W, Schaefer SD. Modern concepts of frontal sinus surgery. Laryngoscope. 2001; 111(1):137–146

[2] Korban ZR, Casiano RR. Standard endoscopic approaches in frontal sinus surgery: technical pearls and approach selection. Otolaryngol Clin North Am. 2016; 49(4):989–1006

[3] Vázquez A, Baredes S, Setzen M, Eloy JA. Overview of frontal sinus pathology and management. Otolaryngol Clin North Am. 2016; 49 (4):899–910

[4] Folbe AJ, Svider PF, Eloy JA. Anatomic considerations in frontal sinus surgery. Otolaryngol Clin North Am. 2016; 49(4):935–943

[5] Eloy JA, Vázquez A, Liu JK, Baredes S. Endoscopic approaches to the frontal sinus: modifications of the existing techniques and proposed classification. Otolaryngol Clin North Am. 2016; 49(4):1007–1018

[6] Eloy JA, Marchiano E, Vázquez A. Extended endoscopic and open sinus surgery for refractory chronic rhinosinusitis. Otolaryngol Clin North Am. 2017; 50(1):165–182

[7] Silverman JB, Prasittivatechakool K, Busaba NY. An evidence-based review of endoscopic frontal sinus surgery. Am J Rhinol Allergy. 2009; 23(6):e59–e62

[8] Saini AT, Govindaraj S. Evaluation and decision making in frontal sinus surgery. Otolaryngol Clin North Am. 2016; 49(4):911–925

[9] Selleck AM, Desai D, Thorp BD, Ebert CS, Zanation AM. Management of frontal sinus tumors. Otolaryngol Clin North Am. 2016; 49 (4):1051–1065

[10] Liu JK, Mendelson ZS, Dubal PM, Mirani N, Eloy JA. The modified hemi-Lothrop procedure: a variation of the endoscopic endonasal approach for resection of a supraorbital psammomatoid ossifying fibroma. J Clin Neurosci. 2014; 21(12):2233–2238

[11] Friedel ME, Li S, Langer PD, Liu JK, Eloy JA. Modified hemi-Lothrop procedure for supraorbital ethmoid lesion access. Laryngoscope. 2012; 122(2):442–444

[12] Eloy JA, Friedel ME, Murray KP, Liu JK. Modified hemi-Lothrop procedure for supraorbital frontal sinus access: a cadaveric feasibility study. Otolaryngol Head Neck Surg. 2011; 145(3):489–493

[13] Eloy JA, Kuperan AB, Friedel ME, Choudhry OJ, Liu JK. Modified hemi-Lothrop procedure for supraorbital frontal sinus access: a case series. Otolaryngol Head Neck Surg. 2012; 147(1):167–169

[14] Eloy JA, Friedel ME, Kuperan AB, Govindaraj S, Folbe AJ, Liu JK. Modified mini-Lothrop/extended Draf IIB procedure for contralateral frontal sinus disease: a case series. Int Forum Allergy Rhinol. 2012; 2 (4):321–324

[15] Eloy JA, Friedel ME, Kuperan AB, Govindaraj S, Folbe AJ, Liu JK. Modified mini-Lothrop/extended Draf IIB procedure for contralateral frontal sinus disease: a cadaveric feasibility study. Otolaryngol Head Neck Surg. 2012; 146(1):165–168

[16] Eloy JA, Liu JK, Choudhry OJ, et al. Modified subtotal Lothrop procedure for extended frontal sinus and anterior skull base access: a cadaveric feasibility study with clinical correlates. J Neurol Surg B Skull Base. 2013; 74(3):130–135

[17] Eloy JA, Mady LJ, Kanumuri VV, Svider PF, Liu JK. Modified subtotal-Lothrop procedure for extended frontal sinus and anterior skull-base access: a case series. Int Forum Allergy Rhinol. 2014; 4(6):517–521

[18] Javer AR, Alandejani T. Prevention and management of complications in frontal sinus surgery. Otolaryngol Clin North Am. 2010; 43 (4):827–838

[19] Eloy JA, Svider PF, Setzen M. Preventing and managing complications in frontal sinus surgery. Otolaryngol Clin North Am. 2016; 49 (4):951–964

7 The Frontal Sinus Rescue Procedure

Fahad Alasousi, Anali Dadgostar, and Amin Javer

Abstract

Mastering the endoscopic frontal sinusotomy technique is one of the defining features of an advanced endoscopic sinus surgeon. Being attentive to the principles of mucosal preservation and to the resection and clearance of remnant bony shelves with the ultimate result of reestablishing the natural mucociliary clearance pathway should be the aim of every endoscopic frontal sinus procedure. However, there continues to be a lack of agreement in the literature with regard to the appropriate approach to the frontal sinus resulting in higher-than-acceptable numbers of revision surgeries, and more recently drill-outs, by tertiary rhinologists.[1,2] Even though there are good supporting data against the resection of the middle turbinate, it continues to be a source of controversy.[3] Many advanced endoscopic surgeons and teachers continue to promote very conservative anterior inferior resections of the middle turbinate in difficult sinus cases. Such statements by key opinion leaders are often misinterpreted by the general otolaryngologists as an allowance to resect the entire middle turbinate. As the medial boundary of the frontal recess, the middle turbinate provides the endoscopic surgeon with a pathway into the frontal recess proper. Resection of the anterior aspect of the middle turbinate can result in the collapse and scarring of the middle turbinate remnant against the orbit, thereby closing off the frontal recess outflow tract. This leads to suboptimal outcomes and this eventually resulted in the development of the frontal sinus rescue procedure, more formally described as the revision endoscopic frontal sinusotomy with mucoperiosteal flap advancement.

Keywords: frontal sinus, revision, middle turbinate, rescue

7.1 Indications

It is critical that the frontal sinus anatomy be conceptualized in the surgeon's mind during perioperative review and preparation for the surgery. According to the International Frontal Sinus Anatomy Classification (IFAC) and Classification of the Extent of Endoscopic Frontal Sinus Surgery (EFSS) documents, the space into which the frontal sinus drains is called the frontal recess. It is bounded by the space posterior to the frontal beak (nasal process of the frontal bone) anteriorly. The lateral boundary consists of the lamina papyracea of the orbit. The vertical lamella of the middle turbinate (MT) anterior to the basal lamella, and continuing on to the lateral wall of the olfactory fossa, forms the medial boundary. The narrowest area of the transition zone from the frontal sinus to the frontal recess is defined as the frontal sinus ostium. The anterior edge of the ostium is formed by the frontal sinus beak, and the posterior edge by the anterior skull base. The lateral boundary of the frontal ostium is the upward extension of the lamina papyracea, while the medial boundary is the upward extension of the vertical lamella of the MT and the lateral wall of the olfactory fossa.[4] When these anatomical sites are obstructed secondary to poor surgical technique and/or resection of the MT, reestablishing and maintaining a pathway of drainage can be accomplished by carrying out the frontal sinus rescue (FSR) procedure. Citardi et al developed the FSR in 1997 and the initial results of this procedure were published in 2001. Long-term relief from frontal recess scar and frontal ostium stenosis was achieved in 14 of 16 sides (87.5%) in 12 patients with average follow-up of 8.5 months.[5] In another publication by the same group, frontal recess patency and complete resolution of symptoms was reported in 29 of 32 operative sides in 24 patients. In their cohort, 18 sides were successfully treated with the FSR on the first attempt, 7 sides required a revision FSR procedure, and 4 sides required 2 revision FSR procedures for complete resolution. The mean follow-up was 9.6 months, and one patient had long-term patency at 37 months.[6] These results were achieved when the procedure was newly developed. It is expected that as surgeons develop more experience with the procedure, the results are likely to continue to improve.

In order to properly evaluate a diseased frontal sinus for a potential FSR procedure, assessment should naturally begin with a thorough history and endoscopic evaluation. The patient will typically present with a past history of sinus surgery with postoperative nonimprovement or worsening of frontal sinusitis symptoms (i.e., frontal headache, pressure symptoms, etc.). Endoscopic examination of the nasal cavity and frontal recess with angled endoscopes (30, 45, 70 degrees) will reveal an obstructed frontal recess and collapsed medial wall of the frontal recess: the lateralized stump of a remnant MT in the majority of cases. A high-resolution computed tomography (CT) of the paranasal sinuses will confirm the findings of (1) diseased frontal sinus and (2) obstructed pathway secondary to a lateralized, scarred stump of the MT remnant against the lamina papyracea.

7.2 Surgical Steps

The relationship of the MT remnant to the medial orbital wall must be identified. In addition, it is important to determine the relative position of the skull base, including the cribriform plate as the posterior limit of dissection.

Being inattentive of this detail could lead to a cerebrospinal fluid (CSF) leak during removal of the posterior vertical bony lamellae remnant of the stump of the MT.

The initial description of the technique recommended infiltration with local anesthetic (1% lidocaine with 1:100,000 epinephrine). However, after 15 years of experience in performing this procedure, the authors have found little use for this step. Distortion of the anatomy from overinflation is a risk, as is the risk of inadvertent injection into the orbital cavity in the case of a small bony dehiscence in the lamina papyracea. Also, increased mucosal bleeding usually follows a few minutes into the procedure secondary to vasodilatation, once the effect of local epinephrine wears off. Instead, the authors prefer to use a topical Neuro Pattie Sponges (Medtronic, United States) soaked in oxymetazoline against the site of surgery for 3 to 4 minutes prior to making the initial incision. Also, other techniques to reduce bleeding such as a 15-degree elevation of the head of the bed are very useful in keeping the field dry.

7.2.1 Step 1

After locating and confirming the site of the anterior aspect of the MT remnant (▶ Fig. 7.1a), a parasagittal incision is performed. A sharp sickle knife or a no. 15 blade may be utilized to perform the incision as described previously. However, a 45-degree through-cutting instrument (e.g., the Heuwieser by Karl Storz GmbH & Co. KG, Tuttlingen, Germany) is often found to be safer and more effective in resecting the scar between the MT remnant and the lateral nasal wall. Due to the fairly superior location of the MT stump attachment, the through-cutting instrument often has to be placed above the angled endoscope for adequate reach and performance. Alternatively, one of the longer neck through-cut instruments can be used to make this initial incision. The primary goal of this initial but important step is to release the scar band causing lateralization of the MT and obstruction of the frontal recess outflow tract.

7.2.2 Step 2

The remnant MT vertical segment stump can be well appreciated at this point (▶ Fig. 7.1b). The mucosal covering on either sides of the MT stump is gently dissected and elevated off of the bone (▶ Fig. 7.1c) with fine instrumentation (frontal sinus seekers, frontal sinus curettes). If possible, methylene blue on a needle tip can be used to mark the mucosal aspect of the lateral flap. This will assist in correctly repositioning the lateral flap in step 4. In order to properly position the advancement flap, the medial mucosal segment, as well as a small area of the adjacent frontal sinus floor mucosa, is resected and discarded (▶ Fig. 7.1d). The lateral mucosal flap that was already elevated and preserved is left within the frontal sinus in order to prevent any trauma or damage to it (▶ Fig. 7.1e). This flap will eventually form "the mucoperiosteal flap."

7.2.3 Step 3

The skeletonized MT vertical segment (▶ Fig. 7.1e) is then carefully resected with a side-to-side through-cutting instrument. Kuhn Rhinoforce Frontal Sinus side opening through-cutting forceps (Karl Storz GmbH & Co. KG) or the Serpent through-cutting instruments (Smith and Nephew, London, United Kingdom) are ideally suited for this step.

7.2.4 Step 4

The mucoperiosteal flap previously prepared and preserved within the frontal recess in step 2 is relocated and placed in position to drape over the skeletonized MT segment and over the previously denuded frontal recess (▶ Fig. 7.1f). The unmarked inner surface is positioned facing the denuded bone in order to ensure correct placement. A small piece of Gelfoam or Surgicel can be used to hold the flap in place during the healing process.

7.3 Reverse Frontal Rescue Procedure

The initial reasoning for utilizing the lateral flap as the mucoperiosteal advancement flap was to preserve and utilize the original mucosa and cilia within the frontal recess so that the mucociliary outflow tract would be preserved for proper frontal sinus drainage. However, the past decade has seen a significant increase in the use of drills within the frontal recess by inexperienced surgeons. This often leads to damaged mucus membrane on the lateral aspect of the MT stump and within the frontal recess. Such cases often have relatively thick and nonfunctional lateral mucoperiosteal flaps. For these patients, the medial flap may be preserved instead and the thick diseased and nonfunctional lateral mucosal flap may be resected. The remaining procedural steps are followed as described earlier. Figs. 7.2 and 7.3 demonstrate the post operative endoscopic appearance of the frontal sinus at 12 weeks and 1 year, respectively.

7.4 Complications

- During manipulation and resection of the vertical stump of the MT at its weakest insertion point of the skull base, that is, the cribriform plate, a CSF leak may occur. Careful attention should be paid during resection and manipulation of the MT stump, particularly at its posterior insertion point to the skull base.
- Mucoperiosteal flap tear is a potential risk. Powered instrumentation should be avoided within the frontal

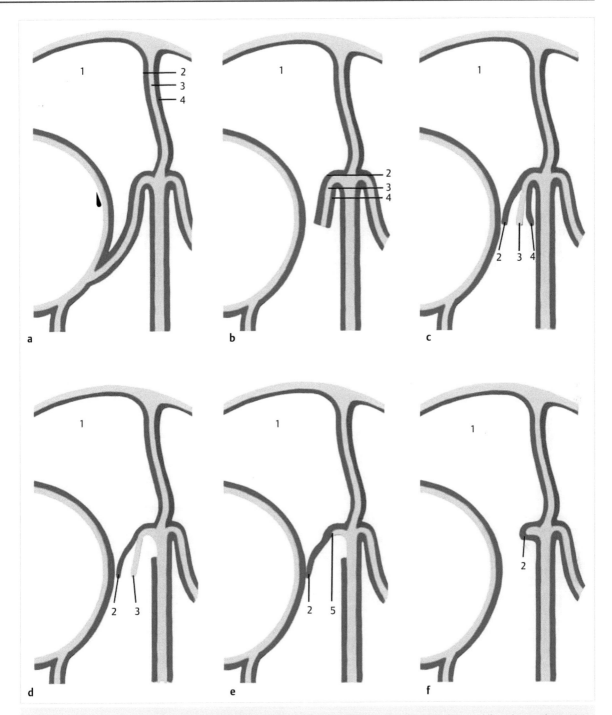

Fig. 7.1 Coronal views of the right paranasal sinuses at the level of the frontal recess. **(a)** Remnant of the middle turbinate obstructing the frontal recess. **(b)** The middle turbinate vertical segment stump is detached from the lamina papyracea. **(c)** Dissection of the medial and lateral mucoperiosteal flaps of the middle turbinate. **(d)** Resection of the medial mucoperiosteal flap. **(e)** Resection of the middle turbinate vertical segment stump. **(f)** The lateral mucoperiosteal flap drapes the skeletonized middle turbinate segment. 1. Frontal sinus. 2. Lateral mucosal covering. 3. Middle turbinate remnant. 4. Medial mucosal covering. 5. Horizontal attachment of middle turbinate to lateral nasal wall.

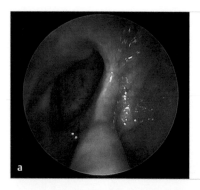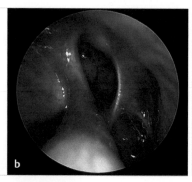

Fig. 7.2 Pictures showing a right and left postoperative frontal sinus 12 weeks after a rescue procedure.

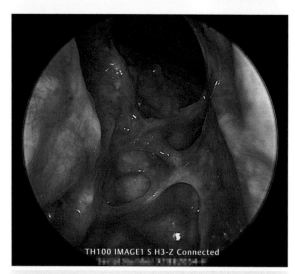

Fig. 7.3 Picture showing a healed frontal sinus ostium 1 year postoperatively.

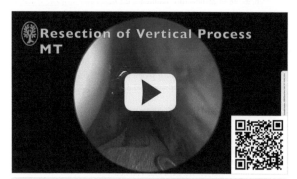

Video 7.1 Frontal sinus rescue procedure

recess. Gentle handling of the tissue with appropriate choice of instrumentation is important.

- Improper placement or malpositioning of the mucoperiosteal advancement flap can lead to an area of exposed bone resulting in neo-osteogenesis and crust formation. Good planning prior to flap preparation and dissection

is necessary. In the cases of a shorter-than-necessary flap with a large area of exposed bone, a free mucosal graft from the nasal floor can be utilized for adequate bony coverage.

- Failure and re-scarring have been reported in the original publications as mentioned earlier. Revision of this procedure may be needed later especially for the novice frontal sinus surgeon going through a sharp learning curve early on.

7.5 Tips and Tricks

- Sharp through-cut angled instrumentation works best to remove the bone together with the mucus membrane until the desired resection level to the skull base has been achieved.
- Forty-five-degree side-to-side through-cut giraffe forceps are our favorites to carry out the procedure.
- The mucosal advancement flap does not need to be large or long. It only needs to be long enough to cover the free bony edge of the resected upper MT.
- In revision cases, image guidance is highly recommended to determine the posterior extension of the turbinate stump resection. Going too far posteriorly risks a CSF leak complication.
- Avoid powered instrumentation to reduce the risk of mucosal membrane trauma.
- If there is exposed bone due to inadequate amount of mucosal membrane, a free mucosal graft from the nasal floor is always a good option for obtaining adequate coverage.

7.6 Conclusion

The frontal sinus rescue procedure has the benefit of providing a significantly less invasive option to an obstructed frontal sinus recess in comparison to the traditional modified Lothrop approach. It also facilitates natural mucociliary clearance and has less risk of developing future neo-osteogenesis as compared to traditional modalities.

Acknowledgments

We would like to recognize the efforts of our research coordinator, Christopher Okpaleke, for his assistance with this paper.

References

[1] Philpott CM, McKiernan DC, Javer AR. Selecting the best approach to the frontal sinus. Indian J Otolaryngol Head Neck Surg. 2011; 63 (1):79–84

[2] Eloy JA, Vázquez A, Liu JK, Baredes S. Endoscopic approaches to the frontal sinus: modifications of the existing techniques and proposed classification. Otolaryngol Clin North Am. 2016; 49(4):1007–1018

[3] Sowerby LJ, Mann S, Starreveld Y, Kotylak T, Mechor B, Wright ED. A comparison of radiographic evidence of frontal sinusitis in middle-turbinate sacrificing versus middle-turbinate sparing approaches to the sella. Am J Rhinol Allergy. 2016; 30(4):306–309

[4] Wormald P-JJ, Hoseman W, Callejas C, et al. The International Frontal Sinus Anatomy Classification (IFAC) and Classification of the Extent of Endoscopic Frontal Sinus Surgery (EFSS). Int Forum Allergy Rhinol. 2016; 6(7):677–696

[5] Citardi MJ, Javer AR, Kuhn FA. Revision endoscopic frontal sinusotomy with mucoperiosteal flap advancement: the frontal sinus rescue procedure. Otolaryngol Clin North Am. 2001; 34(1):123–132

[6] Kuhn FA, Javer AR, Nagpal K, Citardi MJ. The frontal sinus rescue procedure: early experience and three-year follow-up. Am J Rhinol. 2000; 14(4):211–216

8 Draf III (Endoscopic Modified Lothrop)— Inside-Out and Outside-In Approaches

Christos Georgalas, Vasileios Chatzinakis, Klementina Avdeeva, Georgiy A. Polev, and Anshul Sama

Abstract

In 1991 in Fulda, Professor Wolfgang Draf developed the type 3 median drainage procedure[1] (endoscopic modified Lothrop,[2] bilateral frontal sinus drillout,[3] nasofrontal approach IV[4]) as a valid alternative to frontal sinus obliteration. Compared with the osteoplastic flap approach, Draf III avoids problems such as cutaneous scarring, cosmetic deformity as well as late-onset mucoceles while preserving the natural drainage of the frontal sinus. Initial reports showed significant complications including rates of cerebrospinal fluid (CSF) leak as high as 11%.[5] However, over time and in experienced hands it was a safe procedure with minimal and rare complications,[6] and in appropriately selected cases, it results in significant improvement in the patients' quality of life.[7]

Draf III is the complete drillout of the floor of the frontal sinus, frontal beak, intersinus septum, and, importantly, an adjacent part (anterosuperior) of the nasal septum. Resection of the anterosuperior part of nasal septum allows binostril intraoperative manipulation and provides access to lateral areas of the frontal sinus. If the surgery does not include the maximally possible drainage (i.e., when intersinus septum is not completely removed), the term modified Draf III could be used.

In the following chapter indications and surgical techniques of both standard Draf III and outside-in frontal sinus drillout are described. It also includes possible complications and the ways of avoiding them and dealing with them, if any occurred. Photos of step-by-step dissection and some relevant cases are illustrated.

Keywords: Draf III, modified endoscopic Lothrop procedure, frontal sinus floor drillout, frontal sinus, endoscopic sinus surgery, indications, complications

8.1 Indications

- Symptomatic patients with recalcitrant chronic frontal rhinosinusitis who have failed maximum medical therapy as well as functional endoscopic frontal sinus procedures and/or external frontal sinus drainage
- Patients with mucoceles or benign tumors (osteomas, inverted papillomas, ossifying fibromas, etc.) or carefully selected malignant frontal sinus tumors
- Patients with idiopathic, post-traumatic, or postsurgical cerebrospinal fluid (CSF) leak from the posterior frontal plate
- Patients undergoing transcribriform or transfrontal approaches for anterior skull base tumors accessible endonasally (olfactory neuroblastomas, adenocarcinomas, meningiomas)
- Primarily in patients with chronic rhinosinusitis (CRS) and severely impaired mucociliary clearance:
  - Samter's triad
  - Severe polyposis
  - Severe scarring of frontal recess
  - Cystic fibrosis
  - Immunodeficiency

8.1.1 Relative Contraindications

- Less than 1 cm anteroposterior distance between the anterior nasal beak and skull base
- Hypoplastic or aplastic frontal sinus
- Frontal sinus tumors involving the anterior frontal plate or very lateral tumors especially involving the lateral orbital roof

(*specifically tumors or lesions that include and obliterate the frontal recess may be approached in a more oncological way by directly entering the frontal sinus while bypassing the frontal recess—i.e., outside-in/medial-to-lateral approach*).

8.2 Surgical Steps

The surgery is performed under general anesthesia (preferably total intravenous anesthesia [TIVA], with reduced heart rate and controlled hypotension). We use the 30-degree endoscope from the start to the end of the procedure (only rarely using the lateral view of a 70-degree endoscope for extreme lateral lesions). However, some colleagues prefer 0-degree endoscope for the early parts of the procedure with the option of using a 45-degree endoscope for the more advanced steps. We use image-guided navigation in almost all cases.

8.3 Lateral-to-Medial/Inside-Out Technique[8]

Anatomical landmarks:
- Axilla of middle turbinate
- Agger nasi and frontal (anterior and posterior) cells
- Anterior ethmoid artery
- Bulla ethmoidalis
- Subcutaneous tissue over the nasion and nasal beak
- Lamina papyracea
- Posterior frontal plate

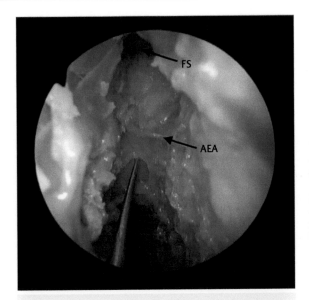

Fig. 8.1 Complete anterior and posterior ethmoidectomy (left nasal cavity). AEA, anterior ethmoid artery; FS, frontal sinus.

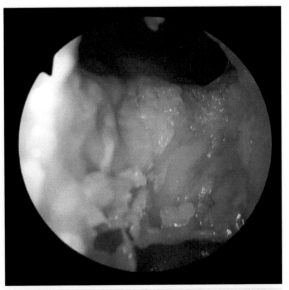

Fig. 8.2 Completed frontal sinusotomy (Draf IIa, left side).

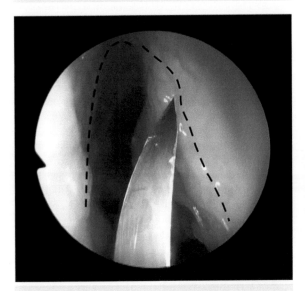

Fig. 8.3 Anterior incisions of laterally based flap.

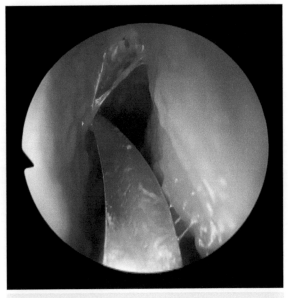

Fig. 8.4 Medially based middle turbinate flap.

Step 1: Bilateral Draf IIa: Although it is debatable, in cases of chronic rhinosinusitis with or without nasal polyps, we usually perform a complete anterior and posterior ethmoidectomy, including all frontoethmoidal cells, as their remnants can compromise the operation's success, both by limiting frontal sinus outflow pathway as well as by acting as a nidus of persisting inflammation (▶ Fig. 8.1). The most anterior aspect of the axilla of the middle turbinate is removed bilaterally, up to the level of the posterior frontal plate bilaterally (▶ Fig. 8.2).

Step 2: Harvesting of flaps: Before removing the middle turbinate axilla, harvest laterally based flaps, as described in the relevant chapter (Section 35.1 The Use of Flaps in Frontal Sinus Surgery), starting just anteriorly to the axilla of the middle turbinate, and proceeding antero-superiorly before reaching the roof of the nose and crossing over the nasal septum (▶ Fig. 8.3). Alternatively, a flap based on the middle turbinate and septal branch of the anterior ethomoid artery can be used (▶ Fig. 8.4).

Step 3: Partial anterior septectomy: Using a number 15 blade or a monopolar cutting needle diathermy, an incision through the anterosuperior septum is performed. This originates just anteriorly to the posterior frontal plate at the level of the frontal ostium and extends

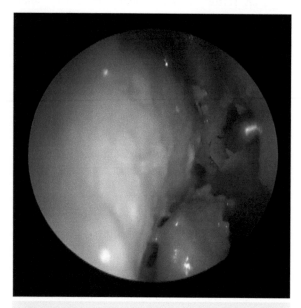

Fig. 8.5 Anterior septectomy.

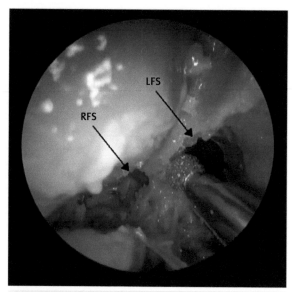

Fig. 8.6 Frontal sinus ostia visualized bilaterally. LFS, left frontal sinus ostium; RFS, right frontal sinus ostium.

vertically 2 cm at the same coronal plane, before turning 90 degrees anteriorly and then superiorly until it reaches the roof of the nasal cavity. The mucosa of the septum can incorporated into the lateral pedicled flap described above, or harvested for use as a free graft subsequently or be removed with a shaver and the underlying cartilage with a cutting Blakesley and/or scissors. The posterior limit of this opening is the first olfactory fiber/anterior skull base on each side and the opening itself should be wide enough for visualization of both frontal ostia up to the stump of the contralateral middle turbinate (▶ Fig. 8.5).

Step 4: The axilla of the middle turbinate and the mucosa and soft tissue between two frontal ostia are then removed exposing the bone of the nasal beak (▶ Fig. 8.6).

Step 5: The bone of the nasal beak is drilled in antero-medial direction, keeping in mind that the skull base extends anteriorly in the midline. Bone drilling is done caudally to cephalically and in a smooth fashion, so as to create a wide, saucerized cavity, with no sharp edges and continuous visibility into the frontal sinus. Subsequently the intersinus septum is drilled and lowered. During this stage it is important to remove any intersinus and high anterior or superior frontal (Kuhn type 4) cells as their remnants may lead to frontal sinus stenosis[9] (▶ Fig. 8.7).

Drilling continues anteriorly until all nasal beak is removed up to periosteum and skin, both anteriorly and anterolaterally. Drilling of anterior border is continued until the drill could be felt under the skin of the nasal bridge, aiming for a largest cavity possible (▶ Fig. 8.8). At the end of the procedure the anterior frontal wall should be easily visualized with a 0-degree endoscope with no ledges (▶ Fig. 8.9).

Lateral borders (▶ Table 8.1) of the final common outflow pathway should be the lacrimal bones and the periosteum under the skin laterally—anteriorly, the periosteum of the frontal beak and posteriorly, the anterior skull base (specifically, the most anterior olfactory fibers posteriorly—not to be confused with the septal branch of the anterior ethmoid artery or the anterior ethmoid nerve, which often penetrate together; ▶ Fig. 8.10, ▶ Fig. 8.11, and ▶ Fig. 8.12).

In our current practice we routinely use flaps—mostly laterally based flaps but also middle turbinate flaps and sometimes free mucosal grafts—to cover the exposed bone. (For more details, see the relevant chapter—Section 35.1, Use of Flaps in Frontal Sinus Surgery). We do not normally use dressings or drains but we leave a thin (0.25 mm) rolled silastic sheet, which is removed after 2 to 3 weeks, to keep the flap in place (▶ Fig. 8.13).

8.4 Outside-In/Medial-to-Lateral Technique

Although the planned final outcome of the neo-ostium is the same, the corridor used to approach the floor of the frontal sinus is different. The inside-out/lateral-to-medial approach uses the transethmoidal corridor to the natural frontal drainage pathway, whiel the medial-to-lateral/outside-in approach uses the transnasal corridor to drill through the frontal sinus floor before combining laterally with the natural drainage pathway. This corridor can be beneficial when there is considerable scarring in the frontal recess or lateral wall dehiscence from previous surgery, there is a tumor occupying or involving the frontal recess/sinus, or there is a very vascular and inflamed pathology in the frontal recess.[10]

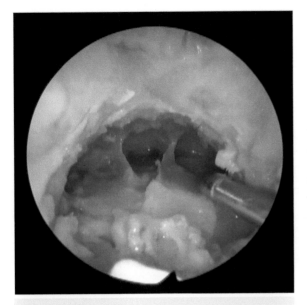

Fig. 8.7 Complete drillout of nasal beak and removal of all frontal sinus cells.

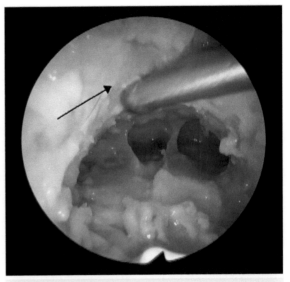

Fig. 8.8 Drillout continues until reaching subcutaneous tissue anterolaterally (black arrow).

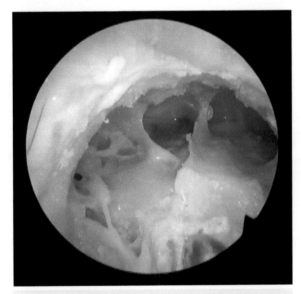

Fig. 8.9 Complete visualization of anterior frontal sinus wall with a 0-degree endoscope.

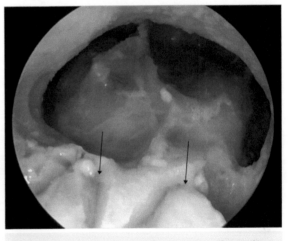

Fig. 8.10 Drillout of posterior wall until the first olfactory fibers (black arrows).

Anatomical landmarks and sequence:
- Axilla of middle turbinate
- First penetrations of skull base—first olfactory fila/septal branch of anterior ethmoid artery
- Posterior frontal plate
- Anterior frontal plate/periosteum
- Lamina papyracea
- Bulla ethmoidalis and anterior ethmoidal artery

Table 8.1 Landmarks for the borders of Draf III neo-ostium

Landmarks for Draf III	
Lateral	Orbital plates of the frontal bone and periosteum of the skin over frontal process of the maxilla
Posteriorly	First olfactory fiber (shows the forward projection of the olfactory bulb)
Anteriorly	Plane of anterior table of frontal sinus and periosteum over frontal process of maxilla

Note: The anterior ethmoid nerve and the septal branch of the anterior ethmoid artery should not be mistaken for the olfactory fascicles!

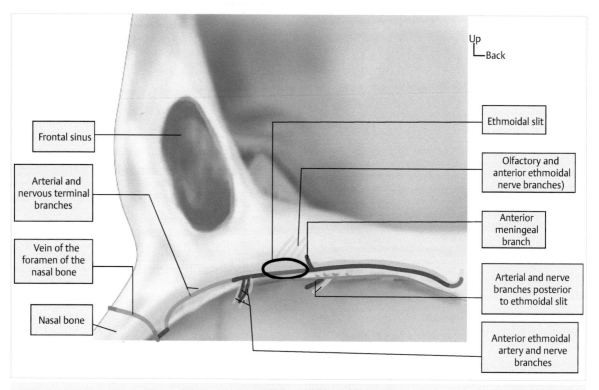

Fig. 8.11 Branches of the anterior ethmoidal nerve and artery with regard to the frontal sinus.

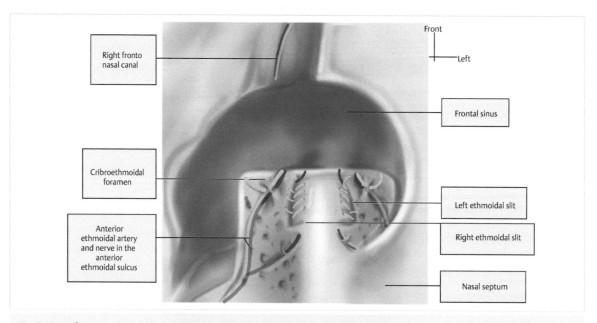

Fig. 8.12 Draf III procedure with regard to the ethmoidal slit and cribroethmoidal foramen.

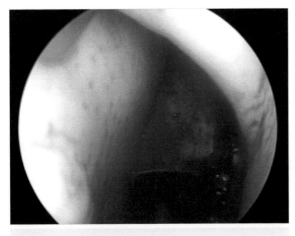

Fig. 8.13 Placement of silastic sheet.

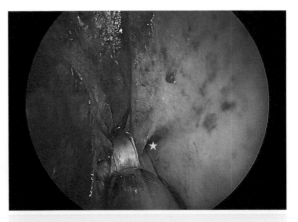

Fig. 8.14 Right nasal cavity, intraoperative endoscopic view showing the nervous and arterial branches defining the posterior limits of Draf III: yellow star (Medially) showing the ethmoidal cleft with olfactory filia passing through and blue oval, showing the cribroethmoidal foramen with external and posterior nasal branches of the anterior ethmoidal artery and nerve.

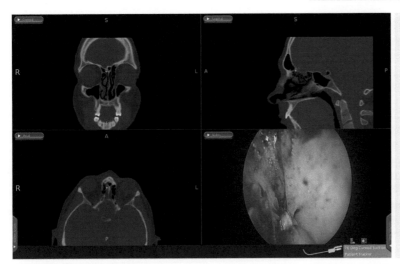

Fig. 8.15 Computed tomography (CT) correlations of first olfactory filia as seen in neuroguidance system (navigation).

Step 1: Harvesting mucosal flaps: As per the inside-out/lateral-to-medial approach, it is valuable to raise and harvest the mucosal flaps early in the procedure to avoid damaging the precious mucosa and exposing the bone that needs to be drilled to achieve the final neo-ostium. As previously described, there is an opportunity to raise the laterally pedicled mucosal flap based on the inferior maxillary process encompassing the lateral wall, roof of the nasal cavity, and septal window mucosa. This flap is often tucked away into the maxillary sinus for protection from instruments and the drill. The mucosa on the medial wall of the middle turbinate and the roof of the nasal cavity can be raised as a posteriorly based mucosal flap fed by the septal branch of the anterior ethmoid artery. This flap remains protected by tucking posteriorly between the middle turbinate and septum. This process is undertaken bilaterally.

Step 2: Identifying the first penetration of the anterior skull base: The posteriorly based mucosal flap is raised over the roof of the nasal cavity till the anterior-most structures entering the nasal cavity through the anterior-most aspect of the crista gali are identified—first olfactory filia, septal branch of anterior ethmoid artery, and the accompanying anterior ethmoid nerve (▶ Fig. 8.14 and ▶ Fig. 8.15). Usually there are three distinct penetrations identifiable. Once these are identified, they define the posterior limit of the drilling and the coronal plane of the posterior wall of the frontal sinus.

Step 3: Septal window: If bilateral lateral flaps have been raised together with the posterior flap, the area of the septal window is denuded of mucosa on both surfaces. A 2-cm window is created in the septum using the coronal plane of the first penetrations as the posterior limit. The endoscopic view should now be able to see both first penetrations of the skull base posteriorly and axilla of the middle turbinate from the contralateral side. It is important to ensure you make an adequate window to allow bilateral instrumentation and reduce the possibility of postoperative stenosis.

It is also often convenient to enter the frontal recess at this point. Although no dissection has been undertaken in the ethmoid complex, penetrating and removing the middle turbinate caudal to the first penetrations lateral will allow access to the frontal recess and anterior or posterior frontal cells.

Step 4: Drilling floor of the frontal sinus: Unlike the traditional approach, medial-to-lateral/outside-in approach enters the frontal sinus floor before reaching the frontal ostium/drainage pathway laterally into the ethmoid complex. By keeping the first skull base penetrations in site, any drilling caudal to this landmark is safe. As there is greater room for instrumentation than with the lateral-to-medial approach, the frontal floor can be drilled away quickly. Saucerization is much safer than tunnelling with your drilling technique, keeping the first skull base penetrations in site at all times, drilling in to out and wide, always moving the drill away from the danger area of the critical landmark.

Once the floor of the frontal sinus has been penetrated from below, the landmark of the posterior plate is identified and the thick frontal beak drilled away to reveal the anterior plate of the frontal sinus.

Step 5: Joining up with the natural ostium: Once the floor of the frontal sinus has been drilled away with anterior wall, posterior wall, and skull base in vision, it is relatively easy to enter the ethmoid complex to join this neo-ostium with the natural drainage pathway. It is the authors' preference to dissect from above down—frontal sinus–frontal recess–anterior ethmoid cells–maxillary ostium. The reasoning being the dissection plane is always moving away from the danger areas with the skull base and ethmoid roof always in vision.

It is paramount that the dissection around the drainage pathway is undertaken with care to preserve the mucosa in this area and the natural mucocilary drainage pathway for the frontal sinuses.

Step 6: Maximize the neo-ostium: As per any Draf III procedure, it is important to maximize the new opening to ensure all bones are drilled away between the periosteum of the nasion and the frontal projection of the skull in the sagittal plane and the lacrimal bone to lacrimal bone on opposite side in the coronal plane. It is important to cover all/as much of the drilled exposed bone as possible with the mucosal flaps raised in the start of the procedure to minimize postoperative stenosis and optimize healing.

8.5 Tips and Tricks

- One should keep in mind that a degree of stenosis is inevitable. Hence, aim to create the absolute maximum ostium possible, including laterally all of the nasal beak (up to the skin) as well as the posterior plate up to the first olfactory fibers.
- In cases of an acutely inflamed sinus think of postponing surgery (if at all possible) until the acute inflammation has subsided.

8.6 Case Examples

8.6.1 A Case of Allergic Fungal Rhinosinusitis with Fronto-orbital Mucocele

A 17-year-old young woman presents with proptosis and an episode of periorbital cellulitis. She has been complaining of nasal obstruction, anosmia, and thick nasal secretions affecting her quality of sleep and associated tiredness. She suffers from asthma and is hypersensitive to aspirin. Total IgE is 1000 and on skin prick tests (SPT) she shows reactivity to house dust mite, cat, and dog. Sinonasal outcome test (SNOT 22) is 20. On examination there is evidence of grade 4 polyps (more on the right than the left) while imaging, including computed tomography (CT) and magnetic resonance imaging (MRI), of sinus showed complete opacification of the right

Point of difficulty	Technical solution
Obstruction of view by blood and dust on the endoscope	Use of rinsing sheath or rinsing of the nose with warm water and using three-hand technique with suction
"Sword-fighting" between endoscope and curved instruments in the frontal sinus	Alternate nostrils and try different combinations of endoscope/instrument and nostril (either in the same or different nostrils) Ensure an adequate septal window
Difficulty in visualizing the most lateral or anterior parts of frontal sinus	Maximize bone removal proximally and try to use more angled endoscope
Inability to reach lateral roof of orbit	Try to mobilize the orbit ("orbital transposition" technique)
Extensive osteitis and/or very thick nasal beak	Use faster curved (30000 rpm) or skull base (60,000) drills
High risk of stenosis	Use flaps and/or grafts to cover all exposed bone

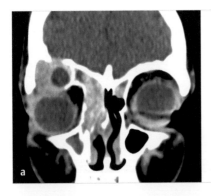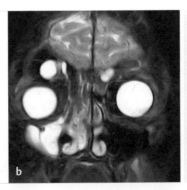

Fig. 8.16 (a, b) Coronal computed tomography (CT) and coronal T2 magnetic resonance imaging (MRI). Note the complete opacification of the right anterior ethmoids and right frontal sinus and the presence of a mucocele, eroding the orbital roof laterally and displacing the orbit inferiorly.

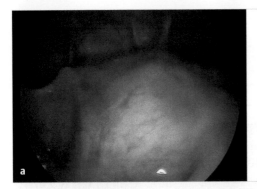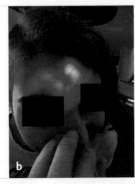

Fig. 8.17 (a, b) Endoscopic view of the Draf III open cavity, 6 months after surgery, and transillumination of the frontal sinus in the outpatient department (OPD).

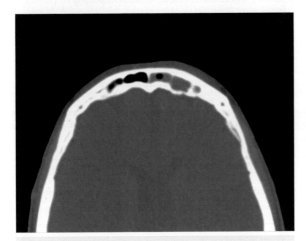

Fig. 8.18 Left frontal sinus obstructed by Kuhn type 3 cell.

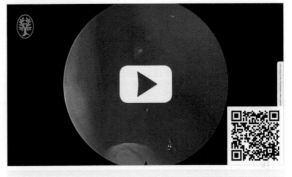

Video 8.1 Lateral fronto-orbital mucocele Draf III approach (Case 8.6.1)

ethmoids, frontal sinus, and sphenoid with a secondary supraorbital mucocele pushing the orbit inferomedially (▶ Fig. 8.16a, b).

Diagnosis was made of allergic fungal rhinosinusitis. Following a short course of steroids, a Draf III procedure was undertaken. Nasal douching with topical steroids as well as a short course of oral steroid was prescribed post-operatively (Video 8.1).

Following surgery, the patient's nasal symptoms improved significantly while her proptosis resolved. On examination, there was no evidence of pus or polyps and the frontal sinus neo-ostium was patent (▶ Fig. 8.17a, b; Video 8.2).

8.6.2 A Case of Chronic Frontal Sinusitis with a High Posterior Frontal (Type 3) Cell

A 60-year-old female presented with frontal headache associated with mucopurulent discharge of 3 months duration. She had undergone two endoscopic sinus procedures, one middle meatal antrostomy and a Draf IIa elsewhere, as well as multiple courses of oral steroids and targeted antibiotics, with no improvement of her symptoms. She has no allergies and does not have asthma. Her CT of sinus showed an incomplete ethmoidectomy with a high posterior (Kuhn type 3) cell obstructing the left frontal sinus which is opacified (▶ Fig. 8.18). A Draf III was performed with the use of a laterally based flap (Video 8.3).

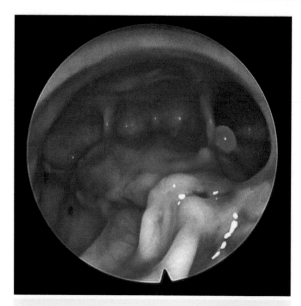

Fig. 8.19 Intraoperative endoscopic view of ▸ Fig. 8.18.

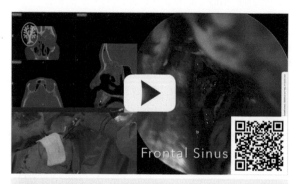

Video 8.3 Live surgery – Inside out Draf III with laterally based flap (Case 8.6.2)

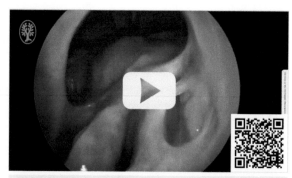

Video 8.2 Outpatient endoscopic view after Draf III for fronto-orbital mucocele (Case 8.6.1)

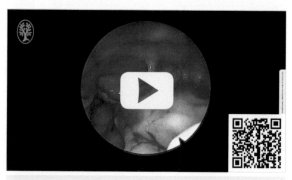

Video 8.4 Outpatient endoscopic view after Draf III for recurrent frontal sinusitis (Case 8.6.2)

Following surgery her symptoms resolved completely. Her endoscopic appearance is shown in ▸ Fig. 8.19 and Video 8.4.

8.6.3 A Case of Chronic Frontal Sinusitis—Riedel's Procedure Reversal

A 58-year-old male was presented with a few months history of severe nasal obstruction, headaches, mucopurulent nasal discharge, and hyposmia, symptoms matching acute rhinosinusitis. On examination, he had evidence of excessive frontal bone defect. He mentioned he had undergone multiple undefined endoscopic operations in the past and an open procedure 2 years ago. CT scan revealed that despite the fact the patient had undergone a Riedel's procedure, frontal sinuses were opacified and their drainage path was blocked by remaining high ethmoid cells. The symptoms of the patient were refractory to medical treatment so a decision was taken for surgical management, i.e., Draf III procedure. Three days postoperatively, the

patient's symptoms had improved significantly and he was discharged from hospital. Aesthetic correction of the forehead contour with autogenous materials was scheduled for 6 months later, once the original infectious process was fully eradicated (▸ Fig. 8.20).

8.7 Postoperative Management

The patient is discharged the day after the surgery. In case of pus in the frontal sinus, culture-guided antibiotics are prescribed, while in cases of chronic rhinosinusitis with nasal polyps (CRSwNP) a course of systemic steroids is given. The patient is advised to start nasal rinsing from the first postoperative day and instructed to gradually increase the frequency of nasal douching up to eight times a day. Topical nasal steroids (budesonide or fluticasone nasal drops) are added in nasal douching twice daily. The first follow-up visit is approximately 2 weeks after the surgery, when the rolled silastic sheet is removed and the neo-ostium is gently debrided. Subsequent visits depend on pathology and the healing process but usually include a visit at 6 weeks and 3 months postsurgery for gentle endoscopic debridement and removal of clots and crusts until healing is complete, which, depending on the amount of bare bone, can be anywhere between 2 and 3 months or even longer.

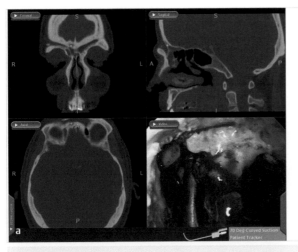
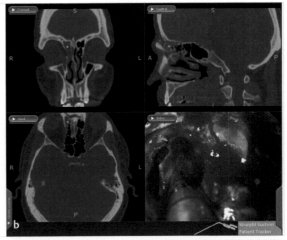

Fig. 8.20 (a, b) Removal of remaining ethmoid cells obstructing frontal sinuses' drainage path. Note the results of previous Riedel's procedure.

It has been shown that during the first year after Draf III, neo-ostium tends to narrow by 33%.[11] Patients with asthma, allergy, cystic fibrosis, Samter's triad,[6] previous frontal sinus surgery, osteitis,[12] allergic fungal sinusitis,[13] and eosinophilic mucin chronic rhinosinusitis[11] are at a higher risk of developing re-stenosis, although there are indications that free musosal grafts[14,15] (e.g., of the resected septum) or pedicled mucosal flaps[16] may improve healing and prevent postoperative stenosis. In cases when grafts or flaps are used it is recommended not to debride the nose for 2 to 3 weeks after the surgery as it takes some time for collagen fibers to fix the transplant.[15]

8.8 Complications and their Management

Specific complications of Draf III (in addition to general surgical complications such as deep vein thrombosis, postoperative atelectasis, and pneumonia) can be divided into intraoperative, and early and late postoperative (▶ Fig. 8.21). A diligent review of the preoperative CT scans and detection of certain anatomical variants (asymmetry of anterior skull base, anterior ethmoid artery hanging on "mesenterium," bony dehiscence, defects of lamina papyracea, etc.) and preoperative planning can help to avoid complications.

8.8.1 Skull Base Injury and Cerebrospinal Fluid Leak

The most serious complication of Draf III is CSF leak, which, if left unrecognized and untreated, can lead to meningitis, epidural or subdural abscess, or pneumocephalus. The most vulnerable area is the thin lateral lamella from the level of the first olfactory fibers to the anterior ethmoidal artery (during the first steps of the procedure). Additionally, the use of drill during the final parts of the procedure to lower the posterior frontal plate at the area of crista galli can also be associated with CSF leak. If unrecognized, theoretically the intracranial breach can lead to intracranial injury including cerebral vasculature or brain tissue. Although rare[6,12,17] (we have not yet had one during a Draf III procedure) compared to early series,[5] the operating surgeon must always keep in mind this potential complication and the ways of preventing and dealing with it.

The risk of creating a CSF leak is higher in patients who had multiple previous sinus surgeries and extensive osteitis as well as in those with low or asymmetric anterior skull base, a deep olfactory recess (Keros types 2 and 3), and laterally rather than vertically inclined lateral lamella.[18]

If recognized, repair is usually straightforward: Various repair techniques have been described, including grafts (fat, fascia, nasal mucosa), flaps (nasoseptal,[19,20] flip-flap[21]), bath-plug,[22,23] etc. Usually in cases of small CSF leaks, the use of small, free mucosal grafts, with or without underlay fascia lata, works very well.

8.8.2 Hemorrhage

Excessive bleeding may occur both in the intra- and postoperative periods. Intraoperative bleeding is usually more of a hindrance than any hemodynamic issue as it distorts the visual field making it difficult to recognize anatomical landmarks and thus may increase the risk of complications and extend the duration of the surgery. Causes of the bleeding may be surgery- or patient-related, although clinically significant bleeding is rarely seen after Draf III. Patient-related risk factors could be divided into local (e.g., inflammation, infection, osteitis, previous surgery) and systemic (e.g., hypertension, clotting factors and vitamin K deficiency,

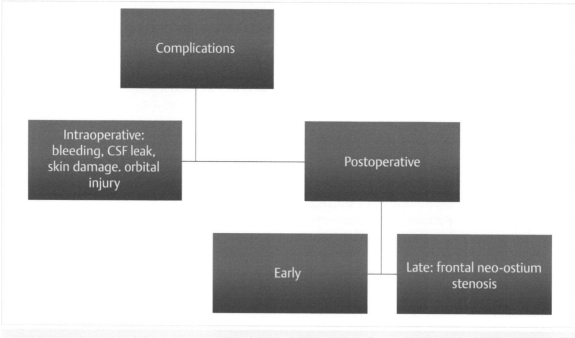

Fig. 8.21 Complications of Draf III.

platelet dysfunction, inherited blood vessel and collagen abnormalities, usage of aspirin, antiplatelet agents, etc.).

Measures taken in all surgeries to prevent excessive bleeding include anti-Trendelenburg positioning, application of topical and local vasoconstrictors, and controlled hypotension achieved through total intravenous anesthesia. If polyposis is present, preoperative systemic steroids help in reducing the size of polyps and degree of inflammation and thus reduce intraoperative bleeding.[24] Intraoperatively, bipolar coagulation and irrigation with warm saline can also help to reduce bleeding. Topical or systemic tranexamic acid can be beneficial.

8.8.3 Orbital Injury

The anterior ethmoid artery is well behind the field of the Draf III neo-ostium—usually one cell posterior to the posterior limit of the frontal recess. If the surgeon damages the anterior ethmoid artery and it is recognized immediately, then it may be coagulated with bipolar diathermy. However, it may evade recognition: In such cases the distal end of the artery may retract into the orbit and produce an intraorbital hematoma, manifesting as proptosis, eyelid edema and ecchymosis, subconjunctival hemorrhage, and mydriasis/reduced reactivity of the pupil. Tonometry, if available, will confirm increased intraocular pressure.

If the patient is awake, he or she may complain of orbital pain, diplopia, loss of color vision, or vision acuity up to blindness. Once intraorbital hematoma is suspected, ophthalmology consultation should be obtained and any nasal

packing must be immediately removed. If intraorbital pressure does not decrease after conservative measures, lateral canthotomy and inferior cantholysis must be immediately performed. Alternatively, endoscopic orbital decompression may be performed together with canthotomy—cantholysis: lamina papyracea is removed and periorbita is incised to release orbital fat.

8.8.4 Skin Injury

Damage of the skin of nasal bridge may occur during exposure of the most lateral aspects of neo-ostium. Damage may be mechanical or thermal. Skin may be perforated when a cutting burr is applied to a certain area for several seconds, so it is recommended to continuously move the burr throughout the procedure. Also, continuous irrigation is recommended to prevent thermal injury. However, the use of diamond drills makes such injuries extremely unlikely and at most the patient may complain of a mild edema of the bridge of the nose.

8.8.5 Stenosis of the Frontal Sinus Neo-ostium

Stenosis of the neo-ostium of frontal sinus is seen most often within the first 12 to 24 months,[12,16] that is why the follow-up is crucial during this period. Following first year after the surgery the ostium stabilizes and then increases marginally, which could be explained by further stabilization and thinning of the mucosa of the neo-ostium.[12] Major risk factors include: allergic fungal sinusitis, recalcitrant *S. aureus* infections, polyposis and cystic fibrosis, Samter's traid, asthma, and multiple environmental allergies.[6,12,16] However, a more recent study identified the presence of osteitis preoperatively as the single-most important factor in predicting neo-ostium stenosis.[11]

References

[1] Draf W. Endonasal micro-endoscopic frontal sinus surgery: the Fulda concept. Oper Tech Otolaryngol–Head Neck Surg. 1991; 2(4):234–240

[2] Gross WE, Gross CW, Becker D, Moore D, Phillips D. Modified transnasal endoscopic Lothrop procedure as an alternative to frontal sinus obliteration. Otolaryngol Head Neck Surg. 1995; 113(4):427–434

[3] Metson R, Gliklich RE. Clinical outcome of endoscopic surgery for frontal sinusitis. Arch Otolaryngol Head Neck Surg. 1998; 124 (10):1090–1096

[4] May M, Schaitkin B. Frontal sinus surgery: endonasal drainage instead of an external osteoplastic approach. Oper Tech Otolaryngol Head Neck Surg. 1995; 6(3):184–192

[5] Close LG, Lee NK, Leach JL, Manning SC. Endoscopic resection of the intranasal frontal sinus floor. Ann Otol Rhinol Laryngol. 1994; 103 (12):952–958

[6] Georgalas C, Hansen F, Videler WJM, Fokkens WJ. Long terms results of Draf type III (modified endoscopic Lothrop) frontal sinus drainage procedure in 122 patients: a single centre experience. Rhinology. 2011; 49(2):195–201

[7] Georgalas C, Detsis M, Geramas I, Terzakis D, Liodakis A. Quality of life outcomes in frontal sinus surgery. J Clin Med. 2020; 9(7):E2145

[8] Georgalas C, Fokkens WJ. Rhinology and Skull Base Surgery: From the Lab to the Operating Room—An Evidence-Based Approach. Thieme; 2013

[9] Casiano RR, Livingston JA. Endoscopic Lothrop procedure: the University of Miami experience. Am J Rhinol. 1998; 12(5):335–339

[10] Chin D, Snidvongs K, Kalish L, Sacks R, Harvey RJ. The outside-in approach to the modified endoscopic Lothrop procedure. Laryngoscope. 2012; 122(8):1661–1669

[11] Tran KN, Beule AG, Singal D, Wormald P-J. Frontal ostium restenosis after the endoscopic modified Lothrop procedure. Laryngoscope. 2007; 117(8):1457–1462

[12] Ye T, Hwang PH, Huang Z, et al. Frontal ostium neo-osteogenesis and patency after Draf III procedure: a computer-assisted study. Int Forum Allergy Rhinol. 2014; 4(9):739–744

[13] Naidoo Y, Bassiouni A, Keen M, Wormald PJ. Long-term outcomes for the endoscopic modified Lothrop/Draf III procedure: a 10-year review. Laryngoscope. 2014; 124(1):43–49

[14] Conger BT , Jr, Riley K, Woodworth BA. The Draf III mucosal grafting technique: a prospective study. Otolaryngol Head Neck Surg. 2012; 146(4):664–668

[15] Hildenbrand T, Wormald PJ, Weber RK. Endoscopic frontal sinus drainage Draf type III with mucosal transplants. Am J Rhinol Allergy. 2012; 26(2):148–151

[16] Seyedhadi S, Mojtaba MA, Shahin B, Hoseinali K. The Draf III septal flap technique: a preliminary report. Am J Otolaryngol. 2013; 34 (5):399–402

[17] Shirazi MA, Silver AL, Stankiewicz JA. Surgical outcomes following the endoscopic modified Lothrop procedure. Laryngoscope. 2007; 117(5):765–769

[18] Preti A, Mozzanica F, Gera R, et al. Horizontal lateral lamella as a risk factor for iatrogenic cerebrospinal fluid leak. Clinical retrospective evaluation of 24 cases. Rhinology. 2018; 56(4):358–363

[19] Zanation AM, Carrau RL, Snyderman CH, et al. Nasoseptal flap reconstruction of high flow intraoperative cerebral spinal fluid leaks during endoscopic skull base surgery. Am J Rhinol Allergy. 2009; 23 (5):518–521

[20] Kassam AB, Thomas A, Carrau RL, et al. Endoscopic reconstruction of the cranial base using a pedicled nasoseptal flap. Neurosurgery. 2008; 63(1) Suppl 1:ONS44–ONS52, discussion ONS52–ONS53

[21] Battaglia P, Turri-Zanoni M, De Bernardi F, et al. Septal flip flap for anterior skull base reconstruction after endoscopic resection of sinonasal cancers: preliminary outcomes. Acta Otorhinolaryngol Ital. 2016; 36(3):194–198

[22] Wormald PJ, McDonogh M. Bath-plug" technique for the endoscopic management of cerebrospinal fluid leaks. J Laryngol Otol. 1997; 111 (11):1042–1046

[23] Wormald PJ, McDonogh M. The bath-plug closure of anterior skull base cerebrospinal fluid leaks. Am J Rhinol. 2003; 17(5):299–305

[24] Pundir V, Pundir J, Lancaster G, et al. Role of corticosteroids in functional endoscopic sinus surgery—a systematic review and meta-analysis. Rhinology. 2016; 54(1):3–19

9 Transseptal Approach

Bobby A. Tajudeen and Pete S. Batra

Abstract

The transseptal frontal sinusotomy (TSFS) utilizes the unique relationship of the nasal septum to the medial frontal sinus floor and allows for entry into the midline frontal sinus floor where the bone is thinnest. This technique is especially advantageous in the cases of extensive neo-osteogenesis that preclude identification and cannulation of the frontal recess. Similar to the Draf III and the endoscopic modified Lothrop procedure, TSFS provides good access to the midline frontal sinus floor and permits but does not require intersinus septum removal. In addition, TSFS offers several theoretical advantages over frontal sinus obliteration including decreased morbidity, improved cosmesis, and ease of endoscopic and radiographic surveillance postoperatively. A concise review of the indications, procedural steps, and complications will be presented. An illustrative example with be shown and potential points of difficulty during the procedure will be addressed.

Keywords: transseptal frontal sinusotomy, frontal sinus surgery, Draf III, modified Lothrop, frontal sinusitis

9.1 Background and CT Review

Candidacy for transseptal frontal sinusotomy (TSFS) is based on careful consideration of all surgical options. Generally, patients with significant osteoneogenesis not amenable to standard endoscopic frontal techniques are considered candidates. Furthermore, TSFS may also be considered an adjunct approach in patients with benign or malignant neoplasms involving the frontal sinus or the anterior skull base. Consent is also obtained for adjunct open approaches (endoscopic frontal trephination, osteoplastic flap without obliteration) in the cases where strict endoscopic approaches may not achieve the desired surgical objective.

A detailed computed tomography (CT) review is performed prior to considering surgical intervention. Review of triplanar CT images on an image-guidance computer workstation facilitates understanding of the complex three-dimensional relationships of the frontal recess. Images are evaluated to determine the frontal sinus pneumatization pattern, including the nature of agger nasi pneumatization, presence of frontal cells, supraorbital ethmoid cells, supra- and frontal bullar cells, and/or intersinus septal cells, and frontal sinus mucocele formation. "Y-shaped" nasal septal attachment to the floor of the frontal sinus is assessed (▶ Fig. 9.1). Imaging is also reviewed for the relationship of the middle turbinate to the frontal sinus and the integrity of the skull base in the area of the proposed dissection. The width and depth of the frontal sinus floor are estimated in either direct coronal or reconstructed sagittal plane on CT images. An anteroposterior diameter of approximately 1.0 cm is considered an important requisite for safe endoscopic drilling; a diameter less than this is considered a relative contraindication and limitation to successfully performing the TSFS.

9.2 Indications and Contraindications

- Chronic frontal sinusitis after failed endoscopic sinus surgery, especially in the setting of "neo-osteogenesis" or middle turbinate resection.
- Frontal sinus mucocele formation.
- Inverted papilloma.
- Sinonasal or skull base malignancy.
- Fibro-osseous lesion.
- Trauma.

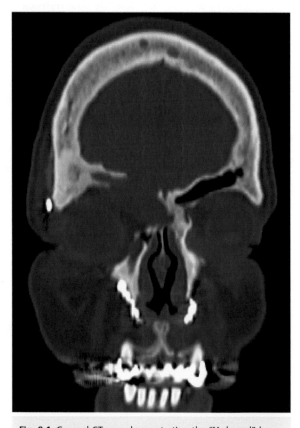

Fig. 9.1 Coronal CT scan demonstrating the "Y-shaped" bony attachment of the nasal septum to the floor of the frontal sinus. Note the presence of mucocele in the right frontal sinus and relationship to the frontal sinus floor.

Contraindications include the following:

- Lack of requisite expertise with extended endoscopic frontal sinus approaches.
- Unavailability of required specialized surgical instrumentation, including drills and image guidance.
- Frontal sinus floor with anteroposterior diameter less than 1.0 cm (relative).

9.3 Advantages

- Functional approach with restoration of frontal sinus drainage pathway.
- Permits mucosal preservation of the frontal recess.
- Utilizes inherent anatomic landmarks to facilitate surgery.
- Allows for endoscopic and radiographic surveillance postoperatively.
- Improved cosmesis through avoidance of facial incisions.
- Decreased morbidity compared to open frontal sinus approaches.
- May resort to open approaches if required.

9.4 Disadvantages

- Requirement of endoscopic expertise and specialized surgical instrumentation.
- Risk of inadvertent cerebrospinal fluid (CSF) leak and skull base injury greater than with routine frontal sinus surgery.
- Possible bone loss at radix.
- Drill-related trauma to adjacent sinonasal tissues.
- Controlled septal perforation with potential for chronic crusting.

9.5 Surgical Steps

- All surgery is performed under general anesthesia. The patient is positioned, prepped, and draped as for routine endoscopic sinus surgery.
- Although this technique was first applied without a computer-aided surgery, it is now typically performed using image guidance. This helps confirm critical anatomic landmarks throughout a technically challenging procedure.
- At the outset of the procedure, image guidance is properly registered and verified. Oxymetazoline is instilled in each nasal cavity. Injections with 1% lidocaine with 1:200,000 epinephrine are performed bilaterally on the septum, lateral nasal wall (agger nasi region), and middle turbinate remnant. Alternately, 1:1,000 topical epinephrine may be applied to these areas to achieve appropriate vasoconstriction.
- Because most of these patients have undergone previous endoscopic sinus surgery, the adjacent paranasal sinus disease, if present, is addressed first since

superiorly created bleeding with TSFS can result in difficulty in performing the remainder procedures.

- A 1.5- to 2-cm iatrogenic septal perforation is created just across from the leading edge of the middle turbinate/agger nasi region below the skull base. This permits further exposure, ventilation, future endoscopic inspection, and sinus debridement through the nasal cavity. The incisions for the perforation are created utilizing an ophthalmic crescent knife. Thru-cutting endoscopic forceps or soft-tissue shaver is helpful in completing the controlled perforation. Exposed areas of bone or cartilage are minimized throughout the procedure.
- The floor of the frontal sinus is identified by intraoperative surgical navigation or, alternately, by using surgical landmarks that are helpful in gauging the position of the frontal sinus relative to the cribriform plate. The midline position of the floor of the frontal sinus is typically localized posterosuperior to the most anterosuperior aspects of the septal bony–cartilaginous junction. This location is approximated adjacent to the most anterior remnant or root of the middle turbinate and the agger nasi (ascending process of the maxilla). This is considerably more anterior than the position of the naturally occurring frontal recess. In patients with a Y-shaped septum at the floor of the frontal sinus, the midline floor of the frontal sinus has an appearance similar to that of the anterior wall of the sphenoid sinus that has been described during trans-septal sphenoid surgery. It appears as the "prow of a ship," albeit in a much narrower region (▶ Fig. 9.1).
- After careful inspection of the roof of the nasal vault, the frontal sinus is entered. The evolution of surgical instrumentation has permitted the use of angled drills with concurrent suction/irrigation (▶ Fig. 9.2). Larger burs can give a critical advantage while drilling around corners anteriorly but may also pose a hazard by permitting inadvertent drilling of the posterior table of the

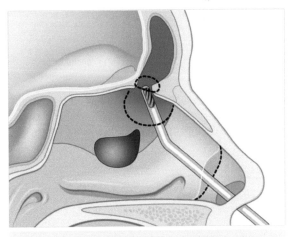

Fig. 9.2 Sagittal illustration demonstrates drilling of the frontal sinus floor through a superiorly created septal window.

frontal sinus. Concurrent saline irrigation is essential to avoiding inadvertent heat injury to bone and surrounding tissue. If straight drills are used without concurrent suction irrigation, irrigation can be applied through a 5-Fr ureteral catheter with the help of an assistant and are positioned through the contralateral nares into the operative field. Alternatively, depending upon the thickness of the floor of the sinus, curetting may be sufficient to enter the frontal sinus (▶ Fig. 9.3a).

- After successful entry into the lumen of the frontal sinus, the opening can be enlarged further by drilling anteriorly and laterally. Depending on the extent of the disease, dissection can be carried laterally to include the frontal recess. Note that the frontal recess is located posteriorly and drilling directly across from one frontal recess to the other should not be performed. This straight path of drilling will traverse the olfactory fossa and anterior cranial vault and place the patient at risk for CSF leak or even intracranial injury. All efforts are made to preserve the mucosa throughout the procedure, especially in the frontal recess. By reducing mucosal injury, bone exposure is minimized and risk of delayed stenosis is reduced. When drilling anteriorly, care must be taken to preserve the integrity of the radix. The inferior aspect of the intersinus septum may be resected in order to provide a common outlet for both right and left frontal sinuses at the midline. In this fashion, a "neo-ostium" is created as illustrated in ▶ Fig. 9.3b.

9.6 Tips and Tricks

9.6.1 Case Example

A 50-year-old man with history of facial trauma and frontal sinus obliteration presented with persistent frontal headache and right eye swelling. On imaging, a large frontal mucocele with hyperdense foreign bodies was noted (▶ Fig. 9.4). Marked neo-osteogenesis of the frontal recess bilaterally precluded standard entry into the frontal sinus through the frontal recess and thus a TSFS approach was utilized to enter the frontal sinus in the midline. The mucocele was successfully evacuated and retained metallic screws were removed (Video 9.1). The patient had resolution of his headache and eye swelling. Postoperative endoscopy revealed a well-healed frontal neo-ostium at 2 years (▶ Fig. 9.5).

9.7 Complications

McLaughlin et al presented the initial results of TSFS.[1] Twenty patients were included with mean follow-up of 16 months. The primary indication of surgery was frontal recess stenosis after a previously failed endoscopic frontal sinusotomy. Endoscopic patency was reported in all 20 patients, with a diameter of 3 mm confirmed by passage of a curved suction in 19/20 (95%) patients. Of the patients evaluated by telephone questionnaire, 17/19 patients (89.5%) reported symptom improvement and 12/18 patients (67%) reported reduction in medication requirements.

Lanza et al reported a follow-up study on 29 patients undergoing TSFS between 1995 and 1999.[2] The main indication for TSFS was chronic frontal sinusitis in the setting of a previously failed endoscopic surgery; other indications included mucocele formation and nasofacial trauma. Twenty-four patients (83%) were available for telephone interview postoperatively with a mean follow-up period of 45 months (range 9–69 months). In this subset of patients, 18 of 24 (75%) reported at least 50% improvement of symptoms, while 14 of 24 (58%) reported ≥ 80%

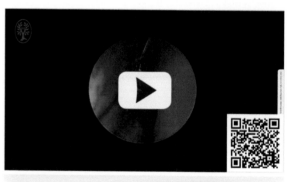

Video 9.1 Transeptal frontal sinus approach for frontal sinus mucocele with osteogenesis (Case 9.6.1)

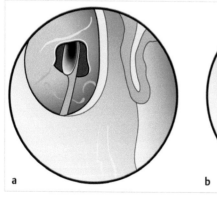
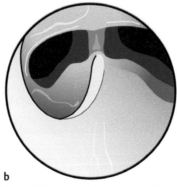

Fig. 9.3 (a) Entry into the frontal sinus utilizing a frontal sinus curette. (b) "Neo-ostium" created via transseptal frontal sinusotomy.

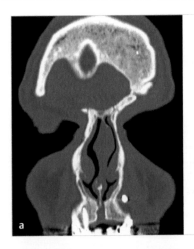
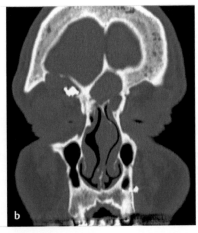

Fig. 9.4 (a) Coronal CT scan demonstrating a frontal mucocele. (b) A hyperdense foreign body is visualized in the mucocele cavity (*right panel*).

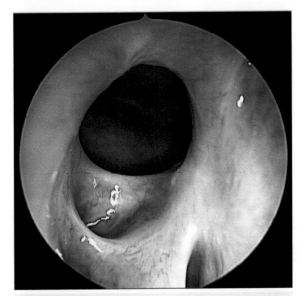

Fig. 9.5 Endoscopic appearance of healed "neo-ostium."

Table 9.1 Potential points of difficulty and proposed solutions while performing the transseptal frontal sinusotomy

Point of difficulty	Technical solution
Difficulty accessing and visualizing frontal sinus floor	1. Use of a shoulder roll to extend neck. This creates extra space between the nose and chest to manipulate instruments and endoscopes. 2. Boundaries of the septal window will govern access. Enlarge the window sufficiently to permit visibility and access for the drill. 3. Septal translocation can aid in widening the working corridor.
Hemostasis	1. Topical 1:1,000 epinephrine can provide additional hemostasis. 2. Warm saline irrigation will aid with bleeding mucosal edges.
Patency of the neo-ostium	1. Reduce mucosal injury and exposed bone. 2. All inflammatory diseases should be removed from the frontal sinus. 3. Meticulous postoperative care and close follow-up. 4. Prolonged frontal stenting may aid in maintaining patency.

improvement of their symptoms. Four (16.6%) patients underwent further frontal sinus surgery with three having frontal sinus obliteration. Complications included CSF leaks (two cases), unplanned anterior inferior septal perforation (one case), and chronic crusting at the planned perforation (one case). One leak was attributable to surgical trauma from the drill in a patient with narrow anteroposterior dimensions, and the second occurred during debridement of scarred mucosa within the frontal sinus in a patient with history of severe maxillofacial trauma. Both CSF leaks were identified and repaired intra-operatively without further sequelae. Both patients with septal issues had undergone prior septoplasty. A recent study by Nishiike et al reported on 16 patients undergoing TSFS with mean follow-up of 16 months.[3] In their study, a patent neo-ostium was reported in all cases without intracranial or orbital complications. ▶ Table 9.1 outlines potential points of difficult and surgical solutions for TSFS.

References

[1] McLaughlin RB, Hwang PH, Lanza DC. Endoscopic trans-septal frontal sinusotomy: the rationale and results of an alternative technique. Am J Rhinol. 1999; 13(4):279–287

[2] Lanza DC, McLaughlin RB, Jr, Hwang PH. The five year experience with endoscopic trans-septal frontal sinusotomy. Otolaryngol Clin North Am. 2001; 34(1):139–152

[3] Nishiike S, Yoda S, Shikina T, Murata J. Endoscopic transseptal approach to frontal sinus disease. Indian J Otolaryngol Head Neck Surg. 2015; 67(3):287–291

Suggested Readings

Batra PS, Cannady SB, Lanza DC. Surgical outcomes of drillout procedures for complex frontal sinus pathology. Laryngoscope. 2007; 117(5):927–931

Lanza DC, McLaughlin RB, Jr, Hwang PH. The five year experience with endoscopic trans-septal frontal sinusotomy. Otolaryngol Clin North Am. 2001; 34(1):139–152

McLaughlin RB, Hwang PH, Lanza DC. Endoscopic trans-septal frontal sinusotomy: the rationale and results of an alternative technique. Am J Rhinol. 1999; 13(4):279–287

Wormald PJ. Salvage frontal sinus surgery: the endoscopic modified Lothrop procedure. Laryngoscope. 2003; 113(2):276–283

10 Endoscopic Endonasal Orbital Transposition for Lateral Frontal Sinus Lesions

Paolo Castelnuovo, Mario Turri-Zanoni, Enrico Fazio, Paolo Battaglia, and Apostolos Karligkiotis

Abstract

In the era of endonasal endoscopy, the frontal sinus disease management still remains the most difficult challenge for rhinologists. Despite the great strides made in surgical techniques and technology in recent years, some cases require the use of external approaches. Recently, the growing experience in endoscopic sinus surgery along with significant technological advances have allowed the expansion of indications for selected lesions located more and more laterally in the frontal sinus as inverted papilloma, fibro-osseous lesions, and mucoceles. In selected cases, a complete radical surgery can be obtained by conservative approaches using the so-called endoscopic endonasal orbital transposition. Keep in mind that this type of approach should not be understood as totally substitute, but rather as an additional solution to the traditional approaches in order to ensure optimal treatment in different situations. This chapter explains the indications and contraindications to this type of approach, the surgical steps, and some tips and tricks to avoid intraoperative complications.

Keywords: frontal sinus, far lateral, orbital transposition, Draf IIb/III, inverted papilloma, mucoceles, osteomas

10.1 Indications

Nowadays, the endoscopic endonasal technique represents a valid alternative to the traditional external approaches in the treatment of several frontal sinus lesions, localized medially to a virtual sagittal plane that passes through the lamina papyracea. Draf et al described a well-known classification system for endoscopic approaches to the frontal sinus known as the Draf type I, II (IIa and IIb), and III procedures, which are commonly used to expose the frontal sinus. However, adequate visualization with proper management of disease when approaching the lateral aspect of the frontal sinus may not always be feasible and remains one of the most difficult endoscopic sinonasal procedures and a great challenge for modern rhinologists. Thus, in some conditions involving the frontal sinus, such as mucoceles and tumors, an external osteoplastic approach with or without frontal sinus obliteration or a frontal sinus trephination is still necessary. Recently, the introduction of the so-called endoscopic endonasal orbital transposition allowed expansion of the indications of the techniques described by Draf et al for selected lesions localized more laterally into the frontal sinus. The lesions amenable to this technique are laterally based frontal sinus mucoceles as well as benign tumors such as inverted papillomas and fibro-osseous lesions (osteomas, fibrous dysplasia, and ossifying fibromas) involving the supraorbital recess and the lateral frontal sinus.

Accessing the lateral portion of the frontal sinus through an exclusive transnasal approach can be very challenging because of some critical aspects that should be carefully considered. One of the most important factors is the anatomy of the frontal sinus. In case of a very pneumatized frontal sinus, it may not be possible to reach lesions localized in the superior portion or in the far lateral aspect of the sinus. Another limit to access the frontal sinus laterally is the convexity of the orbital roof. The anteroposterior diameter of the frontal recess must be adequate (minimum distance should be 1 cm) to allow the passage of the surgical instruments. The interorbital distance is another fundamental aspect because the access to the frontal sinus is restricted laterally by the orbital walls. The relatively large distance allows adequate access to the surgical instruments, whereas the opposite is true for a narrow nasal inlet.

Other factors to consider are related to the lesion to be treated; the key points are the consistence (based on biology), the medial extension of the lesion, and the site of the lesion's attachment. In the case of osteomas and inverted papillomas, what really matters is the site of attachment of the lesion; those that extend laterally but with a more medial attachment can be removed with curved drills and instruments. The more laterally the attachment of the lesion is located, the more difficult will be its complete removal. A mucocele that extends laterally in the far lateral portion of the frontal sinus but reaches medially to the lamina papyracea can be easily marsupialized through the frontal recess; its lateral extension is not a difficult issue to manage because, when the medial wall of the mucocele is perforated, all the contents of the mucocele are drained. When a lateral or supraorbital mucocele extends medially as far as the sagittal plane that passes through the mid-orbit, or even more laterally, the difficulty to reach this area is higher, although feasible in some cases, with double-curved instruments. However, multiple mucoceles of the lateral aspect of the frontal sinus that are separated one from the other by bony septations (multilobulated mucoceles) are challenging to be treated through the transnasal corridor. In these cases, perforating the medial wall of each far lateral mucocele may be impossible or not adequate, with high risk of persistent or recurrent disease.

Regarding the contraindications for an endoscopic endonasal orbital transposition, it should be clearly stated that a massive lateral supraorbital attachment of the lesion in a laterally pneumatized frontal sinus or a massive involvement of the mucosa of the frontal sinus and/or of a supraorbital cell by an inverted papilloma are contraindications for an exclusive endoscopic endonasal approach. The more laterally the attachment is located, the more difficult it is to remove the lesion by a pure endoscopic approach.

Moreover, the erosion of the posterior wall of the frontal sinus with intracranial extension of the lesion and/or extension of the lesion through the anterior frontal plate, the presence of abundant scar tissue from previous surgery or relevant posttraumatic anatomic changes of the frontal bone, and the histological evidence of squamous cell carcinoma in inverted papilloma or primary malignant tumors that involve the far lateral portion of the frontal sinus should be considered absolute contraindications of a pure endoscopic endonasal approach.

Conversely, the high solidity of an osteoma (e.g., ivory type osteomas), which may require a long drilling time due to the low speed of the angled drills, may represent a relative contraindication; in this case, an osteoplastic flap through a coronal approach could be more suitable to reduce the operating time (by using straight drills) and the risks associated with a prolonged general anesthesia.

10.2 Surgical Steps

The operative setting requires general hypotensive anesthesia and hyperextension of the head of the patient. It is crucial to obtain optimal nasal decongestion; thus, both nasal cavities should be packed with pledges soaked in 2% oxymetazoline, 1% oxybuprocaine, and epinephrine (1/100,000) solution for 10 minutes. Meanwhile, the setting of the navigation system is performed in order to prevent the risk of skull base and orbital complications. Both optic and magnetic systems permit real-time tracking of images with three-dimensional reconstruction, which is very useful to laterally transpose the orbit and to drill out the boundaries of the frontal sinus. However, only the newest magnetic navigation systems, as opposed to the optical one, do not require a line of sight between the field generator and the instruments, which avoids conflicts for space due to the presence of four hands in the binostril approach.

In terms of surgical equipment, the new multiangled high-speed intranasal drills (12.000–30.000 rpm) and shavers (straight, 40- and 60-degree curved shaver, 15-, 40-, and 70-degree standard and diamond drills), along with 0-, 45-, and 70-degree telescopes are necessary to achieve complete control of the lesion's boundaries, even if located in the far lateral portion of the frontal sinus or into the supraorbital recess. Nevertheless, double-bended endoscopic instruments are required for dissection.

To approach the far lateral aspect of the frontal sinus and the supraorbital recess with an endoscopic endonasal approach, it is essential to start creating enough space

allowing the use of curved instruments. This is achieved by performing adequate frontal sinusotomy, such as Draf type IIb and III (known as the "modified Lothrop procedure" or "median drainage") procedures. The choice varies case by case and depends on the anatomy of the frontal sinus. The Draf type IIb entails the removal of the frontal sinus floor from the lamina papyracea to the nasal septum and it provides access to the ipsilateral frontal sinus recess, offering a limited surgical freedom related to the mononostril dissection. By adding a frontal intersinus septectomy to the Draf IIb and maintaining an intact nasal septum, a modified mini-Lothrop procedure is created. This modification allows access to both the posterior frontal sinus walls but has limited surgical freedom due to mononostril access. The addition of a superior septectomy to the Draf IIb creates a modified hemi-Lothrop procedure that significantly increases surgical freedom by allowing "two nostrils, four hands" technique and provides a better far lateral access through the superior septotomy window from the contralateral nasal cavity. The modified subtotal Lothrop procedure includes the addition of a superior septectomy and frontal intersinus septectomy to a Draf IIb and preserves the contralateral frontal sinus recess. These modifications of the standard Draf IIb would provide adequate exposure and surgical maneuverability in accessing complex frontal sinus pathology and also allow the preservation of the integrity of the contralateral frontal recess. However, the majority of the cases require a Draf type III sinusotomy, obtained by removing the frontal sinus floor from the lamina papyracea of one side to the contralateral lamina papyracea, together with the removal of the interfrontal septum, in order to create a wide median drainage of the frontal sinuses. The Draf type III procedure allows a greater angle of inclination and a better maneuvering of curve instruments, which are crucial to reach lesions localized in the far lateral region of the frontal sinus. Moreover, it also permits use of, similarly to the techniques previously discussed, the contralateral fossa for the "two nostrils, four hands technique," in which different surgical instruments work simultaneously through both the nasal cavities. After creating space by performing one of the previously mentioned frontal sinusotomies, the anterior ethmoidal artery is identified, coagulated, and transected in its middle portion, in order to prevent its retraction into the orbit and to avoid a retrobulbar hemorrhage. At this point, the lamina papyracea is completely exposed, then fractured and removed in its upper portion, paying attention to maintain intact the underlying periorbital layer. A flexible retractor is used to transpose laterally the orbit; in this way, the bony floor of the supraorbital recess is exposed and drilled out with a diamond bur. A recent modification of the technique permits fracturing the lamina papyracea but not removing it from the periorbit. This preservation of the bony lamina papyracea attached on the periorbit will permit the second surgeon to place the curved suction or a flexible retractor on it and displacing laterally the orbital content without

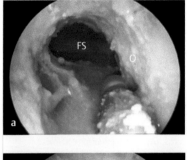
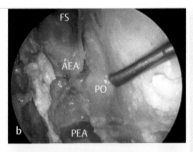
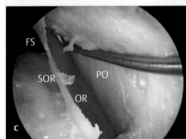
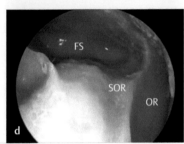

Fig. 10.1 (a) Cadaveric dissection performing a Draf type IIb with drilling out of the maxillary branch. (b) The anterior ethmoidal artery is skeletonized until its exit point from the orbit. (c) The periorbit is detached from the orbital roof, which is subsequently drilled out. (d) Final view with the orbital roof, the supraorbital recess, and the far lateral aspect of the frontal sinus completely exposed. (Abbreviations: AEA, anterior ethmoidal artery; FS, frontal sinus; OR, orbital roof; PEA, posterior ethmoidal artery; PO, periorbit; SOR, supraorbital recess.)

risk of damaging the periorbit and/or herniation of the orbital fat into the surgical field. Once the bony floor of the supraorbital recess is exposed, the orbital roof can be drilled out paying attention not to cross the coronal plane passing through the posterior table of the frontal sinus, this in order to avoid dural exposure and/or cerebrospinal fluid (CSF) leaks. When detaching the periorbit and removing the superomedial bony angle of the orbit, it is crucial to maintain the integrity of the troclea-periorbit as a unit. In this way, proper extraocular muscles balance and motility will be ensured. With this manoeuver, the surgeon will obtain more space and will be able to reach the far lateral aspect of the frontal sinus by passing over the orbit with double-bended surgical instruments, as well as with curved shavers or drills (▶ Fig. 10.1). At the end of the procedure, the retractor is removed, which allows the re-expansion of the orbit to its natural position (▶ Fig. 10.2). Moreover, in the cases characterized by a very narrow supraorbital recess, it is possible to enlarge the milling, with the cleverness to use a temporary silastic sheet covering the periorbit. In the past, these cases were approached regularly through an osteoplastic flap. To note, the surgical expedients herein described (Draf type IIb/III, access through the contralateral nasal fossa, endonasal orbital transposition, and double-curved instruments) are differently and complementarily used in order to create a custom surgery for every case, tailored to the frontal sinus anatomy, to the lesion's biology, and its extension.

10.3 Tips and Tricks

▶ Table 10.1 provides summary of the commonest pitfalls a surgeon may encounter and the ways to deal with them.

10.4 Case Example

Endoscopic endonasal orbital transposition for a left fronto-ethmoidal inverted papilloma. A 78-year-old man was referred to our department after a partial resection of a left sinonasal tumor, histologically compatible with inverted papilloma. The pathology review of the slides performed at our institute highlighted the presence of inverted papilloma associated with squamous metaplasia. There were no signs of invasive squamous cell carcinoma. The patient complained of left anterior and posterior rhinorrhea and recurrent frontal headache. The CT scan and the contrast-enhanced MRI scan showed a bulky tumor, occupying entirely the left nasal fossa, the ethmoidal compartment, and the maxillary and frontal sinuses, and protruding into the nasopharynx (▶ Fig. 10.3). Multiple areas of hyperostosis were detectable in the ethmoid. Due to the extension of the disease in the left frontal sinus, the possibility of performing an osteoplastic flap was planned and discussed with the patient preoperatively. The patient underwent an endoscopic endonasal approach. Intraoperative frozen sections confirmed involvement of the anterior wall of the frontal sinus. Nonetheless, a complete endoscopic resection was possible through a Draf type IIb frontal sinusotomy associated with the orbital transposition, avoiding the need of an external procedure (▶ Fig. 10.4). Intraoperatively, a CSF leak on the left olfactory fissure occurred during the drilling out of the bony skull base and it was repaired with an overlay mucosal graft (single-layer technique). The last clinical and radiological follow-up performed 1 year after surgery was negative for recurrence of disease (▶ Fig. 10.5).

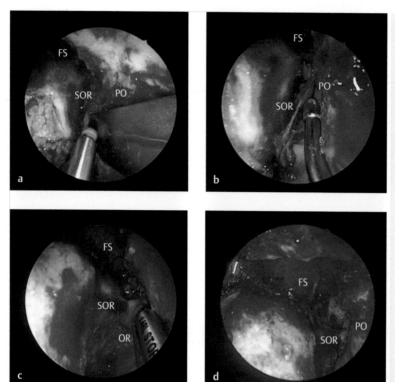

Fig. 10.2 **(a)** Intraoperative endoscopic view after exposure of the ethmoidal roof; the periorbit is kept protected with a flexible retractor and the superomedial angle of the orbit is drilled out. **(b)** During the procedure, the periorbit is progressively detached from the most cranial portion of the superomedial angle in order to expose the orbital roof. **(c)** The orbital roof is reached and drilled until the supraorbital recess. **(d)** Final view after complete exposure of the far lateral portion of the frontal sinus. (Abbreviations: FS, frontal sinus; OR, orbital roof; PO, periorbit; SOR, supraorbital recess.)

Table 10.1 List of difficulty points and their technical solutions

Point of difficulty	Technical solution
1. Narrow frontal recess' space	1. Drill anteriorly the frontal branch of the maxilla
2. Avoid orbital lesion and fat blowout	2. Gentle removing of papyracea
3. Preserve the periorbital layer and the trochlea	3. Use silastic sheet to cover the orbit when drilling
4. Avoid the anterior ethmoidal artery shrinking	4. Coagulate the artery and then cut it in the middle
5. Reach the most lateral portion of the frontal sinus	5. Use double curved instruments and drills
6. Use the "two nostrils, four hands" technique	6. Perform Draf type IIB/IIB modified vs. Draf type III

10.5 Complications

- *CSF leak.* A serious complication when approaching the frontal sinus using the endoscopic endonasal orbital transposition is the iatrogenic CSF leak. Usually, it occurs at the posterior frontal sinus wall or at the level of the lateral lamella of the *cribriform plate* of the ethmoid at the entry point of the anterior ethmoidal artery, while drilling the skull base or during the detachment of a lesion attached at this level. If a skull base defect is evident intraoperatively, a concomitant

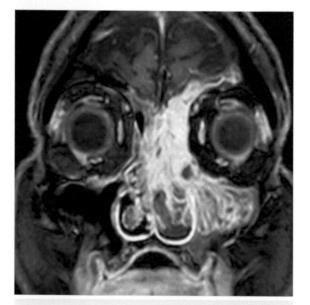

Fig. 10.3 MRI in T1 sequence with contrast enhancement showing a left sinonasal lesion compatible with inverted papilloma (contrast enhancement with cerebriform appearance) involving the left nasal fossa, the maxillary sinus, the ethmoid, the frontal recess, and the frontal sinus.

reconstruction is mandatory. There are different techniques to repair a skull base defect based on its position and dimension. The reconstruction methods can be

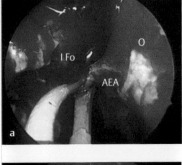
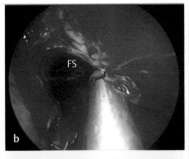
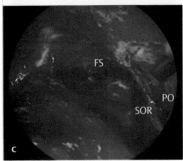
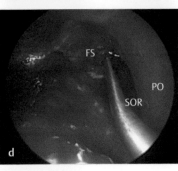

Fig. 10.4 (a) Intraoperative endoscopic view of the ethmoidal roof with the anterior ethmoidal artery crossing it in a lateral-to-medial direction, from posterior to anterior. The artery is cauterized with bipolar forceps and sectioned at its midpoint. (b) The frontal branch of the maxilla is then drilled in order to widen the frontal sinusotomy and to expose the periorbit. (c) The periorbit is then gently lateralized with a smooth tool to expose the superomedial angle of the orbit. (d) After drilling the superomedial angle of the orbit, the far lateral portion of the frontal sinus is well visualized and explorable. (Abbreviations: AEA, anterior ethmoidal artery; FR, frontal recess; FS, frontal sinus; I fov, first ethmoidal fovea; O, orbit; PO, periorbit; SOR, supraorbital recess.)

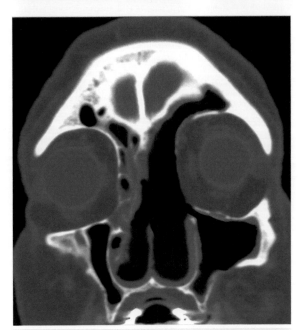

Fig. 10.5 Postoperative CT scan showing the drainage pathway of the far lateral portion of the left frontal sinus and the nasal fossa, with the bony superomedial angle of the orbit completely removed.

divided into free grafting techniques (which include the "multilayer technique") and pedicled flaps. These options can also be combined when needed. No matter what type of technique is used, the preparatory stage must include an appropriate exposure of the bony margins of the defect, undermining the dural margins (when possible) in the epidural space and smoothing of the defect edges to ensure a better engraftment of the flap or graft. It is important to use a graft/flap larger than the dural defect in order to compensate for its shrinking during the healing process. The free graft techniques include the overlay placement of a free graft (mucoperichondrium or mucoperiosteum harvested from the nasal septum or nasal floor) to repair and consolidate a small defect when the dura is not involved. The underlay technique uses intracranial intradural grafts (e.g., fascia lata or fascia temporalis) that are combined afterward with overlay grafts, representing the so-called multilayer technique, which is appropriate for repairing larger defects. This technique usually involves the positioning of three layers: the first one is usually made up of fascia or dural substitutes placed intracranially and intradurally as an underlay layer and serve as a guide for fibroblast migration. This first layer must be 30% larger than the dural defect. The second layer is placed in an intracranial extradural (underlay) fashion, inserted in the epidural space, in order to get stability to the duraplasty. Any difficulties encountered during the insertion of the edge of the strip in the epidural space can be overcome by using autologous cartilage or bone fragments removed from the nasal septum or ear concha. In these cases, the suitably shaped fragments are used to push the layer in an appropriate way. The third and last layer, consisting of fascia or free grafts such as mucoperichondrium or mucoperiosteum, is placed extracranially intranasally (overlay) to facilitate the sealing capacity of the duraplasty by guiding the repair mechanisms of the nasal mucosa.

the layer in an appropriate way. The third and last layer, consisting of fascia or free grafts such as muco-perichondrium or mucoperiosteum, is placed extracra-nially intranasally (overlay) to facilitate the sealing capacity of the duraplasty by guiding the repair mechanisms of the nasal mucosa.

- *Retrobulbar hemorrhage.* It is a possible complication that occurs, during frontal sinus surgery, when the anterior ethmoidal artery is not identified and carefully cauterized with bipolar forceps. The anterior ethmoidal artery, collateral branch of the ophthalmic artery, after passing into the eponymous canal of the ethmoid bone, exits at level of the ethmoidal roof and runs obliquely from lateral to medial and from posterior to anterior, behind the first fovea of the ethmoid. It is usually covered with a light shell bone, but it can be occasionally dehiscent. If the artery is accidentally striped or sectioned without having been properly cauterized, it can retract inside the orbit and cause a retrobulbar hemorrhage, which is difficult to manage, causing fatal consequences such as visual impairment or blindness, which may require orbital decompression through an endoscopic approach or external surgery (e.g., lateral canthotomy and cantholysis). Therefore, the accurate exposure of the roof of the ethmoid and the detection of the artery is crucial to prevent its accidental injury and its retraction.
- *Damage of the trochlea.* The superior oblique muscle determines the rotation of the eye downward and sideways. It originates from the medial edge of the optic canal and goes forward on the roof of the orbit, giving rise to a tendon that passes through the trochlea, a

small fibrocartilaginous ring placed in the superomedial orbital roof. After the trochlea, the tendon changes direction and heads back and sideways, fitting on the back of the eyeball. If a lesion of the trochlea occurs, strabismus may not be evident but diplopia can be present when the patient turns to look below the horizontal plane, when the action of the inferior rectus muscle will be no longer counterbalanced by the action of the superior oblique muscle. To avoid its damage during the drilling out of the superomedial bony portion of the orbit, it is important to preserve the integrity of the periorbit. In fact, the opening of the periorbit with herniation of the orbital fat in the operative field not only makes the procedure more difficult but also increases the risk of damages to the trochlea. Therefore, the surgeon should remove the papyracea gently, then, while drilling out the orbital wall, it is recommended to protect the periorbit with a silastic sheet or pushing it sideways using a malleable retractor.

Suggested Readings

Karligkiotis A, Pistochini A, Turri-Zanoni M, et al. Endoscopic endonasal orbital transposition to expand the frontal sinus approaches. Am J Rhinol Allergy. 2015; 29(6):449–456

Liu JK, Mendelson ZS, Dubal PM, Mirani N, Eloy JA. The modified hemi-Lothrop procedure: a variation of the endoscopic endonasal approach for resection of a supraorbital psammomatoid ossifying fibroma. J Clin Neurosci. 2014; 21(12):2233–2238

Poczos P, Kurbanov A, Keller JT, Zimmer LA. Medial and superior orbital decompression: improving access for endonasal endoscopic frontal sinus surgery. Ann Otol Rhinol Laryngol. 2015; 124(12):987–995

11 The Role of Frontal Sinus in Anterior Skull Base Surgery and the Transcribriform Approach

E. Ritter Sansoni, Raymond Sacks, and Richard J. Harvey

Abstract

Addressing the frontal sinus is an important component of anterior skull base surgery and the transcribriform approach. Opening the frontal sinus improves endoscopic visualization and surgical access to the anterior aspect of the ventral skull base, which facilitates resecting the lesion and reconstructing the skull base. Additionally, widely opening the sinus helps mitigate the sinonasal dysfunction resultant of the surgery. The location of the surgical target along the anterior skull base dictates whether a Draf IIa or III is most appropriate. The anterior ethmoidal artery is the anatomic landmark that helps determine which frontal sinus procedure to employ. A Draf III is done if the lesion involves or is anterior to the area of the anterior ethmoidal artery. However, if the lesion is posterior to the anterior ethmoidal, a Draf IIa is typically sufficient. A technical modification to the Draf III procedure, the outside-in approach, increases surgical efficiency and does not require navigation of the frontal recess when creating a common frontal sinusotomy. This approach only requires a 0-degree endoscope and straight instruments, and provides a panoramic view of the entire cribriform plate and posterior table of the frontal sinus.

Keywords: frontal sinus, Draf IIa, Draf III, Lothrop, outside-in Lothrop, transcribriform approach, anterior skull base surgery

11.1 Indications

Consideration of the frontal sinus is an essential component of anterior skull base surgery and the transcribriform approach. Opening the frontal sinus provides an endoscopic view of the ventral skull base and allows for improved surgical access. Additionally, addressing the frontal sinuses simplifies postoperative care and surveillance. Although the location of the pathology will dictate the extent of frontal sinus dissection, postoperative care of the patient and surveillance also contribute to decision-making.

The two frontal sinus approaches that are most commonly employed in combination with the transcribriform approach are the Draf IIa and III, or modified endoscopic Lothrop procedure (MELP). The anatomic landmark we use to determine which procedure to employ is the anterior ethmoid artery (▶ Fig. 11.1). If the lesion is posterior to and does not involve the area around the anterior ethmoidal artery, then a Draf IIa should provide sufficient surgical access. However, a MELP is performed if the

lesion approximates or is anterior to the anterior ethmoidal artery. The rationale for doing this is twofold: first, it permits the use of a 0-degree endoscope and straight instrumentation and, second, it creates a simple, common neosinus that is easy to maintain in the postoperative period.

An inherent challenge with resecting lesions that extend or are based more anteriorly on the skull base is the angle of approach. The posterior table of the frontal sinus and nasofrontal beak limit anterosuperior exposure. Creating a common frontal sinusotomy by removing the nasofrontal beak and floor of the frontal sinus significantly improves surgical exposure and gives the surgeon a panoramic view of the entire cribriform plate and posterior table of the frontal sinus, which is the anterior limit of the resection[1] (▶ Fig. 11.2). The use of a 0-degree endoscope and straight instruments facilitates bilateral triangulation of instruments during the resection of the lesion.[2] Alternatively, angled endoscopes and instruments can be used to navigate this issue by accessing the posterior table of the frontal sinus through the frontoethmoidal recess, but this is cumbersome and adds unnecessary difficulty. Wide exposure of the posterior table also helps during skull base reconstruction since it acts as a shelf to support subdural underlay grafts.[3] Additionally, the improved surgical exposure during the initial resection of malignancies translates to easier tumor surveillance in the clinic postoperatively by providing an expansive view of the entire sinonasal cavity (▶ Fig. 11.3).

Endoscopic endonasal approaches to the skull base create significant sinonasal dysfunction in the postoperative period by disrupting mucociliary clearance, creating surgical trauma and edema, and leaving large areas to heal by secondary intention. This is further compounded if adjuvant radiotherapy is required. Creating a common frontal sinusotomy helps minimize the risk of postoperative frontal sinus stenosis and iatrogenic mucocele formation.[3] Furthermore, maximally opening the frontal sinus has been shown to improve the delivery of nasal irrigations to the frontal sinus when compared to more limited dissections.[4] This is important to help overcome the acquired mucostasis and clear retained secretions and debris, which may negatively impact postoperative healing.[5]

There are two approaches for creating a common frontal sinusotomy: the traditional approach in which bony removal commences after the frontal recess is first dissected and an outside-in approach where bone is first removed away from the frontal recess. A benefit of using the outside-in MELP as opposed to the inside-out approach is that it does not require navigation of the

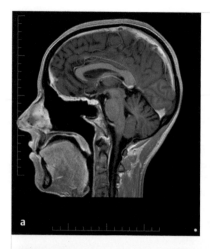
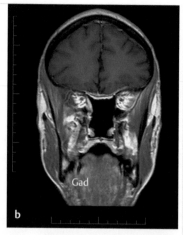

Fig. 11.1 T1-weighted MRI of a large olfactory groove meningioma in the sagittal plane. The approximate location of the anterior ethmoidal artery (*white asterisk*) delineates whether a Draf IIa or III should be performed in conjunction with the transcribriform approach.

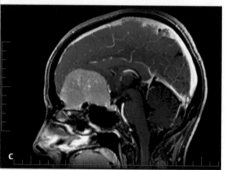
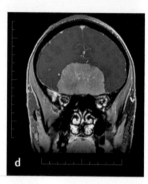

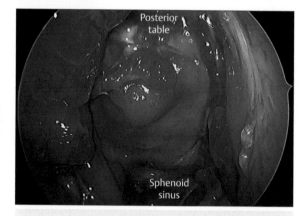

Fig. 11.3 Endoscopic view of the entire ventral skull base 2 months following resection of the olfactory groove meningioma. A minimal amount of surgical edema remains, but the cavity is otherwise very healthy.

Fig. 11.2 Endoscopic view of the ventral skull base after resection of the olfactory groove meningioma. The frontal sinus (*black arrow*) and posterior table (*dashed line*) are easily seen using a 0-degree nasal endoscope.

complex and varied frontal recess anatomy. Rather, it relies on known anatomical landmarks that serve as the boundaries for creating the common frontal sinusotomy cavity.[6] This is especially useful in situations where the frontal recess has significant disease or tumor burden, neo-osteogenesis, or scarring from prior interventions. Additionally, this method only requires a 0-degree endoscope and is more efficient than the standard approach, thus adding little time to the overall operation.[6] The following section details the surgical steps of the outside-in MELP when being used in conjunction with a transcribriform approach.

11.2 Surgical Steps

1. Patient positioning and preparation:
   - The patient is placed in the standard supine position with a shoulder roll to extend the neck, which permits improved and more comfortable surgical access to the frontal sinus and the ventral skull base.
   - The endotracheal is secured to the right lower lip.
   - The surgical bed is placed at 15 to 20 degrees in a reverse Trendelenburg position to improve venous drainage.
   - Cotton pledgets soaked in 1% ropivacaine and 1:2,000 adrenaline should be placed into the nasal cavities as soon as possible.
   - The image guidance system is then set up.
   - One-percent ropivacaine with 1:100,000 adrenaline is infiltrated into the head and axilla of the middle turbinate, the nasal septum near the swell body and insertion of the anterior ethmoid artery, and laterally into the mucosa overlying the frontal process of the maxilla. Additionally, prepare for raising the most appropriate vascularized flap.
   - The anesthesiologist should use total intravenous anesthesia and maintain the patient's bradycardia (55–65 bpm) with mean arterial pressures near 60 throughout the case.

2. Anterior ethmoid dissection and defining the medial orbital wall:
   - Depending on the indications for surgery, this sequence of steps may vary.
   - Bilateral maxillary antrostomies and complete sphenoethmoidectomies are completed. If a nasoseptal flap is to be used, do not make a large sphenoidotomy until after the flap is raised.
   - The middle turbinates are removed near their insertion at the skull base.
   - Raise an appropriately sized nasoseptal flap, or another vascularized flap, and place it in the nasopharynx or the maxillary sinus.

3. Exposing the nasofrontal beak and the first olfactory neuron:
   - The mucosa overlying the nasofrontal beak, frontal sinus floor, frontal process of the maxilla, and septum is raised as a single mucosal flap on both sides.
   - Use a monopolar electrocautery with a needle tip bent at a 45-degree angle and a setting of 12 on coagulation mode to make the mucosal incisions.
   - Starting at the apex within the nasal cavity at a point in line with the anterior table, make a lateral mucosal incision inferiorly along the frontal process of the maxilla to the parasagittal plane of the medial orbital wall. A similar medial incision is made inferiorly along the septum, slightly more anterior to stagger the cuts. The septal incision should incorporate any septal swell body or upper deviation (▶ Fig. 11.4).
   - The mucosal flaps are raised using a Cottle elevator. This is initiated at the apex, then along the lateral wall, and finally the septum. The flaps are reflected posteriorly until the first olfactory neuron is reached. This is often heralded by a small emissary vein that tends to course laterally (▶ Fig. 11.5).
   - Remove the flaps with a microdebrider and cauterize the bleeding mucosa with a COBLATOR (Smith & Nephew, London, United Kingdom) or bipolar electrocautery.

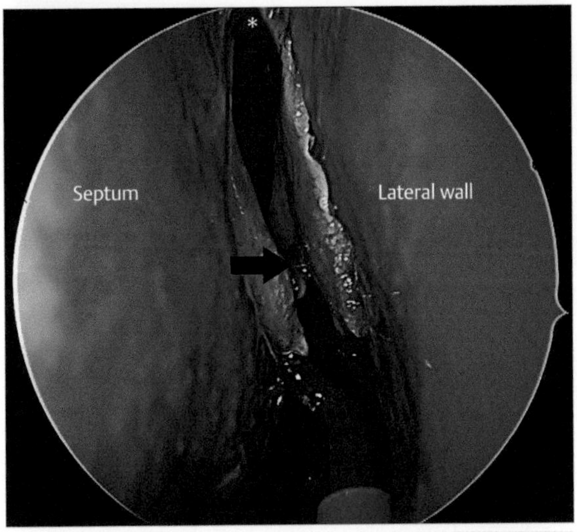

Fig. 11.4 Endoscopic view of the mucosal incisions used to raise the mucosal flaps. The superior starting point (*white asterisk*) is below the anterior table of the frontal sinus. The superior aspect of the previously resected middle turbinate (*black arrow*) gives a sense of the incision length.

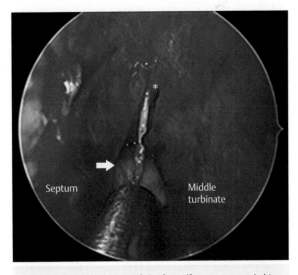

Fig. 11.5 Endoscopic view of the first olfactory neuron (*white arrow*). A small emissary vein (*asterisk*) is typically seen anterior to the true fascicle.

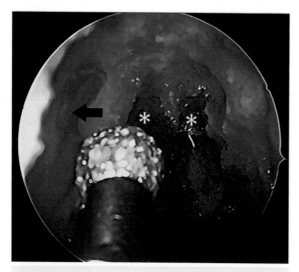

Fig. 11.6 Endoscopic view of the exposed periosteum of the frontal process of the maxilla (*black arrow*). Note the white color compared to the surrounding bone. The locations of the first olfactory neurons are seen posteriorly (*white asterisks*).

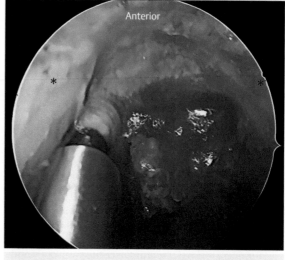

Fig. 11.7 Endoscopic view of drilling away the nasofrontal beak in an arcing motion between the exposed periosteum (*asterisks*) and anterior to the first olfactory neurons.

- A septectomy is then performed leaving an adequate caudal strut for support.
4. Drilling to define the lateral limits:
   - A high-speed, 15-degree, self-irrigating drill with a rough diamond bur should be used. A drill that is capable of 30,000 rpm and has an integrated distal suction will allow for improved surgical efficiency. The bur size should be 4 mm or greater.
   - The small, remaining crest of bony septum inferior to the frontal sinus is drilled away first. Then, the bone of both lateral walls is drilled down to expose the periosteum superiorly.
   - The periosteum is whiter in color compared to the overlying bone and bleeds more noticeably (▶ Fig. 11.6).
   - This defines the lateral limits of the future frontal sinusotomy.
5. Drilling away the nasofrontal beak and frontal sinus floor:
   - This portion of the procedure can be disconcerting since it requires drilling through thick bone. However, it is important to recognize that frontal sinus or the frontal recess is always between the drill and the skull base.
   - Starting centrally, drill between the lateral limits in an arcing motion through the nasofrontal beak (▶ Fig. 11.7).
   - Remove bone along a broad front from the nasofrontal beak and anterior to the frontal recess. This will prevent "tunneling" into the frontal sinus.
   - As the mucosa of the frontal sinus becomes visible, avoid the temptation to enter the sinus until the remainder of the overlying bone is thinned. Entering

prematurely will cause bleeding that will disrupt the visual field.
   - Once the sinus is entered, bone can be quickly removed enlarging the sinusotomy.
   - Using a 2-mm Kerrison rongeur, connect the frontal recess frontal sinusotomy and remove any remaining partitions in the frontal recess.
   - Drill away any frontal sinus partitions. Also, follow the orbital wall as it turns into the orbital roof. Doing so will "square off" the cavity and maximize its dimensions.
   - The surgeon now has a panoramic view of the anterior projection of the olfactory fossa and the posterior table of the frontal sinus (▶ Fig. 11.8).
6. Obtaining anterior vascular control and removing the crista galli:
   - Coblator the mucosa covering the ventral skull base to help with hemostasis.
   - Use a Cottle elevator to remove the lamina inferior to the anterior ethmoidal arteries and a curette to remove the skull base surrounding the arteries. The periorbital will "tent" around the anterior ethmoid canal.
   - With the arteries free of surrounding bone, cauterize them with bipolar electrocautery and divide them medially.
   - Drill away the upper septum into the crista galli.
   - Use a Cottle elevator to elevate the dura off both sides of the crista to expose the bone.
   - Remove the posterior table on either side of the crista galli with a 2-mm Kerrison rongeur working superior.
   - Drill away the anterior attachment of the crista galli and the posterior table of the frontal sinus. This should entirely free the crista from any remaining

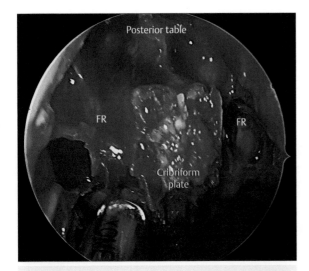

Fig. 11.8 Endoscopic view of the exposure afforded by the Draf III cavity after the frontal recesses (FR) have been connected up to the cavity. The posterior table and entire length of the cribriform plate are seen with a 0-degree nasal endoscope.

attachments. Use straight Blakesley forceps to remove the crista galli.

- The entire length and width of the ventral skull base is now exposed and the remainder of the resection can commence.

11.3 Tips and Tricks

- As with any surgical procedure, many pitfalls of the Draf III are avoided with attention to detail and proper technique (▶ Table 11.1).
- Patient positioning and setup are critical for this procedure. Ensure that the neck is extended and that the endotracheal tube and circuit are not on the patient's chest.
- Hemostasis greatly improves the visual field and consequently surgical efficiency. Place the topical vasoconstrictor in the nose as soon as possible and put the bed in reverse Trendelenburg to help venous drainage. The role of the anesthesiologist cannot be overstated in maintaining hemostasis throughout the case.
- Use a high-speed (30,000 rpm), self-irrigating drill with distal suction. The nasofrontal beak can be quite thick and slower, less aggressive drills can add a significant amount of time to the case.
- Maximize the dimensions of the frontal sinusotomy. This will lessen the chance of postoperative stenosis.
- A silastic sheet should be placed into the frontal sinusotomy and over the exposed bone to optimize wound healing and prevent significant crusting. This may be removed after 3 weeks.
- High-volume nasal irrigations should be started 1 week following surgery. Do not use any nasal spray in the

Table 11.1 Solutions to common surgical challenges

Surgical challenges	Technical solutions
Frontal sinus access	• Extend the patient's neck • Ensure the circuit and endotracheal tube are secured at the corner of the right lower lip and are off the patient's neck and chest
Hemostasis	• Place the surgical bed at 15–20 degrees in a reverse Trendelenburg position • Use 1:2,000 adrenaline as a topical vasoconstrictor • Keep the mean arterial pressures in the 60 s and the heart rate between 55 and 65 bpm • Avoid mucosal stripping. Coblate the mucosa that will be removed during the resection prior to removing it
Creating the common frontal sinusotomy	• Clearly expose and trust the surgical limits of dissection • Use a high-speed, self-irrigating drill with distal suction and a coarse diamond bur • Remove the bone broadly and drill in a steep anterior vector toward the frontal sinus • Remove the bone anterior to the frontal recess to maximize the width of the Draf III cavity
Postoperative stenosis and crusting	• Maximize the dimensions of the Draf III cavity to the limits of the dissection • Use mucosal grafts to cover the exposed bone of the frontal process of the maxilla • Cover the exposed bone of the nasofrontal beak with a silastic sheet • Start large-volume irrigations 1 wk after surgery and see the patient for routine postoperative debridement at 3 wk

first week as this may confound the signs of an early postoperative cerebrospinal fluid leak.

11.4 Complications

- Stenosis of the frontal sinusotomy is best avoided by widely opening the sinus. There is also evidence to support the use of mucosal grafts.[7] Additionally, postoperative irrigations and debridement are important.
- It is common for patients to get swelling around the nasion several days following surgery. This is caused by inflammation of the periosteum and does not indicate infection. It responds well to nonsteroidal anti-inflammatory drugs.

References

[1] Khan OH, Raithatha R, Castelnuovo P, Anand VK, Schwartz TH. Draf III extension in the endoscopic endonasal transethmoidal,

transcribriform approach through the back wall of the frontal sinus: a cadaveric study. World Neurosurg. 2016; 85:136–142

[2] Liu JK, Christiano LD, Patel SK, Tubbs RS, Eloy JA. Surgical nuances for removal of olfactory groove meningiomas using the endoscopic endonasal transcribriform approach. Neurosurg Focus. 2011; 30(5):E3

[3] Batra PS, Kanowitz SJ, Luong A. Anatomical and technical correlates in endoscopic anterior skull base surgery: a cadaveric analysis. Otolaryngol Head Neck Surg. 2010; 142(6):827–831

[4] Barham HP, Ramakrishnan VR, Knisely A, et al. Frontal sinus surgery and sinus distribution of nasal irrigation. Int Forum Allergy Rhinol. 2016; 6(3):238–242

[5] Jo HW, Dalgorf DM, Snidvongs K, Sacks R, Harvey RJ. Postoperative irrigation therapy after sinonasal tumor surgery. Am J Rhinol Allergy. 2014; 28(2):169–171

[6] Chin D, Snidvongs K, Kalish L, Sacks R, Harvey RJ. The outside-in approach to the modified endoscopic Lothrop procedure. Laryngoscope. 2012; 122(8):1661–1669

[7] Illing EA, Cho Y, Riley KO, Woodworth BA. Draf III mucosal graft technique: long-term results. Int Forum Allergy Rhinol. 2016; 6(5):514–517

12 Extended Endonasal Anterior Skull Base Approaches

Soma Subramaniam, Guillermo Maza, Daniel M. Prevedello, and Ricardo L. Carrau

Abstract

Open and expanded endoscopic endonasal approaches (EEAs) may be utilized for resection of anterior cranial fossa tumors based on the stage, histology, and patient's specific needs and characteristics (i.e., body habitus, severe sleep apnea), as well as the surgical team's training and preference. Traditional open craniofacial approaches require a craniotomy and maxillofacial osteotomies that may include those necessary for a subfrontal approach. Despite the development of minimal access approaches (endonasal, transorbital, and minicraniotomy), a subfrontal technique remains one of the primary strategies to manage anterior cranial base lesions, especially those with significant lateral or anterior extension or those involving critical neurovascular structures. Endoscopic, endoscopic-assisted, and open approaches afford advantages and disadvantages and have different indications and limitations; therefore, skull base surgeons and their teams must be versed in all techniques. However, the EEA has been increasingly applied for the resection of select anterior cranial base lesions. Benefits of EEAs include its enhanced visualization, the minimal manipulation of the brain (no retraction), avoidance of maxillofacial osteotomies, and lack of facial scars or cosmetic deficits. In this chapter, we will review all aspects of EEAs to the anterior cranial fossa. We include two case examples to illustrate how EEAs are used in two different scenarios.

Keywords: expanded endonasal approach, reconstruction, anterior skull base, vascularized flap, craniofacial resection

12.1 Indications

Expanded endoscopic endonasal approaches (EEAs) play an important role in both neoplastic and non-neoplastic conditions involving the anterior skull base. Neoplastic lesions typically include median lesions with or without an intradural component: olfactory neuroblastoma, olfactory groove meningiomas, and benign or malignant paranasal sinus neoplasms with anterior skull base involvement. Non-neoplastic indications include fractures, cerebrospinal fluid (CSF) leaks and meningoencephaloceles.

EEAs have been shown to be viable and safe alternatives to surgically expose the rostrocaudal ventral skull base.[1,2,3] In well-selected patients, an EEA can be successfully employed to treat complex midline lesions, regardless of its proximity to cranial nerves, presence of a intradural extension, or even if intimately associated with major vascular structures.[4] As with other techniques, the intricacies of every clinical scenario may influence the outcome; however, the latter is dependent mostly on an appropriate selection of cases and the surgical team's experience, with an important contribution by institutional resources.

In general, anatomical boundaries for EEA to the anterior skull base includes rostrocaudally from the posterior table of the frontal sinus to the posterior end of the planum sphenoidale and laterally extending to the midplane of the orbital roof and the inferomedial extent of both optic nerves. These anatomical boundaries mark the area that is accessible and are safe to remove via EEA.

Whenever the procedure requires posterior or lateral dissection outside of these boundaries, one must consider an open technique (e.g., transcranial, transfacial), either in combination with the EEA or as the sole surgical corridor. Combinations of open and an endoscopic approach can be planned as separate, staged surgical acts (e.g., when managing benign tumors of significant size), or simultaneously.[4,5]

Some of the limitations associated with EEAs are inherently linked to the anatomic extension of the targeted lesion. It should be recognized that some areas are not amenable to an oncological resection via EEA. Among others, these include the facial skin, the lateral recess and anterior table of the frontal sinuses, the lateral aspect of the infratemporal fossa, the lateral wall of the maxillary sinus, and orbital soft tissues (especially if an orbital exenteration or a total maxillectomy is indicated for complete tumor extirpation).[6] Relative contraindications include intracranial involvement of neural structures encompassing extensive invasion of the brain parenchyma, bilateral invasion of optic nerves, or chiasm. In addition, lymphoreticular neoplasias do not benefit from a surgical resection unless surgery is conducted to palliate compression of adjacent structures.[5,7] Presence of an acute bacterial or fungal infection of the sinonasal tract requires delaying a transdural resection until this is addressed with proper antibiotics.

12.2 Surgical Steps

12.2.1 Principles

Endoscopic approaches can be classified according to the anatomical location of the surgical target in median (sagittal plane) and paramedian (coronal plane). Median approaches extend from the frontal sinus to the second cervical vertebra, following the sagittal plane. Paramedian approaches extend in the coronal plane and can be subdivided into three different levels according to the involved cranial fossa. At the anterior cranial fossa, they extend laterally to the midline of the roof of the orbit and the optic nerve canal, whereas in the middle cranial fossa they extend to the internal carotid canal and in the posterior cranial fossa to the jugular foramen.[1,2,3]

In this chapter, we focus on the sagittal plane approaches to the anterior cranial fossa, namely, *the transcribriform, transplanum,* and *transtuberculum approaches.* A lateral extension over the roof of the orbits (most anterior coronal plane) is also pertinent as this is often necessary to control the extension of both benign (e.g., meningiomas) and malignant (e.g., esthesioneuroblastoma or adenocarcinoma). These modules can be employed separately, jointly, or even in conjunction with further ventral approaches (e.g., trans-sellar module), according to the pathology at hand. An endoscopic endonasal corridor must incorporate several important concepts to be reliable, practical, and effective including the creation of a unicameral nasal access that incorporates both nasal cavities to allow for a two-surgeon four-hand technique (i.e., bimanual instrumentation) and a wide surgical corridor that allows unhindered visualization and instrumentation, preferably using a 0-degree endoscope (i.e., straight line of sight).

These approaches are generally contraindicated when their pathways cross a critical structure (cranial nerve or major vessel). In this regard, one can visualize that EEAs allow access to the ventral skull base for select benign and malignant tumors within the anatomical boundaries formed by cranial nerves and internal carotid arteries laterally and the cerebral circulation superiorly and posteriorly. The principles of tumor dissection for endoscopic approaches are similar to those used during microscopic dissection and include early identification of critical neurovascular structures, control of the tumor blood supply, and early tumor debulking to facilitate its mobilization. This latter technical nuance allows the preservation of crucial vasculature adjacent to the tumor and a precise dissection of the lesion from the pia mater.

12.2.2 Operative Setup

Following the induction of general anesthesia, the patient remains in supine position, with the head resting on a horseshoe or a three-pin head fixator and tilted to the left, with the neck extended and turned to the right to facilitate the visualization of the most anterior skull base. We prefer a three-pin fixator for prolonged procedures, for those where significant drilling over the internal carotid artery (ICA) or cranial nerves is anticipated, or when paralysis is contraindicated due to the need to monitor cranial nerves (i.e., electromyography). Most commonly, the procedure is performed under neurophysiological monitoring (somatosensory evoked potentials) and assisted by frameless stereotactic navigation.

The patient's face, abdomen (for fat harvest), and the lateral thigh (for fascia lata harvesting) are prepared in standard fashion. To maximize hemostasis, cottonoids soaked with adrenaline 1/10,000 to 1/20,000 are inserted in both nasal cavities and a solution of lidocaine 1% and epinephrine 1/100,000 is infiltrated at the lateral wall (anterior to the middle turbinates) and nasal septum.

12.2.3 Surgical Technique

We will describe the technique involved in the endonasal endoscopic transcribriform approach to large anterior cranial fossa tumor resections. For tumors limited to the posterior section of the anterior cranial fossa that require a less steep trajectory, we use a transplanum/transtuberculum approach. Important variations of the approach will be discussed at the end of this section.

Transcribriform Approach

The initial approach is usually performed through the nostril with predominant involvement of the tumor, thus facilitating its debulking. Inferior turbinates are lateralized by an in- and outfracturing maneuver. An ipsilateral middle turbinectomy gains further space for instrumentation and allows a better assessment of the tumor. If the tumor involves the nasal cavity bilaterally, both middle turbinates are resected. Wide bilateral sphenoidotomies and nasoantral windows are completed, thus allowing the visual identification of the skull base (i.e., roof of sphenoid) and lamina papyracea, and combining the posterior nasal cavities into a single chamber. Bilateral ethmoidectomies further expose the superior aspect of the septum and its attachment to the anterior cranial base.

For benign tumors and select malignancies, not involving the nasal septum, a Hadad–Bassagaisteguy flap (HBF) is raised on the unaffected side and is then stored in the nasopharynx. This is followed by a posterior bony septectomy (vomer and perpendicular ethmoid plate) and a Caicedo reverse septal flap (CRSF). It is of utmost importance that the superior and posterior margins of the flaps (HBF and CRSF) are sent for histological ("frozen section") analysis to confirm the absence of tumor involvement. Once the reverse septal flap is sutured in place, we suture silicone septal splints to prevent intraoperative trauma to the reverse septal flap. The remaining soft tissue at the skull base includes the tumor "stump," which is removed before drilling the bone of the anterior fossa floor.

Bilateral frontal sinusotomies (Draf III), followed by the drilling of the crista galli, help establish the anterior resection margin, whereas wide sphenoidotomies establish the posterior margin. Lateral margins are marked by the medial walls of the orbits; however, the exposure can be extended to the midline of each orbit by the removal of the laminae papyracea and the lateral displacement of the soft tissues of the orbit. Following the exposure of these boundaries, the roof of the ethmoid sinuses and cribriform plate are drilled thin and dissected off the dura bilaterally. The planum sphenoidale is removed posteriorly, as needed.

The anterior ethmoidal arteries (AEAs) and posterior ethmoidal arteries (PEAs) are identified, coagulated with a bipolar electrocautery, and divided. This step effectively devascularizes anterior skull base tumors. Once the bones of the fovea ethmoidalis, crista galli, and cribriform are drilled until eggshell thin, they are elevated with a combination of Cottle elevator, Kerrison rongeurs, and forceps to expose the dura of the anterior fossa. As aforementioned, bone removal can be extended laterally to include the lamina papyracea to obtain a clear margin or to facilitate control of the ethmoidal arteries. The dura is opened as an "inverted U" starting at the lateral margins to avoid injury of the median frontopolar, fronto-orbital, and parafalcine arteries. The crista galli is dissected superiorly and the cerebral falx is then incised under direct visualization in a ventrocaudal direction. This allows inferoposterior displacement of any residual tumor, cribriform plate, dura, and olfactory tracts en bloc. Using gentle suction (e.g., using 6-Fr graded suction tip) as traction, and a combination of blunt and sharp dissection, all arachnoid adherences are freed. In the case of esthesioneuroblastoma resection, both olfactory bulbs are resected for margins. Great care is taken to preserve the frontopolar arteries and the integrity of the frontal lobes.

Most commonly, the final defect extends from orbit to orbit and from crista galli to planum sphenoidale. An important olfaction-sparing variation may be possible in select patients with unilateral tumors. In this technique, the olfactory cleft (i.e., cribriform plate with olfactory bulb, tract, and nerves) as well as the middle and superior turbinates of the uninvolved side are preserved (i.e., the contralateral nasal septum olfactory strip—i.e., olfactory epithelium—is removed as there are bilateral connections between the olfactory nerves).

Transplanum/Transtuberculum Approach

Tumors in this region primarily comprise meningiomas, craniopharyngiomas, and large pituitary suprasellar tumors. They involve differences in the technique:

- Patients' olfactory function should be tested (likely be intact if the tumor does not involve the cribriform plate). If present, olfactory sparing techniques should be considered.
- As the plane of dissection is more posterior than the transcribriform approach, there is no need for extensive dissection of the frontal sinus (e.g., Draf III) or anterosuperior ethmoid air cells (unless a transfrontal pericranial flap is anticipated for reconstruction). One must note that the required surgical exposure will still include a posterior septectomy, wide sphenoidotomy, posterior ethmoidectomy, with exposure of the posterior (and middle, if present) ethmoidal vessels for early control and devascularization of the tumor.
- We expose the intrasellar dura (remove its rostrum) to allow wide exposure of the surgical site of concern.

12.2.4 Reconstruction

Once adequate resection margins are confirmed by intraoperative histological analysis ("frozen sections"), and hemostasis is achieved, we proceed with the reconstruction of the defect using an inlay sheet of collagen matrix or autologous fascia lata. The HBF, which had been previously harvested and stored in the nasopharynx, is retrieved and positioned to cover the defect overlapping the raw surfaces that comprise its boundaries. Autologous fat graft is sometimes inserted in the sphenoid sinus to obliterate significant dead space prior to positioning the HBF, thereby permitting optimal flap positioning. Finally, the reconstruction is bolstered in place using nonadherent material, followed by sponge packing.

In patients where the HBF is not available (due to tumor invading the nasal septum, sphenoid rostrum, or pterygopalatine fossa, or due to previous surgical resection of the septum), a transfrontal pericranial flap should be considered as an alternative.[8,9] To harvest the latter, the scalp hair is parted in alignment with a coronal incision but no hair is shaved. After sterile preparation and injection with lidocaine 1% with epinephrine 1/100,000, a coronal incision is carried down to the calvarium (between the temporalis muscles) or down to the temporalis fascia superficial to the temporalis muscle. Alternatively, a subgaleal dissection posterior to the coronal plane of the incisions may be used to maximize the length of the pericranial flap. The scalp is elevated from the skull in a caudal direction to reach the orbital rims, and to identify the supraorbital and supratrochlear neurovascular bundles. Once the neurovascular bundles have been dissected from their corresponding notches or foramina, the scalp dissection continues to expose the nasion and nasal bones. The pericranium (i.e., loose areolar tissue and periosteum) are subsequently elevated from the galea (unilateral) following a cephalocaudal direction and narrowing down to about 3 cm at the level of the pedicle (unilateral).

A high-speed drill with a 4-mm coarse diamond bur is used to open a window at the level of the nasion into the nasofrontal recesses. The pericranial flap is then transposed through this bony window under endoscopic visualization, preventing torsion of the vascular pedicle. The pericranial flap is gently pressed down and flattened to cover the inlay fascia lata graft, exposed dural edges, and the surrounding bony framework of the defect with an extradural extracranial onlay technique.

12.2.5 Postoperative Considerations

Postoperative care after an endoscopic resection is similar to that after open craniofacial resection. An immediate postoperative noncontrast CT scan is performed to rule out any significant intracranial hemorrhage, contusion, or tension pneumocephalus. A contrasted MRI within

24 hours of surgery confirms the completeness of surgical resection. In addition, the contrast uptake assists in confirming the vascularity of the reconstructive flap, as well as its position. Indwelling lumbar spinal drainage is not utilized routinely. It is only reserved for patients who are considered a high risk for increased intraventricular pressure or those with a high-flow leak (defined as a leak that communicates with either the third ventricle or at least two cisterns).

12.3 Tips and Tricks

- It is imperative to review the preoperative imaging (both MRI and CT) to assess for tumor extent, and its relationship to important neurovascular structures, and to assess for anatomical variants.
- Wide exposure of the anterior and posterior ethmoidal vascular bundles is advisable. Bipolar cautery should be utilized medially, away from the lamina papyracea to avoid inadvertent transection and retraction of the vessels into the orbit resulting in orbital hematoma.
- Warm saline irrigation to clear the lens of the endoscope helps reduce delays in maintaining good visualization throughout this potential lengthy surgery (as opposed to utilizing telescope sleeves for irrigation).
- Plan for the harvesting of abdominal fat to bolster the reconstruction or to fill surrounding dead space, thus increasing the "reach" of the nasoseptal flap.

12.4 Case Examples

12.4.1 Esthesioneuroblastoma (Transcribriform Approach)

A 55-year-old woman presents with a history of nasal congestion for about 1 year, worse on the left side, associated with hyposmia and recurrent epistaxis. She has a background history of recurrent rhinosinusitis. She underwent endoscopic endonasal sinus surgery and septoplasty at an outside facility with presumed diagnosis of rhinosinusitis. Intraoperative biopsies of a reddish polypoid mass confirmed esthesioneuroblastoma (Hyams grade 3). MRI (▶ Fig. 12.1a, b) showed tumor involving the left vault of the nasal cavity, but not crossing the midline. A nuclear PET imaging confirmed the absence of metastatic disease. The patient underwent an endoscopic endonasal unilateral anterior cranial fossa tumor resection with preserving the contralateral middle and superior turbinates and olfactory cleft (▶ Fig. 12.1c–f). The skull base reconstruction was performed with underlay collagen matrix followed by a right pedicled nasoseptal flap onlay. Postoperative imaging confirmed complete resection of tumor and HBF enhancement (▶ Fig. 12.1g).

12.4.2 Tuberculum Sellae Meningioma: Endoscopic Transtuberculum/Transplanum Approach

A 53-year-old woman presents with a history of reduced vision in the left eye associated with headaches. MRI imaging revealed a tuberculum sellae meningioma in contact with the left optic nerve (▶ Fig. 12.2a, b). In view of these findings, the patient underwent endoscopic endonasal transtuberculum/transplanum approach for endonasal resection of the tumor (▶ Fig. 12.2d–i). Tumor was completely excised and the skull base was reconstructed with an underlay collagen matrix, followed by a pedicled nasoseptal flap. Postoperative imaging confirmed tumor resection (▶ Fig. 12.2c).

12.5 Complications and Management

The skull base is distinct by its intimate association with a high density of vascular and neural structures, confined to a relatively small space. This spatial arrangement renders it especially vulnerable to surgical trauma (e.g., direct or due to exertion of undue force) or collateral tissue injury from powered tools (thermal and mechanical trauma). Intraoperative navigation and a progressive surgical experience somewhat diminished the incidence of complications, but they still occur, thus requiring the surgical team to be vigilant and prepared to confront them.

12.5.1 Vascular Complications

The EEA involves systematic clipping and coagulation of vessels that are progressively exposed. Proper hemostasis preserves the visualization of the surgical field and promotes early devascularization of tumors, thereby reducing the patient's morbidity.[1]

Low-flow oozing (capillary or venous) from bone and mucosa responds well to irrigation with warm saline (40–42 °C),[10] inducing platelet activation and interstitial edema narrowing the lumen of the vessels. Bipolar diathermy may be helpful to control focal bleeding. Bleeding from a venous sinus can be controlled by topical application of absorbable biomaterials such as a gelatin-thrombin matrix.[11] However, high-flow arterial bleeding requires prompt identification and isolation of the responsible vessel with the help of suctions, and then cauterizing the vessel (if not critical) with bipolar diathermy. Injury to a large vessel is best managed by the application of crushed muscle.

Prevention of vascular complications starts with a proper evaluation of the preoperative imaging, to identify

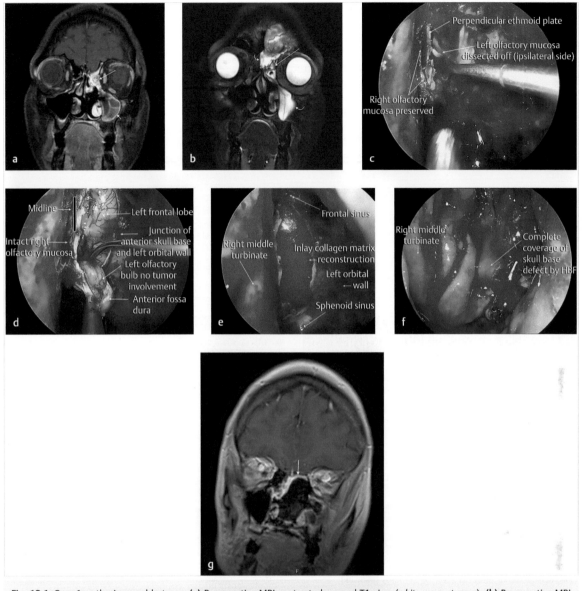

Fig. 12.1 Case 1: esthesioneuroblastoma. **(a)** Preoperative MRI contrasted coronal T1 view (*white arrow*: tumor). **(b)** Preoperative MRI contrasted coronal T2 view (*long white arrow*: tumor; *short curved arrow*: mucus within sinuses). **(c)** Endoscopic endonasal unilateral anterior cranial fossa tumor resection with preserving the contralateral middle and superior turbinates and olfactory cleft. **(d)** Excision of the dura. **(e)** Duragen repair. **(f)** Nasoseptal flap repair. **(g)** Postoperative MRI contrasted (+ c) coronal T1 view (*white arrow*: nasoseptal flap). Tumor completely resected.

vascular malformations, aneurysms, and dehiscences in the bony structure. CT angiography highlights the vascular anatomy and is preferred when the lesion is intimately associated with large and critical vessels.[12]

Neurophysiological monitoring of cortical and brainstem function should be performed to monitor cerebral perfusion. Controlled hypotensive anesthesia can be used in extradural cases, maintaining a mean arterial pressure

(MAP) of 65 to 70 mmHg to reduce bleeding while preventing neural ischemia.[11] Conversely, caution is advised with hypotensive techniques during intradural surgery, for an increased risk of hypoperfusion of neural structures.

Management of iatrogenic injury of the ICA is difficult; thus, prevention is the best option. Statistically, injuries are more common on the cavernous segment and on the left side compared to the right side.[13] Massive hemorrhage

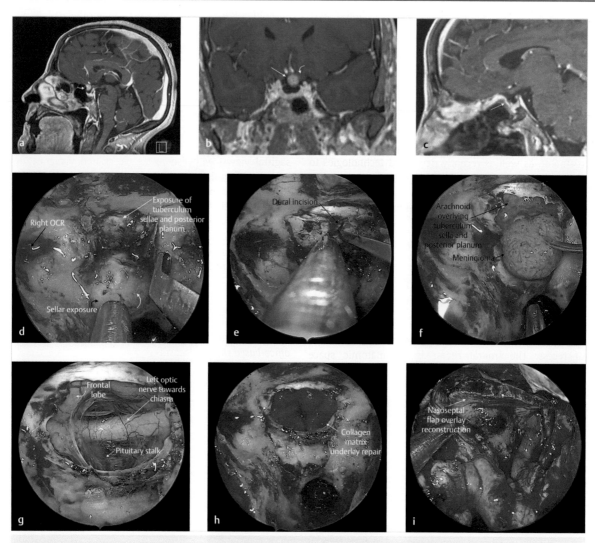

Fig. 12.2 Case 2: tuberculum sellae meningioma: Endoscopic transtuberculum/transplanum approach and reconstruction. **(a)** Preoperative MRI contrasted (+c) sagittal T1 view (*white arrow*: tuberculum sellae meningioma). **(b)** Preoperative MRI contrasted (+c) coronal T1 view (*straight white arrow*: tumor; *curved white arrow*: left optic nerve in contact with tumor). **(c)**. Postoperative MRI contrasted (+c) sagittal T1 view (white arrow: nasoseptal flap). Tumor completely resected. Collagen matrix filling the space. **(d)** Meningioma exposure. **(e)** Dural incision. **(f)** Tumor resection. **(g)** Exposed suprasellar space. **(h)** Duragen repair. **(i)** Nasoseptal flap repair.

is best handled by two-surgeon four-hand technique with dynamic endoscopic visualization. Two large bore suction tips offer the best chance of identifying the injury site. Flow preservation maneuvers are challenging, whereas suture repair is near impossible; alternatives such as reconstruction with aneurysm clips may be attempted if proximal and distal vascular controls have been previously obtained. A suggested "best" option is the application of crushed muscle patch.[14] In addition, although it seems counterintuitive, administration of heparin is important to avoid embolic phenomena.[15]

Muscle is best harvested from the lateral thigh (other sites may yield inadequate muscle or present the opportunity for other complications) and placed directly over

the injury site, applying enough pressure to stop the bleeding while allowing blood flow.[16] Once hemostasis is obtained, the patient can be transported to an endovascular unit for interventional angiography. If used, packing must be applied with caution, as overpacking has been associated with increased comorbidity.[17] Nasal packing should not be used when the dura has already been opened, because blood can flow back into the subdural space.[14]

If the clinical condition allows it, an assessment of collateral cerebral circulation and occlusion balloon tests should be undertaken, to identify patients who would not tolerate ICA occlusion, benefitting instead from bypass surgery or endovascular covered stents.[18]

Furthermore, when managing tumors, the vasculature is habitually pushed to the periphery, or sometimes is embedded in the tumor capsule. In these cases, careful retraction is required to avoid vessel avulsion, with internal tumor debulking and extracapsular sharp dissection. Other strategies may also be considered, like preoperative embolization.

Another well-known complication is retrobulbar hematomas, which may occur if AEAs/PEAs are injured and retract into the retrobulbar space, resulting in rapid proptosis and high intraorbital pressure that could lead to optic nerve ischemia. If the pressure surpasses the capillary perfusion pressure (25 mm Hg), an emergency lateral canthotomy and cantholysis will relief the intraorbital pressure and save vision. An orbital decompression is an acceptable alternative, but it may lead to postoperative enophthalmos.

The presence of postoperative bleeding after an otherwise uncomplicated EEA is frequently self-limited and easy to control with topical vasoconstrictors, hemostatic biomaterials, or self-expanding sponges. Significant postoperative epistaxis is rare, but may arise from branches of the internal maxillary artery or the AEAs. The offending site should be cauterized or the vessel be clipped. Angiography and embolization are advisable for patients who are not surgical candidates, when injury to the ICA is suspected or when surgery cannot be performed expeditiously.

12.5.2 Cranial Nerve Injury

Cranial nerves do not readily tolerate manipulation; thus, the key strategy in the prevention of neural lesions depends almost entirely on an appropriate selection of cases where the required corridor does not cross the path of a cranial nerve, and a surgical technique that avoids undue traction on the nerves. Thermal injury from any powered device is also a concern. This may occur from extensive drilling alongside the nerves, or the use of electrocautery adjacent to these structures. Regular and profuse irrigation may help reduce thermal injury. Olfactory impairment has been discussed previously in this chapter.[19] Orbital complications, such as ophthalmoplegia, diplopia, or even vision loss, may be a consequence of cranial nerve disruption, damage to the extraocular muscles, and postoperative edema. Intraoperative monitoring using electromyography is useful to identify and avoid injury to cranial nerves III to VII and IX to XII.

In patients presenting with severe visual impairment before surgery, blood pressure must be maintained at a minimum MAP of 85 mm Hg to avoid further ischemia of the optic nerves.[20] This precautionary measure may be applied to any cranial nerve affected by compression. Caution must be exercised when using nasal packing (especially Foley balloons) after decompression of optic canals, as they can transmit pressure and cause visual deterioration due to optic nerve ischemia.[21] Any delayed postoperative neurological deficit demands careful evaluation.

12.5.3 Cerebrospinal Fluid Fistulas

CSF leaks are the most frequent major complication of EEA; however, the increase in surgical experience and the adoption of multilayered techniques with vascularized tissue flaps for the reconstruction of skull base defects have decreased their incidence to less than 5%.[14] A combination of good intraoperative reconstructive techniques coupled with vigilant postoperative care is of utmost importance for their prevention. Patients must be instructed to avoid any activity that may increase their intracranial pressure (e.g., lifting, straining) or nose blowing. A lumbar spinal drain is only considered in some patients at high risk for failure of closure such as those with high-flow leaks, previous radiotherapy, or recurrent CSF leaks.

If present, a CSF leak may not be evident in the early postoperative period, but the patient may manifest some early clinical clues such as salty taste in the throat, the presence of an increasing pneumocephalus on imaging, or clear fluid leaking through the nasal packing. If detected, the patient must be taken back to the operating room for immediate repair, usually requiring repositioning of the flap or augmentation with a fascial or fat graft.

12.5.4 Postoperative Infection

After surgery, normal saline irrigations are indicated to promote nasal hygiene and diminish crusting, which in association with interruption of airflow and tissue edema may lead to excessive bacterial growth and possible local infection. Intracranial infections such as meningitis or brain abscesses are fortunately rare, with an estimated incidence of 1.8% and more commonly seen in the presence of a CSF fistula (odds ratio [OR]: 12.99; $p < 0.001$) or a CSF shunt (OR: 6.38; $p = 0.005$). Their treatment requires IV antibiotics, surgical drainage, and repair of the fistula.[21]

12.5.5 Other Complications

Complications such as subarachnoid bleeding, tension pneumocephalus, stroke, and scalp necrosis (after reconstruction with a galeal or galeopericranial flap) are extremely rare. immediate CT after surgery helps detect these before they become clinically evident.

Local nasal morbidities such as crusting and hypoesthesias usually resolve within 6 months after the surgical procedure.[22,23] In order to avoid synechiae, it is preferably to use nasal splints until the seventh postoperative day.

Overall, the most significant development supporting the prevention of complications in EEA has been the establishment of a multidisciplinary surgical team, working synergistically to enhance technical efficiency and the quality of surgical decisions.[24]

References

[1] Kassam A, Snyderman CH, Mintz A, Gardner P, Carrau RL. Expanded endonasal approach: the rostrocaudal axis. Part I. Crista galli to the sella turcica. Neurosurg Focus. 2005; 19(1):E3

[2] Kassam A, Snyderman CH, Mintz A, Gardner P, Carrau RL. Expanded endonasal approach: the rostrocaudal axis. Part II. Posterior clinoids to the foramen magnum. Neurosurg Focus. 2005; 19(1):E4

[3] Kassam AB, Gardner P, Snyderman C, Mintz A, Carrau R. Expanded endonasal approach: fully endoscopic, completely transnasal approach to the middle third of the clivus, petrous bone, middle cranial fossa, and infratemporal fossa. Neurosurg Focus. 2005; 19(1):E6

[4] Dhandapani S, Negm HM, Cohen S, Anand VK, Schwartz TH. Endonasal endoscopic transsphenoidal resection of tuberculum sella meningioma with anterior cerebral artery encasement. Cureus. 2015; 7 (8):e311

[5] Bhatki AM, Carrau RL, Snyderman CH, Prevedello DM, Gardner PA, Kassam AB. Endonasal surgery of the ventral skull base: endoscopic transcranial surgery. Oral Maxillofac Surg Clin North Am. 2010; 22 (1):157–168

[6] Kasemsiri P, Carrau RL, Prevedello DM, Otto B, Ditzel L. Principles of anterior skull base resection: open and endoscopic techniques. Oper Tech Otolaryngol Head Neck Surg. 2013; 24(4):197–207

[7] Ong YK, Solares CA, Carrau RL, Snyderman CH, Snyderman CH. New developments in transnasal endoscopic surgery for malignancies of the sinonasal tract and adjacent skull base. Curr Opin Otolaryngol Head Neck Surg. 2010; 18(2):107–113

[8] Zanation AM, Snyderman CH, Carrau RL, Kassam AB, Gardner PA, Prevedello DM. Minimally invasive endoscopic pericranial flap: a new method for endonasal skull base reconstruction. Laryngoscope. 2009; 119(1):13–18

[9] Patel MR, Shah RN, Snyderman CH, et al. Pericranial flap for endoscopic anterior skull-base reconstruction: clinical outcomes and radioanatomic analysis of preoperative planning. Neurosurgery. 2010; 66(3):506–512, discussion 512

[10] Kassam A, Snyderman CH, Carrau RL, Gardner P, Mintz A. Endoneurosurgical hemostasis techniques: lessons learned from 400 cases. Neurosurg Focus. 2005; 19(1):E7

[11] Thongrong C, Kasemsiri P, Carrau RL, Bergese SD. Control of bleeding in endoscopic skull base surgery: current concepts to improve hemostasis. ISRN Surg. 2013; 2013:191543

[12] Gardner PA, Kassam AB, Rothfus WE, Snyderman CH, Carrau RL. Preoperative and intraoperative imaging for endoscopic endonasal approaches to the skull base. Otolaryngol Clin North Am. 2008; 41 (1):215–230, vii

[13] Chin OY, Ghosh R, Fang CH, Baredes S, Liu JK, Eloy JA. Internal carotid artery injury in endoscopic endonasal surgery: a systematic review. Laryngoscope. 2016; 126(3):582–590

[14] Valentine R, Boase S, Jervis-Bardy J, Dones Cabral JD, Robinson S, Wormald PJ. The efficacy of hemostatic techniques in the sheep model of carotid artery injury. Int Forum Allergy Rhinol. 2011; 1 (2):118–122

[15] Solares CA, Ong YK, Carrau RL, et al. Prevention and management of vascular injuries in endoscopic surgery of the sinonasal tract and skull base. Otolaryngol Clin North Am. 2010; 43(4):817–825

[16] Rajiv S, Rodgers S, Bassiouni A, Vreugde S, Wormald PJ. Role of crushed skeletal muscle extract in hemostasis. Int Forum Allergy Rhinol. 2015; 5(5):431–434

[17] Raymond J, Hardy J, Czepko R, Roy D. Arterial injuries in transsphenoidal surgery for pituitary adenoma; the role of angiography and endovascular treatment. AJNR Am J Neuroradiol. 1997; 18(4):655-665

[18] Kim BM, Jeon P, Kim DJ, Kim DI, Suh SH, Park KY. Jostent covered stent placement for emergency reconstruction of a ruptured internal carotid artery during or after transsphenoidal surgery. J Neurosurg. 2015; 122(5):1223–1228

[19] Kassam AB, Prevedello DM, Carrau RL, et al. Endoscopic endonasal skull base surgery: analysis of complications in the authors' initial 800 patients. J Neurosurg. 2011; 114(6):1544–1568

[20] Ditzel Filho L, de Lara D, Prevedello DM, et al. Expanded endonasal approaches to the anterior skull base: a review. Otorhinolaryngology Clinics: An International Journal.. 2011; 3(3):176–183

[21] Kono Y, Prevedello DM, Snyderman CH, et al. One thousand endoscopic skull base surgical procedures demystifying the infection potential: incidence and description of postoperative meningitis and brain abscesses. Infect Control Hosp Epidemiol. 2011; 32(1):77–83

[22] Pant H, Bhatki AM, Snyderman CH, et al. Quality of life following endonasal skull base surgery. Skull Base. 2010; 20(1):35–40

[23] de Almeida JR, Snyderman CH, Gardner PA, Carrau RL, Vescan AD. Nasal morbidity following endoscopic skull base surgery: a prospective cohort study. Head Neck. 2011; 33(4):547–551

[24] Snyderman CH, Pant H, Carrau RL, Prevedello D, Gardner P, Kassam AB. What are the limits of endoscopic sinus surgery?: the expanded endonasal approach to the skull base. Keio J Med. 2009; 58(3):152–160

13 Revision Endoscopic Frontal Sinus Surgery

Salil Nair and Peter John Wormald

Abstract

Revision endoscopic frontal sinus surgery for recurrent or persistent sinus disease is a significant challenge owing to the close proximity of vital structures, the complexity of the frontal sinus outflow tract, and the predilection in the frontal recess for scarring and stenosis. This chapter aims to provide a stepwise guide on how to approach such patients, including identifying predisposing factors that may predict poorer outcomes. We examine the indications for surgery and discuss the importance of patient selection. Using careful analysis of the imaging available, one should be able to assess the complexity of each case and formulate a surgical plan that best suits the case scenario to achieve the optimal results. An up-to-date stepwise surgical approach to the frontal sinus, with key steps highlighted, will be used to tackle various scenarios. The chapter will specifically cover the axillary flap technique, mini-frontal sinus trephination and the frontal drillout procedure (also known as the grade 6 extent of frontal sinus surgery, endoscopic modified Lothrop, or Draf III). With this approach and an aggressive postoperative regimen of debridement, excellent results can be achieved when managing this difficult clinical problem.

Keywords: frontal sinus, endoscopic revision surgery, modified Lothrop, drillout, Draf, EFSS grade 6, mini-trephine, axillary flap

13.1 Introduction

In endoscopic sinus surgery, the management of the frontal sinus remains a challenge. This is in part due to the complex and variable anatomy, the narrow confines, and difficult angles in which to manipulate instruments. The frontal ostium, with its recess below, is situated behind the frontal beak, bound medially by the middle turbinate and olfactory fossa and laterally by the lamina papyracea.

These technical and anatomical issues are amplified in revision endoscopic frontal sinus surgery, where normal landmarks may be absent or distorted. Other factors that influence surgical complexity include the extent of polyp disease, increased vascularity, scarring, and the presence of neo-osteogenesis.[1,2]

Primary endoscopic frontal sinus surgery has a long-term success rate, defined as a patent frontal ostium, of over 90% in the best tertiary rhinology centers.[3] Patients requiring revision frontal sinus surgery are a subset of patients with advanced or poorly controlled disease often with a narrow frontal ostium. This may represent recurrent, persistent, or iatrogenic disease. The key to successful revision endoscopic frontal sinus surgery is careful patient selection, preoperative planning, and appropriate trial of medical therapy. In addition, a thorough knowledge of the anatomy, appropriate surgical skill, and choice of the right surgical approach are important. A meticulous attention to detail, using mucosal sparing techniques, and careful postoperative care are clearly important in minimizing scarring and adhesion formation.[4]

13.2 Indications

A number of factors may predispose a particular patient to revision frontal sinus surgery (▶ Table 13.1). These may be related to the disease process, the previous surgery, or the underlying anatomy. The initial complexity of the frontal sinus anatomy is an important factor. In an attempt to better categorize and anticipate the complexity of frontal sinus surgery, a classification has recently been proposed—the International Classification of Complexity (ICC; ▶ Table 13.2).[5]

Additional factors identified as important causes of failure include persistent mucosal disease (polyps and mucosal edema), retained cells due to incomplete dissection, adhesions, and neo-osteogenesis.[6]

Table 13.1 Factors that may predispose to failure in frontal sinus surgery

Surgical (iatrogenic)	Anatomical	Pathological
Scarring and adhesions in the frontal recess	Narrow AP diameter of the frontal ostium	Persistent mucosal edema within the frontal recess (CRSsNP)
Lateralized middle turbinate	A small or poorly pneumatized frontal sinus	Recurrent nasal polyps obstructing the frontal sinus (CRSwNP)
Retained cells: ethmoidal, agger nasi, and frontal cells	Prominent frontal cells (supra agger or supra bulla frontal cells)	Presence of neo-osteogenesis
Retained uncinated process		Extensive disease associated with asthma, aspirin sensitivity, and fungal disease

Abbreviations: AP, anteroposterior; CRSsNP, chronic rhinosinusitis without nasal polyps; CRSwNP, chronic rhinosinusitis with nasal polyps.

Table 13.2 The International classification of complexity of frontal sinus surgery

	Wide AP diameter (≥ 10 mm)	Narrow AP diameter (9–6 mm)	Very narrow AP diameter (≤ 5 mm)
Cells below ostium (AN, SAC, SBC)	Less complex (grade 1)	Moderate complexity (grade 2)	High complexity (grade 3)
Cells encroaching into the ostium (SAFC, SBFC, SOEC, FSC)	Moderate complexity (grade 2)	High complexity (grade 3)	Highest complexity (grade 4)
Cells extending significantly into the frontal sinus (SAFC, SBFC, SOEC, FSC)	High complexity (grade 3)	Highest complexity (grade 4)	Highest complexity (grade 4)

Abbreviations: AN, agger nasi; FSC, frontal septal cell; SAC, supra agger cell; SAFC, supra agger frontal cell; SBC, supra bulla cell; SBFC, supra bulla frontal cell; SOEC, supraorbital ethmoid cell.
Source: Data from Wormald et al.[5]
Note: AP refers to the frontal ostium anteroposterior diameter as measured from the frontal beak to the skull base at its narrowest distance on the parasagittal CT scan. Classification of the cells is in accordance to the International Frontal Sinus Classification.[30]

In a symptomatic patient who has completed a course of optimum medical therapy, indications for revision frontal sinus surgery include ongoing mucosal disease, incomplete dissection, lateralization of the middle turbinate, scarring and synechiae, and neo-osteogenesis, which are discussed in details in the following sections.

13.2.1 Ongoing Mucosal Disease

One of the major factors identified in patients undergoing revision frontal sinus surgery is inflammatory mucosal disease. Persistent or recurrent nasal polyps frequently obstruct the sinuses and are associated with high rates of symptom recurrence.[6] Risk factors for recurrence include eosinophilic mucin chronic rhinosinusitis (CRS) with polyps and patients with asthma and polyps.[7] The commonest site of recurrence of nasal polyps is the frontal recess and ostium (▶ Fig. 13.1). Mucosal inflammatory disease in the frontal recess, in the absence of anatomical reasons for obstruction, may require intensive medical treatment to control. However, studies suggest that more aggressive surgery such as a frontal sinus drillout may be useful in gaining better long-term disease control and improving patient outcomes.[8]

13.2.2 Incomplete Dissection

Retained sinus cells, incomplete uncinate resection, or septations in the frontal recess can impede drainage and exacerbate ongoing mucosal inflammation.[9,10] One of the most frequent findings is the presence of agger nasi cells, followed by supra agger, supra bulla, and supraorbital cells[6] (▶ Fig. 13.2a). A recent study suggested that, with the exception of mucosal disease, all identified causes of failure of frontal sinus surgery were as a result of surgical technique. The study highlights the importance of complete dissection in the frontal recess if this area is entered.[11]

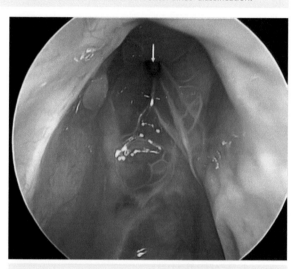

Fig. 13.1 Recurrent mucosal disease in the frontal recess. Edematous mucosa narrows the postoperative frontal ostium (*arrow*).

13.2.3 Lateralization of the Middle Turbinate

Whether partial resection of the middle turbinate predisposes to frontal sinusitis is unclear (▶ Fig. 13.2b). Although middle turbinate lateralization has not been shown to be associated with patient-reported symptoms, it may be associated with a more rapid need for revision surgery, possibly due to impaired drainage of the frontal sinus.[12] The incidence of lateralized middle turbinates in revision surgery is high (36–78%).[10,13] It is unlikely that middle turbinate lateralization alone would necessitate revision frontal sinusotomy, but it is often associated with scarring and retained cells.

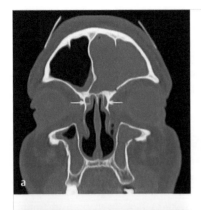
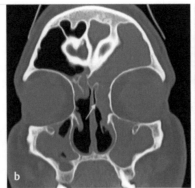
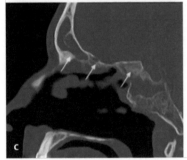

Fig. 13.2 Radiological findings associated with recurrent frontal sinus disease. **(a)** *White arrows* indicate bilateral retained agger nasi cells. **(b)** *White arrow* indicates an amputated middle turbinate with adhesions to the lateral nasal wall. **(c)** Neo-osteogenesis seen in the region of frontal ostium, skull base, and sphenoid (*white arrows*). Anteroposterior distance measured from the frontal beak to the skull base.

13.2.4 Scarring and Synechiae

Meticulous attention to detail can help minimize unnecessary trauma and subsequent scarring. Scar formation can occur as the result of mucosal trauma, exposed bone, persistent inflammatory disease, or retained air cells. To minimize this, one should adopt the all-or-nothing approach when considering surgery in the frontal recess. It is better to avoid any or partial manipulation in the frontal recess as adhesions are likely to form where residual cells are left in close proximity to each other. However, in some patients synechia and scarring, when present, may not always be symptomatic.[7,13]

13.2.5 Neo-Osteogenesis

Failure to preserve mucosa results in scarring and neo-osteogenesis.[14] This is poorly understood, but inflammation-induced osteoblastic activity in the periosteum leads to sclerotic bone formation[15] (▶ Fig. 13.2c). The incidence of neo-osteogenesis is higher in patients who have undergone sinus surgery. It may occur secondary to a combination of factors such as persistent mucosal inflammation, ongoing infection, and surgical trauma. The ongoing osteitis promotes mucosal inflammation and edema and may contribute to frontal recess stenosis.[16]

13.3 Patient Selection

When considering revision endoscopic frontal sinus surgery, patient selection is a critical step in optimizing outcomes. The key question is whether the patients' signs and symptoms are attributable to ongoing frontal sinus disease. A careful history and endoscopic examination should be performed. Underlying conditions that may have contributed to failure of the primary surgery need to be actively sought and managed. If necessary, investigations to exclude immunodeficiency, allergies, aspirin sensitivity, respiratory diseases (including asthma), granulomatous diseases, and disorders of ciliary function should be considered. Swabs of mucopus and debris from the nose should be submitted for both histological and microbiological analysis. The patient should be assessed in clinic with details of any previous sinus surgery and imaging available. A careful review of the imaging and operative records will help indicate whether one is dealing with recurrent, residual, or iatrogenic disease. Symptomatic disease, despite adequate surgery, should be managed by appropriate maximum medical therapy. This may consist of both topical and oral corticosteroids, saline irrigations, and culture directed antibiotics.[17,18]

As with primary surgery, one should be cautious when considering revision surgery where frontal pain is the predominant symptom. Symptoms of headache correlate poorly with CRS.[19,20] Not all patients who have disease within the frontal sinus are symptomatic. Conversely, frontal pain and headaches should not be considered the only surgical indication for revision endoscopic frontal sinusotomy. Mucosal disease in the frontal sinus without specific frontal symptoms can contribute to ongoing symptoms of CRS such as nasal obstruction, rhinorrhea, hyposmia, and postnasal drip. Symptom improvement following surgery may be attributable to resolution of pathological changes in any of the paranasal sinuses. Postsurgical stenosis of the frontal ostium correlates significantly with persistence of symptoms, infection, and polyp recurrence.[3]

13.4 Preoperative Planning

Once the decision has been made to progress to revision surgery, a careful analysis should be performed to identify the causes for the failure of the previous surgery. These are highlighted above. Apart from reviewing relevant previous imaging, a repeat CT imaging is required to study the anatomy and compare the studies to identify the extent of previous surgery.

Ideally, multiplanar CT imaging is used to reconstruct a three-dimensional (3D) image of the frontal sinus and recess. Axial images acquired at 0.625- to 1-mm sections are easily reformatted on a workstation to give sagittal and coronal views. There are a number of free software programs available for both Windows PC and MacIntosh platforms that allow image manipulation. Alternatively, the images can be loaded and studied on a surgical navigation platform if this is being used.

13.4.1 Analyzing the Computed Tomography Imaging

Prior to surgery, it is helpful to identify less favorable anatomical variations such as a narrow anteroposterior (AP) distance of the frontal sinus, a poorly pneumatized frontal sinus, extensive neo-osteogenesis, a prominent frontal beak, and extensive frontal cells, so that the appropriate surgical procedure can be planned. A narrow AP distance is best viewed on either the axial or the parasagittal view. It is defined as the distance from the frontal beak to the anterior projection of the skull base, and it gives the surgeon an indication of maneuverability in this area (▶ Fig. 13.2c).

Recognizing potential difficulties can aid the surgeon in counseling the patient regarding the potential success of the procedure, the need for additional surgery in the future, and the likelihood of a possible ancillary procedure such as a mini-trephine of the frontal sinus.

13.4.2 Computer-Assisted Navigation during Surgery

The use of surgical navigation during sinus surgery has increased as systems become increasingly more accurate and affordable. At present, image guidance systems are either optical (infrared) or electromagnetic (EM) based. The former uses light-emitting diodes (LEDs) attached to the patient via a headframe and on the instruments. EM systems utilize radiofrequency to track markers placed on the patient's head and within instruments used.

Navigation systems are particularly useful in revision sinus surgery where important landmarks such as the middle turbinate may be absent or significantly distorted. The ability to identify critical structures such as the orbit, skull base, and structures within the sphenoid in all three orthogonal planes is important to minimize complications.

13.4.3 Endoscopes and Equipment

Of all the sinuses, it is the frontal sinus that requires the most specialized equipment and instruments. Classically, angled endoscopes, 30, 45, and 70 degrees, with appropriate lens washing systems have been used in frontal sinus surgery. However, the more angled the scope, the greater the degree in difficulty of the dissection due to the use of increasingly angulated instruments. The axillary flap approach was designed to improve access to the frontal recess while using a 0-degree scope for as long as possible.[21] The aim was to reduce collateral damage and trauma to surrounding mucosa while providing better ergonomics. The key steps to the approach are described later. It is useful to have a range of angled (15, 40, and 70 degrees) cutting and diamond head drills with suction and irrigation incorporated. Fine giraffe cutting and noncutting forceps along with a set of Wormald frontal sinus malleable instruments (including a suction curette and frontal sinus probe; Integra, MicroFrance) are very useful. Additionally, Hajek-Koffler, Cobra, and Hosemann (Storz, Tuttlingen) frontal sinus punches should be available.

13.5 Choice of Procedure

The choice of surgical procedure used to manage recurrent frontal sinus disease will depend on a number of factors outlined (▶ Table 13.1). The surgeon needs to take into account the extent and completeness of the previous surgery, the anatomy of the frontal sinus, and the overall burden of disease. An assessment of the surgical complexity based on the anatomy alone is available in ▶ Table 13.2.

A variety of surgical approaches have been described. Procedures range from an anterior ethmoidectomy without manipulation of the frontal recess or frontal ostium to entire removal of the floor of the frontal sinus, frontal beak, and intersinus septum (▶ Table 13.3). While the former is rarely used in revision frontal sinus surgery, the latter is indicated to manage failure of less extensive approaches and is the final step in the endoscopic management algorithm.

The general principles of revision surgery are to complete a full ethmoidectomy, sphenoidotomy (if diseased or to identify the level of the skull base), and to remove osteitic bony partitions along the skull base and frontal recess. The aim is to maximize the frontal sinus opening without bone removal. The concept of when to enlarge

Table 13.3 Extent of frontal sinus surgery (EFSS)

Draf classification[22]	International classification of the extent of EFSS[30]	
	0: no bone or tissue removal. Balloon dilatation	No tissue removal
Draf I: ethmoidectomy and removal of cells below the frontal sinus	1: removal of cells in the frontal recess not directly obstructing the frontal ostium	Removal of cells
	2: removal of cells obstructing the ostium but not extending through the ostium	
Draf IIa: enlargement of the frontal ostium between the lamina papyracea and the middle turbinate	3: removal of cells extending through the frontal ostium (no widening of the frontal ostium)	
	4: removal of cells extending through the frontal ostium with enlargement of the ostium (bone removal, usually frontal beak)	Removal of bone
Draf IIb: enlargement of the frontal ostium from the LP and the nasal septum	5. Enlargement of the frontal ostium from the LP to the nasal septum	
Draf III: bilateral enlargement of the frontal ostia, resection of the superior nasal septum, floor of the frontal sinus, and intersinus septum	6. Bilateral enlargement of the frontal ostia into a common ostium, with resection of the superior nasal septum, intersinus septum, and floor of the frontal sinus	

Note: A comparison between the Draf frontal sinus surgery classification and a new proposed international classification of extent of frontal sinus surgery.

an ostium is controversial. Our philosophy is that if a drill is to be used to enlarge an ostium, one should consider performing a wide opening such as a frontal drillout, Draf III,[22] or a modified endoscopic Lothrop. Unilateral enlargement of a frontal ostium by removal of bone provokes an intense fibroblastic response that rapidly obstructs the neo-ostium, and any intraoperative gain in the size of the ostium is rapidly lost postoperatively. However, removal of bony cells, and septations with appropriate punches, is necessary to achieve the largest possible frontal ostium without the use of a bur. Drilling tends to stimulate an intense reaction within bone with fibrin deposition and a predisposition to postoperative scarring.[4]

13.6 Surgical Steps

Where the middle turbinate is present, an axillary flap may be used to aid access the frontal sinus.

13.6.1 The Axillary Flap Technique

- An incision is made 8 mm above and 8 mm anterior to the axilla of the middle turbinate using a no. 15 scalpel blade (see ▶ Fig. 13.3).
- The incision is then carried under the root of the middle turbinate.
- The mucosal flap is elevated using a suction Freer elevator ensuring that the inferior edge of the flap is freed from the axilla of the middle turbinate by using a sickle knife.

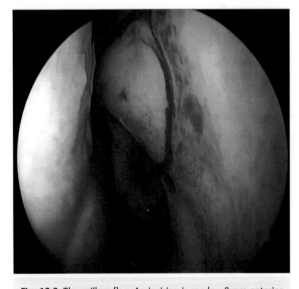

Fig. 13.3 The axillary flap. An incision is made ~8 mm anterior and superior to the attachment of the middle turbinate (MT) on the lateral nasal wall (LW).

- The flap is then tucked away between the middle turbinate and septum using the tip of the sickle knife.
- A Hajek-Koffler punch is used to remove the bone of the axilla of the middle turbinate, which corresponds to the anterior wall of the agger nasi cell.
- Bone removal will be dictated by the degree of pneumatization of the agger nasi cell. More extensive bone removal allows better access to the frontal recess.

- Once the agger nasi is exposed and identified, the 3D anatomy of the frontal recess pathway should be confirmed by reviewing the CT imaging.
- Once the frontal ostium has been cleared of any obstructing cells, the flap can be folded back to cover the exposed bone of the middle turbinate and residual anterior wall of the agger nasi cell.

13.6.2 Frontal Sinus Mini-Trephine

A modified frontal trephine technique, the mini-trephine (Medtronic, Jacksonville, Florida) is useful when the natural frontal drainage pathway is not easily visible. Cannulas are placed, through the anterior table, into the sinus and irrigated with fluorescein-stained saline. This fluorescein-stained pathway can then be followed with a probe to aid dissection and identify the natural drainage pathway.

Prior to placing the mini-trephine, the CT imaging is reviewed to check the presence, size, and depth of the frontal sinus. After local anesthetic injection, a stab incision is made in the medial aspect of the eyebrow or in a frown crease line. It is important not to place the incision too high and to keep the incision along an imaginary line joining the medial ends of the eyebrows corresponding to the supraorbital ridge. The CT scan will confirm that the sinus is sufficiently pneumatized above this rim for safe penetration. If not, the incision can be lowered.

- The incision is made 1 to 1.5 cm from the midpoint along the imaginary line. The landmarks are depicted in ▶ Fig. 13.4.
- Gently widen the incision with a pair of Iris scissors.
- Place the drill guide through the incision ensuring that skin is not trapped and that the guide teeth sit flush on the anterior table. This may require some adjustment of the guide.
- Ensure that once drilling commences, the drill bit is withdrawn entirely each time it comes in contact with the bone so that the end may be directly irrigated. Constant irrigation is required to prevent the bur from heating up and burning both the skin and the bone.
- The trephine bur is 11 mm in length and is designed not to penetrate the posterior table of the frontal sinus.
- As the bur enters the sinus, there is a characteristic "give." Remove the bur and place the guidewire through the guide. Holding the guidewire in place, withdraw the guide.
- Railroad the cannula over the guidewire and remove the guide. Ensure the cannula is secure.
- Using a 10-mL syringe with only 2 to 3 mL of saline, aspirate to ensure correct placement of the cannula.

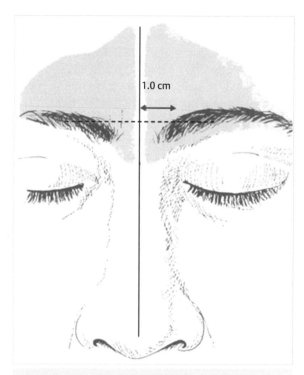

Fig. 13.4 Landmarks for the frontal sinus mini-trephine. A vertical incision can be hidden within the eyebrow line or in a forehead crease just medial to the eyebrow.

Aspiration should yield air, pus, mucus, or blood. Clear fluid indicates intracranial penetration. The trephine should be removed and the wound sutured.

- Initial irrigation can be with saline. Following confirmation, fluorescein-stained saline can be used.
- Prior to irrigation, be cautious when a dehiscence of the orbit or posterior table of the frontal sinus is present. Complications such as intracranial penetration with cerebrospinal fluid (CSF) leak, periorbital trauma, and incision-related infection have been reported.[23,24,25]
- If the cannulas are removed and not kept in for postoperative irrigation, the wound is closed with a Steri-strip applied.

Reasons for failure to aspirate and appropriate solution are as follows:

- Incomplete penetration of the anterior table of the frontal sinus—reposition the cannula (never superiorly —always inferiorly).
- Contents of the sinus are too thick to be aspirated— instill 1 mL of saline and reaspirate.

- The cannula is through the anterior table bone but remains submucosal in the sinus—reposition the cannula.
- The cannula is blocked—remove the cannula, flush, and try again.

13.7 Specific Scenarios

13.7.1 Retained Cells in the Frontal Recess or Extending into the Frontal Sinus (Draf I or International Classification of Extent of Endoscopic Frontal Sinus Surgery Grades 1–3)

Retained cells due to incomplete surgery are a common anatomical cause for revision frontal sinus surgery. These include a retained agger nasi cell, superior uncinate process, cap of the ethmoid bulla, or a lateralized middle turbinate remnant.[6,11]

- Neuropatties soaked in a solution of adrenaline, cocaine, and saline are placed in the middle meatus, along the middle and inferior turbinate posteriorly.
- Local anesthetic is injected into the axilla of the middle turbinate and the lateral attachment of the middle turbinate.
- Using a double-ended ball probe any residual uncinate is fractured medially and removed with a 45-degree through-cutting Blakesley forceps (Storz).
- The maxillary antrostomy is inspected with a 30-degree angled endoscope.
- In revision cases where the anterior ethmoidal cells have been partially or completely removed, 3D reconstruction of the frontal anatomy is not possible. In these cases, the junction between the horizontal and vertical ground lamella of the middle turbinate is identified.
- This is punctured in the inferomedial corner, and staying medial, the endoscope is advanced to identify the superior turbinate.
- The natural ostium of the sphenoid lies medial to the lower third of the superior turbinate.
- The sphenoid can be opened medially initially along the nasal septum and floor until the roof is identified.
- A revision ethmoidectomy is performed using the roof of the sphenoid as a guide to the skull base.
- An axillary flap, as described earlier, is performed. Using a frontal sinus suction curette, the frontal ostium is identified by walking the curette along the skull base and into the frontal ostium. The drainage pathway is confirmed. Any remaining or obstructing cells can be gently removed. The bone fragments are removed with giraffe forceps or debrided.
- The frontal sinus ostium must be visualized.

13.7.2 A Narrow Frontal Ostium and/or Extensive Supra Agger/Bulla Frontal Cells, or Ongoing Significant Burden of Disease (CRSwNP, Aspirin-Sensitive Asthma, Allergic Fungal Disease [Draf III/EFSS 6])

Studies suggest that there is a higher rate of failure in primary frontal sinus surgery when the ostium is less than 5 mm in maximum dimension.[3] The size of the natural frontal ostium is even more critical in revision surgery. Patients who have undergone a good clearance of their frontal recess and exposure of the natural frontal ostium and have a disease recurrence are best managed with a frontal drillout/Draf III/extent of endoscopic frontal sinus surgery (EFSS) 6 procedure.

- Preoperative preparation of the nose is the same as for the patients discussed earlier.
- In order to define the skull base, frontal sinus minitrephines are placed as described earlier. The fluorescein-stained saline marks the posterior limit of the dissection. As long as the dissection is anterior and lateral to the Fluorescein, the skull base should be safe. This should be augmented with regular use of image guidance. Alternatively, image guidance alone can be used regularly throughout the case to define the position of the skull base.
- The first step is to create a septal window. The landmarks for the septal window are posteriorly the middle turbinate, superiorly the roof of the nose, inferiorly so an instrument can be placed over the lower edge of the septal window, and under the axilla of the middle turbinate on the opposite side of the nose. The anterior landmark is so that 1 cm of frontal process of the maxilla anterior to the middle turbinate can be seen with a 0-degree scope through the septal window on the opposite side of the nose (▶ Fig. 13.5).
- To create the septal window, the mucosa overlying the septum between these landmarks is harvested. This free graft is taken in a submucosal plane rather than in the subperiosteal plane (▶ Fig. 13.6). We have found that the take rate for submucosal grafts is better than that for subperiosteal grafts.

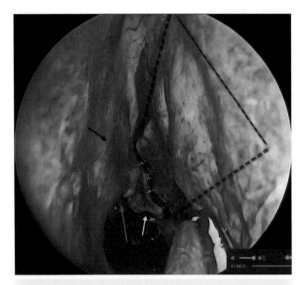

Fig. 13.5 The *white arrow* indicates the middle turbinate, which is the posterior landmark for the septal window. The *red arrow* indicates the axilla—the scalpel blade makes the inferior incision for the septal window along the *black dotted line*—this is ~5 mm below the axilla and forms the inferior landmark for the septal window. The *superior dotted line* indicates the superior incision as high as possible on the septum and the *anterior dotted line* indicates the vertical incision that marks the anterior limit of the septal window allowing the frontal process of the maxilla of the opposite nasal cavity to be seen. The *black arrow* marks the frontal process of the maxilla on the right side.

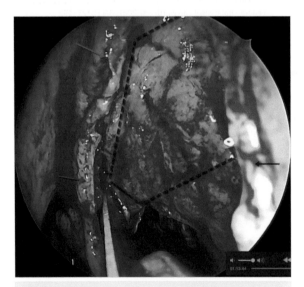

Fig. 13.7 The posterior edge of the septal window is marked by the *blue arrow* and the anterior edge by the *black arrow*. The *red arrow* indicates the superior edge. The scalpel makes the incisions for the anterior-based pedicled flap on the frontal process of the maxilla (*black dotted line*).

- Next, anterior-based pedicled flaps are created and rolled back toward the nasal vestibule. Initial incisions are made through the septal window (▶ Fig. 13.7). The

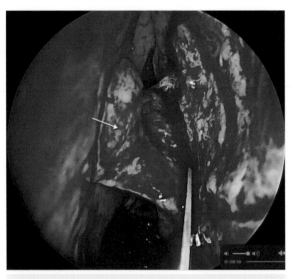

Fig. 13.6 The free mucosal graft (*white arrow*) is harvested from the area of the septal window in a plane above the perichondrial layer. This gives a thin graft that takes better on exposed bone.

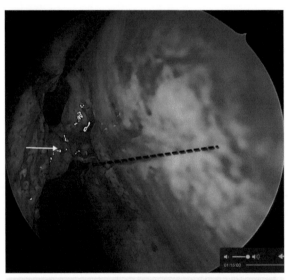

Fig. 13.8 The scope is placed on the same side as the pedicled flap and the initial rolled flap (*white arrow*) is seen. *Black dotted lines* mark out further scalpel incisions to allow this flap to be rolled far enough anteriorly that it is no longer in the surgical field.

scope is then placed on the ipsilateral side and the incisions continued anteriorly allowing the flaps to be rolled anteriorly (▶ Fig. 13.8). These are used at the end of the procedure to give mucosal covering to the bone forming the frontal neo-ostium.

- Using a zero endoscope and working from the right nostril across the septal window onto the left side, the bone of the frontal process of the maxilla is drilled away until the underlying skin is exposed (▶ Fig. 13.9). Initially, drill laterally and then superiorly. The frontal ostium is the landmark guiding this drilling with bone

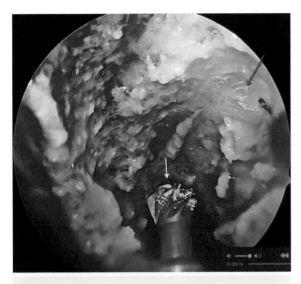

Fig. 13.9 Drilling is performed with a 0-degree endoscope starting in the axilla (*white arrow*) and in proceeding laterally until a small area of skin (*red arrow*) is exposed.

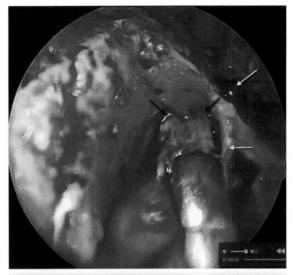

Fig. 13.10 The *black arrows* indicate the olfactory neurons, the *white arrow* the frontal ostium, and the *yellow arrow* the middle turbinate.

removal directly above and lateral to the natural ostium at all times.

- This is continued until the level of the first olfactory neuron (▶ Fig. 13.10). The first olfactory neuron is identified by pushing back the cut edge of the mucosa from the posterior edge of the septal window until the neuron can be seen tenting down from the skull base.
- Once the dissection has proceeded to the point where the bone removal around the new frontal ostium is above this olfactory neuron, the dissection can be brought medially anterior to the skull base (▶ Fig. 13.11).
- This is done on both sides and the two sides are joined up forming a new frontal ostium.
- Next, the frontal T formed by the middle turbinates and septum is lowered onto the first olfactory neuron. Regular checking with image guidance is required to ensure that the anteriorly projecting skull base is protected (▶ Fig. 13.12).
- Now the endoscope is changed to a 30-degree scope and using an angled bur the anterior lip of the frontal neo-ostium is removed until the anterior wall of the frontal sinus runs smoothly out into the nasal cavity without any lip (▶ Fig. 13.13).
- The pedicled free flaps are rolled back into the neo-ostium and any remaining exposed bone covered with the free flaps. No stents or packing is put in place. If mini-trephines had been placed, they are now removed (▶ Fig. 13.14).
- Nasal douches are commenced the following day with follow-up in 2 weeks in outpatients.

13.8 Tips and Tricks

- Although headaches may be one of the symptoms associated with recurrent frontal sinus disease, one should be cautious in offering surgery when this is the only complaint.
- Careful postoperative care, including medical management, with topical and, if necessary systemic steroids, and meticulous debridement, is necessary to maintain patency of the frontal sinus opening.
- Multiplanar CT is essential in reconstructing a 3D image of the anatomy of the frontal recess.
- When assessing the complexity, pay particular attention on the CT imaging to the thickness of the frontal beak (coronal and sagittal views), the anteroposterior dimension of the frontal ostium (axial and sagittal views), and accessory cells extending into the frontal sinus (coronal and parasagittal views).
- Total intravenous anesthesia maintaining hypotensive, bradycardic (< 60 hear rate)[26] parameters is essential in optimizing the best surgical field.

13.9 Case Example

This patient is a 55-year-old man who presents with a history of nasal polyps and having undergone two previous surgeries at other centers (*white arrow* on the parasagittal scan in ▶ Fig. 13.15). He has significant nasal obstruction post nasal discharge and recurrent infections. He complains of a constant fullness and pressure over his frontal sinuses, which become very painful during

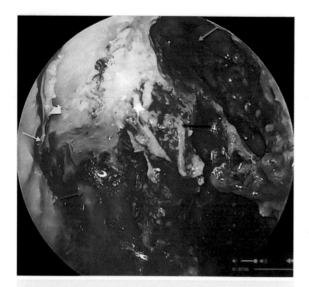

Fig. 13.11 The *black arrow* indicates the frontal T, while the *red arrow* indicates the fluorescein-stained saline marking the frontal ostium and posterior limit of the dissection. The *yellow arrow* indicates skin exposed on the right side. Note how the left dissection (*green arrow*) has being brought medially over the olfactory neurons and frontal T.

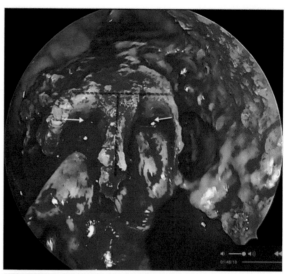

Fig. 13.12 The *white arrows* indicate the olfactory neurons and the *dotted black line* indicates the frontal T.

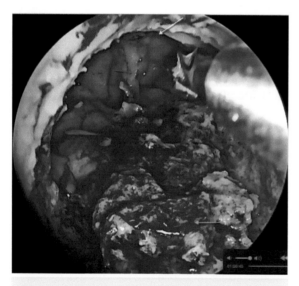

Fig. 13.13 The anterior lip of the frontal ostium is lowered (*white arrow*). The intersinus septum (*red arrow*) has being taken right to the top of the sinus. The *green arrow* indicates the frontal T. This dissection maximizes the frontal ostium.

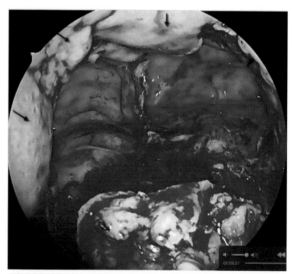

Fig. 13.14 The flaps lining the frontal neo-ostium are indicated by the *black arrows*. The central (12 o'clock position) and right (10 o'clock position) *arrows* indicate the free mucosal grafts, while the remaining grafts are pedicled grafts.

infections. On endoscopy, his nose was full of polyps on the left (*red arrow* on the parasagittal CT in ▶ Fig. 13.15). He had adhesions on the right side with discharge in the nasal cavity. The frontal recesses on both sides appeared completely blocked with scar tissue. He underwent a full course of medical treatment and then had a CT scan of his sinuses (▶ Fig. 13.15). He has bilateral frontal septal cells with quite thick septations (crosshairs on ▶ Fig. 13.15). In addition, he has new bone formation on the right frontal recess (*black arrow* on the coronal CT in ▶ Fig. 13.15). As the patient has extensive polyposis, previous failed surgery with scar tissue obstructing the frontal ostia with new bone formation in the frontal recesses and obstructive frontal septal cells with thick septations, he is not

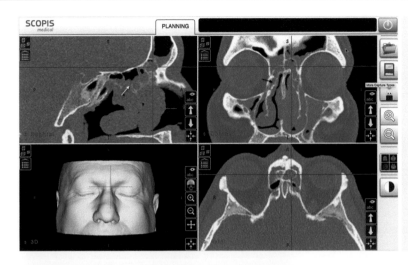

Fig. 13.15 The crosshairs indicate the frontal septal cell in all three planes. The *black arrow* in the coronal planes indicates neo-osteogenesis, while the *white arrow* on the parasagittal plane indicates previous ethmoid surgery and the *red arrow* the large nasal polyps.

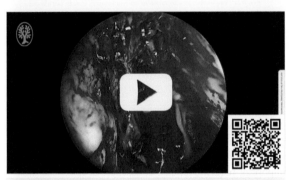

Video 13.1 Frontal drillout

suitable for a standard revision sinus surgery. The failure rate for a further standard functional endoscopic sinus surgery (FESS) would be unacceptably high. He underwent a frontal drillout (EFSS 6, Draf III, or modified Lothrop). Video 13.1 demonstrates the surgical steps for this procedure. He is now 2 years postsurgery and has a healthy clean cavity with patent sinus ostia for all his sinuses and his frontal ostium measures 20 × 18 mm.

13.10 Complications: Management

The major complications that can result from revision frontal sinus surgery include scarring and restenosis, trauma to the anterior ethmoidal artery, orbital penetration, and damage to the skull base with CSF leak.

13.10.1 Scarring and Restenosis

The narrow confines of the frontal recess predispose this area to scarring and adhesion formation. To minimize this, one needs to pay particular attention to mucosal preservation with avoidance of circumferential mucosal stripping. The use of a curved Rad 60-degree debrider

blade (Medtronic, ENT) and through-cutting instruments can reduce the risk of mucosal loss. Controlling intraoperative hemostasis and a regime of careful postoperative debridement are helpful in reducing adhesion formation. The use of chitosan gel as a dressing has demonstrated promising results in reducing postoperative ostial stenosis and may have a role in the future.[27]

13.10.2 Anterior Ethmoid Artery

The anterior ethmoidal artery usually lies one cell posterior to the frontal ostium on the skull base. It is more likely to lie in a mesentery if the lateral lamella of the cribriform plate is deep (>4 mm) or in the presence of supraorbital ethmoid cells.[28] This can be identified prior to surgery by reviewing the CT images carefully. The artery can be identified intraoperatively by finding the frontal ostium and by carefully dissecting posterior to this using a malleable suction curette. It is most often located just posterior to the ethmoid bulla lamella on the skull base. Alternatively, by identifying the roof of the sphenoid (the lowest part of the anterior skull base), one can carefully dissect anteriorly toward the frontal ostium. Using a suction curette, in between the skull base septations, it is possible to gently remove diseased mucosa. The artery can be visualized traversing the skull base in its characteristic posterolateral-to-anteromedial path in the roof of the ethmoid.

If the anterior ethmoid artery (AEA) is injured during the surgery, it can usually be managed by initially placing a surgical neuropattie with a topical vasoconstrictor agent over it to aid hemostasis and visualization. Using suction bipolar forceps, the artery can be cauterized. Suction monopolar cautery should be used with extreme caution as it may penetrate the skull base, resulting in a CSF leak. A transected artery may retract into the orbit causing an orbital hematoma. This will require an emergency decompression of the orbit.

13.10.3 Orbital Injury

Fracture of the lamina papyracea can occur while dissecting in the frontal recess. This may be minor with little consequence. However, if the periorbita is breached, periorbital fat may prolapse into the surgical field, making further dissection difficult and hazardous. In experienced hands, one may be able to complete the dissection by avoiding manipulation of the fat or covering the exposed area with a small piece of silastic film. The decision as to whether to abandon the procedure or not will depend on the individual surgeon's experience and the amount of fat exposed.

13.10.4 Cerebrospinal Fluid Leak

Fracture through the lateral lamella of the cribriform plate or roof of the ethmoid can result in a CSF leak. A particularly vulnerable area is at the point where the AEA pierces the lateral lamella. Intraoperatively a CSF can be recognized by the "washout" sign. Observing an area where a CSF leak is suspected will reveal that the blood is diluted and constantly washed away. If a leak is confirmed, this will require a repair. Inform the anesthetist of the situation and cover the area with a surgical neuropattie to aid hemostasis and visualization. Review the imaging, which may help confirm the site of the leak. Most intraoperative CSF leaks are small and can be managed with a layered closure (using a free or pedicled mucosal graft) or a "bathplug" technique.[29] The site of the leak needs to be exposed by gently clearing away the mucosa to expose the defect. Judicious use of low-power bipolar cautery can help with hemostasis. Dural substitutes are rarely required, but fibrin glue is useful to secure the graft in place.

References

[1] Lund VJ, Stammberger H, Fokkens WJ, et al. European position paper on the anatomical terminology of the internal nose and paranasal sinuses. Rhinol Suppl. 2014; 24(24):1–34

[2] Wormald PJ. Endoscopic Sinus Surgery: Anatomy. Three Dimensional Reconstruction and Surgical Technique. 3rd ed. New York, NY: Thieme; 2012

[3] Naidoo Y, Wen D, Bassiouni A, Keen M, Wormald PJ. Long-term results after primary frontal sinus surgery. Int Forum Allergy Rhinol. 2012; 2(3):185–190

[4] Chiu AG, Goldstein GH, Kennedy DW. Revision endoscopic frontal sinus surgery. In: Kountakis SE, Senior BA, Draf W, eds. The Frontal Sinus. 2nd ed. Berlin: Springer-Verlag; 2016:301–314

[5] Wormald PJ, Bassiouni A, Callejas CA, et al. The International Classification of the radiological Complexity (ICC) of frontal recess and frontal sinus. Int Forum Allergy Rhinol. 2016

[6] Otto KJ, DelGaudio JM. Operative findings in the frontal recess at time of revision surgery. Am J Otolaryngol. 2010; 31(3):175–180

[7] Friedman M, Bliznikas D, Vidyasagar R, Joseph NJ, Landsberg R. Long-term results after endoscopic sinus surgery involving frontal recess dissection. Laryngoscope. 2006; 116(4):573–579

[8] Bassiouni A, Wormald PJ. Role of frontal sinus surgery in nasal polyp recurrence. Laryngoscope. 2013; 123(1):36–41

[9] Meyer TK, Kocak M, Smith MM, Smith TL. Coronal computed tomography analysis of frontal cells. Am J Rhinol. 2003; 17(3):163–168

[10] Chiu AG, Vaughan WC. Revision endoscopic frontal sinus surgery with surgical navigation. Otolaryngol Head Neck Surg. 2004; 130 (3):312–318

[11] Valdes CJ, Bogado M, Samaha M. Causes of failure in endoscopic frontal sinus surgery in chronic rhinosinusitis patients. Int Forum Allergy Rhinol. 2014; 4(6):502–506

[12] Bassiouni A, Chen PG, Naidoo Y, Wormald PJ. Clinical significance of middle turbinate lateralization after endoscopic sinus surgery. Laryngoscope. 2015; 125(1):36–41

[13] Musy PY, Kountakis SE. Anatomic findings in patients undergoing revision endoscopic sinus surgery. Am J Otolaryngol. 2004; 25 (6):418–422

[14] Ling FT, Kountakis SE. Important clinical symptoms in patients undergoing functional endoscopic sinus surgery for chronic rhinosinusitis. Laryngoscope. 2007; 117(6):1090–1093

[15] Kocak M, Smith TL, Smith MM. Bone involvement in chronic rhinosinusitis. Curr Opin Otolaryngol Head Neck Surg. 2002; 10:49–52

[16] Lee JT, Kennedy DW, Palmer JN, Feldman M, Chiu AG. The incidence of concurrent osteitis in patients with chronic rhinosinusitis: a clinicopathological study. Am J Rhinol. 2006; 20(3):278–282

[17] Fokkens WJ, Lund VJ, Mullol J, et al. EPOS 2012: European position paper on rhinosinusitis and nasal polyps 2012. A summary for otorhinolaryngologists. Rhinology. 2012; 50(1):1–12

[18] Orlandi RR, Kingdom TT, Hwang PH, et al. International consensus statement on allergy and rhinology: rhinosinusitis. Int Forum Allergy Rhinol. 2016; 6 Suppl 1:S22–S209

[19] Lal D, Rounds AB, Rank MA, Divekar R. Clinical and 22-item Sino-Nasal Outcome Test symptom patterns in primary headache disorder patients presenting to otolaryngologists with "sinus" headaches, pain or pressure. Int Forum Allergy Rhinol. 2015; 5(5):408–416

[20] Jones NS. Sinus headaches: avoiding over- and mis-diagnosis. Expert Rev Neurother. 2009; 9(4):439–444

[21] Wormald PJ. The axillary flap approach to the frontal recess. Laryngoscope. 2002; 112(3):494–499

[22] Weber R, Draf W, Kratzsch B, Hosemann W, Schaefer SD. Modern concepts of frontal sinus surgery. Laryngoscope. 2001; 111(1):137–146

[23] Bartley J, Eagleton N, Rosser P, Al-Ali S. Superior oblique muscle palsy after frontal sinus mini-trephine. Am J Otolaryngol. 2012; 33(1):181–183

[24] Lee AS, Schaitkin BM, Gillman GS. Evaluating the safety of frontal sinus trephination. Laryngoscope. 2010; 120(3):639–642

[25] Seiberling K, Jardeleza C, Wormald PJ. Minitrephination of the frontal sinus: indications and uses in today's era of sinus surgery. Am J Rhinol Allergy. 2009; 23(2):229–231

[26] Nair S, Collins M, Hung P, Rees G, Close D, Wormald PJ. The effect of beta-blocker premedication on the surgical field during endoscopic sinus surgery. Laryngoscope. 2004; 114(6):1042–1046

[27] Ngoc Ha T, Valentine R, Moratti S, Robinson S, Hanton L, Wormald PJ. A blinded randomized controlled trial evaluating the efficacy of chitosan gel on ostial stenosis following endoscopic sinus surgery. Int Forum Allergy Rhinol. 2013; 3(7):573–580

[28] Floreani SR, Nair SB, Switajewski MC, Wormald PJ. Endoscopic anterior ethmoidal artery ligation: a cadaver study. Laryngoscope. 2006; 116(7):1263–1267

[29] Wormald PJ, McDonogh M. The bath-plug closure of anterior skull base cerebrospinal fluid leaks. Am J Rhinol. 2003; 17(5):299–305

[30] Wormald PJ, Hoseman W, Callejas C, et al. The International Frontal Sinus Anatomy Classification (IFAC) and classification of the extent of endoscopic frontal sinus surgery (EFSS). Int Forum Allergy Rhinol. 2016; 6(7):677–696

14 Complications of Frontal Sinus Surgery

David Morrissey and Alkis J. Psaltis

Abstract

The frontal sinus is an anatomically complex region in which to perform sinus surgery and presents a challenge to the sinus surgeon. It has a higher incidence of surgical complications when compared to other sinuses due to this complexity and the access difficulties it can present. This chapter describes in detail the potential complications associated with endoscopic approaches to the frontal sinus. It describes how these complications may occur along with the management and care necessary to address such complications. The frontal sinus surgeon should gain an appreciation of how to perform safe surgery in the frontal sinus region and develop an understanding of the relationship between good technique and safe surgery. This will help the surgeon to maximize frontal patency outcomes and minimize the risk of adverse outcomes. The complications discussed in this chapter include the immediate perioperative complications of cerebrospinal fluid leak, orbital injury, pain, hemorrhage and infection, as well as the more delayed postoperative complications of frontal stenosis and mucocele. Emphasis is placed on prevention of such complications through considered preoperative surgical planning and review of imaging, via the use of meticulous surgical technique and by employing a comprehensive approach to the postoperative management of the patient.

Keywords: frontal sinus, endoscopic sinus surgery, complication, pain, hemorrhage, infection, stenosis cerebrospinal fluid leak, mucocele, orbital injury

14.1 Introduction

Frontal sinus surgery is considered to be among the more technically demanding techniques employed during endoscopic sinus surgery.[1,2,3] This is due to its narrow confines, the possibility for significant variations in the cellular anatomy, and the close proximity to vital structures, such as the skull base, orbit, anterior ethmoid artery, and olfactory neurons. Successful frontal sinus surgery therefore requires a comprehensive understanding of the frontal recess anatomy, superb endoscopic visualization, appropriate instrumentation, and in some cases navigation systems to compliment the skills of the endoscopic sinus surgeon. Complications may occur with endoscopic approaches to the frontal sinus and their management is similarly complicated by the complex anatomy of the region.

14.2 Epidemiology and Etiology

Major complications from endoscopic sinus surgery have been estimated to occur in 0.20 to 0.40% of patients. The frontal sinus is more likely than all other sites to be the region of concern when a major complication occurs with an adjusted odds ratio of 1.53 to 2.14.[4] This is likely to reflect the increased complexity of endoscopic sinus surgery in the frontal sinus region. ▶ Table 14.1 summarizes the different incidence of frontal sinus complications according to the extent of frontal sinus surgery performed.

14.3 Specific Complications of Endoscopic Approaches to the Frontal Sinus

14.3.1 Failure to Accomplish the Specific Aim of the Procedure

Chronic rhinosinusitis with or without nasal polyposis is by far the most common reason to operate in the frontal sinus region, but other indications may include benign or malignant neoplasms as well as mucoceles. In some instances, endoscopic approaches to the frontal sinus can fail to achieve the desired surgical outcome. Indeed the presence of disease involving the frontal sinus at the time of the primary sinus procedure has been shown to be an independent risk factor for the need to have future revision sinus surgery.[5]

The nature of the surgical failure can be defined in a number of ways, but may include a failure to alleviate symptoms as expected, stenosis of the frontal sinus drainage pathway, recurrence of disease, or the need for further or revision surgery. It is important to recognize that procedural failure is by no means absolute and the above definitions provide an imperfect measure of failure.

Table 14.1 Incidence of endoscopic frontal sinus surgery complications

Complication	Incidence
Stenosis of the neo-ostium	8.2–10.0% Draf IIa (primary) 20.7% Draf IIa (revision) 35.9% unilateral drillout (Draf IIb) 5–32% in EMLP (Draf III) 21% in revision EMLP
Hemorrhage	1% standard sinus surgery 3.9% EMLP
CSF leak	1.9% EMLP
Infection	4.9% EMLP
Orbital injury	0.32%

Abbreviations: CSF, cerebrospinal fluid; EMLP, endoscopic modified Lothrop procedure.

There may be instances where the patient has experienced significant symptomatic improvements despite the development of a stenosis or the return of their original disease. In these situations, revision surgery may be indicated despite symptomatic improvements, in order to provide additional gains after primary surgery.

Multiple authors have described failure rates of specific endoscopic frontal sinus procedures. Draf IIa frontal sinusotomy fails as a primary procedure in 8.2 to 10%, while revision is less successful with a failure rate of 20.7%.[6,7] Draf IIb procedures have been reported to have an even higher failure rate of up to 35.9% of cases.[8] Draf III or endoscopic modified Lothrop procedure (EMLP) has a historically reported failure rate of up to 32%, but more recent series suggest a failure rate of around 8 to 10%.[1,6,8,9,10] Revision EMLP failures requiring further surgery occur in 21%.[11] It is important to recognize that failure of endoscopic frontal sinus surgery can also present many years after the original procedure and therefore the current literature may underestimate the true rate of long-term failure.[8]

Patient- and surgeon-related factors may influence frontal sinus surgical success. Naidoo et al demonstrated that the presence of multiple adverse patient and surgical factors increases the risk of failure in frontal sinus surgery.[6] The complexity of the individual's anatomy can increase the difficulty of the surgery and limit the ability of the surgeon to access and address the pathology. The inherent nature of the condition being addressed may also increase the chance of disease recurrence and need for further surgery. Underlying systemic medical conditions may adversely influence wound healing or be associated with an increased risk of postoperative infection and consequent scarring. Bleeding diathesis or the need for continued anticoagulation intraoperatively can increase intraoperative bleeding and impair surgical visualization. Compliance with postoperative care can also impact on the success of the surgery, if clots and debris are not removed in the postoperative period.

Factors pertaining to the surgeons themselves can also influence postoperative outcomes. Surgical experience and appropriate frontal sinus surgical training is a particularly important determinant in ensuring success when operating in this region. Surgical decision-making and consequent choice of endoscopic approach can influence the access and ultimate success of the surgery as well as the possible complications encountered. Critical to success in frontal sinus surgery is adequate visualization. Therefore, techniques aimed at minimizing bleeding and improving hemostasis are essential. Meticulous tissue handling and avoidance of mucosal stripping and tissue trauma are likely to not only minimize bleeding but also significantly impact on long-term postoperative outcomes.

The development of technical skills and an understanding of the frontal sinus anatomy can be attained via adequate frontal sinus training during residency and through undertaking postresidency sinus surgery courses. This enables the surgeon to form an intimate and comprehensive knowledge of frontal sinus anatomy and the possible variations that may be encountered. The use of preoperative planning software and intraoperative image guidance may further improve a surgeon's appreciation of the relevant frontal anatomy enabling a complete and atraumatic dissection of the frontal recess. It should be noted, however, that such navigational tools are never a substitute for anatomical knowledge and that the data examining the impact of navigation tools upon the incidence of complications in sinus surgery are conflicting.[4,12] Navigation tools are typically utilized when more complex cases are undertaken, which may also confound the research outcomes.

Prior to undertaking endoscopic approaches to the frontal sinus patient comorbidities should be addressed, with optimization of the patient's health status prior to surgery. Unnecessary medications that increase the risk of bleeding should be discontinued and the need for anticoagulant medications should be rationalized on a case-by-case basis. Infections should be detected early and treated appropriately. The use of perioperative corticosteroids may reduce inflammation and the risk of bleeding intraoperatively while also improving wound healing postoperatively. Intraoperative management of blood pressure and pulse rate have been shown to be important factors in improving the surgical field and ultimately influence long-term outcomes.[13,14,15]

Where endoscopic approaches to the frontal sinus do fail, the operating surgeon can often reflect upon the case and identify factors that may have contributed. The authors routinely record their procedures, which enables cases to be reviewed retrospectively. Such a habit enables the surgeon to identify technical and intraoperative factors that may have contributed to a less optimal outcome, in some instances many years after the initial surgery.

Some of the more common technique errors that may contribute to surgical failure include poor tissue handling with consequent mucosal stripping and wide exposure of bone. This leads to prolonged healing and is thought to contribute to stenosis and neo-osteogenesis. Similarly, incomplete clearance of cells in the frontoethmoidal region will narrow the surgically created ostium and where the frontal ostium diameter is less than 4 mm, it leaves the sinus more likely to stenose[6,9] (▶ Fig. 14.1). Creating surgical ostia with maximal dimensions is important in reducing the chance of a postoperative surgical stenosis. Middle turbinate lateralization (▶ Fig. 14.2a, b) can lead to obstruction of the frontal sinus outflow tract, reduced ability to inspect the frontal region, and additionally reduces access of topical medications to the region. This may also play a role in the failure of some endoscopic frontal sinus procedures.

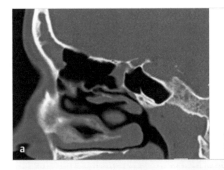
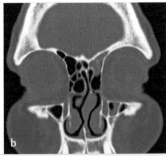

Fig. 14.1 (a,b) Incomplete dissection of the frontal recess is noted in these CT images. The remnant bulla ethmoidalis is compromising the frontal sinus outflow tract.

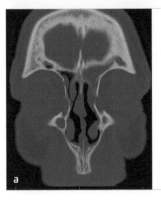
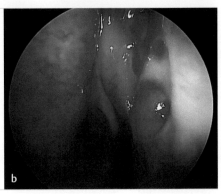

Fig. 14.2 (a) This CT scan demonstrates a lateralized left middle turbinate following surgery with consequent obstruction of the frontal sinus outflow tract. (b) An intraoperative image of the same patient with the middle turbinate lateralization clearly visible and associated infection present.

14.3.2 Pain

The sinuses are relatively insensate to pain, with most patients reporting minimal pain following endoscopic sinus surgery. Procedures that involve extensive bone drilling may, however, result in subjectively more pain than a standard sinus operation. An EMLP or Draf III involves the removal of a significant amount of bone from the frontal beak region, with reactive postoperative inflammation that can typically lead to an increase in pain approximately 1 week after surgery. Patients undergoing this procedure should be warned of the possibility of this occurrence and provided with adequate analgesia to address the issue. The authors find the use of a selective cyclooxygenase-2 (COX-2) inhibitor useful in these circumstances. When patients experience pain that seems out of proportion to the procedure performed, the surgeon must consider the possibility of a surgical complication contributing to the pain. Orbital pain may reflect increasing intraorbital pressure from a delayed hematoma, while an unremitting headache, particularly in association with other neurological signs, may reflect an intracranial breach causing meningitis or pneumocephalus. Postural headaches, aggravated by standing and relieved by the supine position, may indicate cerebrospinal fluid (CSF) hypotension from an undetected CSF leak at the time of surgery. Consequently, it is critical that the surgeon consider these possibilities in circumstances where a patient is experiencing more pain than is typically expected.

The provision of adequate analgesia is a key aspect in the care provided to patients by their sinus surgeon. Intraoperative administration of intravenous paracetamol, opioid and nonopioid analgesia, as well as intraoperative corticosteroids enables the patient to awaken from the surgery with minimal discomfort. The subsequent provision of regular simple analgesia as well as pro re nata (prn) analgesia as required allows the patient to control their pain and titrate their own analgesia to their specific needs.

14.3.3 Bleeding

All endoscopic sinus surgery involves tissue trauma and thus a degree of bleeding is anticipated. Typically, the bleeding is minor and leads to little in the way of discomfort for the patient. It may require the use of a nasal bolster for the first 48 hours after surgery and will typically reduce in frequency and volume as the recovery progresses.

Significant epistaxis is an uncommon event following frontal sinus surgery. Major hemorrhage following standard endoscopic sinus surgery is seen in approximately 1% of cases.[16] Epistaxis following EMLP requiring intervention is seen in up to 3.9%.[8] There are two major vessels at risk in the frontal sinus region. The first is the anterior ethmoidal artery (AEA), which is situated in the frontoethmoidal recess and can be inadvertently damaged during dissection of the region. At the time of surgery, an injury to the AEA is likely to result in profuse pulsatile bleeding, but if transected adjacent to the lamina papyracea, there is a significant risk of retraction into the orbit and the subsequent development of an orbital hematoma, which will be discussed in the orbital injury section. Delayed bleeding of this vessel can lead to a profuse epistaxis, in some instances a number of hours following the procedure. Critical to the avoidance of injury to the AEA is preoperative assessment of its position relative to the skull base. In up to 36% of cases, the vessel can be suspended upon a mesentery (usually in combination with a supraorbital cell) within the paranasal sinuses and is consequently at higher risk of injury.[17,18] Careful review of the coronal CT scan will usually identify the site of the vessel as it exits the orbit, where it forms a "nipplelike" projection into the sinus cavity (▶ Fig. 14.3). Intraoperatively, the surgeon should take great care as the frontoethmoidal recess is approached. Powered and cutting instruments should be avoided and careful dissection of the region will often allow identification of the vessel. As an AEA on a mesentery often represents a small superior dehiscence of the lamina papyracea, ballottement of the eye when operating in this area may help further delineate its position. Additionally, the surgeon should work from a medial-to-lateral direction during dissection. This further protects the patient from an orbital hematoma as should the vessel be inadvertently transected in the frontoethmoidal recess, it is less likely to retract into the orbit.

The second vessel at risk in this region is a more distal branch of the AEA as it passes beneath the nasal bones to emerge as the dorsal nasal artery. The creation of a septal window during EMLP and removal of the bone of the frontal beak will typically and unavoidably expose the vessel. Careful control of this vessel via bipolar electrocautery should be addressed during or at the conclusion of the EMLP.

Should bleeding occur from either vessel during endoscopic frontal sinus surgery, the bleeding is best controlled with bipolar electrocautery. Use of monopolar electrocautery in the region of the skull base and lamina papyracea presents a risk of electrical current transmission via delicate structures such as the orbital contents and the thin bone and dura of the lateral lamella of the cribriform plate. This could lead to orbital injury or CSF leak and thus should be avoided. In the instances where the bleeding is not well controlled via the measures outlined earlier, then the surgeon should return to basic principles to attain control of the bleeding and hence the surgical field. Initially, the surgeon should ensure the patient is positioned head up and that the mean arterial pressure is approximately 60 to 70 mm Hg if age and comorbidities permit. A relative bradycardia should be maintained. The region bleeding can be temporarily packed with topical vasoconstricting agents soaked onto a pledget. Patience at this step will often control minor bleeding points and help identify the primary vessels of concern. It would be unusual to need to employ further hemostatic measures; however, in very rare circumstances, an external ligation of the AEA within the orbit may be necessary.

14.3.4 Infection

As with all surgical sites, there is the potential for postoperative infection following endoscopic sinus surgery. The increased burden of inflammation associated with such an occurrence presents a risk of increased scarring and possible stenosis. There are little data on the rate of postoperative infection in the 30 days following frontal sinus surgery. Of interest is a report of infection requiring antibiotics in 4.9% of EMLP cases.[8] The proximity of the frontal sinus to the orbit and cranial contents presents the potential for transmission of localized infection to either of these regions. While rare, infection of the frontal sinus region following surgery should be managed aggressively to limit further complications.

Basic surgical principles should be applied to sinus surgery to minimize the risk of infection. Sterile technique should always be employed and intraoperative antibiotics are advocated. Any obvious infective material at the time of surgery should be collected and assessed via microscopy, culture, and sensitivity as this information could prove helpful in the event of a postoperative infection. Although antibiotics are commonly used in the first 1 to 2 weeks post sinus surgery, there is no high-level evidence supporting this practice, or the fact that they reduce the frequency of postoperative infection. Antibiotics should always be considered, however, if packing material is left in the nose postsurgery.

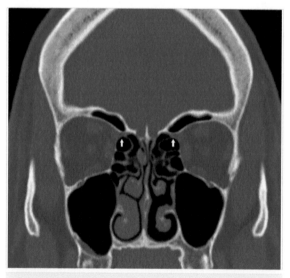

Fig. 14.3 The anterior ethmoidal artery in this patient is present on a mesentery bilaterally (*arrows*).

14.3.5 Scar/Stenosis

Perhaps the most common reason for surgical failure in endoscopic frontal sinus surgery is scarring and stenosis of the frontal region following the procedure (▶ Fig. 14.4).

Of critical importance to the prospects of avoiding stenosis are the maximal dimensions of the frontal sinus ostium at the conclusion of the procedure. The size of the frontal ostium at the conclusion of a Draf IIa frontal sinus-otomy has been demonstrated to be an important risk factor for restenosis and persistence of symptoms, with an ostium size of less than 4 mm being an important marker of possible failure.[6,9] The same principle applies to EMLP. Tran et al utilized a linear regression model to predict restenosis of the frontal neo-ostium following EMLP and found that the size of the frontal ostium created at surgery was a significant factor in predicting post-operative area and hence emphasized the importance of maximizing the size of the neo-ostium.[19] In the authors' experience, it is critical that the frontal ostium be enlarged in all directions. In particular, the bone of the posterior table of the skull base as it merges with the nasal septum and middle turbinate insertions inferiorly, referred to as the "frontal T" due to its endoscopic appearance, is critical to maximizing the anterior-to-posterior dimensions. When the "frontal T" is left intact (▶ Fig. 14.5a), the neo-ostium takes an inverted "U" or horseshoe configuration, whereas its removal (▶ Fig. 14.5b) leads to a more oval shape.

Stenosis of the frontal ostium following EMLP is a common phenomenon. Tran et al observed that the EMLP ostium narrowed at 1 year by an average of 33%, with a greater than 50% stenosis seen in approximately 40% of patients 12 months after surgery. Indeed, nearly one-fifth may develop what appears to be an obliterated ostium.[8,19] Restenosis is thought to occur due to a combination of scarring, adhesions, and neo-osteogenesis.[19,20,21,22] Interestingly, the presence of stenosis or even apparent obliteration of the frontal sinus neo-ostium is not in itself an indication for revision surgery as some of these patients may remain asymptomatic.[8,19,21,23]

It is postulated that stenosis of the frontal neo-ostium, especially in the case of EMLP, is related to the circumferential exposure of bone and subsequent inflammation and neo-osteogenesis. The use of mucosal flaps and free grafts (▶ Fig. 14.6) has been suggested as a possible remedy for this issue with some early though small studies suggesting promise.[24]

14.3.6 Mucocele Formation

The primary etiological factor associated with the development of a mucocele is the obstruction of normal sinus drainage.[25,26] The continued production of mucous in the obstructed sinus leads to accumulation of secretions and the gradual enlargement of the mucocele. This expansion of the mucocele in the frontal sinus can result in demineralization of the neighboring bone resulting in intraorbital and intracranial extension (▶ Fig. 14.7a–c). Endoscopic approaches to the frontal sinus place the patient at risk of mucocele development secondary to obstruction of sinus drainage following surgery.

Frontal sinus mucocele presents one of the more difficult pathological entities to manage in the frontal sinus region. Failure rates of surgery directed at addressing mucoceles are reported to be up to 38.9%.[8] This pathology

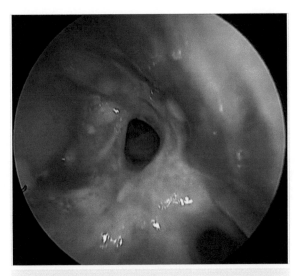

Fig. 14.4 Stenosis of the frontal ostium following endoscopic modified Lothrop procedure.

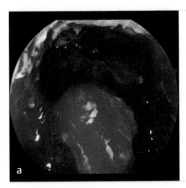
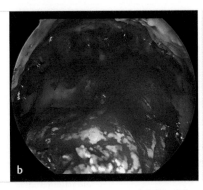

Fig. 14.5 (a) A traditional horseshoe-shaped drillout where the frontal T has not been lowered and consequently adhesions between the anterior and posterior margins are more likely. (b) A large endoscopic modified Lothrop procedure cavity maximizing the anterior to posterior and lateral dimensions via maximal bone removal from the frontal process of the maxilla, intersinus septum, and importantly the "frontal T." Note the oval shape at conclusion.

is also a very indolent one and may become apparent many years following the original surgery.

The only curative treatment available for mucoceles is surgical drainage.[25] Marsupialization of the mucocele has been demonstrated to be critical to its successful management. In the region of the frontal sinus, the endoscopic approach and ability to access the mucocele can present significant problems for the operating surgeon. A mucocele lateral to the mid-pupillary line is often considered to be inaccessible via standard endoscopic approaches and usually requires an endoscopic modified Lothrop procedure for long-term success. Innovative approaches such as the transblepharoplasty approach described by Knipe et al have also shown to have had some success in treating such mucoceles.[27]

Critical to the avoidance of mucocele formation is meticulous tissue handing. Avoiding stripping the mucosa

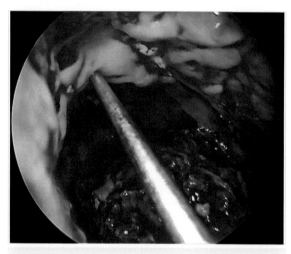

Fig. 14.6 A mucosal graft is being positioned over the exposed bone following the endoscopic modified Lothrop procedure.

from bone and careful preservation of normal mucosa where possible will help limit the risk of postoperative sinus obstruction and subsequent mucocele formation.

14.3.7 Anterior Skull Base Injury/ Cerebrospinal Fluid Leak

The frontal sinus is the site of CSF fistula in 7% of all CSF fistula cases[28] and with respect to frontal surgery it occurs as an iatrogenic complication in 0.1 to 1.9% of cases.[4,8,29]

When there is intracranial injury and CSF leak occurs and is recognized intraoperatively, it should be immediately repaired. The specific type of repair may vary, but the basic principles apply to all repairs. Initially, the site of leak should be clearly identified and the adjacent mucosa removed around its margin. In most instances, an underlay will be placed, which may take the form of a fat graft, fascia, septal cartilage, or bone, and in some instances allograft materials. A free mucosal graft should then be placed across the site of the leak and the bare adjacent bone with support provided from below with packing materials. It is the authors' preference to use absorbable packing materials adjacent the free mucosal graft with nonabsorbable packing supporting the absorbable ones. The nonabsorbable packing materials are typically removed a week after surgery.

If the injury and CSF leak are not recognized at the time of surgery, there is a risk of serious sequelae including meningitis, pneumocephalus, and possibly coma or death.[30] Where there is delay in the diagnosis, any suspicious fluid can be collected and assessed for the presence of Beta-2 transferrin. Once confirmed, high-resolution CT imaging should be utilized to identify the likely site of the injury and for planning of the surgical repair. Typically, the repair will follow the same principles outlined earlier.

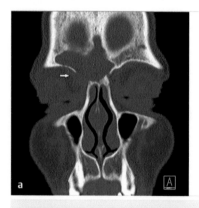
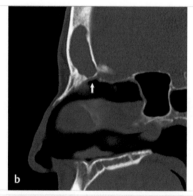
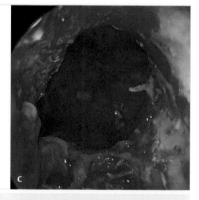

Fig. 14.7 This patient had frontal sinus surgery 18 years before presenting with a frontal mucocele. **(a)** Coronal CT image of the right frontal mucocele with erosion of the bone of the medial orbital roof (*white arrow*). **(b)** A representative parasagittal image of the same patient where the complete obstruction of frontal drainage pathway was present (*white arrow*). **(c)** An intraoperative image of the widely patent neo-ostium created during an endoscopic modified Lothrop procedure.

14.3.8 Orbital Injury

Major orbital complications are rare when performing endoscopic approaches to the frontal sinus. Krings et al reported a rate of major orbital complication in this setting of 0.32%.[4]

Injury to the orbit can take a number of forms. At its simplest, it involves a breach of the lamina papyracea with exposure of orbital fat. Rarely it can also involve injury to the orbital musculature and may potentially involve orbital nerve injury and consequent blindness. The presence of a dehiscence of the orbital lamina and exposure of orbital fat can usually be confirmed with intraoperative ballottement of the eye, which leads to movement of the periorbital and orbital fat. Should exposure of orbital fat occur, it is essential that the surgeon refrain from using powered instrumentation at and around the site of exposure in order to limit further injury.

Orbital hematoma can occur as a result of venous or arterial injury. Retraction of the transected AEA into the bony orbit may lead to rapid intraoperative proptosis and compression of the optic nerve within the bony confines of the orbit. The critical consideration in the management of this complication is decompression of the optic nerve, which typically requires an immediate lateral canthotomy with upper and/or lower cantholysis. This increases the orbital volume and reduces intraorbital pressure. In some instances, endoscopic orbital decompression may be necessary to reduce intraocular pressures and avoid injury to the optic nerve. Simultaneous medical management with mannitol (1 g/kg IV) is also recommended.[30] Prompt ophthalmology review is critical in maximizing the outcome for the patient. Venous orbital hematoma is a more slowly progressive complication occurring over hours. Gradually, there is an increase in proptosis and a progressive visual loss. Red color vision should be assessed as this is typically lost early in the pathogenesis of this complication. Any nasal packing should be removed to alleviate its contribution to the increasing pressure. Medical and surgical management may also be required as described earlier.

An injury to the medial rectus muscle can be a devastating complication and will require the assistance of an oculoplastic surgeon. This injury typically occurs with the use of powered instrumentation in the region of the lamina papyracea. Medial rectus injury typically leads to diplopia and treatment is seldom successful.[31] When an injury occurs to the medial rectus muscle, the patient will usually demonstrate an adduction deficit, diplopia, and conjunctival hemorrhage. An ophthalmology consultation should be urgently sought with tonometry and fundoscopy performed. Management should initially be directed toward maintaining intraocular pressures of less than 30 mm Hg. In some instances, surgical management coupled with botulism toxin injection may be necessary to address diplopia, but unfortunately the prognosis for these injuries remains poor.[31]

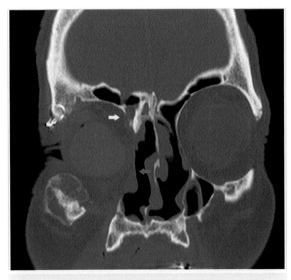

Fig. 14.8 This patient experienced facial trauma in a motor vehicle accident many years prior to his presentation. Of note is the presence of an encephalocele (*red arrow*), and orbital dehiscence into the frontal recess (*white arrow*) and a broad area with absent lamina papyracea (*blue arrow*).

Injury to the trochlear is a rare orbital complication seen when performing EMLP. The trochlea is situated on the superomedial wall of the orbit and can be traumatized while drilling the lateral bone during an EMLP. In the event of this injury, the patient experiences vertical diplopia, which is typically transient. Endoscopic approaches to the frontal sinus have not been formally reported to be associated with this injury; however, in the era of open approaches to the frontal sinus, it has been reported to lead to permanent, disabling vertical diplopia.[32]

In order to minimize orbital complications in endoscopic frontal sinus surgery, it is critical that the surgeon assess the patient for potential risk factors. A history of maxillofacial trauma, previous surgery, sinonasal tumor, and primary orbital pathology should alert the surgeon to the possibility of unusual orbital anatomy (▶ Fig. 14.8). Preoperative CT scans should be carefully inspected for breaches of the orbital lamina, prolapse of orbital contents into the sinonasal cavity, and the location and associated anatomy of the anterior ethmoidal arteries.

During the procedure, the surgeon should identify the orbital lamina early and skeletonize it to provide a consistent anatomic landmark. Instruments in the region of the lamina papyracea should be directed away from the lamina to avoid inadvertent injury.

14.4 Prevention of Complications

The prevention of complications when operating in the frontal sinus and its drainage pathway requires a multifaceted approach. There are numerous perioperative tasks and techniques upon which the operating surgeon can focus in order to predict and prevent complications of frontal sinus surgery.

14.4.1 Preoperative Planning

Attention should be directed toward optimizing the condition of the patient prior to undertaking surgery. Infection leads to inflammation and increased vascular flow. This can lead to hemostasis issues intraoperatively and thus any overt infection should be addressed prior to surgery with culture-directed antibiotics.

The presence of inflammation and extensive polyposis within the paranasal sinuses prior to surgery also leads to an increase in the bleeding risk during the procedure. Perioperative oral and intranasal corticosteroids can aid in reducing inflammation and consequently the intraoperative bleeding.[30] Similarly, preparation of the nasal cavity with topical and injected anesthesia and vasoconstriction leads to reductions in bleeding.

A thorough review of the preoperative imaging will allow the surgeon to anticipate regions of potential concern during surgery while facilitating planning for the surgical approach to minimize these issues. In particular, complex anatomy can be identified and the frontal sinus drainage pathway can be predicted. The need for adjuvant procedures such as mini-trephination can be ascertained and the surgeon may also elect to utilize navigation technology to aid the surgery.

14.4.2 Perioperative Technique

The success of surgery in the frontal sinus region is highly reliant upon the quality of the surgical field and consequent visualization that the surgeon can obtain while completing the surgery. Anesthetic techniques including hypotensive anesthesia help reduce intraoperative blood loss and consequently improve visualization. The patient should be elevated to minimize vascular congestion in the paranasal sinuses. A relative bradycardia and the utilization of total intravenous anesthesia have also been demonstrated to aid in surgical field optimization.

Access to appropriate equipment to complete the surgery is an obvious but critical element of safe endoscopic frontal sinus surgery. Surgeons operating in the frontal sinus region require appropriate angled instrumentation in order to complete the task at hand while also minimizing complications. Inadequate instrumentation will lead to inferior surgical results and also places the patient at higher risk of complications. In many instances, the utilization of navigation systems can aid the surgeon in orientation and intraoperative assessment of anatomy. It is critical to appreciate that all navigation systems have an inherent margin of error and thus should not be considered anything more than a surgical aid. The surgeon should trust their own anatomy knowledge and instincts

when it comes to assessment of the critical structures within the paranasal sinuses.

Where identification of the frontal sinus and its drainage pathway becomes difficult, it is helpful to utilize frontal mini-trephination. This technique involves the placement of a mini-trephine into the frontal sinus. Upon successful placement, the surgeon should be able to aspirate into a syringe air, blood, or pus to confirm the position. Subsequently, fluorescein-stained saline can be irrigated into the frontal sinus and its drainage into the nose observed from below, thus identifying the frontal drainage pathway.

The operating surgeon should also endeavor to employ gentle tissue handling techniques.

The preservation of native mucosa and the minimization of bone exposure facilitate more rapid healing and reduce neo-osteogenesis.[30]

14.4.3 Postoperative Care

Just as the preoperative and perioperative care is critical in attaining a successful surgical outcome, so too is the postoperative care essential in the success of frontal sinus surgery. Saline irrigation of the postoperative sinus cavity helps remove clot and debris, which in turn reduces scar and synechia formation. Topical corticosteroids have been demonstrated to be effective in reducing recurrence of disease and symptoms following endoscopic sinus surgery in general and the incorporation of the steroid into high-volume saline irrigations aids the penetration of the steroid into the frontal sinus region.[33] Debridement of the sinonasal cavity following endoscopic sinus surgery expedites healing and recovery while also reducing the formation of scar and adhesions.

References

[1] Friedman M, Landsberg R, Schults RA, Tanyeri H, Caldarelli DD. Frontal sinus surgery: endoscopic technique and preliminary results. Am J Rhinol. 2000; 14(6):393–403

[2] Valdes CJ, Bogado M, Samaha M. Causes of failure in endoscopic frontal sinus surgery in chronic rhinosinusitis patients. Int Forum Allergy Rhinol. 2014; 4(6):502–506

[3] Wormald P-J, Hoseman W, Callejas C, et al. The International Frontal Sinus Anatomy Classification (IFAC) and classification of the extent of endoscopic frontal sinus surgery (EFSS). Int Forum Allergy Rhinol. 2016; 6(7):677–696

[4] Krings JG, Kallogjeri D, Wineland A, Nepple KG, Piccirillo JF, Getz AE. Complications of primary and revision functional endoscopic sinus surgery for chronic rhinosinusitis. Laryngoscope. 2014; 124(4):838–845

[5] Mendelsohn D, Jeremic G, Wright ED, Rotenberg BW. Revision rates after endoscopic sinus surgery: a recurrence analysis. Ann Otol Rhinol Laryngol. 2011; 120(3):162–166

[6] Naidoo Y, Wen D, Bassiouni A, Keen M, Wormald P-J. Long-term results after primary frontal sinus surgery. Int Forum Allergy Rhinol. 2012; 2(3):185–190

[7] Chandra RK, Palmer JN, Tangsujarittham T, Kennedy DW. Factors associated with failure of frontal sinusotomy in the early follow-up period. Otolaryngol Head Neck Surg. 2004; 131(4):514–518

[8] Ting JY, Wu A, Metson R. Frontal sinus drillout (modified Lothrop procedure): long-term results in 204 patients. Laryngoscope. 2014; 124(5):1066–1070

[9] Hosemann W, Kühnel T, Held P, Wagner W, Felderhoff A. Endonasal frontal sinusotomy in surgical management of chronic sinusitis: a critical evaluation. Am J Rhinol. 1997; 11(1):1–9

[10] Anderson P, Sindwani R. Safety and efficacy of the endoscopic modified Lothrop procedure: a systematic review and meta-analysis. Laryngoscope. 2009; 119(9):1828–1833

[11] Morrissey DK, Bassiouni A, Psaltis AJ, Naidoo Y, Wormald P-J. Outcomes of revision endoscopic modified Lothrop procedure. Int Forum Allergy Rhinol. 2016; 6(5):518–522

[12] Dalgorf DM, Sacks R, Wormald P-J, et al. Image-guided surgery influences perioperative morbidity from endoscopic sinus surgery: a systematic review and meta-analysis. Otolaryngol Head Neck Surg. 2013; 149(1):17–29

[13] Boonmak P, Boonmak S, Laopaiboon M. Deliberate hypotension with propofol under anaesthesia for functional endoscopic sinus surgery (FESS). Cochrane Database Syst Rev. 2016; 10:CD006623

[14] Ha TN, van Renen RG, Ludbrook GL, Wormald P-J. The effect of blood pressure and cardiac output on the quality of the surgical field and middle cerebral artery blood flow during endoscopic sinus surgery. Int Forum Allergy Rhinol. 2016; 6(7):701–709

[15] Ha TN, van Renen RG, Ludbrook GL, Valentine R, Ou J, Wormald P-J. The relationship between hypotension, cerebral flow, and the surgical field during endoscopic sinus surgery. Laryngoscope. 2014; 124(10):2224–2230

[16] Halderman AA, Sindwani R, Woodard TD. Hemorrhagic complications of endoscopic sinus surgery. Otolaryngol Clin North Am. 2015; 48(5):783–793

[17] Jang DW, Comer BT, Lachanas VA, Kountakis SE. Aspirin sensitivity does not compromise quality-of-life outcomes in patients with Samter's triad. Laryngoscope. 2014; 124(1):34–37

[18] Floreani SR, Nair SB, Switajewski MC, Wormald P-J. Endoscopic anterior ethmoidal artery ligation: a cadaver study. Laryngoscope. 2006; 116(7):1263–1267

[19] Tran KN, Beule AG, Singal D, Wormald P-J. Frontal ostium restenosis after the endoscopic modified Lothrop procedure. Laryngoscope. 2007; 117(8):1457–1462

[20] Wormald PJ. Salvage frontal sinus surgery: the endoscopic modified lothrop procedure. Laryngoscope. 2003; 1; 13(2):276–283

[21] Schlosser RJ, Zachmann G, Harrison S, Gross CW. The endoscopic modified Lothrop: long-term follow-up on 44 patients. Am J Rhinol. 2002; 16(2):103–108

[22] Rajapaksa SP, Ananda A, Cain TM, Oates L, Wormald P-J. Frontal ostium neo-osteogenesis and restenosis after modified endoscopic Lothrop procedure in an animal model. Clin Otolaryngol Allied Sci. 2004; 29(4):386–388

[23] Georgalas C, Hansen F, Videler WJM, Fokkens WJ. Long terms results of Draf type III (modified endoscopic Lothrop) frontal sinus drainage procedure in 122 patients: a single centre experience. Rhinology. 2011; 49(2):195–201

[24] Wei CC, Sama A. What is the evidence for the use of mucosal flaps in Draf III procedures? Curr Opin Otolaryngol Head Neck Surg. 2014; 22(1):63–67

[25] Barrow EM, DelGaudio JM. In-office drainage of sinus mucoceles: an alternative to operating-room drainage. Laryngoscope. 2015; 125(5):1043–1047

[26] Scangas GA, Gudis DA, Kennedy DW. The natural history and clinical characteristics of paranasal sinus mucoceles: a clinical review. Int Forum Allergy Rhinol. 2013; 3(9):712–717

[27] Knipe TA, Gandhi PD, Fleming JC, Chandra RK. Transblepharoplasty approach to sequestered disease of the lateral frontal sinus with ophthalmologic manifestations. Am J Rhinol. 2007; 21(1):100–104

[28] Psaltis AJ, Schlosser RJ, Banks CA, Yawn J, Soler ZM. A systematic review of the endoscopic repair of cerebrospinal fluid leaks. Otolaryngol Head Neck Surg. 2012; 147(2):196–203

[29] Eloy JA, Svider PF, Setzen M. Preventing and managing complications in frontal sinus surgery. Otolaryngol Clin North Am. 2016; 49(4):951–964

[30] Javer AR, Alandejani T. Prevention and management of complications in frontal sinus surgery. Otolaryngol Clin North Am. 2010; 43(4):827–838

[31] Bleier BS, Schlosser RJ. Prevention and management of medial rectus injury. Otolaryngol Clin North Am. 2010; 43(4):801–807

[32] Rosenbaum AL, Astle WF. Superior oblique and inferior rectus muscle injury following frontal and intranasal sinus surgery. J Pediatr Ophthalmol Strabismus. 1985; 22(5):194–202

[33] Thomas WW, III, Harvey RJ, Rudmik L, Hwang PH, Schlosser RJ. Distribution of topical agents to the paranasal sinuses: an evidence-based review with recommendations. Int Forum Allergy Rhinol. 2013; 3(9):691–703

15 Delivery of Topical Therapy to the Frontal Sinus

John R. Craig and Nithin D. Adappa

Abstract

Optimizing topical delivery to inflamed or infected frontal sinuses is important when managing patients with chronic rhinosinusitis with or without polyps. Evidence suggests that better topical delivery leads to better outcomes after sinus surgery. Surgical state has been shown to be the most important factor in determining the degree of frontal sinus topical delivery. Before frontal sinus surgery, minimal to no topical delivery to the frontal sinus can be achieved. Topical delivery to the frontal sinus improves after a Draf IIa frontal sinusotomy, and further improves following a Draf III procedure. Topical therapies should be delivered by high-volume devices (≥ 100 mL) to account for nasal dead space. Patients should be instructed to irrigate in at least a vertex-to-wall head position to optimize topical delivery of high-volume irrigations to the frontal sinus. If patients are flexible enough to assume a vertex-to-floor position, this may further optimize topical delivery to the frontal sinus. Early data suggest that the improved topical penetration of the frontal sinuses with a Draf III procedure may lead to decreased polyp recurrence and revision surgery rates in select cases.

Keywords: chronic rhinosinusitis, nasal polyps, topical delivery, head position, frontal sinus surgery, Draf IIa, Draf III

15.1 Introduction

One of the major roles of endoscopic sinus surgery (ESS) in the setting of chronic rhinosinusitis (CRS) is to optimize the topical delivery of saline and other medications to inflamed or infected sinus mucosa.[1] The frontal sinus has received significant attention in the literature with regard to topical delivery, due to its location making it difficult to reach with various topical delivery methods, as well as its preponderance for recurrent disease and postoperative stenosis. The main factors affecting topical delivery to the frontal sinus include the surgical state of the ostium, the type of delivery device used, and patient head positioning.[1,2] Common head positions discussed in the literature regarding frontal sinus topical delivery include vertex-to-ceiling (or Frankfort horizontal position), vertex-to-wall (or nose-to-floor), and vertex-to-floor (▶ Fig. 15.1, ▶ Fig. 15.2, ▶ Fig. 15.3). Both basic science and clinical research studies have been conducted in attempts to answer the questions of how best to deliver topical therapy to the frontal sinuses, and this research will be described in the following sections of this chapter.

15.2 Basic Science Research on Topical Distribution to the Sinuses

Most studies evaluating topical distribution to the sinuses have utilized cadavers before and after ESS, and have evaluated the effects of different macroscopic factors on

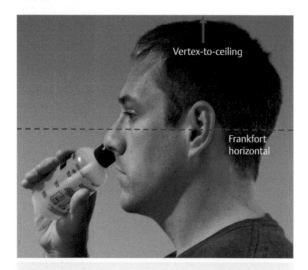

Fig. 15.1 Example of a vertex-to-ceiling (Frankfort horizontal) head position when performing sinonasal irrigations with a squeeze bottle. This position has been associated with poorer penetration of the frontal sinus compared to the vertex-to-wall and vertex-to-floor head positions.

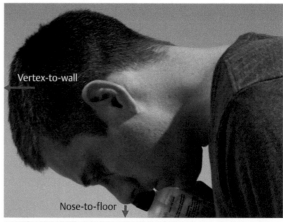

Fig. 15.2 Example of a vertex-to-wall (nose-to-floor) head position when performing sinonasal irrigations with a squeeze bottle. This position has been associated with improved penetration of the frontal sinus compared to the vertex-to-ceiling position.

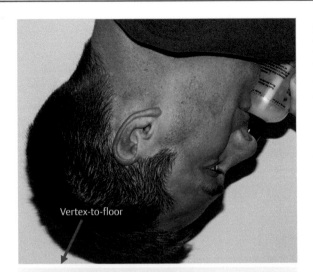

Fig. 15.3 Example of a vertex-to-floor head position when performing sinonasal irrigations with a squeeze bottle. This position has been associated with improved penetration of the frontal sinus compared to the vertex-to-ceiling position.

delivery to the sinuses (surgery state, irrigation volume, head position). First, topical delivery to all the sinuses has been shown to be minimal before ESS. ESS has been shown to improve distribution to each of the paranasal sinuses, including the frontal sinuses.[3,4,5,6] It has also been shown that ostial diameters of at least 4 to 4.7 mm are necessary to allow reliable penetration of topical irrigation fluid to each of the sinuses.[5,6] Harvey et al showed improved delivery to the frontal sinus after a Draf IIa was performed in 10 cadavers, compared to the unoperated state. They evaluated multiple delivery devices as well, and found that the high-volume devices outperformed nasal sprays. They only irrigated the heads in what they described as a bent-over-the-sink head position.[3] Singhal et al performed Draf I, IIa, or III frontal sinusotomies on 10 cadavers, and evaluated the effects of surgery and head position on topical distribution. They found that Draf IIa and III were superior to Draf I for frontal topical delivery, and delivery was improved when the head was turned downward compared with when the head was upright. The best delivery based on head position was found when the nose was pointed directly to the floor, termed the 90-degree position in the paper, which is synonymous with the vertex-to-wall position.[6]

Head position does appear to affect frontal sinus topical delivery. Multiple papers have shown that topical delivery is improved when the frontal sinus is placed in a more gravity-dependent position. This generally refers to a vertex-to-floor or vertex-to-wall head position. Beule et al evaluated the effect of vertex-to-wall versus vertex-to-floor head position, as well as irrigation volume on topical delivery in cadaver heads with Draf III drillouts. While they found that irrigations of at least 100 mL achieved

adequate penetration of the Draf III cavity regardless of head position, they also found that frontal penetration was more pronounced in the vertex-to-floor position.[7] Volume of delivery is another major factor affecting topical distribution to the frontal sinus. High-volume irrigations (≥ 100 mL per side) by a squeeze bottle, NetiPot, or a pulse irrigator have been shown to provide better sinus distribution than low-volume sprays, drops, or nebulizers.[3,8,9,10] While higher volumes of irrigation appear to be more important than head position, frontal sinus penetration has been shown to be improved further in a vertex-to-wall or vertex-to-floor head position, compared with vertex-to-ceiling (Frankfort horizontal) head position.[6,7,11]

A recent cadaveric study by Barham et al evaluated the effects of the following factors on topical distribution to the frontal sinus: surgical opening (Draf IIa vs. Draf III), head position (vertex-to-wall vs. Frankfort horizontal), and low- vs. high-volume devices (60 vs. 120 mL per side). They used a grading system to classify the degree of penetration of the frontal sinus, but considered distribution "poor" if irrigations were not visualized penetrating the frontal sinus at all. A Draf IIa frontal sinusotomy resulted in poor distribution to the frontal sinus in 50% of irrigations, regardless of head position and irrigation volume. On the contrary, the Draf III procedure provided delivery to the frontal sinus in 91% of irrigations, with 50% of irrigations providing complete filling, regardless of head position and irrigation volume. This study demonstrated that surgical state was the main determinant of topical delivery to the frontal sinus, and specifically the Draf III procedure was superior to the Draf IIa frontal sinusotomy for topical delivery. While head position and volume were less important than surgical state, there were trends toward improved delivery with the vertex-to-wall position and high-volume irrigations, though these effects did not reach statistical significance.[11]

Another new and very exciting area of topical therapy research has been computational fluid dynamic (CFD) modeling of sinonasal irrigations. The authors have published two papers recently on this topic. Zhao et al published on the use of CFD modeling of sinonasal irrigations, detailing the technique, and presenting the differences in topical irrigation distribution to each of the paranasal sinuses before and after sinus surgery in a single patient. In the study case example, CFD models were created based on preoperative and postoperative computed tomography scans. Surgery had included a complete ESS with a Draf III procedure. In that case, the CFD models demonstrated no frontal sinus penetration by the irrigations before ESS, but rapid penetration and complete filling of the frontal sinuses after the Draf III procedure. Representative still images of the preoperative and postoperative CFD models from that patient are presented in ▶ Fig. 15.4.[12] Craig et al published a cadaveric validation study of CFD modeling of sinonasal irrigations.

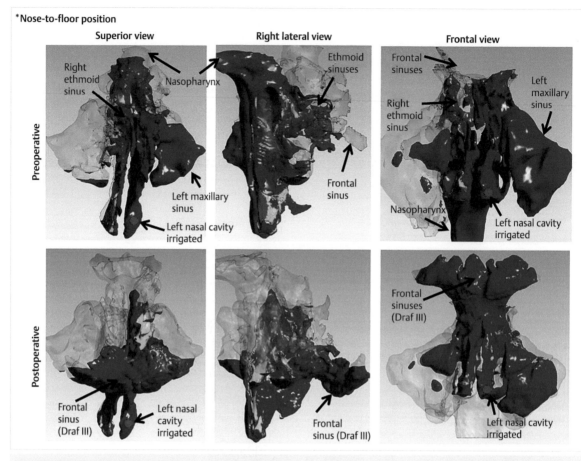

*Nose-to-floor position

Fig. 15.4 Preoperative and postoperative computational fluid dynamic models before and after a Draf III procedure. Simulations were performed in the vertex-to-wall (nose-to-floor) head position, and 120 mL of irrigation fluid had been irrigated through the left nasal cavity at a rate of 60 mL/s. Before sinus surgery, neither of the frontal sinuses was penetrated by the irrigation. After the Draf III procedure, both frontal sinuses were rapidly and completely filled by the irrigation.

In that study, sinus irrigation patterns were compared between endoscopically recorded irrigations in cadavers and simulated irrigations in CFD models, both preoperatively and postoperatively. Irrigation patterns were nearly identical between the CFD models and those visualized endoscopically in cadaver sinuses.[13] The results of these early studies are very encouraging for furthering our understanding of sinonasal irrigations. CFD modeling has the ability to study the moment-to-moment dynamic flow of irrigations from initiation to completion, which is unique from other published methods. CFD modeling is also significantly less labor intensive than previously published methods, with the ability to test effects of various parameters on irrigation distribution (surgical status, irrigation velocity, and head position). A more thorough CFD study will be performed in the future to assess the effects of different degrees of frontal sinus surgery (Draf I, IIa, IIb, III) and head positioning on topical delivery to the frontal sinuses.

15.3 Clinical Research on Topical Distribution to the Sinuses

Clinical evidence has generally supported the concepts of wider surgical openings and higher volume irrigations as means to improve frontal sinus topical delivery. Studies have shown that high-volume steroid irrigations are more effective than nasal steroid sprays in patients with CRS in preventing postoperative symptom or polyp recurrence.[14,15,16] These studies suggest that the improved distribution of high-volume steroid irrigations compared with nasal sprays is responsible for the improved patient outcomes. Snidvongs et al reviewed 48 studies and performed a meta-analysis to assess the effect of sinus surgery and low- versus high-volume intranasal steroids on symptom and polyp endoscopy scores in patients with CRS with nasal polyps. They found that both symptom scores and polyp recurrences were lower in patients who had had sinus surgery and who had used high-volume steroid delivery.[17] This study suggested that improved topical delivery led to improved long-term postoperative outcomes. Bassiouni and Wormald evaluated polyp recurrence patterns in patients with CRS with nasal polyps who had undergone Draf IIa frontal sinusotomies. They found that the frontal recess and frontal sinus were among the most common areas of polyp recurrence. Reviewing 338 surgical cases, they found that Draf III surgery led to a lower revision surgery rate compared with Draf IIa ($p < 0.05$).[18] They also showed that Draf III led to lower polyp recurrence rates than Draf IIa, but these differences were not statistically significant. The decreased revision surgery and polyp recurrence rates with Draf III over Draf IIa may be the result of improving delivery of topical steroids to the frontal recess and sinus, the most common areas of polyp recurrence.

15.3.1 Tips and Tricks

- Wide endoscopic Draf II or III frontal sinusotomies and meticulous postoperative care to maintain sinus patency are essential for optimizing topical frontal sinus delivery.
- High-volume irrigations provide the most reliable penetration of the frontal sinuses, in both vertex-to-wall and vertex-to-floor head positions.
- Educating patients on proper irrigation technique may help with compliance and outcomes.

15.4 Conclusion

Performing frontal sinus surgery is the main determinant of improving topical delivery to the frontal sinus. The Draf III procedure allows for more reliable penetration of the frontal sinus compared with a Draf IIa frontal sinusotomy, which may provide a lower polyp recurrence and revision surgery rates (further investigation is necessary). High-volume devices and either vertex-to-wall or vertex-to-floor head position further optimize topical distribution to the operated frontal sinus.

References

[1] Thomas WW, III, Harvey RJ, Rudmik L, Hwang PH, Schlosser RJ. Distribution of topical agents to the paranasal sinuses: an evidence-based review with recommendations. Int Forum Allergy Rhinol. 2013; 3 (9):691–703

[2] Harvey RJ, Schlosser RJ. Local drug delivery. Otolaryngol Clin North Am. 2009; 42(5):829–845, ix

[3] Harvey RJ, Goddard JC, Wise SK, Schlosser RJ. Effects of endoscopic sinus surgery and delivery device on cadaver sinus irrigation. Otolaryngol Head Neck Surg. 2008; 139(1):137–142

[4] Snidvongs K, Chaowanapanja P, Aeumjaturapat S, Chusakul S, Praweswararat P. Does nasal irrigation enter paranasal sinuses in chronic rhinosinusitis? Am J Rhinol. 2008; 22(5):483–486

[5] Grobler A, Weitzel EK, Buele A, et al. Pre- and postoperative sinus penetration of nasal irrigation. Laryngoscope. 2008; 118(11):2078–2081

[6] Singhal D, Weitzel EK, Lin E, et al. Effect of head position and surgical dissection on sinus irrigant penetration in cadavers. Laryngoscope. 2010; 120(12):2528–2531

[7] Beule A, Athanasiadis T, Athanasiadis E, Field J, Wormald PJ. Efficacy of different techniques of sinonasal irrigation after modified Lothrop procedure. Am J Rhinol Allergy. 2009; 23(1):85–90

[8] Wormald PJ, Cain T, Oates L, Hawke L, Wong I. A comparative study of three methods of nasal irrigation. Laryngoscope. 2004; 114 (12):2224–2227

[9] Valentine R, Athanasiadis T, Thwin M, Singhal D, Weitzel EK, Wormald PJ. A prospective controlled trial of pulsed nasal nebulizer in maximally dissected cadavers. Am J Rhinol. 2008; 22(4):390–394

[10] Abadie WM, McMains KC, Weitzel EK. Irrigation penetration of nasal delivery systems: a cadaver study. Int Forum Allergy Rhinol. 2011; 1 (1):46–49

[11] Barham HP, Ramakrishnan VR, Knisely A, et al. Frontal sinus surgery and sinus distribution of nasal irrigation. Int Forum Allergy Rhinol. 2016; 6(3):238–242

[12] Zhao K, Craig JR, Cohen NA, Adappa ND, Khalili S, Palmer JN. Sinus irrigations before and after surgery-Visualization through computational fluid dynamics simulations. Laryngoscope. 2016; 126(3):E90–E96

[13] Craig JR, Zhao K, Doan N, et al. Cadaveric validation study of computational fluid dynamics model of sinus irrigations before and after sinus surgery. Int Forum Allergy Rhinol. 2016; 6(4):423–428

[14] Neubauer PD, Schwam ZG, Manes RP. Comparison of intranasal fluticasone spray, budesonide atomizer, and budesonide respules in patients with chronic rhinosinusitis with polyposis after endoscopic sinus surgery. Int Forum Allergy Rhinol. 2016; 6(3):233–237

[15] Snidvongs K, Pratt E, Chin D, Sacks R, Earls P, Harvey RJ. Corticosteroid nasal irrigations after endoscopic sinus surgery in the management of chronic rhinosinusitis. Int Forum Allergy Rhinol. 2012; 2 (5):415–421

[16] Jang DW, Lachanas VA, Segel J, Kountakis SE. Budesonide nasal irrigations in the postoperative management of chronic rhinosinusitis. Int Forum Allergy Rhinol. 2013; 3(9):708–711

[17] Snidvongs K, Kalish L, Sacks R, Sivasubramaniam R, Cope D, Harvey RJ. Sinus surgery and delivery method influence the effectiveness of topical corticosteroids for chronic rhinosinusitis: systematic review and meta-analysis. Am J Rhinol Allergy. 2013; 27(3):221–233

[18] Bassiouni A, Wormald PJ. Role of frontal sinus surgery in nasal polyp recurrence. Laryngoscope. 2013; 123(1):36–41

16 Postoperative Management: Dressings and Toilet

Neil Cheng-Wen Tan and Peter John Wormald

Abstract

Effective postoperative care following frontal sinus surgery promotes rapid wound healing and the return of normal mucociliary function within the paranasal sinuses. Nasal dressings have been used for a number of functions, namely, their hemostatic properties, their ability to stent open the middle meatus and frontal ostium, and as a surface covering to promote wound healing. More recently, dissolvable packings have been introduced that maintain surgically widened ostia and deliver topical therapies to surrounding tissues. Nasal debridement has an important role in the removal of blood clot, crusts, and debris that may contribute to the formation of adhesions. Finally, medical treatments are also important and include saline nasal irrigations and topical intranasal corticosteroids aimed at reducing the postsurgical inflammatory burden, undissolved packing materials, and retained secretions. With a wide range of treatment options, some controversy exists on the best practice available. The aim of this chapter is to discuss the existing evidence base and give recommendations for each of these treatments.

Keywords: postoperative, packing, absorbable, nonabsorbable, debridement, irrigation, stent, intranasal steroid

16.1 Natural History of Sinus Ostia after Surgery

Trauma to mucosal surfaces from endoscopic sinus surgery initiates the classic wound response and healing pattern of hemostasis, inflammation, proliferation, and maturation. Intraoperative and postoperative steps can be taken to reduce the risk of scarring and adhesion formation. It is well recognized that the principle of mucosal preservation surgery rather than mucosal stripping surgery leads to better outcomes; however, the surgeon should nevertheless expect a degree of sinus ostia stenosis following surgery. The frontal sinus ostium will reduce in size by between 31 and 46%[1,2] through a combination of bony and soft-tissue stenosis. A wide frontal ostium and maintenance of the soft tissues will reduce the risk of local granulations, circumferential scarring, and subsequent soft-tissue stenosis. Exposed bone will contribute to granulations and therefore cutting instruments should be employed in the frontal recess and drilling of the ostial region avoided if at all possible. Where drilling of the neo-ostium is required, for example, during a frontal drillout (modified Lothrop/Draf III), exposed bone can lead to stenosis of the frontal drillout ostium (▶ Fig. 16.1). Therefore, the concept of mucosal flaps has been

introduced to cover exposed bone. A combination of anterior-based pedicled mucosal flaps and free mucosal grafts harvested from the superior septostomy can be placed on the exposed bone of the frontal neo-ostium (▶ Fig. 16.2).[3] This technique has been reported in a number of uncontrolled case series and can lead to excellent mucosal healing with wide ostia (▶ Fig. 16.3); however, further studies are required before this can be considered routine practice.

16.2 Intranasal Packing

In the past, the nasal pack has been considered indispensable after endoscopic sinus surgery (▶ Fig. 16.4). The intent is to control postoperative hemorrhage and as a physical barrier to prevention of adhesion formation and middle turbinate lateralization. In more recent years, novel substances and devices have been marketed that promote hemostasis, faster wound healing, or deliver topical medication with a view to improve outcomes. Despite their widespread use, there is no consensus on many factors regarding nasal packs in terms of using nonabsorbable or absorbable packs, their constituent material, how long they should remain in situ, and if they should even be used at all.

16.2.1 Nonabsorbable Packs

A wide range of materials have been used for short-term nasal packing including simple Vaseline-soaked ribbon

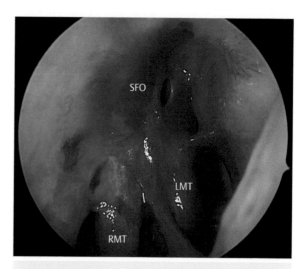

Fig. 16.1 In-office endoscopic view of frontal neo-ostium through the superior septostomy demonstrating significant soft-tissue stenosis. (SFO, stenosed frontal ostium; LMT, left middle turbinate; RMT, right middle turbinate.)

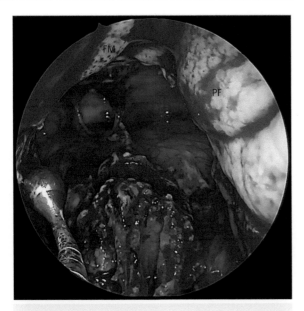

Fig. 16.2 Intraoperative image of frontal drillout cavity with mucosal flaps in position. (FM, free mucosal graft; PF, anterior-based pedicled mucosal flap.)

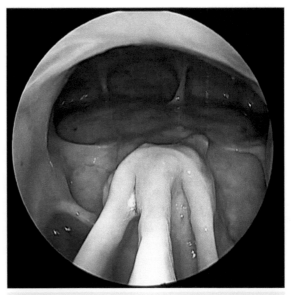

Fig. 16.3 Postoperative endoscopic view demonstrating widely patent neo-ostium with well-healed mucosa.

gauze or preformed spongelike packs made of polyvinyl acetyl (PVA; Merocel, Medtronic, Jacksonville, FL; or Netcell, Network Medical Products, North Ripon, United Kingdom). PVA packs are capable of absorbing up to 20 times their weight in fluid, and thus can absorb blood products as well as provide a suitably moist surface to promote wound healing. Alternatively, balloon tamponade devices can be used, typically with a surface coating designed to promote hemostasis such as the Rapid Rhino with its carboxymethylcellulose (CMC) surface (Smith & Nephew, Andover, MA).

The major drawbacks from nonabsorbable packs are discomfort while in situ and the need for removal, although a number of other risks and complications of nasal packing have been documented. These include septal perforation, pressure necrosis at the nasal margin, pack dislodgement, toxic shock syndrome, and even death.[4] A further concern to the sinus surgeon is that nonabsorbable packs have been found to have caused an increased rate of postoperative adhesions,[5] a factor acknowledged to be important in surgical relapse.

16.2.2 Absorbable Packings

Absorbable packs encompass a range of natural, modified, or synthetic compounds that offer their functions for a short period of time until they dissolve naturally within the nasal cavity or are absorbed and incorporated into the surrounding mucosa during the healing process. They come in a wide range of formats including foams, gels, films, sponges, and powders. A range of commercially available products are detailed in ▶ Table 16.1.

Gelfoam (Pfizer, New York City, NY) and Spongostan (Ferrosan, Copenhagen, Denmark) are porcine-derived gelatin sponges. They act by providing a mechanical barrier as well as having hemostatic properties through platelet activation.[6] When applied to the sinuses, however, they were found to initiate a marked foreign body response with scarring, adhesions, and ostial stenosis in the postsurgical sinonasal cavities.[7,8,9] Gelatin has been mixed with human-derived thrombin to produce foam-like materials that have very strong hemostatic properties, acting at the beginning of the coagulation cascade by platelet activation and at the end of the cascade by promoting fibrinogen to fibrin formation. Floseal (Baxter, Deerfield, IL) and Surgiflo (Ethicon Endo-Surgery, Somerville, NJ) are two such products and they have demonstrated their effectiveness in obtaining hemostasis both during ESS and in the postoperative period.[10] Similarly to gelatin alone, however, the risks of granulations and adhesions have been well highlighted from in vivo animal studies[11] and in clinical trials.[12] As a consequence, the use of gelatin-based products as a packing material must be carefully considered by the surgeon.

Hyaluronic acid (HA) is a key component of extracellular matrix and has an important role in wound healing. Its breakdown products are capable of activating key pathways of wound healing including fibroblast proliferation and angiogenesis.[13] It has found use in other areas of medical practice including plastic surgery and orthopaedics. It can be manufactured as a gel spacer (Sepragel, Genzyme, Cambridge, MA) and clothlike sponge (Merogel, Medtronic) and is designed to be inserted into the nasal cavity to act as both a stent and possible hemostat. Although early in vivo animal studies demonstrated that

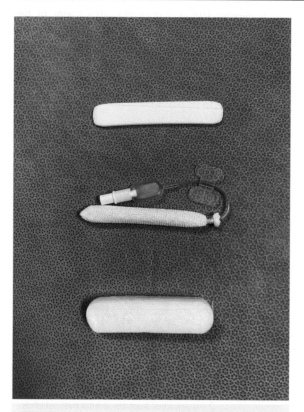

Fig. 16.4 A selection of common packing materials. Top: Merocel (Medtronic). Middle: Rapid Rhino (Smith & Nephew). Bottom: Nasopore (Stryker).

Table 16.1 Commercially available absorbable nasal packing materials

Product	Chemical component	Absorption time
Nasopore	Polyurethane	5–7 d
Chitogel	Polymer of chitin bound to dextrose	10–14 d
FloSeal	Bovine gelatin and thrombin	6–8 wk
Gelfoam	Purified porcine skin	4–6 wk
Merogel	Hyaluronic acid ester	2 wk
Sepragel	Cross-linked hyaluronic acid molecule	2 wk
Seprapack	Hyaluronic acid and carboxy-methylcellulose	2 wk
Spongostan	Porcine gelatin	4–6 wk

they may have a beneficial effect on wound healing,[14] this was not seen when transferred into an animal model of sinusitis.[15] In human studies HA packs were not found to be significantly different from no packing for either healing or hemostasis.[16,17]

Chitosan-dextran gel (Chitogel Pty, Wellington, NZ) is a novel mucoadhesive gel that uses the hemostatic properties of chitosan, a naturally occurring polymer found in squid and shellfish, and is believed to achieve hemostasis through platelet activation and aggregation of erythrocytes[18] (▶ Fig. 16.5). It has been tested in animal models demonstrating improvements in wound healing and a reduction of adhesion formation with good hemostatic activity.[19] These findings were replicated in a human study of 40 patients where it was found to be rapidly hemostatic and led to significantly less adhesions compared to a no-treatment control[20] (▶ Fig. 16.6). To date, it has not been compared to existing packing materials.

Nasopore (Stryker, Kalamazoo, MI) is constructed from polyurethane, a fully synthetic, biodegradable, foamlike material that fragments in an average of 5 to 7 days. It is capable of absorbing 20 times its volume in water without swelling, and thus the risk of mucosal necrosis is theoretically reduced. Studies have noted an improvement in patient symptoms[21] and reduced adhesions with

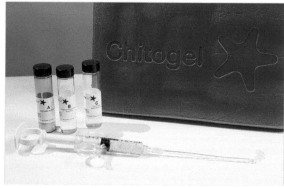

Fig. 16.5 Chitogel (Chitogel Pty); absorbable postsurgical hydrogel comprised of (a) dextran aldehyde, (b) sodium phosphate buffer, and (c) chitosan succinamide.

Nasopore when compared to Merocel packing,[22] but no significant difference in postoperative hemostasis when compared to no packing[23] or nonabsorbable packing.[24]

16.3 To Pack or Not to Pack

Although a wide range of absorbable and nonabsorbable packing materials exist, questions have been raised as to the need for packing at all in the postoperative setting. The risks of packing are well documented and evidence exists that packing does not offer improvements in

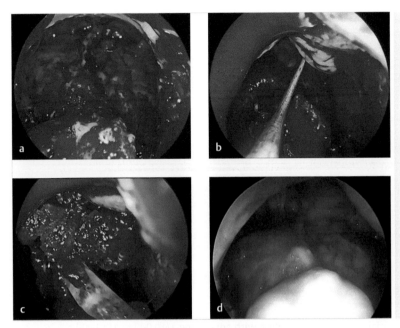

Fig. 16.6 Endoscopic intraoperative and postoperative images of frontal drillout. **(a)** Neo-ostium with significant bone exposure. **(b)** Mucosal flaps in situ. **(c)** Chitogel filling frontal drillout cavity. **(d)** Postoperative.

wound healing or a reduction in postoperative hemorrhage. A range of studies have highlighted in patient cohorts that only 8 to 13% of patients required packing following routine endoscopic sinus surgery[25,26] and a recent meta-analysis of the literature confirmed that there is no advantage in packing.[27] To date, no material has fulfilled the panacea of the perfect pack: well tolerated, effectively hemostatic, and causing minimal inflammatory response, and therefore the decision as to whether to pack or not is up to the treating surgeon.

16.4 Inert Stents

A variety of nonorganic spacers have been used in attempts to maintain patency of sinus ostia in the postsurgical setting with the theory that an inert compound will prevent clot and granulations retention in the ostia, thereby reducing synechia formation. Evidence suggests that the use of silastic spacers can reduce synechiae and are well tolerated by patients[28,29,30] with no evidence of increased infections.[29]

In terms of the frontal sinus, simple inert stents have been fashioned from silastic tubing or using existing stenting devices such as a ureteric stent.[31,32] Small rolls of silastic sheeting can also be inserted into the surgically widened ostium, although care must be taken not to completely occlude the ostium. An important part of postoperative stenting is to maintain a patent communication pathway and therefore drainage of the frontal sinus into the nasal cavity. Obstruction will cause retention of secretions, mucosal hypertrophy, and inflammation that may bear consequences on disease relapse. A drawback of inert stents is that they require office-based removal at between 1 and 2 weeks after surgery. We would caution the use of stents beyond 2 weeks due to the risk of biofilm colonization of the stent.

16.5 Drug-Eluting Stents

Stenting of sinus ostia with delivery of topical medication directly to the surrounding tissues has recently being developed. In 2010, Food and Drug Administration (FDA) approval was granted for a drug-eluting stent that releases 370 µg of mometasone furoate over the course of 30 days in a fully bioabsorbable mesh.[33] The stent itself comes with its own custom-made device for delivery into either the ethmoid cavity or the frontal sinus, after which the meshlike structure expands to fill the cavity or ostium. The original PROPEL (Intersect ENT, Menlo Park, CA) stent has been manufactured for use in ethmoid sinuses, and more recently the PROPEL Mini (Intersect ENT, Menlo Park, CA) gained approval for use in the frontal sinus. This product acts as both a mechanical stent to hold ostia open and a mechanism to facilitate the short- to medium-term delivery of topical corticosteroids, thus reducing postoperative inflammation, granulation, and the risks of poor outcomes.

In recent published studies, the PROPEL stent was compared to the same stent without steroids in the same patient. Using this model, the PROPEL stent has been identified to significantly reduce postoperative inflammation, adhesions, polyp formation, and the need for systemic steroids.[34,35] The PROPEL Mini stent has been examined specifically in the frontal sinus in a randomized trial of patients undergoing bilateral frontal sinusotomy where one side received a stent and the other no implant.[36] This study found a reduction in the need for postoperative intervention, the need for oral steroids, and restenosis rates. However, the cost of the stent remains a concern.

16.6 Postoperative Care

Postoperative care following endoscopic sinus surgery can be categorized into patient-delivered and clinician-delivered treatments. An aspect of patient-delivered care that is considered of paramount importance is saline irrigation throughout the postoperative recovery period. Topical medical therapy can include either steroid or antibiotic treatments, and can be delivered as either a spray, drop, or mixed into a saline wash. Clinician-delivered postoperative treatment is local instrumental debridement of blood clots, nasal crusts, and debris.

16.6.1 Saline Irrigations

Saline irrigation is advocated for reducing of preoperative inflammation, improving mucociliary clearance, and for symptomatic relief in the preoperative management of chronic rhinosinusitis. Further benefits are the removal of debris, clot, and mucoid secretions, all of which may reduce the local inflammatory burden, decrease the risk of postoperative infection, and lead to easier office-based debridement.

A wide range of delivery methods are available including manual plastic squeeze bottles, atomizer sprays, or automated wash bottles, and the volume of saline delivered ranges from a 2-mL spray to 240 mL of wash. Evidence suggests that douching regularly after surgery with a high-volume (240-mL) isotonic irrigation offers improvements in general and specific nasal symptoms compared to no irrigation in a randomized single-blinded trial.[37] Douching with low volumes or saline sprays did not appear to be of benefit.[38,39]

16.6.2 Endoscopic Debridement

The sinonasal cavity after ESS is filled with debris including clot, residual hemostatic dissolvable packing (if placed), and retained secretions. This material is thought to act not only as a perfect culture media for postoperative infections, but also as a potential framework for granulations, scarring, and subsequent ostial stenosis.[40] Convincing evidence exists regarding the benefit of debridement, with numerous trials demonstrating that it offers improvements in symptom scores and endoscopic appearances.[41,42,43] It is recommended that endoscopically assisted cleaning of sinus cavities be performed using appropriate instruments or suction devices at 1 to 2 weeks postsurgery, and then further debridements depending on the individual surgeon's preference and the status of the patient's mucosa.[40] Nonabsorbable stents can be removed during these visits at a time point as per surgeon preference.

16.6.3 Topical Treatments

Intranasal Corticosteroids

Topical intranasal corticosteroids (INCS) reduces tissue edema, promote wound healing,[44,45] and their use in the postoperative setting mirrors that of preoperative treatment. They can be delivered in either spray form, via droplets, or mixed into a high-volume saline douche bottle. The commonly prescribed medications are detailed in ▶ Table 16.2.

INCS sprays delivery their anti-inflammatory effects directly to sinonasal mucosa, and with newer generations of steroids (mometasone and fluticasone) there is a minimum of systemic absorption of steroid (<1%), coupled

Table 16.2 Commonly used intranasal corticosteroid preparations

	Dose	Treatment regime
Nasal sprays		
Beclomethasone dipropionate	50 µg (per spray)	2 sprays, twice daily
Budesonide aqua	100 µg (per spray)	1 spray twice daily or 2 sprays daily
Fluticasone furoate	27.5 µg (per spray)	2 sprays, twice daily
Fluticasone propionate	50 µg (per spray)	2 sprays, twice daily
Mometasone furoate	50 µg (per spray)	2 sprays, daily
Triamcinolone acetonide	55 µg (per spray)	2 sprays, daily
Nasal drops		
Betamethasone sodium phosphate	0.1%	2–3 drops twice daily
Fluticasone propionate	400 µg/vial	200 µg daily or twice daily
Off-label use of intranasal medication		
Dexamethasone ophthalmic	0.1%	2–3 drops twice daily
Prednisolone ophthalmic	1%	2–3 drops twice daily
Ciprofloxacin/ dexamethasone otic	0.3%/0.1%	2–3 drops twice daily
Budesonide respule	0.5 or 1 mg	Diluted into 240 mL saline douche daily or twice daily

with first-pass metabolism of any absorbed giving an excellent safety profile that has been very well investigated.[46] The bioavailability of older corticosteroids (beclomethasone, budesonide, and triamcinolone) may be significantly higher at between 40 and 50%,[47] thus raising a note of caution in their use. The incidence of side effects is low and includes transient local effects such as nasal irritation and epistaxis. Efficacy of INCS is well noted, with randomized trials demonstrating benefits in patient symptoms and endoscopic appearances of the sinonasal cavity.[44,48]

Therefore, their use should be considered routine practice both pre- and postoperatively. A drawback of INCS in the spray form is that delivery to affected sinonasal mucosa is hampered by anatomic factors such as turbinate hypertrophy,[49] septal deviation,[50] and the postoperative field that may have crusts or debris that prevent the steroid from actually reaching the underlying mucosa.

Corticosteroid nasal drops have been utilized to overcome this issue, and when used in either the Moffat head-down position (leaning forward, neck in full flexion) or the Mygind head-hanging (lying flat supine, neck in extension) position, drops may reach the middle meatus and frontal ostium. A step further has been in the off-label use of budesonide respules diluted into high-volume saline irrigation bottles. The safety profile has been well investigated with no evidence of significant systemic absorption, as demonstrated by no hypothalamic-pituitary-adrenal axis suppression even with prolonged courses of more than 2 years.[51] Evidence for this is reported in studies demonstrating improvements in symptom and endoscopic scores.[52,53] However, there is still need for further studies and use of these off-label medications should be guided by clinician preference.

Topical Antibiotic Treatment

The use of topical antibiotic therapies has emerged in recent years with the recognition that bacterial biofilms play an important disease-modifying role in chronic rhinosinusitis. Antibiotics such as tobramycin, vancomycin, gentamicin, and mupirocin have been suggested.[54,55,56] Although effective at elimination of bacteria during and immediately posttreatment, a high relapse rate has been identified,[57] suggesting that topical antibiotics may not penetrate deep enough into a biofilm or be able to reach intracellular or interstitial infection.[57] A recent Cochrane review was unable to identify any high-level evidence supporting topical antibiotics,[58] so they should only be considered by the clinician in the event of treatment failure with standard medical therapies.

16.7 Conclusion

There is evidence both for the use of nasal packs and for no packing after endoscopic sinus surgery. Most materials do not fit the ideal requirements of a nasal pack, namely, being well tolerated, hemostatic, and promoting wound healing without eliciting an inflammatory response. Drug-eluting stents are emerging as a biomaterial that may lead to improved healing of surrounding tissues as well as provide a mechanical scaffold to stent open sinus ostia. There is a wide range of topical therapies available to the clinician in the postoperative period. Saline irrigations improve symptoms by the removal of blood clot, crusts, and proinflammatory debris, and are likely to facilitate delivery of topical corticosteroid to the healing mucosa. Evidence exists for the use of topical corticosteroids either in spray, droplet, or mixed into a saline irrigation after surgery. The evidence for topical antibiotics is less strong, and it is advised that these be reserved for cases that the clinician judges have failed standard topical or systemic treatment.

References

[1] Ye T, Hwang PH, Huang Z, et al. Frontal ostium neo-osteogenesis and patency after Draf III procedure: a computer-assisted study. Int Forum Allergy Rhinol. 2014; 4(9):739–744

[2] Ngoc Ha T, Valentine R, Moratti S, Robinson S, Hanton L, Wormald PJ. A blinded randomized controlled trial evaluating the efficacy of chitosan gel on ostial stenosis following endoscopic sinus surgery. Int Forum Allergy Rhinol. 2013; 3(7):573–580

[3] Hildenbrand T, Wormald PJ, Weber RK. Endoscopic frontal sinus drainage Draf type III with mucosal transplants. Am J Rhinol Allergy. 2012; 26(2):148–151

[4] Fairbanks DN. Complications of nasal packing. Otolaryngol Head Neck Surg. 1986; 94(3):412–415

[5] Weber RK. Nasal packing and stenting. GMS Curr Top Otorhinolaryngol Head Neck Surg. 2009; 8:Doc02

[6] Oz MC, Rondinone JF, Shargill NS. FloSeal Matrix: new generation topical hemostatic sealant. J Card Surg. 2003; 18(6):486–493

[7] Catalano PJ, Roffman EJ. Evaluation of middle meatal stenting after minimally invasive sinus techniques (MIST). Otolaryngol Head Neck Surg. 2003; 128(6):875–881

[8] Tom LW, Palasti S, Potsic WP, Handler SD, Wetmore RF. The effects of gelatin film stents in the middle meatus. Am J Rhinol. 1997; 11 (3):229–232

[9] Rust KR, Stringer SP, Spector B. The effect of absorbable stenting on postoperative stenosis of the surgically enlarged maxillary sinus ostia in a rabbit animal model. Arch Otolaryngol Head Neck Surg. 1996; 122(12):1395–1397

[10] Yan M, Zheng D, Li Y, Zheng Q, Chen J, Yang B. Biodegradable nasal packings for endoscopic sinonasal surgery: a systematic review and meta-analysis. PLoS One. 2014; 9(12):e115458

[11] Maccabee MS, Trune DR, Hwang PH. Effects of topically applied biomaterials on paranasal sinus mucosal healing. Am J Rhinol. 2003; 17 (4):203–207

[12] Shrime MG, Tabaee A, Hsu AK, Rickert S, Close LG. Synechia formation after endoscopic sinus surgery and middle turbinate medialization with and without FloSeal. Am J Rhinol. 2007; 21(2):174–179

[13] Prosdocimi M, Bevilacqua C. Exogenous hyaluronic acid and wound healing: an updated vision. Panminerva Med. 2012; 54(2):129–135

[14] McIntosh D, Cowin A, Adams D, Rayner T, Wormald PJ. The effect of a dissolvable hyaluronic acid-based pack on the healing of the nasal mucosa of sheep. Am J Rhinol. 2002; 16(2):85–90

[15] Rajapaksa SP, Cowin A, Adams D, Wormald PJ. The effect of a hyaluronic acid-based nasal pack on mucosal healing in a sheep model of sinusitis. Am J Rhinol. 2005; 19(6):572–576

[16] Miller RS, Steward DL, Tami TA, et al. The clinical effects of hyaluronic acid ester nasal dressing (Merogel) on intranasal wound healing after

functional endoscopic sinus surgery. Otolaryngol Head Neck Surg. 2003; 128(6):862–869

[17] Wormald PJ, Boustred RN, Le T, Hawke L, Sacks R. A prospective single-blind randomized controlled study of use of hyaluronic acid nasal packs in patients after endoscopic sinus surgery. Am J Rhinol. 2006; 20(1):7–10

[18] Valentine R, Wormald PJ, Sindwani R. Advances in absorbable biomaterials and nasal packing. Otolaryngol Clin North Am. 2009; 42(5):813–828, ix

[19] Athanasiadis T, Beule AG, Robinson BH, Robinson SR, Shi Z, Wormald PJ. Effects of a novel chitosan gel on mucosal wound healing following endoscopic sinus surgery in a sheep model of chronic rhinosinusitis. Laryngoscope. 2008; 118(6):1088–1094

[20] Valentine R, Athanasiadis T, Moratti S, Hanton L, Robinson S, Wormald PJ. The efficacy of a novel chitosan gel on hemostasis and wound healing after endoscopic sinus surgery. Am J Rhinol Allergy. 2010; 24(1):70–75

[21] Wang J, Cai C, Wang S. Merocel versus Nasopore for nasal packing: a meta-analysis of randomized controlled trials. PLoS One. 2014; 9(4): e93959

[22] Piski Z, Gerlinger I, Nepp N, et al. Clinical benefits of polyurethane nasal packing in endoscopic sinus surgery. Eur Arch Otorhinolaryngol. 2017; 274(3):1449–1454

[23] Kastl KG, Reichert M, Scheithauer MO, et al. Patient comfort following FESS and Nasopore® packing, a double blind, prospective, randomized trial. Rhinology. 2014; 52(1):60–65

[24] Shoman N, Gheriani H, Flamer D, Javer A. Prospective, double-blind, randomized trial evaluating patient satisfaction, bleeding, and wound healing using biodegradable synthetic polyurethane foam (NasoPore) as a middle meatal spacer in functional endoscopic sinus surgery. J Otolaryngol Head Neck Surg. 2009; 38(1):112–118

[25] Orlandi RR, Lanza DC. Is nasal packing necessary following endoscopic sinus surgery? Laryngoscope. 2004; 114(9):1541–1544

[26] Eliashar R, Gross M, Wohlgelernter J, Sichel JY. Packing in endoscopic sinus surgery: is it really required? Otolaryngol Head Neck Surg. 2006; 134(2):276–279

[27] Stern-Shavit S, Nachalon Y, Leshno M, Soudry E. Middle meatal packing in endoscopic sinus surgery-to pack or not to pack?: a decision-analysis model. Laryngoscope. 2017; 127(7):1506–1512

[28] Gall RM, Witterick IJ. The use of middle meatal stents post-endoscopic sinus surgery. J Otolaryngol. 2004; 33(1):47–49

[29] Baguley CJ, Stow NW, Weitzel EK, Douglas RG. Silastic splints reduce middle meatal adhesions after endoscopic sinus surgery. Am J Rhinol Allergy. 2012; 26(5):414–417

[30] Chan CL, Elmiyeh B, Woods C, et al. A randomized controlled trial of a middle meatal silastic stent for reducing adhesions and middle turbinate lateralization following endoscopic sinus surgery. Int Forum Allergy Rhinol. 2015; 5(6):517–523

[31] Mirza S, Johnson AP. A simple and effective frontal sinus stent. J Laryngol Otol. 2000; 114(12):955–956

[32] Hughes JP, Rowe-Jones J. Use of a ureteric pigtail stent as a self-retaining frontal sinus stent. J Laryngol Otol. 2004; 118(4):299–301

[33] Wei CC, Kennedy DW. Mometasone implant for chronic rhinosinusitis. Med Devices (Auckl). 2012; 5:75–80

[34] Forwith KD, Chandra RK, Yun PT, Miller SK, Jampel HD. ADVANCE: a multisite trial of bioabsorbable steroid-eluting sinus implants. Laryngoscope. 2011; 121(11):2473–2480

[35] Marple BF, Smith TL, Han JK, et al. Advance II: a prospective, randomized study assessing safety and efficacy of bioabsorbable steroid-releasing sinus implants. Otolaryngol Head Neck Surg. 2012; 146(6):1004–1011

[36] Smith TL, Singh A, Luong A, et al. Randomized controlled trial of a bioabsorbable steroid-releasing implant in the frontal sinus opening. Laryngoscope. 2016; 126(12):2659–2664

[37] Giotakis AI, Karow EM, Scheithauer MO, Weber R, Riechelmann H. Saline irrigations following sinus surgery: a controlled, single blinded, randomized trial. Rhinology. 2016; 54(4):302–310

[38] Pinto JM, Elwany S, Baroody FM, Naclerio RM. Effects of saline sprays on symptoms after endoscopic sinus surgery. Am J Rhinol. 2006; 20(2):191–196

[39] Freeman SR, Sivayoham ES, Jepson K, de Carpentier J. A preliminary randomised controlled trial evaluating the efficacy of saline douching following endoscopic sinus surgery. Clin Otolaryngol. 2008; 33(5):462–465

[40] Rudmik L, Soler ZM, Orlandi RR, et al. Early postoperative care following endoscopic sinus surgery: an evidence-based review with recommendations. Int Forum Allergy Rhinol. 2011; 1(6):417–430

[41] Bugten V, Nordgård S, Steinsvåg S. The effects of debridement after endoscopic sinus surgery. Laryngoscope. 2006; 116(11):2037–2043

[42] Bugten V, Nordgård S, Steinsvåg S. Long-term effects of postoperative measures after sinus surgery. Eur Arch Otorhinolaryngol. 2008; 265(5):531–537

[43] Lee JY, Byun JY. Relationship between the frequency of postoperative debridement and patient discomfort, healing period, surgical outcomes, and compliance after endoscopic sinus surgery. Laryngoscope. 2008; 118(10):1868–1872

[44] Jorissen M, Bachert C. Effect of corticosteroids on wound healing after endoscopic sinus surgery. Rhinology. 2009; 47(3):280–286

[45] Hosemann W, Wigand ME, Göde U, Länger F, Dunker I. Normal wound healing of the paranasal sinuses: clinical and experimental investigations. Eur Arch Otorhinolaryngol. 1991; 248(7):390–394

[46] Sastre J, Mosges R. Local and systemic safety of intranasal corticosteroids. J Investig Allergol Clin Immunol. 2012; 22(1):1–12

[47] Mullol J, Obando A, Pujols L, Alobid I. Corticosteroid treatment in chronic rhinosinusitis: the possibilities and the limits. Immunol Allergy Clin North Am. 2009; 29(4):657–668

[48] Rowe-Jones JM, Medcalf M, Durham SR, Richards DH, Mackay IS. Functional endoscopic sinus surgery: 5 year follow up and results of a prospective, randomised, stratified, double-blind, placebo controlled study of postoperative fluticasone propionate aqueous nasal spray. Rhinology. 2005; 43(1):2–10

[49] Dowley AC, Homer JJ. The effect of inferior turbinate hypertrophy on nasal spray distribution to the middle meatus. Clin Otolaryngol Allied Sci. 2001; 26(6):488–490

[50] Frank DO, Kimbell JS, Cannon D, Pawar SS, Rhee JS. Deviated nasal septum hinders intranasal sprays: a computer simulation study. Rhinology. 2012; 50(3):311–318

[51] Smith KA, French G, Mechor B, Rudmik L. Safety of long-term high-volume sinonasal budesonide irrigations for chronic rhinosinusitis. Int Forum Allergy Rhinol. 2016; 6(3):228–232

[52] Jang DW, Lachanas VA, Segel J, Kountakis SE. Budesonide nasal irrigations in the postoperative management of chronic rhinosinusitis. Int Forum Allergy Rhinol. 2013; 3(9):708–711

[53] Snidvongs K, Pratt E, Chin D, Sacks R, Earls P, Harvey RJ. Corticosteroid nasal irrigations after endoscopic sinus surgery in the management of chronic rhinosinusitis. Int Forum Allergy Rhinol. 2012; 2(5):415–421

[54] Lee VS, Davis GE. Culture-directed topical antibiotic treatment for chronic rhinosinusitis. Am J Rhinol Allergy. 2016; 30(6):414–417

[55] Carr TF, Hill JL, Chiu A, Chang EH. Alteration in bacterial culture after treatment with topical mupirocin for recalcitrant chronic rhinosinusitis. JAMA Otolaryngol Head Neck Surg. 2016; 142(2):138–142

[56] Jervis-Bardy J, Boase S, Psaltis A, Foreman A, Wormald PJ. A randomized trial of mupirocin sinonasal rinses versus saline in surgically recalcitrant staphylococcal chronic rhinosinusitis. Laryngoscope. 2012; 122(10):2148–2153

[57] Jervis-Bardy J, Wormald PJ. Microbiological outcomes following mupirocin nasal washes for symptomatic, Staphylococcus aureus-positive chronic rhinosinusitis following endoscopic sinus surgery. Int Forum Allergy Rhinol. 2012; 2(2):111–115

[58] Head K, Chong LY, Piromchai P, et al. Systemic and topical antibiotics for chronic rhinosinusitis. Cochrane Database Syst Rev. 2016; 4: CD011994

17 Office-Based Frontal Sinus Procedures

Joshua M. Levy and John M. DelGaudio

Abstract

In-office sinonasal procedures represent a rapidly advancing field in otolaryngology, with the potential to surgically impact a patient's disease without assuming the associated risks and costs of general anesthesia. Motivated by an increasing focus on patient satisfaction, physician availability, and resource utilization, the emergence of in-office procedures has also been further supported by technological advances and high patient satisfaction.[1] There are many appealing factors associated with in-office sinonasal procedures. The ability to perform office surgery eliminates the need for a general anesthetic, reduces patient downtime and lost productivity, and eliminates operating room, anesthesia, and recovery room expenses. This can reduce health care expenditures and decrease time to treatment for the appropriately selected patient. A retrospective, matched-pair cost analysis of sinonasal procedures performed in the office versus an ambulatory operating room revealed significantly lower costs for in-office procedures, with mean total charges of $2,737.17 versus $7,329.69 ($p < 0.001$). No significant difference was found in subsequent physician reimbursement.[2] While not for every patient, some frontal sinus disease can be effectively treated in an office-based setting, thereby avoiding a procedure in the operating room. This chapter will review the patient and disease factors that are most amenable to office-based treatment, as well as recently developed technologies to expand indications and improve patient outcomes.

Keywords: office surgery, frontal sinusitis, endoscopic sinus surgery, mucocele

17.1 Indications

17.1.1 Anatomic Considerations

Surgery of the frontal sinus presents a significant challenge due to the varied and complex anatomy of the frontal recess. The frontal recess is an anatomic space immediately inferior to the frontal sinus outflow tract and posterior to the frontal beak of the nasal process of the frontal bone. Additional boundaries include the lamina papyracea (lateral) and vertical lamella of the middle turbinate (medial), as well as the anterior face of the ethmoid bulla (posterior). Patency of the frontal recess may be anatomically compromised by multiple air cells, including the agger nasi cell (ANC), supra agger cell, supra agger frontal cell, supra bulla cell (SBC), supra bulla frontal cell, supraorbital ethmoid cell, or the frontal septal cell.[3] Familiarity with each patient's unique frontal recess anatomy is essential in both understanding their unique disease process and planning a successful procedure. Computed tomography (CT) scan of the sinuses is indispensable in gaining an understanding of this underlying anatomy while evaluating for evidence of acute or chronic inflammation. Thin section axial images (0.5- to 1-mm slice thickness) should be obtained. Reformatted images in the sagittal and coronal planes give additional information regarding the anatomy of the frontal sinus outflow tract.

Prior to any intervention, the surgeon should review imaging with a particular focus on the anatomy of each frontal recess. Patients with simpler configurations are better candidates for office surgical procedures. A larger anteroposterior diameter of the frontal recess, as seen on sagittal views, will also make access and visualization easier in the office. Anatomical factors that may make an office-based approach more difficult include a superior nasal septal deviation, concha bullosa, and a lateralized middle turbinate.

Middle turbinate lateralization and bony obstruction, especially neo-osteogenesis, may make an office frontal sinus procedure difficult (▶ Fig. 17.1a, b).

17.1.2 Patient Selection

Patient selection is the most important consideration in office-based rhinological surgery.[4]

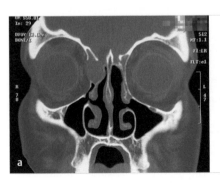
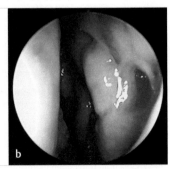

Fig. 17.1 (a) Coronal CT shows a right frontoethmoid mucocele with orbital and skull base erosion that is accessible for office drainage. The left side shows a lateralized, osteitic middle turbinate that is scarred to the lamina papyracea, making it difficult to safely open this frontal sinus in the office. **(b)** Endoscopic view of a scarred, lateralized middle turbinate.

While the underlying disease process or structural anatomy may be amenable to office intervention, the importance of patient tolerance and compliance is paramount. A thorough explanation of the procedure, goals, expectations, and postprocedure care should occur prior to any intervention. Informed consent should discuss all risks associated with the procedure and ample time for questions or patient deliberation should be given. After a candid dialog, the physician should assess the patient's receptiveness to the procedure as well as their associated anxiety level.

Highly nervous patients are poor candidates for in-office procedures. However, apprehension associated with in-office procedures can mitigate after explaining the procedure with the patient.

Patients frequently become more receptive to the in-office procedure when faced with the alternative of going to the OR and having a general anesthesia and more postoperative downtime. One should not exclude those patients whose underlying health and comorbidities may prohibit them from undergoing general anesthesia. In fact, these patients can be excellent candidates for a minimally invasive office-based approach. However, even well-selected patients can experience a vasovagal response, resulting in a self-limited episode of systemic hypotension often associated with bradycardia, peripheral vasodilation, and potential loss of consciousness. The occurrence of vasovagal episodes is rare among patients undergoing office-based rhinological procedures, with a reported incidence of 0.16%.[5] Despite this rare occurrence, the physician and staff should be prepared to manage a patient's symptoms prior to offering in-office procedures.

17.1.3 Frontal Sinusitis

Frontal sinusitis is the result of acute or chronic inflammation and obstruction of the frontal sinus drainage pathway. Patients most likely to benefit from an in-office intervention are those with isolated acute frontal sinusitis with significant symptoms, and those with isolated chronic frontal sinusitis. For a primary frontal sinus procedure in the office, the patient should have a relatively simple frontal recess anatomy. A significant septal deviation to the side of the disease is a relative contraindication. Performing a

primary frontal sinusotomy with cold instruments in the office is difficult and rarely done, but balloon technology can be an appropriate tool to open the frontal recess in these situations.

17.1.4 Frontal Mucoceles

A mucocele is an expanded mucus-filled sinus cavity that results from obstruction of a sinus outflow tract. This is often secondary to chronic inflammation, nasal polyposis, trauma, or a consequence of a prior surgery, such as with lateral scarring of the middle turbinate. Thinning and remodeling of bone, often with areas of dehiscence, can be seen on CT imaging with expansion of the mucocele (▶ Fig. 17.2a, b). A recently published retrospective review evaluated outcomes following in-office drainage of sinus mucoceles, finding the procedure is well tolerated in the appropriately selected patient with 97% undergoing successful drainage.[6] Of note, 14% of patients required additional surgery, with a higher risk of failure among patients with septated mucoceles and neo-osteogenesis of the frontal recess. Septated mucoceles represent a relative contraindication to office-based drainage, with difficult-to-reach segments that are often not accessible in an in-office procedure. Neo-osteogenesis of the frontal recess is a common finding among patients with frontal mucoceles. This finding represents a relative contraindication as thickened bone can be difficult to remove without significant force, which is difficult for the awake patient to tolerate.

17.1.5 Nasal Polyps

Patients with recurrent polypoid obstruction of the frontal recess following endoscopic sinus surgery (ESS) with removal of bony partitions from the frontal recess are good candidates for office-based polypectomy.[7] Polyposis of the frontal recess can be addressed aggressively as long as the anatomy is well understood and only soft-tissue obstruction of the previously opened frontal sinus is present. This can be performed alone or in combination with removal of polyps from the other sinuses. Unilateral sinonasal masses that mimic nasal polyps include such pathologies as meningoencephaloceles and tumors such as inverted papilloma. However, with good preoperative

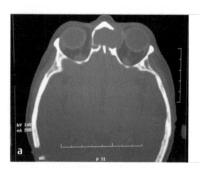
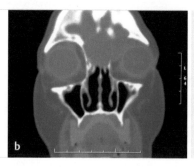

Fig. 17.2 (a) Axial CT shows a left fronto-ethmoid mucocele with orbital and skull base erosion. (b) Coronal view of the same tumor. Notice dehiscence of the lamina papyracea with associated displacement of the globe.

imaging and clinical suspicion, complications and improper diagnosis can be avoided.

As all polyps are not the same, the type of polyps should be considered when deciding to perform an office procedure. While polyps occluding the nasal airway are typically not adjacent to vital structures, those associated with central compartment disease extend from the nasal septum and olfactory fossa medial to the middle turbinates. These types of polyps are harder to adequately remove in the office setting and may be considered better candidates for removal in the operating room.

Patients with recurrent sinonasal polyposis after adequate ESS and failed medical therapy are good candidates for office-based polypectomy.

17.2 Surgical Steps/Anesthesia

After appropriate patient selection, adequate anesthesia is the most important component in performing successful office-based surgery.

Sufficient anesthesia can be obtained with topical agents alone, but injected local anesthetics are sometimes necessary, especially when dissection requires deeper penetration into the sinonasal cavities. As with any nasal endoscopic procedure, mucosal vasoconstriction is important in providing adequate visualization and access, thus reducing unnecessary tissue trauma and pain. Common office decongestants such as oxymetazoline, phenylephrine, or 1:1,000 epinephrine are used topically within the nose to achieve vasoconstriction and minimize bleeding. The former two medications can be applied either through an atomized spray or delivered to the tissue on cotton applicators, while epinephrine can only be applied by cotton applicators. It is important to counsel the patient prior to placing topical vasoconstrictors in anticipation of associated tachycardia.

Topical anesthetic agents are routinely used in nasal endoscopic procedures and are readily available.[8] The most common medications are Pontocaine and lidocaine. These medications provide surface anesthesia and are therefore only effective at the areas of mucosal contact. Each anesthetic has its associated toxicity levels and these should be reviewed prior to use. Often topical anesthetic and decongestant medications are combined to provide both anesthesia and vasoconstriction at the same time. For office procedures, multiple applications of the topical medicine combination spray are necessary, as the distribution of mucosal contact improves with increasing mucosal decongestion. In our practice, we routinely utilize 1:1 oxymetazoline mixed with 4% topical lidocaine, which is extremely safe given the serum toxicity levels of lidocaine > 5 mcg/mL.

In addition to topical anesthetics, local anesthetic injections are frequently employed. These local blocks can provide additional anesthesia to the sinonasal cavity. We use 1% lidocaine with 1:100,000 epinephrine. Longer lasting

agents can be used but are not necessary, as there is no significant pain following the procedure. Injection sites in preparation for frontal sinus procedures include the attachment and caudal edge of the middle turbinate, as well as the superior lateral nasal wall.

The combination of topical anesthetic with decongestant and injected local anesthesia typically provides adequate anesthesia and a cooperative patient.

We do not use sedatives in any of our patients prior to or during the procedure, but this is an option for patients undergoing office-based surgery with the utilization of several sedative anesthetics, such as midazolam or other benzodiazepines. Sedated patients should be monitored during and after the procedure for appropriate recovery, but this is not necessary when using only topical and local anesthetics. Patients receiving oral or intravenous sedation need to be accompanied by another adult and should not be allowed to drive after the procedure.

17.3 Postoperative Management and Procedures

Performing a properly indicated and technically proficient procedure is only part of the required treatment needed to achieve desired outcomes for paranasal sinus disease. Long-term management of chronic rhinosinusitis involves minimizing the mucosal inflammatory process, which requires routine postoperative care and long-term surveillance. If needed, medical and/or surgical interventions are utilized to prevent progression of the underlying inflammatory process.

Routine postoperative care involves an office endoscopy and debridement 1 week after the initial procedure, followed by another additional endoscopy and possible debridement between 2 and 4 weeks later. Frequency of follow-up and endoscopic debridement is determined by the patient's clinical and endoscopic improvement, with compliance and underlying disease process playing major roles. The location of the initial procedure (office vs. OR) should not influence postoperative care.

After any frontal sinus procedure, the frontal sinus should again be visualized in the postoperative period. At the first postoperative visit, the frontal recess should be visualized with an angled endoscope and cleared of debris by gently suctioning with a curved suction. Generally, mucus, crust, dissolvable nasal packing, or blood clot is found at the first visit and should be suctioned and removed. Attention is given to areas of denuded bone, as these areas will be more prone to crusting, granulation, and scarring. Due to the narrow drainage pathway of the frontal recess, circumferential bands can form. If synechiae are noted at the early postoperative visits, they should be lysed to avoid further stenosis. Circumferential scarring or stenosis that is seen at later appointments can still be addressed in the office. Often, these areas of scar can be taken down with frontal cutting instruments while trying to avoid causing further trauma to the frontal drainage pathway. Balloon catheter dilation (BCD) of the frontal ostium may be a good tool to employ in these instances if the scar or stenosis is not from neo-osteogenesis or bony obstruction.[9]

17.3.1 Nasal Irrigations and Topical Therapies

Nasal saline irrigations are recommended for the treatment of chronic rhinosinusitis, both prior to and following surgical intervention.[10] A high-volume, low-pressure system in a squeeze bottle remains the optimal delivery device. The authors' postoperative management commonly includes nasal saline irrigations at least twice daily, generally starting on the operative day.

Topical medical therapies have been added to saline irrigations to optimize healing and control postoperative inflammation and edema. Advantages of topical medical therapies include direct drug delivery onto diseased tissue with the potential for delivering higher local drug concentrations while minimizing systemic absorption. Disadvantages of topical medical therapies include application challenges, local discomfort, epistaxis, and inconsistent sinus penetration.[11]

Nasal steroid irrigations are a frequently utilized topical treatment strategy for patients with recalcitrant chronic rhinosinusitis. A recent Cochrane review of topical steroids used in patients with chronic rhinosinusitis with nasal polyposis showed improved symptoms, reduced polyp size, and decreased polyp recurrence after surgery.[12] A commonly used preparation is budesonide saline irrigations twice daily (0.5 mg/2 mL or 1 mg/2 mL mixed into 240 mL of saline). Topical steroid rinses can be beneficial at any time, but are most effective in patients with residual mucosal inflammation after surgery or recurrent edema or polyps after the first or second postoperative visit.

17.4 Tips and Tricks

17.4.1 Case Examples

Frontal Mucoceles

Wide marsupialization of the mucocele is the recommended treatment.[13] This can be performed in the office if the inferior aspect of the mucocele can be visualized bulging into the nasal cavity and ethmoid sinus (▶ Fig. 17.3), or it can be accessed with dissection through the uncinate process and anterior ethmoid cells. If the frontal recess has previously been opened, then this is usually a very straightforward procedure, as obstructing cells have oftentimes been previously removed. After adequate local anesthesia is obtained, the inferior wall of the mucocele cavity is perforated with a curette under direct endoscopic visualization. This will usually result in

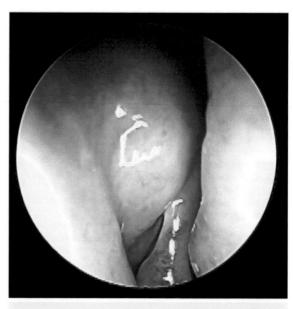

Fig. 17.3 Endoscopic view of a mucocele bulging in the right nasal cavity anterior to the attachment of the right middle turbinate.

mucus draining into the nasal cavity if it hasn't already begun with the local anesthetic injections. The angled curette and cutting forceps can be used to remove the entire inferior wall of the mucocele. The anterior and posterior walls should be removed as widely as possible with cutting instruments such as a frontal mushroom punch, frontal through-cutting forceps, or a frontal Kerrison rongeur. All bone chips and loose mucosa should be removed. Every attempt should be made to minimize trauma and prevent any stripping of frontal sinus or frontal recess mucosa. Even though this is being done in the office, the goal is the same as if it is being done in the operating room, thus creating a large drainage pathway to decompress the mucocele and prevent recurrence, scarring, or stenosis of the frontal recess.

The office-based drainage of frontal mucoceles in the patient who has not had previous sinus surgery is not as straightforward as in the previously operated patient. These patients have normal anatomic structures that oftentimes contribute to their disease process and need to be traversed to access the mucocele. It is essential that the CT scan is thoroughly assessed to understand the frontal recess anatomy and determine the most appropriate location (office vs. OR) and approach for successful drainage.

Frontal mucoceles extending inferiorly to the uncinate process or ANC may often be addressed without disturbing the ethmoid bulla (Video 17.1 and 17.2). However, it may be necessary to open the anterior ethmoidal cells when a frontal mucocele extends posteriorly along the suprabullar recess, above the SBC. The upper portion of the vertical uncinate process and middle turbinate need to be adequately anesthetized to allow for patient comfort and

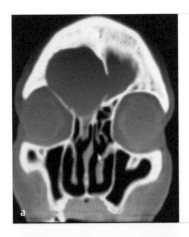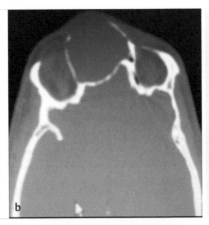

Fig. 17.4 (a, b) Axial and coronal CT scan images displaying right mucocele obstructing the frontal outflow tract with erosion of the orbital wall and skull base. Agger nasi cell is visualized inferior to the right frontal mucocele.

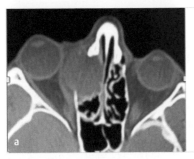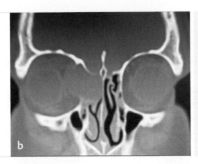

Fig. 17.5 (a, b) Axial and coronal CT scan images displaying right orbital wall dehiscence secondary to mucocele formation.

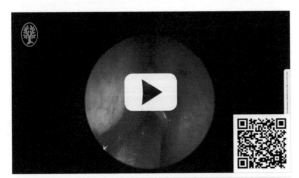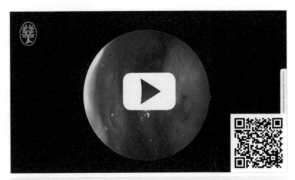

Video 17.1 Frontal mucocele – Intact bulla approach: example 1

Video 17.2 Frontal mucocele – Intact bulla approach: example 2

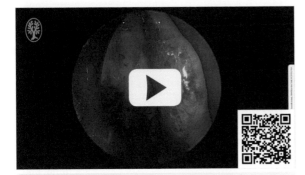

Video 17.3 Frontal sinus mucocele – Trans bulla approach

compliance. The uncinate process is divided with back-biting forceps, and the superior portion removed with 45-degree through-cutting forceps or a straight mushroom punch. The ANC can then be easily accessed through its inferior wall, which should be widely removed. This typically then provides wide access to the frontal recess with direct visualization of the bulging mucocele. Once the inferior wall of the mucocele is identified, it can be marsupialized as mentioned earlier (Video 17.3).

Bony expansion and erosion are common with mucoceles of the frontal sinus and are not contraindications for office-based treatment. The most common areas of bony dehiscence are the orbit, followed by the posterior table

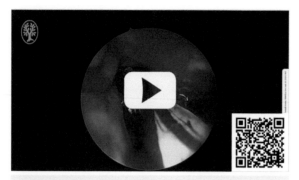

Video 17.4 Outpatient endoscopic frontal polypectomy – example 1

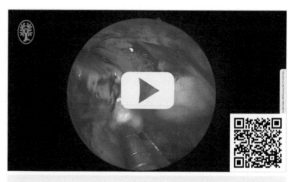

Video 17.5 Outpatient endoscopic frontal polypectomy – example 2

of the frontal sinus and the ethmoid roof.[14] These areas need to be preoperatively identified on the CT scan and accounted for in the surgical approach (▶ Fig. 17.4a, b and ▶ Fig. 17.5a, b). Since the periorbita is usually intact, drainage of the mucocele does not cause prolapse of orbital contents into the mucocele cavity. Lateral dissection in the fronto-orbital recess is to be avoided in these cases until the orbital contents are identified. Additionally, blind passage of instruments into the frontal sinus should be avoided so as not to inadvertently damage the orbital contents or frontal lobe.

Nasal Polyps

The approach for removal of sinonasal polyps is generally the same as in the operating room. The technique involves angled endoscopes and frontal instrumentation. Isolated nasal polyps in the ethmoid cavity and frontal recess can be removed with through-cutting instruments at the mucosal attachment site. For more extensive nasal polyps that are common in patients with prior surgery, 40-, 60-, or 90-degree microdebrider blades can be used conservatively, being mindful to limit mucosal injury. A single-use suction-powered microdebrider (PolypVac) is an option if a microdebrider is not available in the office setting. The removal of all sinonasal polyposis should be attempted. Only pedunculated polyps should be removed in the frontal recess and frontal sinus, and mucosa along the narrow frontal recess should be avoided as circumferential scarring and stenosis is a common cause of surgical failure (Videos 17.4 and 17.5). As polyps are removed, the reapplication of topical and local anesthetic may be necessary to anesthetize deeper tissue. Use of the microdebrider can lead to bleeding from the shearing of polypoid tissue, but this is generally mild. Utilizing topical vasoconstrictive or hemostatic agents and keeping the patient sitting up or in reverse Trendelenburg position can reduce blood loss.[15] Bleeding is typically minimal to mild since the patient is being anesthetized with vasodilating agents. Postoperative treatment with topical corticosteroids is very important in postoperative and long-term management of these patients.

17.5 Controversies

17.5.1 Balloon Catheter Dilation

First described by Lanza in 1993, BCD represents a tissue-sparing technique for the pneumatic widening of sinus ostia for the treatment of paranasal sinus disease.[16] The application of BCD technology to the paranasal sinuses was cleared by the U.S. Food and Drug Administration in April 2005, with subsequently broad utilization approaching 8% of all endoscopic sinus surgeries.[17,18] Recent protocols have described the use of BCD in the office-based setting under local anesthesia,[9,19,20] with great debate regarding appropriate indications and utilization.[21,22,23] BCD systems involve either a flexible guidewire or rigid cannulas over which the balloon is advanced. In general, the protocol for BCD involves topical and local anesthesia, with or without sedation to anesthetize the lateral nasal wall and middle turbinate. The middle turbinate is then medialized, with subsequent positioning of the cannula depending on the anatomy of the frontal recess. The cannula should be placed into the frontal recess, lateral to the middle turbinate, posterior to the agger nasi, and anterior to the ethmoid bulla. The balloon is then advanced and inflated for 10 seconds. The balloon can then be advanced further and reinflated as needed. This results in pneumatic widening of the frontal recess with fracture of the bony lateral and anterior walls of the ethmoid bulla and agger nasi.

Balloon technology can be used in the frontal sinus with the goal of dilating the frontal outflow tract while preserving mucosa.

Multiple industry-sponsored studies have demonstrated the efficacy of BCD for the treatment of paranasal sinus disease, with a recent systematic review and meta-analysis finding that evidence for long-term improvements in quality of life, and sinus opacification is limited to a restricted population of adults with minimal sinus disease.[24] Several studies have prospectively evaluated office-based BCD for the treatment of chronic sinusitis. The optimization and refinement of technique in in-office sinus dilation (ORIOS) series of studies represents a multicenter nonrandomized trial demonstrating safety, patient tolerance, and clinical efficacy with improved 22-item sinonasal outcome test (SNOT-22) and Lund–Mackay scores at last available follow-up.[19,25] In their largest series, Karanfilov et al reported successful BCD of the frontal recess in 93.7% of patients, with 82.3% of the entire cohort reporting that the procedure was well tolerated.[25] Gould et al prospectively evaluated outcomes at 12 months following office-based BCD, with patients reporting an average of 2.3 fewer exacerbations, 2.4 fewer antibiotic courses, and 3.0 fewer physician visits compared to the year preceding intervention.[26] Of note, subgroup analysis demonstrated no difference in outcome between groups with differently treated paranasal sinuses (e.g., maxillary vs. frontal).

Indications for office-based BCD often vary among physicians. Most patients with uncomplicated frontal sinus anatomy and isolated frontal sinusitis are good candidates for BCD. Other possible candidates for a dilation procedure include those with narrowing of the nonbony postoperative frontal sinus outflow tract. Dilations could be performed on these patients, which would minimize trauma and circumferential stenosis.

The technique for office-based balloon dilation of the frontal sinus has been described elsewhere.[27] Balloon dilation of the frontal sinus is performed using an angled endoscope and a 70-degree sinus cannula. The cannula is placed between the uncinate process and the upper face of the ethmoid bulla. A lighted flexible guidewire can then be placed under endoscopic visualization into the frontal recess until cannulation of the frontal ostium is achieved. The lighted guidewire allows for transillumination of the forehead skin overlying the frontal sinus to confirm entrance of the wire into the frontal sinus. The balloon-dilating catheter is then advanced over the guidewire into the frontal recess. The balloon is then inflated for 10 seconds prior to deflation and removal. This can be repeated along the length of the frontal outflow tract as needed.

17.6 Emerging Technologies

Steroid-eluting implants and in-office image-guided surgical systems represent two emerging technologies with the potential to influence office-based frontal sinus surgery. Steroid-eluting implants (Propel, Intersect ENT, Menlo Park, CA) are FDA approved, steroid-releasing dissolvable stents with proven efficacy and prevention of frontal recess stenosis following ESS.[28] While an indication for in-office placement is yet to be demonstrated, active investigation for patients with persistent frontal sinus disease is currently underway.

The ability to utilize image-guidance systems for real-time instrument localization is an important tool for the practicing sinonasal surgeon. This technology is being applied to the office, with the recent release of the Fusion Compact navigation system and NuVent EM Balloon Sinus Dilation System (Medtronic, Dublin, Ireland). While in no way designed to replace knowledge of each patient's unique surgical anatomy, these powerful tools enable the surgeon to utilize image guidance technology while treating patients in an office-based setting.

17.7 Conclusion

Otolaryngologists continue to make great strides in their evaluation and treatment of frontal sinus disease. Attempts to reduce health care expenditures and improve patient satisfaction are reasons to perform office-based surgery. Patient selection is crucial in deciding who will benefit most from an office-based frontal sinus intervention. Office procedures offer the advantage of decreased time off from work, cost advantages for the patients and payers, avoidance of general anesthesia, and comparable reimbursement rates for the physician. With the proper anesthesia, knowledge of the associated anatomy, and surgical technique, office-based frontal sinus surgery can be successfully completed with excellent outcomes.

References

[1] Varshney R, Lee JT. New innovations in office-based rhinology. Curr Opin Otolaryngol Head Neck Surg. 2016; 24(1):3–9

[2] Prickett KK, Wise SK, DelGaudio JM. Cost analysis of office-based and operating room procedures in rhinology. Int Forum Allergy Rhinol. 2012; 2(3):207–211

[3] Wormald P-J, Hoseman W, Callejas C, et al. The International Frontal Sinus Anatomy Classification (IFAC) and Classification of the Extent of Endoscopic Frontal Sinus Surgery (EFSS). Int Forum Allergy Rhinol. 2016; 6(7):677–696

[4] Patel ZM, Wise SK. Patient selection and informed consent for office-based rhinology procedures. In: Patel ZM, Wise SK, DelGaudio JM, eds. Office-Based Rhinology Principles and Techniques. San Diego, CA: Plural Publishing; 2013

[5] Radvansky BM, Husain Q, Cherla DV, Choudhry OJ, Eloy JA. In-office vasovagal response after rhinologic manipulation. Int Forum Allergy Rhinol. 2013; 3(6):510–514

[6] Barrow EM, DelGaudio JM. In-office drainage of sinus mucoceles: an alternative to operating-room drainage. Laryngoscope. 2015; 125 (5):1043–1047

[7] Henriquez OA, DelGaudio JM. Office-based nasal polypectomy. In: Patel ZM, Wise SK, DelGaudio JM, eds. Office-Based Rhinology Principles and Techniques. San Diego, CA: Plural Publishing; 2013

[8] Snidvongs K, Harvey RJ. Nasal and sinus anesthesia for office procedures. In: Patel ZM, Wise SK, DelGaudio JM, eds. Office-Based Rhinology Principles and Techniques. 1st ed. San Diego, CA: Plural Publishing; 2013

[9] Luong A, Batra PS, Fakhri S, Citardi MJ. Balloon catheter dilatation for frontal sinus ostium stenosis in the office setting. Am J Rhinol. 2008; 22(6):621–624

[10] Orlandi RR, Kingdom TT, Hwang PH, et al. International consensus statement on allergy and rhinology: rhinosinusitis. Int Forum Allergy Rhinol. 2016; 6 Suppl 1:S22–S209

[11] Rudmik L, Hoy M, Schlosser RJ, et al. Topical therapies in the management of chronic rhinosinusitis: an evidence-based review with recommendations. Int Forum Allergy Rhinol. 2013; 3(4):281–298

[12] Kalish L, Snidvongs K, Sivasubramaniam R, Cope D, Harvey RJ. Topical steroids for nasal polyps. Cochrane Database Syst Rev. 2012; 12: CD006549

[13] Laury A, DelGaudio JM. Office-based management of mucoceles. In: Patel ZM, Wise SK, DelGaudio JM, eds. Office-Based Rhinology Principles and Techniques. San Diego, CA: Plural Publishing; 2013

[14] Scangas GA, Gudis DA, Kennedy DW. The natural history and clinical characteristics of paranasal sinus mucoceles: a clinical review. Int Forum Allergy Rhinol. 2013; 3(9):712–717

[15] Ko M-T, Chuang K-C, Su C-Y. Multiple analyses of factors related to intraoperative blood loss and the role of reverse Trendelenburg position in endoscopic sinus surgery. Laryngoscope. 2008; 118(9):1687–1691

[16] Lanza DC. Postoperative Care and Avoiding Frontal Recess Stenosis. International Advanced Sinus Symposium, Philadelphia, PA; 1993

[17] Ference EH, Graber M, Conley D, et al. Operative utilization of balloon versus traditional endoscopic sinus surgery. Laryngoscope. 2015; 125 (1):49–56

[18] BlueCross BlueShield Association. Balloon sinus ostial dilation for treatment of chronic rhinosinusitis. Technol Eval Cent Assess Program Exec Summ. 2013; 27(9):1–3

[19] Albritton FD, IV, Casiano RR, Sillers MJ. Feasibility of in-office endoscopic sinus surgery with balloon sinus dilation. Am J Rhinol Allergy. 2012; 26(3):243–248

[20] Eloy JA, Friedel ME, Eloy JD, Govindaraj S, Folbe AJ. In-office balloon dilation of the failed frontal sinusotomy. Otolaryngol Head Neck Surg. 2012; 146(2):320–322

[21] Batra PS. Evidence-based practice: balloon catheter dilation in rhinology. Otolaryngol Clin North Am. 2012; 45(5):993–1004

[22] Kim E, Cutler JL. Balloon dilatation of the paranasal sinuses: a tool in sinus surgery. Otolaryngol Clin North Am. 2009; 42(5):847–856, x

[23] Batra PS, Ryan MW, Sindwani R, Marple BF. Balloon catheter technology in rhinology: Reviewing the evidence. Laryngoscope. 2011; 121 (1):226–232

[24] Levy JM, Marino MJ, McCoul ED. Paranasal sinus balloon catheter dilation for treatment of chronic rhinosinusitis: a systematic review and meta-analysis. Otolaryngol Head Neck Surg. 2016; 154(1):33–40

[25] Karanfilov B, Silvers S, Pasha R, Sikand A, Shikani A, Sillers M, ORIOS2 Study Investigators. Office-based balloon sinus dilation: a prospective, multicenter study of 203 patients. Int Forum Allergy Rhinol. 2013; 3(5):404–411

[26] Gould J, Alexander I, Tomkin E, Brodner D. In-office, multisinus balloon dilation: 1-year outcomes from a prospective, multicenter, open label trial. Am J Rhinol Allergy. 2014; 28(2):156–163

[27] Sillers MJ, Melroy CT. In-office functional endoscopic sinus surgery for chronic rhinosinusitis utilizing balloon catheter dilation technology. Curr Opin Otolaryngol Head Neck Surg. 2013; 21(1):17–22

[28] Smith TL, Singh A, Luong A, et al. Randomized controlled trial of a bioabsorbable steroid-releasing implant in the frontal sinus opening. Laryngoscope. 2016; 126(12):2659–2664

Section III

Open Surgical Approaches to Frontal Sinus Disease

18 Mini- and Maxi-Trephines   142

19 Osteoplastic Flap Approach with and
   without Obliteration   146

20 Riedel's Procedure and
   Cranialization of the Frontal Sinus   150

III

18 Mini- and Maxi-Trephines

David A. Gudis, Charles F. Palmer, and Rodney J. Schlosser

Abstract

The frontal sinus trephine is a minimally invasive external approach to the frontal sinus. For lesions and pathology that extend to the lateral or superior frontal sinus, trephination has proved an invaluable tool for the sinus surgeon. Preoperative imaging review is critical. The surgical technique, herein described, is straightforward and can be readily mastered. Critical sensory nerves are carefully avoided, and generally no reconstruction is required.

Keywords: trephine, lateral frontal sinus, mucocele, inverted papilloma

18.1 Indications

The trephine has long been a mainstay of frontal sinus surgery. Trephination was first described in the medical literature by Ogston in 1884.[1] However, prehistoric skulls excavated in South American villages have demonstrated evidence of surgical trephines performed centuries ago, sometimes following presumed frontal sinus fractures.[2] In the last few decades, endoscopic frontal sinus surgery has largely replaced the trephine for the treatment of frontal sinus disease. The endoscopic frontal sinusotomy has proved an effective treatment for chronic frontal sinusitis while also improving access for postoperative topical irrigation therapies.[3,4] Endoscopic techniques, including the modified endoscopic Lothrop (Draf III), have also enhanced our ability to treat even the majority of lateral frontal sinus inflammatory and neoplastic disease.[5] However, many lesions of the lateral frontal sinus may not be accessible or adequately treated by endoscopic techniques. Specifically, lesions lateral to the mid-orbital point or mid-pupillary line are generally inaccessible by purely endoscopic surgery, even when a trans-septal Draf III approach is used. Likewise, frontal sinus lesions of the frontal sinus floor (orbital roof) may also be similarly inaccessible purely endoscopically.[6] For such lesions, the frontal sinus trephine becomes a critical surgical technique, often in conjunction with standard endoscopic surgery, for an "above-and-below" approach. Common indications for the trephine include frontal osteomyelitis (Pott's puffy tumor), lateral frontal mucoceles, encephaloceles or cerebrospinal fluid (CSF) leaks, fibro-osseous lesions such as osteomas or fibrous dysplasia, and soft-tissue neoplasms such as inverted papilloma or minor salivary gland tumors pedicled in the lateral frontal sinus.

18.2 Surgical Steps

Surgical Planning. The patient should be consented both for trephination and endoscopic surgery, as the joint approach is often critical to successful surgery. Frontal sinus trephination is best performed under general anesthesia. Stereotactic image-guided navigation is an invaluable supplementary tool, and its use is recommended by the authors for confirmation of known anatomic landmarks; dated navigation techniques such as the "6-foot-Caldwell" have been shown to be less reliable.[7]

Incision and Soft Tissue. Several incisions have been described, including the Lynch, transblepharoplasty and various eyebrow incisions. Most patients have enough laxity of the skin and soft tissue over the fronto-orbital periosteum to accommodate safe entry through the anterior table of the frontal sinus regardless of their natural brow position. Therefore, for the optimal cosmetic outcome, the authors recommend an incision just below the hair of the brow, and in general, the incision should not extend medial to the hair of the brow. (Incisions made within the brow, when cut perpendicular to hair follicles, may leave a conspicuous strip of missing hair permanently.) The supratrochlear and supraorbital nerves provide sensory function to the soft tissue of the brow and frontal region. The supratrochlear nerve is a branch of the frontal nerve, which is the largest branch of the ophthalmic nerve (V1), that exits the orbit superior to the trochlea and passes deep to the frontalis muscle near the frontonasal suture. The supratrochlear nerve serves as the medial limit of the trephine incision. The supraorbital nerve, also a branch of the frontal nerve, passes through the supraorbital foramen, whose notch can be palpated in the supraorbital rim approximately one-third to one-half the width of the orbit from the medial canthus. The supraorbital notch serves as the lateral limit of the trephine incision.

After sterile preparation and infiltration of local anesthesia with epinephrine, a no. 15 blade is used to incise epidermis and dermis. To minimize damage to surrounding hair follicles and skin, bipolar cautery should be used if necessary for hemostasis. The subcutaneous fat can be bluntly dissected to expose periosteum, using self-retaining or small hand-held retractors (see ▶ Fig. 18.1). The periosteum should be cut horizontally with the no. 15 blade, and a Freer or periosteal elevator can be used to raise the periosteum superiorly and inferiorly safely. Great care should be used when extending the bony exposure medially and laterally in order to preserve the sensory nerves.

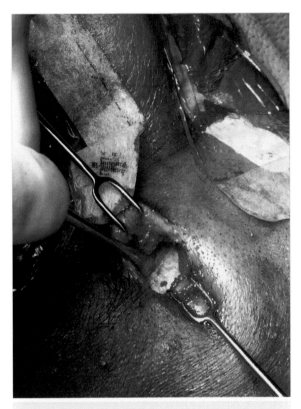

Fig. 18.1 The skin and soft tissue are retracted with skin hooks, and a periosteal elevator is used to expose the anterior table of the frontal sinus in preparation for trephine. (This image is provided courtesy of Medical University of South Carolina Division of Rhinology.)

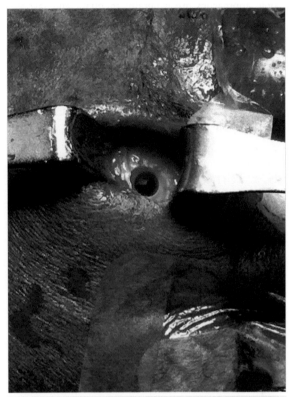

Fig. 18.2 A 5-mm trephine has been created to enter the lumen of the left frontal sinus. (This image is provided courtesy of Medical University of South Carolina Division of Rhinology.)

Frontal Sinus Trephination. With rare exception (see section *Tips and Tricks*), the initial entry into the frontal sinus should aim to be as medial and inferior into the lumen as possible in order to minimize the risk of an inadvertent skull base or orbital injury. Image-guided instruments should be used to confirm a safe point of entry, marked with a marking pen directly on bone. The preoperative CT review should include a measurement of the frontal sinus anterior table thickness, which can then be considered in relation to the bur size used for drilling. For very small "mini-trephines," kits with small burs and drill guides can be useful. These kits typically result in 2-mm trephines that are generally used to flush out the sinus or potentially pass an irrigation catheter into the frontal sinus. Larger "maxi-trephines" can be performed based upon the surgical goals. A 3- or 4-mm round diamond or cutting bur is used to carefully saucerize a 5-mm window through the anterior table (see ▶ Fig. 18.2). The surgeon will notice a color change as the overlying bone becomes very thin and is "egg-shelled" over the mucosa. An image-guided probe or curette can then be used to enter the lumen of the sinus. Once the lumen of the frontal sinus is confirmed, a 2-mm Kerrison rongeur

can be used to widen the trephine as needed for access of an endoscope and/or surgical instruments. Prior to further drilling or tumor resection, the surgeon should carefully identify with direct or endoscopic visualization the limits of the orbital roof and frontal sinus boundaries so that the skull base and orbit can be protected.

Closure. It is very rare for a trephine to cause any cosmetic deformity of the frontal bone. Therefore, no bony reconstruction, cranioplasty, or reconstructive plating is required unless the defect is larger than 2 to 3 cm in diameter or it crosses the supraorbital ridge. The periosteum is closed over the frontal sinus lumen with interrupted 4–0 monocryl or vicryl suture, followed by a cosmetic skin closure. Antibiotic ointment can be used on the incision postoperatively.

When treating severe infectious pathology such as frontal osteomyelitis many surgeons leave an irrigation catheter, such as a red rubber tube, in the sinus. This technique for postoperative frontal sinus antibiotic or saline irrigation has been used since before the development of endoscopic sinus surgery[8]; however, when a trephine is combined with a wide endoscopic frontal sinusotomy and postoperative endonasal irrigations, the additional utility of an irrigation catheter has not been established. For optimal sinus irrigation, the catheter should be placed through the trephine into the lateral or superior limit of the frontal sinus lumen and sutured to the medial limit of the skin incision. After the remainder of the incision has been closed, endonasal endoscopic visualization of the irrigation through the frontal sinusotomy should be confirmed.

18.3 Tips and Tricks

- To avoid neurovascular injury, the surgeon may make the incision only 1 cm initially at the halfway point between the supraorbital and supratrochlear nerves. If the periosteal exposure is inadequate, the incision can then be carefully extended medially and laterally.
- While there is wide anatomic variability among patients, a trephination performed at a distance of 1 cm from the patient's midline has been shown to be safe and cosmetically favorable.[9]
- As in all sinus surgery, preoperative CT review is critical for successful trephination. The thickness of the anterior table of the frontal sinus should be measured preoperatively and is usually around 4 mm. The surgeon can then use a 4-mm bur to readily predict when approaching the lumen of the sinus.
- Note that the anterior table of the frontal sinus is *much* thicker than the posterior table or the orbital roof. Therefore, if using a curette for the trephine, steady pressure must be applied, rather than "leaning" on the instrument, which may result in inadvertently "popping" through the trephine and into a critical structure.
- A common indication for the mini-trephine is the lateral frontal sinus mucocele. These lesions are treated with only marsupialization into the medial frontal sinus cavity rather than wide resection. Therefore, the senior author modifies his trephine approach in this setting. Rather than entering into the inferior aspect of the frontal sinus, the trephine is performed directly over the medial limit of the mucocele so that the bony partition can be directly resected with straight through-cutting forceps.

18.4 Case Example

A 55-year-old man presents with constant left supraorbital pressure and pain. His symptoms are temporarily alleviated by intermittent bursts of oral corticosteroids, but invariably the symptom of pressure returns. ▶ Fig. 18.3 demonstrates a lateral frontal mucocele in a type 4 frontal sinus cell. As the lesion is quite lateral within the frontal sinus, a combined trephine and endonasal endoscopic approach was used to treat the lesion. A trephination (see ▶ Fig. 18.1 and ▶ Fig. 18.2) combined with an endoscopic frontal sinusotomy allows marsupialization of the lesion into the true frontal sinus, with endoscopic visualization and confirmation of drainage and patency.

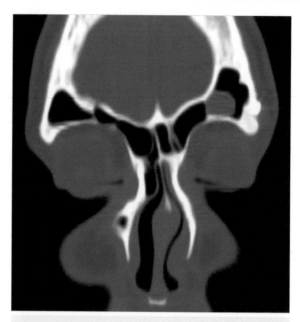

Fig. 18.3 CT scan demonstrating a left lateral frontal sinus mucocele in a type 4 frontal sinus cell. (This image is provided courtesy of Medical University of South Carolina Division of Rhinology.)

18.5 Complications

In 1954, Maxwell Ellis wrote that "surgical treatment of chronic frontal sinusitis is difficult, often unsatisfactory and sometimes disastrous."[10] Despite the advancements in surgical technique and improved outcomes of frontal sinus surgery, serious complications can indeed occur following trephination. There is a wide range of complication rates by published series. Several studies have demonstrated postoperative facial or periorbital cellulitis, occurring in less than 5% of patients.[11,12] CSF leak has been reported to occur in as low as 0.5% of patients with inflammatory disease to up to 20% of patients with lateral frontal inverted papillomas.[11,13] Skin complications, anesthesia complications, and other orbital injuries including proptosis and trochlea injury and superior oblique palsy have also been reported.[11,14,15,16]

Suggested Reading

Patel AB, Cain RB, Lal D. Contemporary applications of frontal sinus trephination: A systematic review of the literature. Laryngoscope. 2015; 125 (9):2046–2053

References

[1] Ogston A. Trephining the frontal sinus for catarrhal diseases. Men Chron Manchester. 1884; 1:235
[2] Canalis RF, Cabieses F, Hemenway WG, Aragon R. Prehistoric trephination of the frontal sinus. Ann Otol Rhinol Laryngol. 1981; 90(2, Pt 1):186–189

[3] DeConde AS, Smith TL. Outcomes after frontal sinus surgery: an evidence-based review. Otolaryngol Clin North Am. 2016; 49(4):1019–1033

[4] Thomas WW, III, Harvey RJ, Rudmik L, Hwang PH, Schlosser RJ. Distribution of topical agents to the paranasal sinuses: an evidence-based review with recommendations. Int Forum Allergy Rhinol. 2013; 3 (9):691–703

[5] Conger BT, Jr, Illing E, Bush B, Woodworth BA. Management of lateral frontal sinus pathology in the endoscopic era. Otolaryngol Head Neck Surg. 2014; 151(1):159–163

[6] Timperley DG, Banks C, Robinson D, Roth J, Sacks R, Harvey RJ. Lateral frontal sinus access in endoscopic skull-base surgery. Int Forum Allergy Rhinol. 2011; 1(4):290–295

[7] Carrau RL, Snyderman CH, Curtin HB, Weissman JL. Computer-assisted frontal sinusotomy. Otolaryngol Head Neck Surg. 1994; 111 (6):727–732

[8] Rogers L. Pott's puffy tumour. Br J Surg. 1949; 36(143):315–316

[9] Piltcher OB, Antunes M, Monteiro F, Schweiger C, Schatkin B. Is there a reason for performing frontal sinus trephination at 1 cm from midline? A tomographic study. Rev Bras Otorrinolaringol (Engl Ed). 2006; 72(4):505–507

[10] Ellis M. The treatment of frontal sinusitis. J Laryngol Otol. 1954; 68 (7):478–490

[11] Seiberling K, Jardeleza C, Wormald PJ. Minitrephination of the frontal sinus: indications and uses in today's era of sinus surgery. Am J Rhinol Allergy. 2009; 23(2):229–231

[12] Batra PS, Citardi MJ, Lanza DC. Combined endoscopic trephination and endoscopic frontal sinusotomy for management of complex frontal sinus pathology. Am J Rhinol. 2005; 19(5):435–441

[13] Walgama E, Ahn C, Batra PS. Surgical management of frontal sinus inverted papilloma: a systematic review. Laryngoscope. 2012; 122 (6):1205–1209

[14] Gallagher RM, Gross CW. The role of mini-trephination in the management of frontal sinusitis. Am J Rhinol. 1999; 13(4):289–293

[15] Bartley J, Eagleton N, Rosser P, Al-Ali S. Superior oblique muscle palsy after frontal sinus mini-trephine. Am J Otolaryngol. 2012; 33(1):181–183

[16] Andrews JN, Lopez MA, Weitzel EK. A case report of intraoperative retroorbital fluid dissection after frontal mini-trephine placement. Laryngoscope. 2013; 123(12):2969–2971

19 Osteoplastic Flap Approach with and without Obliteration

Arjun K. Parasher and James N. Palmer

Abstract

While endoscopic techniques have become the primary approach for management of frontal sinus pathology, the osteoplastic flap with and without obliteration remains a valuable adjunct in the management of complex frontal sinus cases. This chapter will highlight the current indications, surgical steps, potential complications, and case examples to help surgeons optimize this surgical approach in practice.

Keywords: frontal sinus, osteoplastic flap, cranialization, obliteration, frontal sinusitis, frontal sinus tumors

19.1 Indications

First described in 1895 by Schonborn and later modified by Goodale and Montgomery, the osteoplastic flap for the frontal sinus was a mainstay of surgical management of the frontal sinus in the 1950s.[1,2,3] With recent advances in technology and technical ability, endoscopic approaches are now increasingly utilized to address revision frontal sinusitis, neoplasms, and frontal sinus fractures. External approaches including the osteoplastic flap approach are now reserved for cases unable to be adequately or safely addressed via an endoscopic approach. These indications include severe cases of refractory frontal sinusitis, neoplasms with attachments in the frontal sinus or invasion of the orbit or dura impractical for endoscopic resection, posterior table

frontal sinus fractures with cerebrospinal fluid (CSF) leaks, and extensive fibro-osseous lesions.[4]

The indications for obliteration of the frontal sinus remain a clinical challenge with significant controversy. The success of revision endoscopic surgery combined with the long-term risk of failure and the difficulty for tumor surveillance with frontal sinus obliteration has further limited the role of obliteration. In current practice, frontal sinus obliteration is reserved for extreme cases in which no practical way of reestablishing a sustainable frontal sinus outflow tract exists.

Alternative approaches to the frontal sinus with the advantages and disadvantages are included in ▶ Table 19.1.

19.2 Surgical Steps

19.2.1 Osteoplastic Flap without Obliteration

Preparation

- If available, stereotactic surgical navigation registration should be completed prior to incision. Surgical navigation can assist in mapping of the osteoplastic flap; otherwise, a 6-foot Caldwell radiograph template can be used.
- The eyes should be protected with tarsorrhaphy, Tegaderm, or corneal shields to prevent injury during the procedure.

Table 19.1 Surgical approaches, advantages, and disadvantages

Approach	Indication	Advantages	Disadvantages
Endoscopic	Primary workhorse for frontal sinus pathology	Avoid morbidity from external incision Improved visualization of frontal sinus recess	Limited by length and angulation of instruments
Trephine	Acute frontal sinusitis Pathology lateral to mid-pupillary line Additional endoscopic portal	Quick, direct access to frontal sinus	Small external incision
Osteoplastic flap	Neoplasm with frontal sinus attachment or invasion of the orbit or dura Posterior table fracture with cerebrospinal fluid leak Extensive fibro-osseous lesions Refractory frontal sinusitis without possibility of reestablishing frontal sinus outflow tract	Improved visualization of entire sinus Increased range of motion for instrumentation	Large external incision Disruption of frontal sinus mucosa Potential for cerebrospinal leak or orbit injury with osteotomy

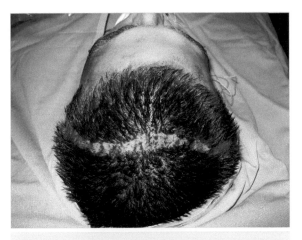

Fig. 19.1 Sinusoidal bicoronal incision marked after shaving of strip of hair.

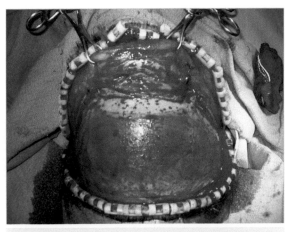

Fig. 19.2 Bicoronal incision elevated in subgaleal plane with subperiosteal dissection limited to frontal sinus osteotomy.

- The incision should be carefully planned based on each specific case. Multiple options exist including the gull wing, mid-brow, pretrichial, or coronal incisions. The coronal incision often provides the least cosmetic deformity and is the mainstay of this procedure. For this chapter, the coronal incision will be utilized and described in detail (▶ Fig. 19.1).
- The hair is carefully parted and the incision line marked with a marking pen from preauricular crease to contralateral preauricular crease. The incision can be marked straight across, in a sinusoidal pattern, or with multiple W incisions. To minimize hair in the incision line, a small strip of hair may be removed with a shaver. Alternatively, hair may be parted with or tied in multiple ponytails away from the incision line. The incision is injected with lidocaine 1% with epinephrine 1:100,000.

Exposure

- Using a no. 15 blade, an incision is made parallel to the hair follicles through the skin, subcutaneous tissue, and galea. If a subperiosteal dissection is used, the incision is carried through the periosteum in the midline. Care is taken not to disrupt the temporalis muscle as this can result in significant pain and trismus postoperatively. Furthermore, care must be taken to avoid injury to the superficial temporal artery and facial nerve as the incision is carried down to the level of the tragus.
- Elevation of the skin flap can be completed in the subgaleal or subperiosteal. In the subgaleal plane, Metzenbaum scissors can be used to blunt dissect and cut any attachments. The pericranium can then be incised along the temporal lines and posteriorly to provide enough length if needed for closure. In the subperiosteal plane, a periosteal elevator or blunt dissection with a sponge

can quickly elevate the flap and pericranium together (▶ Fig. 19.2).
- Laterally, the dissection over the temporalis muscle will occur deep to the temperoparietal fascia but superficial to the temporalis fascia to protect the facial nerve in the subgaleal elevation. In the subperiosteal plane, the dissection will be carried deep to the temporalis fascia, but superficial to the temporalis muscle.
- The supraorbital and supratrochlear neurovascular bundles should be preserved in either the subgaleal or subperiosteal technique. With the subgaleal technique, blunt dissection must be used 1 cm above the supraorbital rim to identify and protect these bundles.
- To gain additional mobility of the flap and improve exposure, the neurovascular bundles may be released from their foramina with an osteotome or high-speed drill.

Removal of Anterior Table

- With exposure complete, the frontal sinus should be carefully mapped out using the 6-foot Caldwell radiograph template, endoscopic illumination, or surgical navigation. In our experience, surgical navigation provides increased safety and precision (▶ Fig. 19.3 and ▶ Fig. 19.4).
- Once marked, an oscillating sagittal saw beveled in toward the frontal sinus cavity is utilized to remove the anterior table. An osteotome may be used to finish incomplete cuts. Alternatively, a high-speed drill can be used to create multiple pilot holes. These pilot holes can then be connected with the oscillating saw.
- The anterior table is removed or reflected if still attached to the periosteum. At this point, exposure of the frontal sinus is complete. The individual pathology

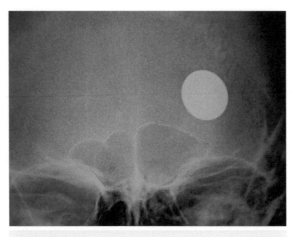

Fig. 19.3 Example of 6-foot Caldwell X-ray used for mapping of frontal sinus osteotomy.

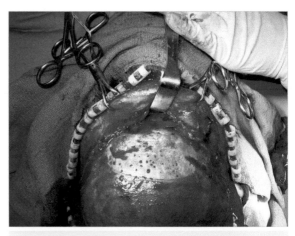

Fig. 19.4 Six-foot Caldwell X-ray placed over frontal sinus to mark prior to osteotomy.

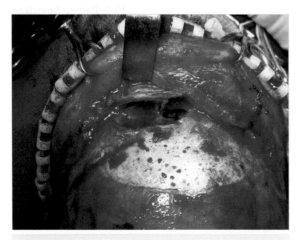

Fig. 19.5 Frontal sinus anterior table reflected forward with view into bilateral frontal sinuses.

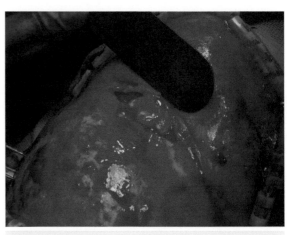

Fig. 19.6 Visualization of frontal sinus osteoma after removal of anterior table.

of the frontal sinus must be addressed depending on each case (▶ Fig. 19.5 and ▶ Fig. 19.6).

- Once the pathology is addressed, a decision must be made on frontal sinus preservation versus obliteration. If the frontal outflow tract cannot be established due to significant trauma or neo-osteogenesis, consideration may be given to obliteration. The steps for frontal sinus obliteration are included in the following section.
- A pericranial flap can now be utilized if a CSF leak is encountered or to separate the sinonasal and intracranial cavity even if the dura remains intact. If the subperiosteal approach is utilized, the flap can now be harvested from the skin flap with Metzenbaum scissors as the surgical assistant provides traction. In the subgaleal approach, the pericranial flap is previously harvested during exposure.

19.2.2 Osteoplastic Flap with Obliteration

- In the cases where a decision is made to proceed with obliteration of the frontal sinus, the surgeon must strip all mucosa from the frontal sinus including the previously removed anterior table. With a high-speed diamond bur, the bone of the frontal sinus should be polished gently to remove any nests of mucosa. Once completed, the frontal sinus cavity should be thoroughly examined to ensure complete removal of the mucosa.
- Next, attention should be paid to the frontal recess. The frontal recess should be sealed with temperoparietal fascia, temporalis muscle, and/or bone pate.
- The frontal sinus cavity should now be filled with fat. Hydroxyapatite can be utilized, but it results in increased difficulty during revision surgery if needed.

- Once the frontal sinus has been obliterated, the anterior table bone should be placed back into position. The bone is plated using a craniofacial thin plates and self-tapping screws.
- The bicoronal flap is then laid back into position and closed in a multilayer fashion. Suction drains are placed under the flap. The hair and bicoronal incision are then washed and a head wrap can then be placed.

19.3 Tips and Tricks

Frontal sinus osteotomy mapping were traditionally completed using a 6-feet Caldwell radiograph. Endoscopic illumination of the frontal sinus can be used, but may underestimate the extent of the frontal sinus due to presents of neoplasm or mucocele. Stereotactic image guidance now enables precise frontal sinus mapping, limiting the potential for complications.

For obliteration of the frontal sinus, attention must be paid to remove all frontal sinus mucosa to reduce risk of subsequent mucocele. After stripping of mucosa, a diamond bur can be used to gently polish the bone of the frontal sinus to remove any remnant nests of mucosa.

In the cases where the posterior table of the frontal sinus has been eroded, frontal sinus mucosa may be adherent to the underlying dura. In these instances, complete removal of the mucosa may be unfeasible and removal attempts can increase the risk of CSF leak.

Given the success of endoscopic sinus surgery in revision sinusitis cases and the improved tumor surveillance without obliteration, frontal sinus obliteration is now rarely utilized in our practice.

The bicoronal dissection can be completed in either a subgaleal or a subperiosteal plane. The subperiosteal plane allows for a quick dissection avoiding risk to the supraorbital or supratrochlear neurovascular bundles. In addition to this technique, a thicker pericranial flap can be subsequently harvested from the skin flap, if needed.

19.4 Complications: Management

Short-term complications from this procedure can include infection, bleeding, damage to the supratrochlear or supraorbital neurovascular bundle, injury to the frontal branch of the facial nerve, and CSF leak. Long-term complications include failure of the osteoplastic flap with development of mucoceles or recurrent frontal sinusitis and aesthetic complications including frontal bossing and loss of the frontal plate, potentially leading to fistula formation. Risk of fistula formation is increased with radiation therapy. When possible, care should be taken to leave the inferior bone flap pedicled to the periosteum and avoid fragmentation of the bone flap itself to preserve blood supply.

Earlier sections have addressed methods to minimize risks to the neurovascular bundles and facial nerve. A CSF leak can occur during the procedure either during tumor resection or during the frontal osteotomy. In these situations, the initial closure steps will depend on the extent of the dural opening. For large defects, a dura substitute may be sutured into place. As described earlier, a pericranial flap can be elevated and laid over the defect via the bicoronal approach. Fibrin glue can be applied over the closure.

Long-term failures, including infection and mucocele formation, present on average 9.7 years after the initial osteoplastic flap.[5] As a result, long-term follow-up is required. Revision rates due to failure are estimated at between 4 and 9%.[6,7] Follow-up magnetic resonance imaging has shown the presence of mucoceles in 10% of cases.[8] In a review, Hwang et al showed that 86% of revisions were addressed endoscopically with an 81% success rate.[5]

19.5 Conclusion

While utilized less frequently, the osteoplastic flap approach to the frontal sinus remains a critical tool in frontal sinus surgery. The need for obliteration has decreased significantly given long-term failure rates, impaired endoscopic and imaging tumor surveillance capacity, and the advances in endoscopic approaches for refractory frontal sinus disease. With appropriate training, the osteoplastic flap can be utilized with limited morbidity to address complex frontal sinus pathology.

References

[1] Schonborn. Ein Beitrag zur Kasuistik der Erkrankungen des Sinus frontalis. In: Wilkop A, ed. Wuzberg, Germany: F. Frome; 1894
[2] Goodale RL. Trends in radical frontal sinus surgery. Ann Otol Rhinol Laryngol. 1957; 66(2):369–379
[3] Goodale RL, Montgomery WW. Experiences with the osteoplastic anterior wall approach to the frontal sinus; case histories and recommendations. AMA Arch Otolaryngol. 1958; 68(3):271–283
[4] Pittman A, Welch K. Osteoplastic flaps with and without obliteration. In: Palmer NJ, Chiu A, eds. Atlas of Endoscopic Sinus and Skull Base Surgery. Philadelphia, PA: Elsevier Saunders; 2013:327–336
[5] Hwang PH, Han JK, Bilstrom EJ, Kingdom TT, Fong KJ. Surgical revision of the failed obliterated frontal sinus. Am J Rhinol. 2005; 19 (5):425–429
[6] Hardy JM, Montgomery WW. Osteoplastic frontal sinusotomy: an analysis of 250 operations. Ann Otol Rhinol Laryngol. 1976; 85(4, Pt 1):523–532
[7] Silverman JB, Gray ST, Busaba NY. Role of osteoplastic frontal sinus obliteration in the era of endoscopic sinus surgery. Int J Otolaryngol. 2012; 2012:501896
[8] Weber R, Draf W, Keerl R, et al. Osteoplastic frontal sinus surgery with fat obliteration: technique and long-term results using magnetic resonance imaging in 82 operations. Laryngoscope. 2000; 110 (6):1037–1044

20 Riedel's Procedure and Cranialization of the Frontal Sinus

Kato Speleman and Anshul Sama

Abstract

Riedel's and Cranialization procedures are external frontal sinus procedures that include the removal of the anterior table and the posterior frontal table, respectively. Both were initially introduced for the management of frontal sinus fractures and have well-established safety and efficacy records when performed appropriately. Their current indications are more narrowly defined but they maintain an important place in frontal sinus surgeon's surgical armamentarium. In the case of Riedel's procedure, indications include ablation of the frontal sinus after failed drainage and failed obliteration, extensive osteomyelitis of the anterior frontal sinus wall, and locally invasive neoplastic disease involving the anterior wall of the frontal sinus. Cranialization indications include treatment of frontal sinus fractures with frontal outflow tract obstruction and, less well documented, as a final treatment option for refractory frontal sinusitis.

Keywords: Riedel's procedure, cranalization, obliteration, osteoplastic flap.

20.1 Riedel's Procedure

20.1.1 Historic Perspective

Riedel's procedure was initially intended as a first-line treatment of extensive frontal sinus fractures. The procedure, as originally described by Riedel in 1898, comprised a complete removal of the anterior table of the frontal sinus as well as the frontal sinus mucosa, the supraorbital rims, and proximal nasal bones.[1] Postoperatively, the forehead skin is left in direct contact with the posterior table. This procedure was later modified by Killian, who preserved a 10-mm bridge of bone along the supraorbital rim in an attempt to improve cosmesis after this disfiguring procedure.[2]

Postoperative disfigurement has always been the main criticism of Riedel's procedure. However, this shortcoming could be reduced to some extent by meticulous chamfering of the frontal sinus margins and supraorbital rims.[3] Also, the contour of the anterior table of the frontal sinus can be reconstructed at a later stage, either by bone grafts or by exogenous material, most commonly titanium mesh. Current 3D printing technology allows a perfect custom-made reconstruction of the frontal sinus anterior table based on pre- and postoperative computed tomography (CT) scans.

A second and equally important criticism is that the removal of the anterior table leaves the frontal lobes largely unprotected in case of head trauma.

Its role in the management of frontal sinus disease today is limited. Riedel's procedure has been abandoned for primary fracture management; however, it has retained a clear place in the treatment of selected cases of complicated frontal sinus disease. The main indications for Riedel's procedure in contemporary sinus surgery are (1) ablation of the frontal sinus after failed drainage and failed obliteration, (2) extensive osteomyelitis of the anterior wall of the frontal sinus (▶ Fig. 20.1), and (3) locally invasive neoplastic disease involving the anterior wall of the frontal sinus.

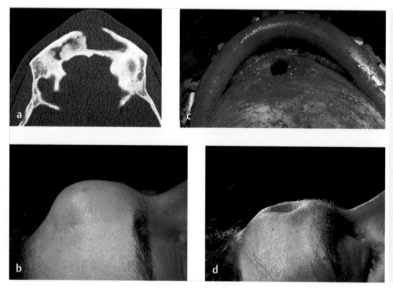

Fig. 20.1 Osteomyelitis of frontal plate of frontal sinus. **(a)** Axial CT showing large dehiscence. **(b)** Frontal abscess associated with osteomyelitis. **(c)** Operative image of the dehiscence and osteomyelitis. **(d)** Defect post evacuation of pus.[3]

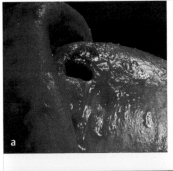
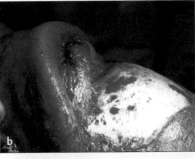
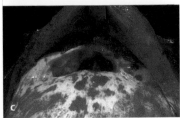
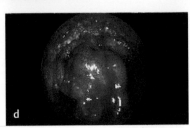

Fig. 20.2 Surgical steps for Riedel's: **(a)** Osteomyelitis defect. **(b)** Post removal of frontal plate of frontal sinus. **(c)** Bevelling of the edges to smoothen transition and ensuring drainage. **(d)** Endoscopic view post repositioning of flap.[3]

20.1.2 Indications

- Failed drainage and failed obliteration.
- Osteomyelitis of the anterior wall.
- Locally invasive neoplastic disease involving the anterior wall.

20.1.3 Technique

The technique of Riedel's procedure is as follows (▶ Fig. 20.2a–d):

- A standard coronal incision is made and the skin flap is raised in a subgaleal plane to the level of the supraorbital rims to adequately expose the frontal bone. The periosteum should be preserved with the exception of the periosteum over the anterior wall of the frontal sinus in case of involvement in the disease process.
- An anteriorly based pericranial flap is raised.
- The presumed margins of the frontal sinus are marked for guidance. Transillumination (if possible) or a (3D printed) template based on a preoperative CT scan or a template cut from a Caldwell view X-ray obtained at a distance of 6 feet can assist the delineation of the sinus margins.
  - In case of osteomyelitis of the anterior wall with the presence of bony defects, these defects can facilitate the identification of the frontal sinus and the removal of the anterior wall.
- The anterior wall is removed with the aid of (curved) chisels or a high-speed cutting drill. A 10-mm bone bridge is preserved along the supraorbital rim. Attention needs to be paid to chamfer the frontal sinus margins and supraorbital rim to improve postoperative aesthetic appearance.
- After removal of the anterior wall, all of the frontal sinus mucosa is removed meticulously with a high-speed diamond drill. To avoid mucosal regeneration, it is important to bur all residual frontal sinus walls past the level of the foramina of Breschet to make sure all mucosal tails that extend along these foramina are adequately removed.
- It is important to ensure adequate intranasal drainage and clearance of the subsupraorbital rim. This is essential as rarely localized disease in this area can persist and require revision endoscopic procedure (▶ Fig. 20.2d).
- As the pericranial flap and skin flap are folded back, the forehead skin is left in direct contact with the posterior table of the frontal sinus.
- The skin incision is closed in layers.

20.2 Cranialization of the Frontal Sinus

20.2.1 Historic Perspective

In 1978, Donald and Bernstein introduced cranialization of the frontal sinus in two patients with compound frontal sinus injuries with intracranial penetration.[4] This procedure involves the removal of the posterior wall of the frontal sinus along with all sinus mucosa and a meticulous closing of the frontal sinus outflow tract. As a result, the space occupied by the frontal sinus is separated from the nasal cavity and becomes part of the intracranial cavity. The former frontal sinus space can initially be left as dead space, or filled up with free fat graft. If left as dead space, the expanding dura and brain will eventually fill the cavity completely over the course of several weeks (▶ Fig. 20.3).[5] A pericranial flap can be used as an extra barrier between the frontal sinus anterior table, the closed-off frontal sinus outflow tract, and the intracranial contents.[6]

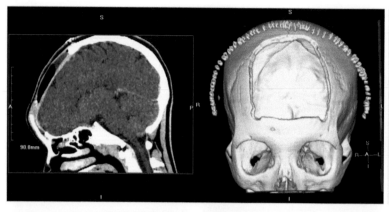

Fig. 20.3 Coronal CT of patient post cranialization. 3D reconstruction of frontal craniotomy

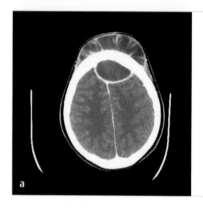
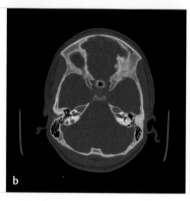

Fig. 20.4 Acute Intracranial sepsis secondary to frontal sinusitis. **(a)** Intracranial and external frontal sepsis. **(b)** Loss of most of the posterior table of frontal sinus due to sepsis

A hermetically closed frontal sinus outflow tract and complete debridement of all sinus mucosa are prerequisites for success and avoidance of late recurrence.

Crucially, in contrast to Riedel's procedure, the anterior frontal sinus wall remains preserved, which offers protection for the frontal lobes and avoids a cosmetic defect.

Cranialization is an established technique in the treatment of frontal sinus fractures with frontal sinus outflow tract obstruction. Its efficacy and safety for this indication have been well documented and an acceptably low complication rate of 6 to 10% is generally reported.[7,8]

In contrast, reports on the use of cranialization for the treatment of refractory chronic frontal rhinosinusitis are scarce.[9,10] Given its efficiency and low complication rate, however, cranialization should be considered the final treatment option for refractory frontal sinusitis after failure of or as an alternative for more conventional treatment options such as endoscopic median drainage procedure and osteoplastic flap frontal sinus obliteration procedure in selected cases.

Cranialization has also proven to be a good treatment option for prevention of secondary mucocele formation in case of open resection of benign frontal sinus lesions (e.g., osteoma, mucocele, fibrous dysplasia, and encephalocele) with an earlier report describing that cranialization of the frontal sinus is noninferior to frontal sinus obliteration for this indication.[11] The commonest current indication for this procedure is the more than 50% loss of the posterior table with acute suppurative intracranial sepsis from frontal sinusitis (▶ Fig. 20.4). In these situations, although the primary management is aimed at evacuation of the intracranial suppurative contents, if the frontal sinus sepsis is not addressed, there is a high risk of recurrence of intracranial sepsis.

As mentioned earlier, complication rates after frontal sinus cranialization are considerably low.[7,8] Possible complications include meningitis, abscess, frontal mucopyocele, frontal lobe laceration, bone flap infection, and epidural pneumocranium.[7,8,9]

20.2.2 Indications

- Frontal sinus fracture with obstruction of the frontal sinus outflow tract.
- Alternative to obliteration for refractory chronic rhinosinusitis.
- Secondary mucocele prevention following open surgery for benign frontal lesions.
- Removal of mucosa or contents in craniofacial resection.
- Extensive loss of posterior table of frontal sinus with intracranial sepsis.

20.2.3 Technique

The technique for cranialization of the frontal sinus is as follows:

- A standard coronal incision is made and the skin flap is raised in a subgaleal plane to the level of the supraorbital rims to adequately expose the frontal bone. The periosteum should be preserved.
- An anteriorly based pericranial flap is designed. Its lateral limits are formed by the superior temporal lines and its posterior limit by the vertex. To raise the flap, a periosteal elevator is used.
- Either a bilateral frontal craniotomy with extension in the superior part of the frontal sinus or an osteoplastic flap is carried out. This allows broad access to the entire frontal sinus and the posterior wall of the frontal sinus.
- The dura mater is carefully dissected free from the posterior wall of the frontal sinus. The latter is then removed completely to the level of the anterior cranial fossa, using a drill or a rongeur.
- Subsequently, all of the frontal sinus mucosa is removed meticulously with a high-speed diamond drill. To avoid mucosal regeneration, it is important to bur all residual frontal sinus walls past the level of the foramina of Breschet to make sure all mucosal tails that extend along these foramina are adequately removed.
- At the level of the frontal sinus outflow tract, the mucosa is inverted.
- Next, the frontal sinus outflow tract is plugged. Available materials for plugging include temporoparietal fascia or muscle, pericranium, or a mixture of cortical bone and pledgets of sterile gelatin sponge (Gelfoam).
- Repair of (posttraumatic) defects in the anterior table or dura, if present.
- In this stage, a pericranial flap can be draped over the frontal sinus anterior table, the closed-off frontal sinus outflow tract, and folded back superiorly over the dura mater of the anterior frontal lobes to serve as an extra layer of protection.
- The bone flap is put back in place and fixated with plates and screws.
- The skin incision is closed in layers.

References

[1] Schenke H. Uber die Stirnhohlen und ihre Erkrankungen. Die Radikal-operation nach Riedel. Inaugural dissertation, Friedrich-Schiller-Universität, Jena, Germany; 1898

[2] Killian G. Die killianischeradikale Operation chronischerStirnhöhleneiterungen: Weitereskasuistisches Material und Zusammenfassung. Arch Laryngol Rhinol. 1903; 13:59–66

[3] Raghavan U, Jones NS. The place of Riedel's procedure in contemporary sinus surgery. J Laryngol Otol. 2004; 118(9):700–705

[4] Donald PJ, Bernstein L. Compound frontal sinus injuries with intracranial penetration. Laryngoscope. 1978; 88(2, Pt 1):225–232

[5] Spinelli HM, Irizarry D, McCarthy JG, Cutting CB, Noz ME. An analysis of extradural dead space after fronto-orbital surgery. Plast Reconstr Surg. 1994; 93(7):1372–1377

[6] Donath A, Sindwani R. Frontal sinus cranialization using the pericranial flap: an added layer of protection. Laryngoscope. 2006; 116 (9):1585–1588

[7] Pollock RA, Hill JL, Jr, Davenport DL, Snow DC, Vasconez HC. Cranialization in a cohort of 154 consecutive patients with frontal sinus fractures (1987–2007): review and update of a compelling procedure in the selected patient. Ann Plast Surg. 2013; 71(1):54–59

[8] Rodriguez ED, Stanwix MG, Nam AJ, et al. Twenty-six-year experience treating frontal sinus fractures: a novel algorithm based on anatomical fracture pattern and failure of conventional techniques. Plast Reconstr Surg. 2008; 122(6):1850–1866

[9] van Dijk JM, Wagemakers M, Korsten-Meijer AG, Kees Buiter CT, van der Laan BF, Mooij JJ. Cranialization of the frontal sinus: the final remedy for refractory chronic frontal sinusitis. J Neurosurg. 2012; 116 (3):531–535

[10] Ameline E, Wagner I, Delbove H, Coquille F, Visot A, Chabolle F. Cranialization of the frontal sinus. Ann Otolaryngol Chir Cervicofac. 2001; 118(6):352–358

[11] Horowitz G, Amit M, Ben-Ari O, et al. Cranialization of the frontal sinus for secondary mucocele prevention following open surgery for benign frontal lesions. PLoS One. 2013; 8(12):e83820

Section IV

Management of Specific Frontal Sinus Conditions

21 Frontal Sinus Barosinusitis — 156

22 Frontal Sinus in Patients with Cystic Fibrosis — 161

23 Pneumosinus Dilatans — 173

24 Frontal Sinusitis in Chronic Rhinosinusitis without Nasal Polyposis — 176

25 Frontal Sinus Surgery in CRSwNP, AFRS, and ASA Triad — 182

26 Frontal Sinus Mucoceles — 188

27 Frontoethmoidal Osteomas — 195

28 Frontal Inverted Papilloma — 205

29 The Frontal Sinus: Fibro-Osseous Lesions — 217

30 Malignant Disease Involving the Frontal Sinus — 226

31 Acute Frontal Osteomyelitis: Intracranial and Orbital Complications — 233

32 Fungal Frontal Sinusitis: Allergic and Nonallergic — 244

33 Frontal Sinus Trauma and Its Management — 250

34 Cerebrospinal Fluid Leak in the Frontal Sinus: Endoscopic Management — 256

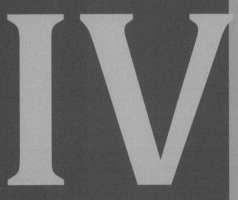

21 Frontal Sinus Barosinusitis

Ioannis I. Diamantopoulos

Abstract

Exposure to ambient pressure changes affects frontal sinus producing a condition called "barosinusitis," also known as "aerosinusitis" in aviation or "squeeze" in diving. With increasing numbers of people exposed, barotrauma of the frontal sinus appears merely as a functional failure of air commuting to and fro the frontal sinus. This chapter deals with etiology, epidemiology, and predisposing factors, and provides guidelines for surgical and medical management of this ambiguous condition affecting air passengers, but more often presenting as an occupational hazard in professionals exposed in fluctuating ambient pressure: pilots (civilian and military), cabin aircrew, divers, parachutists, and extreme sports enthusiasts, among others.

Keywords: frontal sinus barotrauma, sinusitis, aerosinusitis, frontal sinus, barotrauma

> ### Definition
>
> Barotrauma of the frontal sinus (FSB) may be called the adverse effect(s) on the frontal sinus of a subject exposed to surrounding air pressure change, also known as "aerosinusitis" or simply "squeeze."

21.1 Epidemiology and Etiology

Anyone exposed to ambient pressure change may develop sinus barotrauma (SB). The more abrupt the change encountered, the more likely the condition to appear. The most common activities relating to pressure fluctuation include ones with either predictable/controllable or gradual change of pressure, such as flying (air travel, acrobatics, or military flying), parachuting, diving, or ones where unpredictable/rapid changes of pressure are encountered: battle environment, terrorist activities (e.g., blast injury), mechanical ventilation via face mask, or simply forceful nose blowing under certain conditions.[1] Barotrauma may also appear unexpectedly during hyperbaric oxygen therapy[2] and high-attitude chamber training. In a Danish study looking at 948 civilian airline pilots, 12% of pilots have had SB, 70 to 80% of which was solely frontal sinus barotrauma (FSB), not accounting for cases where multiple sinus were affected.[3] With exploding numbers of passengers using air travel, FSB as separate entity started appearing as case reports since 1988.[4,5]

Unlike the eustachian tube communicating air to the middle ear and acting as one-way valve (automatically opening toward the nasopharynx), there is no similar anatomy (e.g., tube) to facilitate equilibration of pressure changes between ambient air and air contained within frontal sinus. These are dependent on the health and patency of their respective osteomeatal complexes,[6] thus on the status of their lining nasal mucosa and anatomical integrity. Therefore, any inflammation, chronic or acute, systemic or local, attributed to allergic, bacterial, viral, environmental causes (toxic, inhaled, postirradiation, etc.) or lifestyle agents (e.g., smoking, cocaine inhalation), all result in local edema, which increases the mechanical resistance on nasal air patency and difficulty in passively achieving air pressure equilibrium between the frontal sinus and ambient air. Likewise, any mechanical compromise of the same air route (congenital, neoplastic, or post-traumatic) will also predispose to FSB.

In spite of care taken by aviation industry to prevent barotrauma by pressurizing passenger-occupied cabins for the majority of civilian transport aircraft to an acceptable compromise (▶ Table 21.1), operational and other reasons may leave aircraft occupants exposed to pressure excursions larger than expected. In general, we may accept that the greater the pressure change, the more common and severe FSB expected, with confirmation derived by experimental animal models.[7]

21.2 Clinical Presentation and Investigations

During ascend in air travel (descent in diving), the gas within the frontal sinus will expand according to Boyle's law of gas under body temperature (i.e., under constant temperature, volume of any gas is inversely related to its surrounding pressure) and any expanding air will passively escape, while during descent (for air travel again) air has to return to the frontal sinus, responding to the increasing of pressure on sea level. If obstructed, air within the frontal sinus will retain its lesser pressure compared to ambient air and will produce symptoms: frontal sinus awareness and/or feeling of pressure, discomfort, persistent dull pain, and occasionally (if the anterior frontal wall is breached) swelling noticeable on the forehead.

Inversely, the same symptoms will present during descend while diving, if any nasal air flow obstruction to the frontal sinus emerges. At this point, remember that every 33 feet (~10 m) of descent, a diver will experience an increase in surrounding pressure by 1 atmosphere (1 atm = 760 mm Hg). Therefore, the commonest symptom prohibiting divers from further descent into depth is acute sinus and/or ear pain, sometimes reflecting to the teeth or head. FSB may also exist during ascent (called "reversed FSB"); intrasinus pathology in turn may impede air from escaping through natural ostia and follow the route of the least resistance, if any, entering adjacent

Table 21.1 Cabin maximum compression and descent rates encountered in common activities

	Activities	Cabin maximum altitude limits (in feet)	Usual rate of descent (feet/min)		Remarks
			Cabin	Aircraft	
Fixed wing aircraft	Airliners/commercial	5,000–8,000	150–500	1.500–2.000	3-degree glideslope (5% descent): "3:1 rule"[b]
	Private/VIP aviation	0–8,500	1.500–2.000	As per airlines	
	General aviation	Unpressurized	150	150	
	Combat transport[a]	5.000–12.000	500	2.500	
	Interceptors[a]	18.000	►3.000	► 10/000	
	Aerobatics	Unpressurised	N/A	N/A	Flight level < 10,000 feet
Rotary wing	Commercial	5,000	300	500	10-degree glideslope Flight level < 5,000 feet
	General/private	Unpressurized	100	100	
Diving	20 m/40 m/free diving	N/A	Depending on depth	N/A	Diving protocols
Parachuting	Civilian/military[a]	N/A	10.000–15000	12,500 feet (drop level)	Fall speed: 115 mph

Note: As noted, pressurized cabins (auto/semi/manual modes) do not allow passenger compression to deviate from comfort levels (150–300 feet/min) despite of aircraft flight levels. Limitations or exceptions to this rule also exist depending on flight parameters.
[a]Oxygen (O_2) supplied via face mask (O_2 mask drop cabin limit is 12.000 feet).
[b]Three miles of travel should be allowed for every 1,000 feet (300 m).[27]

anatomical structures and producing emphysema subcutaneous or orbital emphysema, pneumocephalus, or creating adjacent eye pathology.[8,9]

Occasionally, the full manifestation of acute sinusitis may develop, with mucopurulent discharge, often blood stained, and reduced sense of smell with associated taste disturbances, headache, and malaise. Symptomatology largely depends on preexisting conditions: the usual advice to aircrew is not to fly with an active upper respiratory tract infection (URTI) and refrain from smoking before flying. Slight temperature elevation is to be expected, especially when pain is intense. Nasal bleeding may also be noted originating from ruptured nasal mucosal vessels due to abrupt venous overload, after repeatedly attempted but failed Valsalva maneuvers.

With the exception of these few emergencies, the majority of cases, however, will typically appear sometime after air travel afebrile, with persistent frontal headache, and nasal blockage.

Patient history will disclose any preexisting nasal pathology, which is typically absent in most cases. FBC and blood investigation will then be unremarkable. Nasal endoscopy will affirm blockage and radiography (X-ray or CT) may reveal FS mucosal thickening, fluid accumulation, or intramucosal hematoma formation.[10,11]

Three clinical grades of SBs (► Table 21.2) have been described by Weissman et al[12] and Green Weissman[13] and complemented by Garges:[14]

- Grade I includes cases with mild transient sinus discomfort without changes visible on X-ray.
- Grade II is characterized by severe pain for up to 24 hours, with some mucosal thickening on X-ray.
- Patients with grade III have severe pain lasting for more than 24 hours and X-ray shows severe mucosal thickening or opacification of the affected sinus; epistaxis or subsequent sinusitis may be observed.

If left untreated, affected frontal sinus mucosa without secretion and air communication to nasal cavity will progress to secondary infection, transforming FSB from an acute rhinosinusitis (ARS) to an acute bacterial rhinosinusitis (ABRS).

21.3 Management

Although FSB is attributed to ambient pressure change, it still remains a form of ARS, as defined in the European Position Paper on Rhinosinusitis[15] (EPOS) and should be treated as such. Stage I FSB requires local treatment involving steroids and/or decongestants and may resolve within 2 to 3 days. Stage II FSB will require addition of analgesics, and in severe cases of oral steroids (Visual

Table 21.2 The Weissman/Garges barotrauma classification correlated to radiographic investigation, treatment, aircrew grounding period, and follow-up time, in brief[24,25]

Barotrauma class	I	II	III	Remarks
Intrasinus pressure differential (mm Hg)	100–150	150–250	250–300	
Symptoms	Discomfort	Mild headache, serous rhinorrhea	Nasal congestion, severe pain, hematoma, bloody rhinorrhea	
Radiography	Negative	Thickened mucosa	Sinus opacity (full/partial)	
Underlying lesion	Edema	Mucosa tearing	Open bleeding/intrasinus hematoma formation	
Treatment	Local decongestants	ADDED: local steroids, oral analgesics, oral decongestants,[a] oral steroids	ADDED: oral antibiotics	Treatment fail or repeated FSB: prolong therapy,[a] consider surgery[a]
Days grounded	2–3	1 wk	10	Consider CRSwP
Return to duties	No follow-up	Communicate to airman (self-assessment)	Pending on medical follow-up result	

Abbreviation: CRSwP, chronic rhinosinusitis with polyps.
[a]Allergy involved.

Analogue Scale [VAS] > 7).[15] Stage III FSB with sinus opacification and bloody rhinorrhea will require addition of oral antibiotics. Although stage I and II FSBs may resolve within a week or less, stage III FSB will not be allowed to return to flying duties for a minimum of 10 days. Stage I and II FSBs may fly again depending on self-assessment (e.g., fluent performance of a Valsalva maneuver), but stage III FSB cases will return depending on reevaluation. ▶ Table 21.2 summarizes grades I to III and provides their respective correlation to investigation and treatment.

In real life, however, a case may be not as clear. For example, professional aircrew tend to smoke and fly using over-the-counter local decongestants. A stage III FSB in such a patient may practically be a manifestation of chronic rhinosinusitis without polyps (CRSsP) and should be managed accordingly.

In practice, pressure changes challenge the patency of communication of the frontal sinus to ambient pressure and present a functional test to their integrity. Thus, an occasional sinus airway functional failure may present as FSB. A repeated FSB, however, demands further investigation to account for persistent functional or anatomical issues. When treating an FSB case, treatment should also address any predisposing conditions as described earlier.

Everyone agrees that prophylaxis is critical for prevention of any FSB grade. There are two distinctive patient categories, in need of advice:

- For the general population, air travel should be delayed until nasal blockage has receded. In case there is a need to fly, local nasal decongestants will help during descent, if administered upon aircraft descent initiation

(this usually coincides with arrival announcements by the cabin crew) and accompanied by repeated Valsalva (or any other pressure equalization) procedure, as often as one per minute or 1,000 feet of descend.

- For the professionals, one should note that "grounding" time is a lot longer in case an FSB occurs, rather that postponing their flight. Most aircrew think that if they "fly low" they are less likely to encounter a barotrauma. This is not accurate, as the largest pressure changes occur in the first 10.000 feet of altitude, as shown in ▶ Fig. 21.1, drawn out of values representing International Civil Aviation Organization (ICAO) Standard Atmosphere, same as the ones used by industry to program pressurization facilities onboard their aircraft.[16] If one is able to control descent rate (e.g., pilot-in-command), the most successful way to prevent FSB (as any barotrauma) is to ascend or to lower descent rate to a minimum possible, in order to achieve sinus air pressure equalization.

Divers will usually abandon dives due to intense pain preventing them to continue mission, as supra-atmospheric pressure changes are multiple to the subatmospheric ones. Careless parachutists, however, are rendered unable to continue by the time sea level is obtained.

Surgical intervention for FSB is rarely the case. Patients occupationally exposed to pressure changes are also being medically selected, monitored, and licensed at tactical intervals; therefore, gross pathology is less likely go undetected, compared to the general population. If conservative treatment fails or repeated FSB is noted, surgical

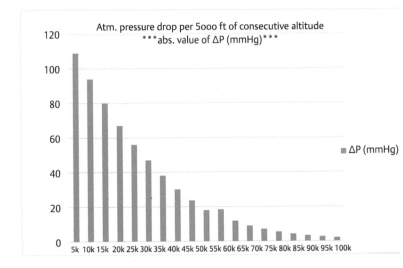

Atm. pressure drop per 5ooo ft of consecutive altitude
abs. value of ΔP (mmHg)

■ ΔP (mmHg)

5k 10k 15k 20k 25k 30k 35k 40k 45k 50k 55k 60k 65k 70k 75k 80k 85k 90k 95k 100k

Fig. 21.1 Atmospheric pressure drop with altitude: values present the difference between 5,000-feet consecutive levels (0–100.000 feet), as derived from ICAO (International Civil Aviation Organization)[16] Standard Atmosphere official tables.

treatment is considered. Endoscopic management methods are preferred[17,18,19] as minimally invasive ones, unless indicated. In several studies, functional endoscopic sinus surgery (FESS) has delivered the best results, allowing most airmen to return to flying duties as compared to prolonged conservative or "classic" sinus surgery. As FESS by principle unifies en route cells of frontal sinus clearance pathway, its efficacy remains without challenge. In specific FSB cases, after carefully identifying though 3D CT study the responsible air cells, one may also try removing just these, thus shortening the 6-week recovery time suggested in earlier studies.[17]

Given the onset of more endoscopic tools, such as endoscopic dilatation balloons (single or combined to image guidance), we should also consider their place as surgical tools in managing FSB, as results still remain controversial.[20,21,22,23,24] Detailed discussion has been presented earlier in Chapter 3.1, Section 2.

21.4 Case Example (Courtesy of Christos Georgalas)

A 35-year-old pilot for a commercial airline has been complaining of acute, sudden-onset left frontal headaches on landing for the past 6 months. The episodes were severe enough to interfere with his work. He has also described episodes of associated nosebleed while denying any other nasal symptoms. These episodes started after an URTI associated with purulent nasal discharge and nasal obstruction. He was otherwise healthy with no allergies or asthma and did not take any medications. He has been taking intranasal steroids for the past 2 months with no apparent improvement in symptoms. On endoscopy, he had a healthy-looking nasal mucosa with minimal secretions. A CT sinus is shown below (▶ Fig. 21.2). A Draf IIa was performed (▶ Fig. 21.3) resulting in complete resolution of his episodes. A postoperative endoscopic

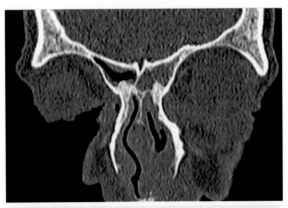

Fig. 21.2 A CT sinus showing obstruction of the left frontal recess with associated opacification of the left frontal sinus. Courtesy: Christos Georgalas

view of his left frontal recess, showing a patent ostium is shown (▶ Fig. 21.3).

References

[1] Hirsch S, Coelho D, Schuman T. Subcutaneous emphysema after vigorous sneezing in the setting of acute frontal sinusitis. Am J Otolaryngol. 2017; 38(2):244–247

[2] Ambiru S, Furuyama N, Aono M, Otsuka H, Suzuki T, Miyazaki M. Analysis of risk factors associated with complications of hyperbaric oxygen therapy. J Crit Care. 2008; 23(3):295–300

[3] Rosenkvist L, Klokker M, Katholm M. Upper respiratory infections and barotraumas in commercial pilots: a retrospective survey. Aviat Space Environ Med. 2008; 79(10):960–963

[4] Rodenberg H. Severe frontal sinus barotrauma in an airline passenger: a case report and review. J Emerg Med. 1988; 6(2):113–115

[5] Singletary EM, Reilly JF, Jr. Acute frontal sinus barotrauma. Am J Emerg Med. 1990; 8(4):329–331

[6] Lund VJ, Stammberger H, Fokkens WJ, et al. European position paper on the anatomical terminology of the internal nose and paranasal sinuses. Rhinol Suppl. 2014; 24 Suppl 24:1–34

[7] Xu X, Wang B, Jin Z, Zhang Y. A dynamic rabbit model of sinus barotrauma and its related pathology. Aerosp Med Hum Perform. 2016; 87(6):521–527

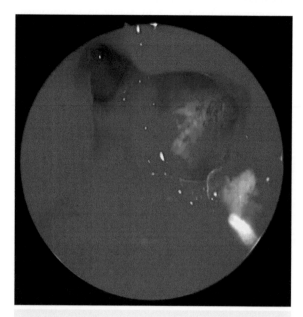

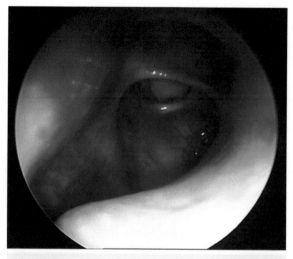

Fig. 21.4 A postoperative endoscopic image of his left frontal recess.

Fig. 21.3 An intraoperative photograph of the left frontal sinusotomy (Draf IIa).

[8] Becker GD, Parell GJ. Barotrauma of the ears and sinuses after scuba diving. Eur Arch Otorhinolaryngol. 2001; 258(4):159–163

[9] Powell MR, Hurley LD, Richardson TC. An unusual complication of barotrauma at altitude. Aerosp Med Hum Perform. 2015; 86(11):994–998

[10] Segev Y, Landsberg R, Fliss DM. MR imaging appearance of frontal sinus barotrauma. AJNR Am J Neuroradiol. 2003; 24:346–347

[11] Vandenbulcke R, van Holsbeeck B, Crevits I, Marrannes J. Frontal sinus barotrauma. J Belg Soc Radiol. 2016; 100(1):60

[12] Weissman B, Green RS, Roberts PT. Frontal sinus barotrauma. Laryngoscope. 1972; 82(12):2160–2168

[13] Green RS, Weissman B. Frontal sinus hematomas in aerospace medicine. Aerosp Med. 1973; 44(2):205–209

[14] Garges LM. Maxillary sinus barotrauma: case report and review. Aviat Space Environ Med. 1985; 56(8):796–802

[15] Fokkens WJ, Lund VJ, Mullol J, et al. EPOS 2012: European position paper on rhinosinusitis and nasal polyps 2012. A summary for otorhinolaryngologists. Rhinology. 2012; 50(1):1–12

[16] International Civil Aviation Organization (ICAO). Manual of the ICAO Standard Atmosphere. 2nd ed. Montreal, Canada: ICAO; 1974

[17] Bolger WE, Parsons DS, Matson RE. Functional endoscopic sinus surgery in aviators with recurrent sinus barotrauma. Aviat Space Environ Med. 1990; 61(2):148–156

[18] O'Reilly BJ, Lupa H, Mcrae A. The application of endoscopic sinus surgery to the treatment of recurrent sinus barotrauma. Clin Otolaryngol Allied Sci. 1996; 21(6):528–532

[19] Parsons DS, Chambers DW, Boyd EM. Long-term follow-up of aviators after functional endoscopic sinus surgery for sinus barotrauma. Aviat Space Environ Med. 1997; 68(11):1029–1034

[20] Andrews JN, Weitzel EK, Eller R, McMains CK. Unsuccessful frontal balloon sinuplasty for recurrent sinus barotrauma. Aviat Space Environ Med. 2010; 81(5):514–516

[21] Bizaki AJ, Taulu R, Numminen J, Rautiainen M. Quality of life after endoscopic sinus surgery or balloon sinuplasty: a randomized clinical study. Rhinology. 2014; 52(4):300–305

[22] Tomazic PV, Stammberger H, Braun H, et al. Feasibility of balloon sinuplasty in patients with chronic rhinosinusitis: the Graz experience. Rhinology. 2013; 51(2):120–127

[23] Hopkins C, Noon E, Roberts D. Balloon sinuplasty in acute frontal sinusitis. Rhinology. 2009; 47(4):375–378

[24] Weiss RL, Church CA, Kuhn FA, Levine HL, Sillers MJ, Vaughan WC. Long-term outcome analysis of balloon catheter sinusotomy: two-year follow-up. Otolaryngol Head Neck Surg. 2008; 139(3) Suppl 3: S38–S46

[25] Weitzel EK, McMains KC, Rajapaksa S, Wormald PJ. Aerosinusitis: pathophysiology, prophylaxis, and management in passengers and aircrew. Aviat Space Environ Med. 2008; 79(1):50–53

[26] Yanagawa Y, Okada Y, Ishida K, Fukuda H, Hirata F, Fujita K. Magnetic resonance imaging of the paranasal sinuses in divers. Aviat Space Environ Med. 1998; 69(1):50–52

[27] Wikipedia. Rule of three (aeronautics). Available at: https://en.wikipedia.org/wiki/Rule_of_three (aeronautics). Accessed November 20, 2016

22 Frontal Sinus in Patients with Cystic Fibrosis

Kiranya E. Tipirneni, Hari Jeyarajan, and Bradford A. Woodworth

Abstract

Cystic fibrosis (CF) is the most common lethally inherited disease in Caucasians. While pulmonary compromise is the primary cause of mortality in this population, up to 100% of these patients invariably develop chronic rhinosinusitis (CRS). Furthermore, CF patients frequently exhibit abnormal sinus anatomy with a high prevalence of underdeveloped frontal sinuses. There is significant evidence supporting the unified airway model in CF, which suggests a bidirectional relationship between the upper and lower airways. As such, adequate management of CRS becomes paramount in minimizing the pulmonary complications of CF patients. However, management of CRS in these patients continues to be limited by the paucity of high-level evidence surrounding CF-related sinus disease. CF is a chronic, systemic disease universally affecting the sinonasal mucosa. As such, it necessitates comprehensive management that includes the frontal sinus.

Keywords: sinusitis, cystic fibrosis, frontal sinus, surgical therapy, drug therapy, endoscopic sinus surgery, Draf III, modified endoscopic Lothrop, Draf IIb, Draf IIa, Draf IIb, Draf III, endoscopic frontal sinusotomy

22.1 Epidemiology and Etiology

First described in 1938, cystic fibrosis (CF) is the most commonly inherited lethal disease among Caucasians, affecting 1 in 2,500 to 3,500 newborns each year.[1,2] The fatal disease is inherited in autosomal recessive fashion and caused by single gene mutations encoding the CF transmembrane conductance regulator (CFTR) protein located on the long arm of chromosome 7.[3] Though several mutations exist, the most common is the F508del, which is responsible for approximately 70% of all CFTR mutations[4] and results in the absence of phenylalanine at position 508.[2] Like all CFTR mutations, F508del causes aberrant chloride (Cl^-) and bicarbonate (HCO_3^-) transport at the apical cell surface and results in multiorgan pathology secondary to increased mucosal viscosity[5] with thick, tenacious secretions and impaired mucociliary clearance (MCC). As such, patients with CF suffer from gastrointestinal obstruction, exocrine pancreatic dysfunction, blockage of biliary ducts, and a myriad of respiratory complications in both the upper and lower airways.[6]

In the upper airways, impaired MCC combined with chronic stasis of inspissated mucous translates to inflammatory sinonasal disease and mucous-filled sinuses with a high propensity for bacterial superinfection.[7,8,9] In fact, nearly 100% of CF patients develop chronic rhinosinusitis

(CRS) as confirmed by clinical or radiographic examination.[10] Despite this, CRS remains a poorly studied manifestation of CF when compared to pancreatic and pulmonary complications, the latter of which is the most common cause of death.[7] Symptoms of CRS continue to be incapacitating and often include headache, facial pain, nasal congestion and obstruction, and chronic rhinorrhea.[11,12,13,14] Sinus anatomy is frequently abnormal in patients with CF and further contributes to the high frequency of abnormal sinus pathology observed in these patients.

Primary treatment of CF historically focused on improving lung function, while management of CRS was considered a secondary, purely quality-of-life (QOL) outcome. However, there is a unique relationship between the upper and lower airways, which is commonly referred to as the unified airway. The unified airway represents a single respiratory unit that consists of the nose, paranasal sinuses, larynx, trachea, and distal lung.[10] As a continuous functional unit consisting of pseudostratified, ciliated, columnar epithelium, the unified airway experiences identical infectious and inflammatory insults, which suggests that CF airway disease is a bidirectional process whereby sinonasal diseases affect disease within the lungs, and vice versa.[2,8,15] Although the average life expectancy has significantly increased over the years due to many improvements in the management of CF-related pulmonary disease, CF patients continue to encounter premature mortality at only 33.4 years in addition to a dramatically reduced QOL in comparison to those without CF.[16] And while a recent meta-analysis highlights that this relationship is not as straightforward as immune-related airway diseases like asthma, there is evidence to suggest that CRS significantly contributes to CF lung disease with bacterial seeding of the upper airways representing the catalyst for the development of lower airway infection and ensuing pulmonary demise.[17,18,19]

22.2 Clinical Presentation and Investigations

CRS in CF is clinically distinct from that exhibited by the general population. CFTR dysfunction leads to defective anion transport and reduced airway surface liquid depth, which results in increased mucosal viscosity by a factor 30 to 60 times greater than that seen in the normal population.[20,21,22,23,24] MCC is further impaired by chronic inflammation and DNA accumulation within the airways that result from extensive neutrophil degradation, both of which congest sinus ostia to cause significant hypoxia and mucosal edema.[25,26] Furthermore, the recurrent inflammatory cycling and remodeling processes promote neutrophil-predominant polyp formation, which is present in approximately 67% of CF patients.[27,28] This is in stark contrast to the eosinophil-dominated nasal polyposis observed in the general population.[29]

While there are no specific criteria to describe CF-related CRS, both the International Consensus Statement on Allergy and Rhinology: Rhinosinusitis (ICAR:RS)[30] and the European Position Paper on Rhinosinusitis and Nasal Polyps (EPOS2012)[31] define the most frequently used criteria for CRS, describing it as persistent inflammation of the paranasal sinuses that lasts a period of 12 weeks or more and often consists of at least two of the following symptoms:

- Nasal blockage.
- Obstruction.
- Congestion.
- Nasal discharge.
- ± Facial pain/pressure.
- ± Olfactory loss or reduction.[30,31]

Despite the high sensitivity of the aforementioned symptoms, they are rather nonspecific for CRS.[30] As such, a definitive diagnosis of CRS must be accompanied by objective findings demonstrating inflammatory and/or mucosal changes.[30] Such changes are often demonstrated by positive endoscopic and/or computed tomography (CT) findings, which often exhibit one or more of the following:

- Nasal polyps.
- Mucopurulent discharge.
- Edema/mucosal obstruction.
- Mucosal changes.[30,31]

Although 67% of CF patients experience a reduction in sense of smell and 80% exhibit CRS as defined by standard criteria, only 10 to 15% freely complain of symptoms.[32] The reason for this is unclear but assumingly attributed to symptom desensitization to chronic disease or lack of severity in relation to other manifestations of CF.[25] Thus, it is particularly critical to use direct questioning with QOL questionnaires, such as Rhinosinusitis Outcome Measure-31 or Sinonasal Outcome Test-22 (SNOT-22) in adults and Sinonasal-5 for children, to adequately assess for sinonasal disease in the CF population.[15]

22.2.1 Radiographic Abnormalities in Cystic Fibrosis and the Frontal Sinus

There is a higher incidence of abnormal radiographic findings, particularly in the form of underdeveloped sinuses, in patients with CF in comparison to the general population.[33] This is relatively unsurprising considering the underlying pathophysiology for CF CRS is appreciably different from that of non-CF CRS. In fact, Orlandi and Wiggins[34] demonstrated that 65.9% CF patients exhibit either frontal sinus hypoplasia (52.6%) or aplasia (13.3%).

In pediatric patients aged 6 to 26 years, Wang et al found that 43% demonstrated frontal sinus aplasia or agensis.[35] In addition, 74.2% of CF patients exhibit poorly developed sphenoid sinuses with 4.4% demonstrating sphenoid aplasia and 69.8% showing sphenoid hypoplasia.[34] While maxillary sinus underdevelopment is more common in CF patients (70 vs. 8% in the non-CF population),[7] it occurs less often than in the sphenoid and frontal sinuses in this population.[7,34] In addition to abnormal sinus development, Orlandi and Wiggins found that sinonasal bony sclerosis occurred with an increased, albeit unequal, frequency in patients with CF.[34] Sclerosis was present with the highest frequency in the maxillary sinuses (81.1%), followed by the sphenoid (73.3%), frontal (35.9%), and ethmoid (8.9%) sinuses.[34] Importantly, there was no significant correlation between bony sclerosis and prior sinus surgery.[34] Another study by Nishioka et al[36] reported three significant differences between CF patients and the non-CF control group: frontal sinus agenesis, medial bulging of the lateral nasal wall, and opacification of the maxilloethmoid sinus. Other CT findings have demonstrated demineralization of the bilateral uncinate processes with medial displacement within the middle meatus for almost all children with CF.[37]

Several studies have attributed chronic inflammation in childhood as the inciting factor for development of sinus hypoplasia or aplasia.[7,38,39] Additionally, some studies have described reduced oxygen saturation and temperature alterations, which themselves may result from CRS or nasal polyposis, as contributing factors for frontal sinus underdevelopment.[39] However, when considering sinonasal development in relation to CF genotypic mutations, one study found that patients homozygous for the F508del mutation had a significantly increased prevalence of underdeveloped sinuses, particularly in the sphenoid (100%) and frontal (98%) sinuses, as compared to CF patients heterozygous for F508del or those with other CFTR mutations (50 and 69%, respectively).[7] Furthermore, these patients also had a significantly increased frequency of aplastic frontal sinuses as compared with the nonhomozygous control group (78 vs. 20%).[7] Importantly, Woodworth et al found no significant difference in the frequency of prior sinus surgeries between study groups, thus suggesting an intrinsic mechanism of aberrant frontal sinus development specific to the homozygous F508del genotype.[7] As such, it is highly probable that F508del homozygosity represents a significant predisposition to pansinus hypoplasia, particularly in the frontal and sphenoid sinuses.[7] Similar findings were demonstrated by Seifert et al, which showed significantly reduced paranasal sinus pneumatization in CF patients homozygous for the F508del mutation.[40] However, the development of the porcine CF animal model indicates, at least in this animal, that sinus hypoplasia predates the onset of sinus infection.[41]

While there are often a myriad of abnormal radiographic findings in patients with CF, patients without CF frequently exhibit normal sinus development despite having a 12.5% prevalence of CRS.[42] Though CT sinonasal opacification is not necessarily indicative of CF rhinosinusitis, it has a rather high sensitivity in that the absence of paranasal sinus opacification virtually excludes a diagnosis of CF to a reasonable degree.[43] Despite the relatively high incidence of frontal sinus abnormalities in CF patients, sphenoid sinus aplasia is probably the most reliable indicator of CF CRS because it very rarely occurs in patients without CF.[44] While uncommon, frontal sinus hypoplasia does occur in 7 to 15% of non-CF patients unilaterally and 2 to 5% bilaterally.[44] Important to consider, however, is that frontal sinus aplasia or hypoplasia in children may be relatively age dependent as a result of its inherently late development.[43] That is, the frontal sinus is the final sinus to develop with initial pneumatization occurring around 2 years of age.[43] As the life expectancy continues to improve, one must consider the cost–benefit ratio of frequent imaging studies and the increased risk associated with cumulative ionizing radiation, particularly in the pediatric CF population.[45] In fact, children and young adults are at the highest risk of facing the carcinogenic effects of radiation due to their developing organs.[46]

22.3 Management

22.3.1 Medical Therapy

While there are no standardized treatment guidelines for CF CRS, management often begins conservatively. While current strategies emphasize symptomatic treatment with a combination of antibiotics, topical irrigations, and surgery, there is a relative paucity of data regarding CF-related CRS particularly pertaining to efficacy and treatment-dosing strategies in CF patients.[5] Nonetheless, the most commonly studied medical regimens consist of nasal saline irrigation, topical and oral antibiotics, topical steroids, dornase alfa, ivacaftor, and ibuprofen.[10,15] Importantly, there is no medical therapy specific to the management of frontal sinus disease in CF patients.

22.3.2 Nasal Saline Irrigations

Nasal saline irrigation helps remove nasal crusting and inspissated mucus from the upper airways.[15,47] While there is little conclusive evidence specific to CF patients, in non-CF patients with CRS, a recent Cochrane review found that nasal irrigation with isotonic (0.9%) saline led to modest improvement in disease-specific QOL and sinonasal symptoms when compared to no treatment.[48,49] Although several delivery options are available, squeeze bottle/neti pot devices achieve the most effective sinus irrigation in both operated and nonoperated sinuses.[15] It should be noted, however, that frontal sinus delivery is almost negligible without surgical access.[50] Some studies have additionally advocated for use of hypertonic saline

due to positive outcomes seen in CF pulmonary disease and in management of CRS in the non-CF population. In these patients, hypertonic saline results in improved MCC, decreased mucus viscosity, and rehydration of thick secretions.[51,52] While there is evidence supporting the use of mildly hypertonic (2%) saline in non-CF patients, a recent study in CF patients demonstrated that nasal irrigation with hypertonic (6%) saline was not, in fact, superior to isotonic (0.9%) saline for the management of CRS.[51] Furthermore, hypertonic (6–7%) nasal saline frequently causes irritation of the sinonasal mucosa and its use is limited by poor patient compliance.[49,53]

22.3.3 Corticosteroids

In patients without CF, topical steroids are the standard of care in decreasing mucosal inflammation, especially in patients with eosinophil-predominant nasal polyposis and allergic CRS.[54] However, both nasal polyposis and CRS in CF patients are characterized by a predominance of neutrophils, which are often less responsive to intranasal steroids.[47] Nevertheless, there is evidence to support the use of topical corticosteroids for management of nasal polyposis in CF patients. In fact, one study showed a significant reduction in nasal polyposis with betamethasone nasal drops when compared to placebo.[55] No studies have shown conclusive evidence in the symptomatic amelioration of CF-related CRS.[31,56] Despite this, low-absorption topical steroid rinses (i.e., mometasone, budesonide) are often prescribed in the treatment of CF CRS due to their well-known anti-inflammatory properties and relatively favorable side effect profiles.[15]

Use of a short, 2- to 4-week course of oral systemic steroids has shown significant improvements for non-CF patients with CRS; however, their use to treat CRS in the CF population is not well studied, as they are frequently reserved for pulmonary exacerbations.[57] Importantly, frequent use of systemic steroids is not routinely recommended as they cause a number of metabolic side effects, especially in patients with CF who experience baseline pancreatic insufficiency.

22.3.4 Topical Antibiotics

Not surprisingly, bacterial pathogens in CF CRS are markedly different than those observed in non-CF CRS. As such, antibiotics should be targeted at common CF pathogens such as *Pseudomonas aeruginosa* and *Staphylococcus aureus*.[47] The addition of antibiotics to nasal lavage in the postoperative period has been shown to decrease the rate of bacterial reseeding in the transplanted lungs of CF patients.[58] Some studies have additionally studied nasal inhalation of tobramycin.[58,59,60] Particularly in the postoperative period, use of inhaled tobramycin has been shown to decrease the frequency of both *P. aeruginosa* infection and CRS exacerbation in CF patients while providing improved symptomatic control for up to 2 years.[58] Other studies have supported the use of topical antibiotics delivered via a large-particle nebulizer for both CF[61] and non-CF[62] patients with recalcitrant CRS. While both studies reported subjective improvements in disease-specific symptoms, the addition of local antibiotics itself appears to be of minimal benefit.[61,62] In fact, it appears that any observed beneficial effects result more from the nebulized delivery method than from the locally administered antibiotics.[61,62] Due to significant variations in evidence-based studies regarding topical antibiotics, their exact role in the management of frontal sinusitis remains unclear, particularly in the CF population, and requires additional high-level evidence.

22.3.5 Oral Antibiotics

Aside from their well-known antibacterial properties, 14- and 15-membered macrolides (i.e., clarithromycin, erythromycin, azithromycin) have the added benefits of improving mucus clearance within the airways, which leads to an overall reduction in inflammatory response.[47] In the lower airways, use of azithromycin has been shown to decrease airway inflammation and reduce lung deterioration.[47,63] While little data are available to support their use in the upper airways of CF patients, patients without CF have demonstrated favorable outcomes with decreased sinonasal secretions, nasal obstruction, and postnasal drip.[64] Still, further studies are necessary to accurately assess their efficacy in the CF population.

22.3.6 Dornase Alfa

Dornase alfa, which consists of recombinant human deoxyribonuclease, is a mucolytic agent that has shown a myriad of improvements in patients with CF, including improvement of CRS symptoms and rhinoscopic findings, as well as overall lung function.[26] In children older than 5 years, it has been shown to significantly improve the forced expiratory volume in 1 second (FEV1) and reduce the frequency of pulmonary exacerbations.[65,66] Furthermore, several studies have demonstrated a reduction in the annual rate of lung deterioration with dornase alfa.[66,67,68,69,70,71] In CF patients with CRS, sinonasal inhalation of dornase alfa, when compared to isotonic saline, has been shown to both reduce symptoms and improve QOL.[72] However, use of dornase alfa for CRS is currently restricted by cost.

22.3.7 Cystic Fibrosis Transmembrane Conductance Regulator modulators

CFTR modulators represent a novel therapeutic strategy that targets the CFTR protein itself rather than attempting to treat the secondary effects of channel dysfunction.[73] One such treatment is the recently Food and Drug Administration (FDA) approved therapy ivacaftor (Kalydeco [VX-770], Vertex Pharmaceuticals, Inc.), a CFTR potentiator that increases the probability of opening faulty chloride channels in patients possessing at least one copy of the defective G551D-CFTR allele.[73,74] Although this mutation is only present in 4 to 5% of the CF population,[75,76] ivacaftor has been shown to cause a 10% improvement in pulmonary function and a significant reduction in the rate of annual lung deterioration when used in combination with routine treatment.[77,78,79] Despite the high cost, which is reported to be upward of $300,000 annually, patients taking ivacaftor are likely to have lower rates of lung transplantation than those receiving routine care due to decreased severity of lung involvement.[80] Furthermore, one case report showed that ivacaftor led to complete reversal of CF sinusitis with resolution of subjective and objective findings.[81]

The next generation of CFTR modulators approved for use in CF patients is aimed at "correcting" the commonest mutation, F508del, while also improving the function of the corrected protein with ivacaftor. The combination drug lumacaftor/ivacaftor (Orkambi [VX809], Vertex Pharmaceuticals, Inc.), was approved by the U.S FDA in 2016.[82] It was shown to significantly improve lung function by causing a 3% increase in the percent predicted FEV1 (ppFEV1) and decreasing the frequency of pulmonary exacerbations in these patients, which can translate in up to a 40% reduction in the annual rate of lung decline.[74,83] This was followed by the combination tezacaftor/ivacaftor (Symdeko®, Vertex pharmaceuticals) which showed similar efficacy but with decreased side effects.[111] More recently, the addition of the corrector elexacaftor to tezacaftor/ivacaftor (Trikafta®, Vertex pharmaceuticals) was approved in 2019 for use in CF patients with at least one copy of the F508del mutation. The blockbuster drug resulted in a 13.8 point improvement in percentage of predicted FEV1 that was 13.8 points higher at 4 weeks and 14.3 points higher through 24 weeks with 63% lower rate of pulmonary exacerbations.[112] While the full breadth of the impact of the new modulators on CF sinusitis has not been evaluated, re-analysis of data from ivacaftor trials for patients with the G551D mutation suggests improvement in sinus related quality of life.[113]

22.3.8 Surgical Therapy

Despite the lack of universal guidelines and often-unpredictable outcomes in CRS management, surgical intervention is frequently reserved for patients who have failed more conservative medical therapy. However, the low incidence of self-reported symptoms complicates the establishment of surgical indications in such a patient population. And while current literature finds that 20 to 60% of CF patients undergo endoscopic sinus surgery for treatment of CRS with good effect, this probably more accurately reflects institutional experience than evidence-based care.[14,15,84,85,86,87,88,89,90,91]

For chronic frontal sinusitis in particular, restoration of normal aeration and MCC by removing diseased frontoethmoidal cells often allows resolution of disease.[92] Wormald's group has established that persistent frontal sinus disease, despite good disease control in all other sinuses, is an independent risk factor for persistent symptoms in non-CF patients.[93] Still, published outcomes for frontal sinus surgery in CF patients are scarce, with the greatest focus on establishment of drainage of maxillary and ethmoid sinuses through modified medial maxillectomies.[94] Nevertheless, CF is a chronic, systemic disease that universally affects all the sinuses equally. Certainly in non-CF patients, refinements in operative techniques and equipment, including focusing on adequate access with 70-degree endoscopes and angled, through-cutting instruments and prioritizing mucosal preservation, have improved functional outcomes in frontal sinus surgery.[95,96] However, it is increasingly recognized that, in non-CF patients, the combination of disease-related (chronic inflammation, active infection, polyposis, smoking) and anatomic (narrow frontal recess and small neo-ostium size) risk factors cumulatively result in a high rate of surgical failure in both primary and salvage settings.[93,97,98] Furthermore, neo-osteogenesis, a significant contributor to neo-ostial stenosis, is strongly associated with the presence of *P. aeruginosa* infection.[99] As such, the surgical approach to frontal sinus disease in CF patients should emulate that taken for non-CF patients at high risk of failure, and additionally appreciate the chronic mucosal inflammation, pseudomonal colonization and infection, poor mucociliary function, and anomalous sinus anatomy unique to CF patients.

22.3.9 Endoscopic Approaches

The ultimate goal in endoscopic frontal sinus surgery is mucosal preservation within the frontal recess in order to minimize the risk of scarring, osteoneogenesis, and subsequent stenosis, while still allowing for both gravity-dependent drainage and access for topical medications through complete removal of the frontal sinus floor.[96] While in non-CF patients, appropriately selected Draf sinusotomies have a low recidivism rate, there is a high propensity for restenosis in CF patients. Thus, creation of larger ostia with Draf IIb and III procedures must be considered but also balanced according to the size of the frontal sinus and subsequent exposed bone that may lead to neo-osteogenesis and further difficulty.[94,100] Visualization is key to safe and effective dissection of the frontal recess in such narrow and poorly developed sinuses. Meticulous division of ethmoidal partitions to expose the anterior skull base and skeletonization of the lamina ensure maximum exposure of the recess. Inflamed, polypoid mucosa can greatly impair visualization and impede

access. The use of through-cutting instruments prevents mucosal stripping, while judicious use of topical vasoconstrictors and selective cautery can significantly improve operative conditions. Communication with anesthesia to ensure adequate head elevation and controlled hypotension and bradycardia are also important considerations. Comfort and proficiency with 70-degree scopes and angled instruments is paramount. Diligent care should be taken medially when resecting the anterior middle turbinate during Draf IIb or III procedures remembering the anterior position of the first olfactory fila can result in an inadvertent cerebrospinal fluid (CSF) leak.

It is the senior author's preference to create a Draf IIb using hand instruments for CF frontal sinuses due to the large amount of bone that requires removal (▶ Fig. 22.1; Video 22.1). Disease burden may not be as high with very small frontal sinuses in CF patients, and a Draf IIb using hand instruments such as the Hosemann punch provides quick healing times with excellent exposure for cleaning with a Van Alyea cannula (▶ Fig. 22.2). A formal Draf III may be more appropriate from the outset if postoperative cleaning will be difficult with a Draf IIb and where the entire sinus cannot be accessed in clinic due to greater pneumatization (▶ Fig. 22.3 and ▶ Fig. 22.4).[101,102,103,104,105,106,107] In such cases where surgical access to the recess is restricted, utilization of an outside-in approach allows for safer use of bigger cutting burs, decreasing operative time, and improving overall bone removal and intraoperative visualization.[108] However, such large areas of exposed bone are susceptible to postoperative osteitis, resulting in significant osteoneogenesis and neo-ostial restenosis.[103] Elevation of inferiorly based lateral nasal mucosal flaps can aid in postoperative mucosal resurfacing. The use of mucosal grafts is an added effort to prevent surgical failure in the frontal recess and has proven to maintain neo-osteal patency at 3 years with a correspondent improvement in subjective outcome measures.[109,110] This can be harvested either from the septum during anterosuperior septectomy or alternatively from the nasal floor or posterior inferior turbinate. A 0.5-mm Silastic stent is then placed

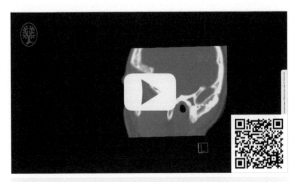

Video 22.1 Frontal sinus surgery in a cystic fibrosis (CF) patient

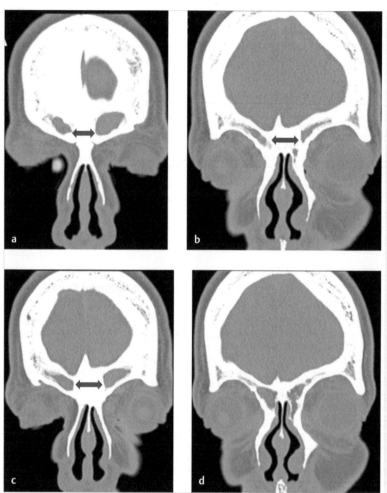

Fig. 22.1 (a–d) Coronal CT scans of the typical pneumatization pattern of a cystic fibrosis frontal sinus. When present, the sinuses are small with an extensive amount of bone between the sinuses (*red arrows*). In this case, a Draf IIb with hand instruments is preferred because a Draf III will create a common sinus that more than double the burden of mucopurulence within the sinus. Furthermore, all recesses of this small sinus can be cleaned through a Draf IIb.

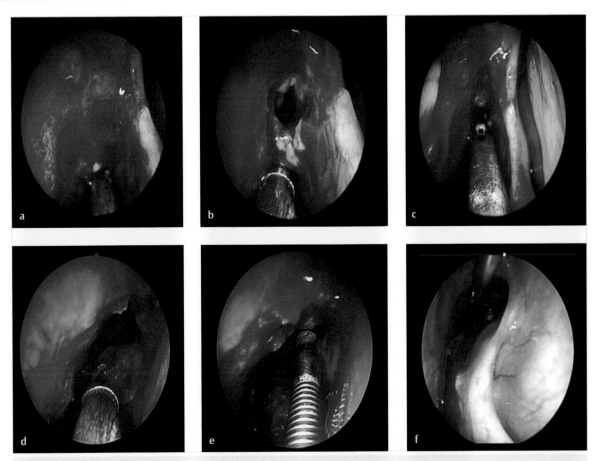

Fig. 22.2 Technical aspects of the hand instrument Draf IIb with 70-degree endoscopic views for the patient in ▶ Fig. 22.1. The frontal recess partitions have not been removed by previous surgeons and the recess is surrounded by polypoid edema. The edema is decompressed with a curved suction **(a)** and the partitions are exposed **(b)**. Thru-cutting angled frontal sinus instruments are used to remove the partitions without stripping the mucosa **(c)**. The medial aspect of the frontal sinus floor is exposed by removal of the anterior aspect of the middle turbinate neck **(d)** and then removed to the septum with a Hosemann punch **(e)**. No drills are used and there is minimal exposed bone. Healing is excellent and allows access to the entire sinus for cleaning with a Van Alyea cannula during routine clinical follow-up **(f)**.

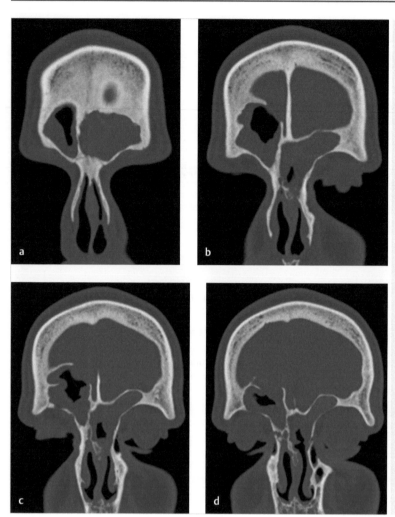

Fig. 22.3 (a–d) Coronal CT scans of a patient with a larger pneumatization pattern and 40 previous operations by previous surgeons. In this case, a Draf III is preferred because the large mucopurulence burden within the frontal sinus requires improved access for rinses and the ability to clean the entire sinus during clinical follow-up.

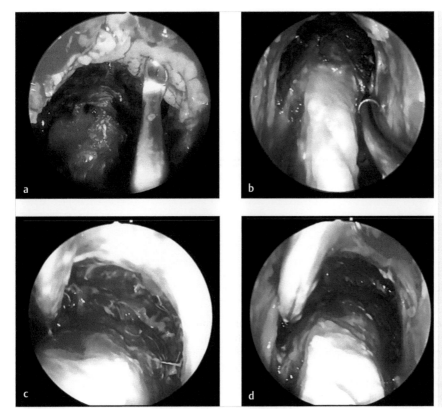

Fig. 22.4 Transnasal endoscopic 70-degree view at the completion of the Draf III showing anteriorly placed mucosal grafts to decrease postoperative neo-osteogenesis **(a)**. The patient has vastly improved access for irrigations, which not only decreases the amount of mucopurulence seen in routine clinical follow-up **(b)**, but also allows cleaning of the entire cavity with a curved suction and 70-degree scope visualization **(c, d)**.

in the frontal sinus drainage pathway (FSDP) to maintain patency as well as prevent inadvertent premature removal of packing. A nonlatex gloved cotton sponge (Merocel, Medtronic, Jacksonville, FL) spacer is then positioned against the front face of the sphenoid, spanning the ethmoid cavity to just anterior of the frontal recess. It is subsequently instilled with saline and secured to the septum via a 2–0 Prolene suture. Culture-directed antibiotics are provided for at least 3 weeks in all CF patients postoperatively.

22.4 Complications: Management

Even with meticulous technique and careful preparation, inadvertent injury can occur to both the ventral skull base and the lamina. While the use of intraoperative navigation can aid in confirming approach and position, it cannot replace operative diligence. Care should be taken at the posteromedial aspect of the recess where inadvertent exposure of the first olfactory fila can result in a CSF leak. In such

narrow recesses, a modified outside-in approach can help safely open the recess without risking skull base injury.

References

[1] Grosse SD, Boyle CA, Botkin JR, et al. CDC. Newborn screening for cystic fibrosis: evaluation of benefits and risks and recommendations for state newborn screening programs. MMWR Recomm Rep. 2004; 53 RR-13:1–36

[2] Chang EH. New insights into the pathogenesis of cystic fibrosis sinusitis. Int Forum Allergy Rhinol. 2014; 4(2):132–137

[3] Sloane AJ, Lindner RA, Prasad SS, et al. Proteomic analysis of sputum from adults and children with cystic fibrosis and from control subjects. Am J Respir Crit Care Med. 2005; 172(11):1416–1426

[4] Welsh MJ, Smith AE. Molecular mechanisms of CFTR chloride channel dysfunction in cystic fibrosis. Cell. 1993; 73(7):1251–1254

[5] Gysin C, Alothman GA, Papsin BC. Sinonasal disease in cystic fibrosis: clinical characteristics, diagnosis, and management. Pediatr Pulmonol. 2000; 30(6):481–489

[6] Derichs N. Targeting a genetic defect: cystic fibrosis transmembrane conductance regulator modulators in cystic fibrosis. Eur Respir Rev. 2013; 22(127):58–65

[7] Woodworth BA, Ahn C, Flume PA, Schlosser RJ. The delta F508 mutation in cystic fibrosis and impact on sinus development. Am J Rhinol. 2007; 21(1):122–127

[8] Tos M. Distribution of mucus producing elements in the respiratory tract. Differences between upper and lower airway. Eur J Respir Dis Suppl. 1983; 128(Pt 1):269–279

[9] Wine JJ, King VV, Lewiston NJ. Method for rapid evaluation of topically applied agents to cystic fibrosis airways. Am J Physiol. 1991; 261(2, Pt 1):L218–L221

[10] Liang J, Higgins T, Ishman SL, Boss EF, Benke JR, Lin SY. Medical management of chronic rhinosinusitis in cystic fibrosis: a systematic review. Laryngoscope. 2014; 124(6):1308–1313

[11] Cepero R, Smith RJ, Catlin FI, Bressler KL, Furuta GT, Shandera KC. Cystic fibrosis: an otolaryngologic perspective. Otolaryngol Head Neck Surg. 1987; 97(4):356–360

[12] Cuyler JP, Monaghan AJ. Cystic fibrosis and sinusitis. J Otolaryngol. 1989; 18(4):173–175

[13] Duplechain JK, White JA, Miller RH. Pediatric sinusitis. The role of endoscopic sinus surgery in cystic fibrosis and other forms of sinonasal disease. Arch Otolaryngol Head Neck Surg. 1991; 117(4):422–426

[14] Ramsey B, Richardson MA. Impact of sinusitis in cystic fibrosis. J Allergy Clin Immunol. 1992; 90(3, Pt 2):547–552

[15] Illing EA, Woodworth BA. Management of the upper airway in cystic fibrosis. Curr Opin Pulm Med. 2014; 20(6):623–631

[16] Mitchell GW, Woodworth BK, Taylor PD, Norris DR. Automated telemetry reveals age specific differences in flight duration and speed are driven by wind conditions in a migratory songbird. Mov Ecol. 2015; 3(1):19

[17] Holzmann D, Speich R, Kaufmann T, et al. Effects of sinus surgery in patients with cystic fibrosis after lung transplantation: a 10-year experience. Transplantation. 2004; 77(1):134–136

[18] Macdonald KI, Gipsman A, Magit A, et al. Endoscopic sinus surgery in patients with cystic fibrosis: a systematic review and meta-analysis of pulmonary function. Rhinology. 2012; 50(4):360–369

[19] Alanin MC, Aanaes K, Høiby N, et al. Sinus surgery postpones chronic gram-negative lung infection: cohort study of 106 patients with cystic fibrosis. Rhinology. 2016; 54(3):206–213

[20] Regnis JA, Robinson M, Bailey DL, et al. Mucociliary clearance in patients with cystic fibrosis and in normal subjects. Am J Respir Crit Care Med. 1994; 150(1):66–71

[21] Zhang S, Blount AC, McNicholas CM, et al. Resveratrol enhances airway surface liquid depth in sinonasal epithelium by increasing cystic fibrosis transmembrane conductance regulator open probability. PLoS One. 2013; 8(11):e81589

[22] Lazrak A, Jurkuvenaite A, Ness EC, et al. Inter-α-inhibitor blocks epithelial sodium channel activation and decreases nasal potential differences in ΔF508 mice. Am J Respir Cell Mol Biol. 2014; 50(5):953–962

[23] Conger BT, Zhang S, Skinner D, et al. Comparison of cystic fibrosis transmembrane conductance regulator (CFTR) and ciliary beat frequency activation by the CFTR Modulators Genistein, VRT-532, and UCCF-152 in primary sinonasal epithelial cultures. JAMA Otolaryngol Head Neck Surg. 2013; 139(8):822–827

[24] Blount A, Zhang S, Chestnut M, et al. Transepithelial ion transport is suppressed in hypoxic sinonasal epithelium. Laryngoscope. 2011; 121(9):1929–1934

[25] Mainz JG, Koitschev A. Pathogenesis and management of nasal polyposis in cystic fibrosis. Curr Allergy Asthma Rep. 2012; 12(2):163–174

[26] Cimmino M, Nardone M, Cavaliere M, et al. Dornase alfa as postoperative therapy in cystic fibrosis sinonasal disease. Arch Otolaryngol Head Neck Surg. 2005; 131(12):1097–1101

[27] Feuillet-Fieux MN, Lenoir G, Sermet I, et al. Nasal polyposis and cystic fibrosis(CF): review of the literature. Rhinology. 2011; 49(3):347–355

[28] Ryan MW. Diseases associated with chronic rhinosinusitis: what is the significance? Curr Opin Otolaryngol Head Neck Surg. 2008; 16(3):231–236

[29] Schraven SP, Wehrmann M, Wagner W, Blumenstock G, Koitschev A. Prevalence and histopathology of chronic polypoid sinusitis in pediatric patients with cystic fibrosis. J Cyst Fibros. 2011; 10(3):181–186

[30] Orlandi RR, Kingdom TT, Hwang PH, et al. International consensus statement on allergy and rhinology: rhinosinusitis. Int Forum Allergy Rhinol. 2016; 6 Suppl 1:S22–S209

[31] Fokkens WJ, Lund VJ, Mullol J, et al. EPOS 2012: European position paper on rhinosinusitis and nasal polyps 2012. A summary for otorhinolaryngologists. Rhinology. 2012; 50(1):1–12

[32] Aanaes K, Johansen HK, Skov M, et al. Clinical effects of sinus surgery and adjuvant therapy in cystic fibrosis patients: can chronic lung infections be postponed? Rhinology. 2013; 51(3):222–230

[33] Hamilos DL. Chronic rhinosinusitis in patients with cystic fibrosis. J Allergy Clin Immunol Pract. 2016; 4(4):605–612

[34] Orlandi RR, Wiggins RH, III. Radiological sinonasal findings in adults with cystic fibrosis. Am J Rhinol Allergy. 2009; 23(3):307–311

[35] Wang X, Kim J, McWilliams R, Cutting GR. Increased prevalence of chronic rhinosinusitis in carriers of a cystic fibrosis mutation. Arch Otolaryngol Head Neck Surg. 2005; 131(3):237–240

[36] Nishioka GJ, Cook PR, McKinsey JP, Rodriguez FJ. Paranasal sinus computed tomography scan findings in patients with cystic fibrosis. Otolaryngol Head Neck Surg. 1996; 114(3):394–399

[37] Nishioka GJ, Cook PR. Paranasal sinus disease in patients with cystic fibrosis. Otolaryngol Clin North Am. 1996; 29(1):193–205

[38] Eggesbø HB, Eken T, Eiklid K, Kolmannskog F. Hypoplasia of the sphenoid sinuses as a diagnostic tool in cystic fibrosis. Acta Radiol. 1999; 40(5):479–485

[39] Eggesbø HB, Søvik S, Dølvik S, Eiklid K, Kolmannskog F. CT characterization of developmental variations of the paranasal sinuses in cystic fibrosis. Acta Radiol. 2001; 42(5):482–493

[40] Seifert CM, Harvey RJ, Mathews JW, et al. Temporal bone pneumatization and its relationship to paranasal sinus development in cystic fibrosis. Rhinology. 2010; 48(2):233–238

[41] Chang EH, Pezzulo AA, Meyerholz DK, et al. Sinus hypoplasia precedes sinus infection in a porcine model of cystic fibrosis. Laryngoscope. 2012; 122(9):1898–1905

[42] Hamilos DL. Chronic rhinosinusitis: epidemiology and medical management. J Allergy Clin Immunol. 2011; 128(4):693–707, quiz 708–709

[43] Kang SH, Piltcher OB, Dalcin PdeT. Sinonasal alterations in computed tomography scans in cystic fibrosis: a literature review of observational studies. Int Forum Allergy Rhinol. 2014; 4(3):223–231

[44] Kim HJ, Friedman EM, Sulek M, Duncan NO, McCluggage C. Paranasal sinus development in chronic sinusitis, cystic fibrosis, and normal comparison population: a computerized tomography correlation study. Am J Rhinol. 1997; 11(4):275–281

[45] O'Connell OJ, McWilliams S, McGarrigle A, et al. Radiologic imaging in cystic fibrosis: cumulative effective dose and changing trends over 2 decades. Chest. 2012; 141(6):1575–1583

[46] Frush DP, Donnelly LF, Rosen NS. Computed tomography and radiation risks: what pediatric health care providers should know. Pediatrics. 2003; 112(4):951–957

[47] Mainz JG, Koitschev A. Management of chronic rhinosinusitis in CF. J Cyst Fibros. 2009; 8 Suppl 1:S10–S14

[48] Harvey R, Hannan SA, Badia L, Scadding G. Nasal saline irrigations for the symptoms of chronic rhinosinusitis. Cochrane Database Syst Rev. 2007(3):CD006394

[49] Elkins MR, Robinson M, Rose BR, et al. National Hypertonic Saline in Cystic Fibrosis (NHSCF) Study Group. A controlled trial of long-term inhaled hypertonic saline in patients with cystic fibrosis. N Engl J Med. 2006; 354(3):229–240

[50] Harvey RJ, Goddard JC, Wise SK, Schlosser RJ. Effects of endoscopic sinus surgery and delivery device on cadaver sinus irrigation. Otolaryngol Head Neck Surg. 2008; 139(1):137–142

[51] Mainz JG, Schumacher U, Schädlich K, et al. Cooperators. Sino nasal inhalation of isotonic versus hypertonic saline (6.0%) in CF patients with chronic rhinosinusitis: results of a multicenter, prospective, randomized, double-blind, controlled trial. J Cyst Fibros. 2016; 15(6):e57–e66

[52] Wark P, McDonald VM. Nebulised hypertonic saline for cystic fibrosis. Cochrane Database Syst Rev. 2009(2):CD001506

[53] Donaldson SH, Bennett WD, Zeman KL, Knowles MR, Tarran R, Boucher RC. Mucus clearance and lung function in cystic fibrosis with hypertonic saline. N Engl J Med. 2006; 354(3):241–250

[54] Fokkens W, Lund V, Mullol J, European Position Paper on Rhinosinusitis and Nasal Polyps group. European position paper on rhinosinusitis and nasal polyps 2007. Rhinol Suppl. 2007; 20(20):1–136

[55] Hadfield PJ, Rowe-Jones JM, Mackay IS. The prevalence of nasal polyps in adults with cystic fibrosis. Clin Otolaryngol Allied Sci. 2000; 25(1):19–22

[56] Mainz JG, Schiller I, Ritschel C, et al. Sinonasal inhalation of dornase alfa in CF: a double-blind placebo-controlled cross-over pilot trial. Auris Nasus Larynx. 2011; 38(2):220–227

[57] Martinez-Devesa P, Patiar S. Oral steroids for nasal polyps. Cochrane Database Syst Rev. 2011(7):CD005232

[58] Davidson TM, Murphy C, Mitchell M, Smith C, Light M. Management of chronic sinusitis in cystic fibrosis. Laryngoscope. 1995; 105(4, Pt 1):354–358

[59] Mainz JG, Schädlich K, Schien C, et al. Sinonasal inhalation of tobramycin vibrating aerosol in cystic fibrosis patients with upper airway Pseudomonas aeruginosa colonization: results of a randomized, double-blind, placebo-controlled pilot study. Drug Des Devel Ther. 2014; 8:209–217

[60] Graham SM, Launspach JL, Welsh MJ, Zabner J. Sequential magnetic resonance imaging analysis of the maxillary sinuses: implications for a model of gene therapy in cystic fibrosis. J Laryngol Otol. 1999; 113(4):329–335

[61] Desrosiers MY, Salas-Prato M. Treatment of chronic rhinosinusitis refractory to other treatments with topical antibiotic therapy delivered by means of a large-particle nebulizer: results of a controlled trial. Otolaryngol Head Neck Surg. 2001; 125(3):265–269

[62] Videler WJ, van Drunen CM, Reitsma JB, Fokkens WJ. Nebulized bacitracin/colimycin: a treatment option in recalcitrant chronic rhinosinusitis with Staphylococcus aureus? A double-blind, randomized, placebo-controlled, cross-over pilot study. Rhinology. 2008; 46 (2):92–98

[63] Jaffé A, Francis J, Rosenthal M, Bush A. Long-term azithromycin may improve lung function in children with cystic fibrosis. Lancet. 1998; 351(9100):420

[64] Majima Y. Clinical implications of the immunomodulatory effects of macrolides on sinusitis. Am J Med. 2004; 117 Suppl 9A:20S–25S

[65] Lindig J, Steger C, Beiersdorf N, et al. Smell in cystic fibrosis. Eur Arch Otorhinolaryngol. 2013; 270(3):915–921

[66] Fuchs HJ, Borowitz DS, Christiansen DH, et al. The Pulmozyme Study Group. Effect of aerosolized recombinant human DNase on exacerbations of respiratory symptoms and on pulmonary function in patients with cystic fibrosis. N Engl J Med. 1994; 331(10):637–642

[67] Shah PL, Conway S, Scott SF, et al. A case-controlled study with dornase alfa to evaluate impact on disease progression over a 4-year period. Respiration. 2001; 68(2):160–164

[68] Konstan MW. Dornase alfa and progression of lung disease in cystic fibrosis. Pediatr Pulmonol. 2008; 43:S24–S28

[69] Jones AP, Wallis C. Dornase alfa for cystic fibrosis. Cochrane Database Syst Rev. 2010; 3(3):CD001127

[70] Quan JM, Tiddens HA, Sy JP, et al. Pulmozyme Early Intervention Trial Study Group. A two-year randomized, placebo-controlled trial of dornase alfa in young patients with cystic fibrosis with mild lung function abnormalities. J Pediatr. 2001; 139(6):813–820

[71] Harms HK, Matouk E, Tournier G, et al. Multicenter, open-label study of recombinant human DNase in cystic fibrosis patients with moderate lung disease. DNase International Study Group. Pediatr Pulmonol. 1998; 26(3):155–161

[72] Mainz JG, Schien C, Schiller I, et al. Sinonasal inhalation of dornase alfa administered by vibrating aerosol to cystic fibrosis patients: a double-blind placebo-controlled cross-over trial. J Cyst Fibros. 2014; 13(4):461–470

[73] Accurso FJ, Rowe SM, Clancy JP, et al. Effect of VX-770 in persons with cystic fibrosis and the G551D-CFTR mutation. N Engl J Med. 2010; 363(21):1991–2003

[74] Deeks ED. Lumacaftor/ivacaftor: a review in cystic fibrosis. Drugs. 2016; 76(12):1191–1201

[75] Woodworth BA, Chandra RK, Hoy MJ, Lee FS, Schlosser RJ, Gillespie MB. Randomized controlled trial of hyaluronic acid/carboxymethylcellulose dressing after endoscopic sinus surgery. ORL J Otorhinolaryngol Relat Spec. 2010; 72(2):101–105

[76] Kaiser J. Personalized medicine. New cystic fibrosis drug offers hope, at a price. Science. 2012; 335(6069):645

[77] Bosch B, De Boeck K. Searching for a cure for cystic fibrosis. A 25-year quest in a nutshell. Eur J Pediatr. 2016; 175(1):1–8

[78] Deeks ED. Ivacaftor: a review of its use in patients with cystic fibrosis. Drugs. 2013; 73(14):1595–1604

[79] Sawicki GS, McKone EF, Pasta DJ, et al. Sustained benefit from ivacaftor demonstrated by combining clinical trial and cystic fibrosis patient registry data. Am J Respir Crit Care Med. 2015; 192(7):836–842

[80] Dilokthornsakul P, Hansen RN, Campbell JD. Forecasting US ivacaftor outcomes and cost in cystic fibrosis patients with the G551D mutation. Eur Respir J. 2016; 47(6):1697–1705

[81] Chang EH, Tang XX, Shah VS, et al. Medical reversal of chronic sinusitis in a cystic fibrosis patient with ivacaftor. Int Forum Allergy Rhinol. 2015; 5(2):178–181

[82] Castellani C, Cuppens H, Macek M, Jr, et al. Consensus on the use and interpretation of cystic fibrosis mutation analysis in clinical practice. J Cyst Fibros. 2008; 7(3):179–196

[83] Woodworth BA, Joseph K, Kaplan AP, Schlosser RJ. Alterations in eotaxin, monocyte chemoattractant protein-4, interleukin-5, and interleukin-13 after systemic steroid treatment for nasal polyps. Otolaryngol Head Neck Surg. 2004; 131(5):585–589

[84] Aanaes K, Rasmussen N, Pressler T, et al. Extensive endoscopic image-guided sinus surgery decreases BPI-ANCA in patients with cystic fibrosis. Scand J Immunol. 2012; 76(6):573–579

[85] Mainz JG, Naehrlich MSL, Kading M, et al. Prevalence of CF-related chronic rhinosinusitis–results from a multicentre interdisciplinary study. J Cyst Fibros. 2010; 9(1):118

[86] Khalid AN, Mace J, Smith TL. Outcomes of sinus surgery in adults with cystic fibrosis. Otolaryngol Head Neck Surg. 2009; 141(3):358–363

[87] Soler ZM, Smith TL. Quality of life outcomes after functional endoscopic sinus surgery. Otolaryngol Clin North Am. 2010; 43(3):605–612, x

[88] Smith TL, Mendolia-Loffredo S, Loehrl TA, Sparapani R, Laud PW, Nattinger AB. Predictive factors and outcomes in endoscopic sinus surgery for chronic rhinosinusitis. Laryngoscope. 2005; 115 (12):2199–2205

[89] Bhattacharyya N. Symptom outcomes after endoscopic sinus surgery for chronic rhinosinusitis. Arch Otolaryngol Head Neck Surg. 2004; 130(3):329–333

[90] Mace JC, Michael YL, Carlson NE, Litvack JR, Smith TL. Correlations between endoscopy score and quality of life changes after sinus surgery. Arch Otolaryngol Head Neck Surg. 2010; 136(4):340–346

[91] Poetker DM, Mendolia-Loffredo S, Smith TL. Outcomes of endoscopic sinus surgery for chronic rhinosinusitis associated with sinonasal polyposis. Am J Rhinol. 2007; 21(1):84–88

[92] Gross WE, Gross CW, Becker D, Moore D, Phillips D. Modified transnasal endoscopic Lothrop procedure as an alternative to frontal sinus obliteration. Otolaryngol Head Neck Surg. 1995; 113(4):427–434

[93] Naidoo Y, Wen D, Bassiouni A, Keen M, Wormald PJ. Long-term results after primary frontal sinus surgery. Int Forum Allergy Rhinol. 2012; 2(3):185–190

[94] Virgin FW, Rowe SM, Wade MB, et al. Extensive surgical and comprehensive postoperative medical management for cystic fibrosis chronic rhinosinusitis. Am J Rhinol Allergy. 2012; 26(1):70–75

[95] Chan Y, Melroy CT, Kuhn CA, Kuhn FL, Daniel WT, Kuhn FA. Long-term frontal sinus patency after endoscopic frontal sinusotomy. Laryngoscope. 2009; 119(6):1229–1232

[96] Ramakrishnan Y, Carrie HVS. Frontal sinus surgery approaches: an evolution. Otorhinolaryngol.. 2015; 8(3):147–153

[97] Tran KN, Beule AG, Singal D, Wormald PJ. Frontal ostium restenosis after the endoscopic modified Lothrop procedure. Laryngoscope. 2007; 117(8):1457–1462

[98] Naidoo Y, Bassiouni A, Keen M, Wormald PJ. Risk factors and outcomes for primary, revision, and modified Lothrop (Draf III) frontal sinus surgery. Int Forum Allergy Rhinol. 2013; 3(5):412–417

[99] Huang Z, Hajjij A, Li G, Nayak JV, Zhou B, Hwang PH. Clinical predictors of neo-osteogenesis in patients with chronic rhinosinusitis. Int Forum Allergy Rhinol. 2015; 5(4):303–309

[100] Draf W, Weber R, Keerl R, Constantinidis J. Current aspects of frontal sinus surgery. I: endonasal frontal sinus drainage in inflammatory diseases of the paranasal sinuses. HNO. 1995; 43(6):352–357

[101] Draf W. Endonasal micro-endoscopic frontal sinus surgery: the Fulda concept. Oper Tech Otolaryngol Head Neck Surg. 1991; 2:234–240

[102] Wormald PJ. Salvage frontal sinus surgery: the endoscopic modified Lothrop procedure. Laryngoscope. 2003; 113(2):276–283

[103] Naidoo Y, Bassiouni A, Keen M, Wormald PJ. Long-term outcomes for the endoscopic modified Lothrop/Draf III procedure: a 10-year review. Laryngoscope. 2014; 124(1):43–49

[104] Wormald PJ, McDonogh M. "Bath-plug" technique for the endoscopic management of cerebrospinal fluid leaks. J Laryngol Otol. 1997; 111(11):1042–1046

[105] Harvey RJ, Debnath N, Srubiski A, Bleier B, Schlosser RJ. Fluid residuals and drug exposure in nasal irrigation. Otolaryngol Head Neck Surg. 2009; 141(6):757–761

[106] Snidvongs K, Kalish L, Sacks R, Craig JC, Harvey RJ. Topical steroid for chronic rhinosinusitis without polyps. Cochrane Database Syst Rev. 2011(8):CD009274

[107] Kalish L, Snidvongs K, Sivasubramaniam R, Cope D, Harvey RJ. Topical steroids for nasal polyps. Cochrane Database Syst Rev. 2012(12): CD006549

[108] Chin D, Snidvongs K, Kalish L, Sacks R, Harvey RJ. The outside-in approach to the modified endoscopic Lothrop procedure. Laryngoscope. 2012; 122(8):1661–1669

[109] Illing EA, Cho Y, Riley KO, Woodworth BA. Draf III mucosal graft technique: long-term results. Int Forum Allergy Rhinol. 2016; 6 (5):514–517

[110] Conger BT, Jr, Riley K, Woodworth BA. The Draf III mucosal grafting technique: a prospective study. Otolaryngol Head Neck Surg. 2012; 146(4):664–668

[111] Taylor-Cousar JL, Munck A, McKone EF, van der Ent CK, Moeller A, Simard C, Wang LT, Ingenito EP, McKee C, Lu Y, Lekstrom-Himes J, Elborn JS.N Engl J Med. 2017 Nov 23;377(21):2013–2023

[112] Middleton PG, Mall MA, Dřevínek P, Lands LC, McKone EF, Polineni D, Ramsey BW, Taylor-Cousar JL, Tullis E, Vermeulen F, Marigowda G, McKee CM, Moskowitz SM, Nair N, Savage J, Simard C, Tian S, Waltz D, Xuan F, Rowe SM, Jain R; VX17-445-102 Study Group. N Engl J Med. 2019 Nov 7;381(19):1809–1819

[113] Int Forum Allergy Rhinol. 2019 Mar;9(3):292–297

23 Pneumosinus Dilatans

Ing Ping Tang, Yves Brand, and Prepageran Narayanan

Abstract

Pneumosinus dilatans (PD) of the frontal sinus is a very rare craniofacial malformation. Less than 150 cases were reported in the literature since 1955. Meyes was the first person to describe this condition in 1898 and later Benjamin renamed it PD in 1918. Urken et al categorized this rare entity into three groups with distinct definitions (hypersinus, PD, and pneumocele) in 1987. The nomenclature and pathophysiology of this rare entity are a continuous controversy as the exact etiology and pathogenesis of the condition still remain unknown. Patients with this condition may be asymptomatic or they can present with cosmetic deformity and nasal, eye, or neurological symptoms. A significant percentage of patients with this condition may have an associated lesion, especially intracranial pathology. Radiological investigations with computed tomography scan and magnetic resonance imaging are crucial to confirm the diagnosis and assess the extent of the disease or any associated lesions. PD can be treated conservatively or surgically, depending on the clinical presentation of the disease. A thorough clinical evaluation is needed to plan for the treatment.

Keywords: pneumosinus dilatans, pneumocele, hypersinus

23.1 Introduction

Pneumosinus dilatans (PD) of the frontal sinus is a very rare condition with less than 150 reported cases in the literature since 1955.[1] The true incidence of this disease is unknown. It is a craniofacial malformation, first described by Meyes in 1898; the term PD was first introduced by Benjamin in 1918.[2] Since then, there have been many reports on the spectrum of clinical presentation. However, there is a continuous controversy on the nomenclature and pathophysiology of this rare entity.[3] Only in 1987, Urken et al categorized this rare entity into three groups with distinct definitions: hypersinus, PD, and pneumocele.[4,5] Hypersinus is defined as an enlarged, aerated frontal sinus with normal walls and without extension beyond the normal boundaries of the frontal bone. PD is defined as an enlarged, aerated frontal sinus with intact sinus walls and extension beyond the normal boundaries of the frontal bone. Pneumocele is defined as focal or generalized thinning of the bony sinus walls and loss of integrity of part of the wall.[5] Frontal sinuses are the most frequently involved paranasal sinuses, followed by sphenoid, maxillary, and ethmoidal sinuses.[6]

23.2 Epidemiology and Etiology

The exact etiology and pathogenesis of the condition still remain unknown. However, several hypotheses have been proposed regarding the possible mechanisms and/or pathogenesis of PD. The proposed pathogenesis consists of the following: (1) the presence of a one-way valve at the frontal recess, (2) spontaneous drainage of a mucocele, (3) hormonal dysregulation, (4) local growth disturbances, (5) trauma, and (6) osteoclastic and osteoblastic activity.[1,7] The ball–valve effect with entrapment of air in affected frontal sinuses under conditions of positive pressure and limited air escape secondary to outflow tract obstruction appears to be the most likely etiology among all.

23.3 Clinical Presentation and Investigations

The usual age of the presentation of PD is between 20 and 40 years with a male predominance. Most of them are asymptomatic or may present with cosmetic deformity with frontal bossing, facial pain, headache, and nasal and eye symptoms.[1,8] Cosmetic deformity is the most common symptom.[6] This condition has also been associated with intracranial tumors, for example, meningioma and arachnoid cyst, orbital tumors, fibrous dysplasia, and bony hyperostosis of the craniofacial skeleton.[2,6,9,10,11] Desai et al reported that 50% of PD patients had an associated condition.[6]

23.4 Diagnosis

The diagnosis of PD can be an incidental finding on imaging studies for an unrelated issue or for the patient's complaints. As the knowledge of this condition is limited, this often leads to incomplete clinical evaluations and inconsistent referral patterns for these patients. Nevertheless, based on the meta-analysis reported by Desai et al,[6] the number of PD cases reported per year is increasing, most likely due to increased availability of imaging services as well as a growing awareness of cosmetic medicine.

A systematic and thorough examination is required whenever PD is suspected. This should include ENT (ear, nose, and throat), eye, and neurological and endocrinological examinations. Computed tomography (CT) scan and magnetic resonance imaging (MRI) are needed to confirm the diagnosis and to assess the extent of the disease and any associated conditions (▶ Fig. 23.1). Literature reviews suggest that an initial plain X-ray should be carried out. With the unusual findings on the initial X-ray

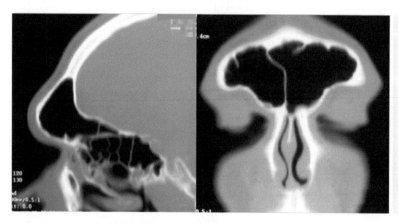

Fig. 23.1 Coronal and sagittal CT scans shows pneumosinus dilatans of frontal sinus.[18]

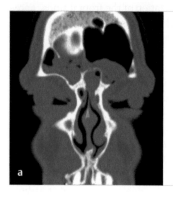
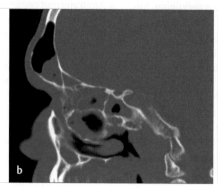

Fig. 23.2 (a, b) Coronal and sagittal scans shows another case of pneumosinus dilatans of frontal sinus with nasofrontal duct obstruction. This case was operated via a Draf IIa approach with subsequent arrest of further expansion. (These images are provided courtesy of C. Georgalas.)

studies, more definite imaging studies such as CT scan and MRI can be considered.[6,12,13]

23.5 Management

The treatment of PD of frontal sinus can be divided into conservative management and surgery.[1] An abnormal expansion of frontal sinus without focal thinning of the wall, without nasofrontal duct obstruction, and without obvious cosmetic deformity can be managed conservatively. Surgical treatment is offered to a patient with PD of frontal sinus if there is nasofrontal duct obstruction with or without cosmetic deformity. Nasofrontal duct obstruction can be relieved via endoscopic surgery (▶ Fig. 23.2). However, open procedure is the only choice to correct cosmetic bony deformity.

Different surgical techniques have been described in the literature to improve cosmesis. Wolfe described his treatment method of burring down the frontal bossing and a forehead lift.[14] Komuro et al removed the outer table of the frontal sinus and drilled the lateral portions of supraorbital rim as well as removed the anterior wall mucosa.[15] Nahabedian et al divided the excised portion of the frontal bone and contoured the frontal bone and fixed with mircoplates.[16] Rehman et al removed the anterior wall of the frontal sinus. The bone was then wrapped in gauze, flattened with a mallet, overlaid, and fixed in position using absorbable sutures.[17] The main aim of these

craniofacial approaches using osteotomies with or without autologous bone is to restore the normal appearance of the forehead especially at the supraorbital rim and the glabellar area.[18]

23.6 Complications

The complications of this rare condition depend on the clinical presentations of the disease. Most of the complications are due to the compression of the surrounding structures by the dilated frontal sinuses. Nasolacrimal duct obstruction and headache are common complications of the dilated frontal sinuses. As this condition may be associated with intracranial lesions, orbital tumors, fibrous dysplasia, and bony hyperostosis of the craniofacial skeleton,[2,6,9,10,11] the complications due to other associated lesions will be higher depending on the structures being compressed.

23.7 Conclusion

PD of the frontal sinus is a very rare condition. It can be asymptomatic or patients can present with cosmetic deformity, and nasal, eye, or neurological symptoms. A significant percentage of patients with this condition may have an associated lesion, especially intracranial pathology. An appropriate clinical evaluation should be carried out when this condition is suspected. The treatment depends on either the obstruction of nasofrontal duct or cosmetic deformity of the frontal bone.

References

[1] Patel AC, Hammoudeh JA, Urata MM. Pneumosinus dilatans: a rare cause of frontal sinus expansion: case report and review of literature. J Oral Maxillofac Surg. 2008; 66(11):2380–2386

[2] Appelt EA, Wilhelmi BJ, Warder DE, Blackwell SJ. A rare case of pneumosinus dilatans of the frontal sinus and review of the literature. Ann Plast Surg. 1999; 43(6):653–656

[3] Tabaee A, Kamat A, Shrivastava R, Buchbinder D. Surgical management of pneumosinus dilatans frontalis in the setting of chronic rhinosinusitis and type III frontal Cell. J Craniofac Surg. 2012; 23 (1):158–160

[4] Walker JL, Jones NS. Pneumosinus dilatans of the frontal sinuses: two cases and a discussion of its aetiology. J Laryngol Otol. 2002; 116 (5):382–385

[5] Urken ML, Som PM, Lawson W, Edelstein D, Weber AL, Biller HF. Abnormally large frontal sinus. II. Nomenclature, pathology, and symptoms. Laryngoscope. 1987; 97(5):606–611

[6] Desai NS, Saboo SS, Khandelwal A, Ricci JA. Pneumosinus dilatans: is it more than an aesthetic concern? J Craniofac Surg. 2014; 25 (2):418–421

[7] Breidahl AF, Szwajkun P, Chen YR. Pneumosinus dilatans of the maxillary sinus: a report of two cases. Br J Plast Surg. 1997; 50(1):33–39

[8] Stretch JR, Poole MD. Pneumosinus dilatans as the aetiology of progressive bilateral blindness. Br J Plast Surg. 1992; 45(6):469–473

[9] Dhillon RS, Williams DC. Pneumosinus dilatans. J Laryngol Otol. 1987; 101(8):828–832

[10] Tellado MG, Méndez R, López-Cedrún JL, et al. Pneumosinus dilatans of the frontal and ethmoidal sinuses: case report. J Craniomaxillofac Surg. 2002; 30(1):62–64

[11] Miller NR, Golnik KC, Zeidman SM, North RB. Pneumosinus dilatans: a sign of intracranial meningioma. Surg Neurol. 1996; 46(5):471–474

[12] Pospisil OA, Balmer MC. Pneumosinus dilatans. Br J Oral Maxillofac Surg. 1988; 26(5):375–380

[13] Suryanarayanan R, Abbott G. Pneumosinus dilatans: demonstrated by sinus expansion on serial sinus X-rays with discussion of possible aetiology. J Laryngol Otol. 2007; 121(1):96–99

[14] Wolfe SA. Correction of the "Simian" forehead deformity. Aesthetic Plast Surg. 1978; 2(1):373–374

[15] Komuro Y, Nishida M, Imazawa T, Koga Y, Yanai A. Combined frontal bone reshaping and forehead lift for frontal sinus hypertrophy. Aesthetic Plast Surg. 1999; 23(5):361–363

[16] Nahabedian MY, Al-Shunnar B, Manson PN. Correction of frontal bone hypertrophy with setback osteotomy and hydroxyapatite cement. Ann Plast Surg. 2000; 44(5):567–572

[17] Rehman KU, Johnston C, Monaghan A, Dover S. Management of the giant frontal sinus: a simple method to improve cosmesis. Br J Oral Maxillofac Surg. 2009; 47(1):54–55

[18] Galiè M, Consorti G, Clauser LC, Kawamoto HK. Craniofacial surgical strategies for the correction of pneumosinus dilatans frontalis. J Craniomaxillofac Surg. 2013; 41(1):28–33

24 Frontal Sinusitis in Chronic Rhinosinusitis without Nasal Polyposis

Kristine A. Smith, Jeremiah A. Alt, and Richard R. Orlandi

Abstract

The frontal sinus is one of the most difficult sinuses to manage in chronic rhinosinusitis without nasal polyposis (CRSsNP). Its anatomic location, proximity to vital structures, and varied anatomy make it challenging to deliver medical therapy and perform safe and successful endoscopic sinus surgery (ESS). The objective of this chapter is to review the epidemiology, pathophysiology, and management of the frontal sinus in CRSsNP. Understanding the etiology of the issues unique to this population is important to allow clinicians to utilize the most appropriate medical and surgical strategies. Initial and continued medical therapy is essential for long-term control. Delivery of medications to the frontal recess is limited in unoperated sinuses and is improved following ESS. Identifying the cause of frontal recess obstruction is important to aid clinicians in deciding the optimal extent of surgery to perform. While ESS is technically challenging in this area and is associated with the highest rates of stenosis, the majority of patients experience improved quality of life and long-term frontal recess patency.

Keywords: chronic rhinosinusitis, sinusitis, frontal, medical therapy, endoscopic sinus surgery, chronic rhinosinusitis without nasal polyposis

24.1 Introduction

The frontal sinus is the most complex sinus to manage in patients with chronic rhinosinusitis (CRS). Medication delivery to the frontal recess can be difficult due to its anterosuperior position as well as the labyrinth of frontal cells, which may partially or completely obstruct the frontal recess. In addition, endoscopic sinus surgery (ESS) involving the frontal recess is challenging due to its highly varied anatomy, narrow confines, and the close proximity of several vital structures including the orbit and the skull base. The frontal sinus also has the highest rate of postoperative stenosis relative to the other sinuses. Successful outcomes require meticulous technique, patience, and experience. In chronic rhinosinusitis without nasal polyposis (CRSsNP), frontal sinusitis is primarily associated with obstructed drainage through the frontal recess, the drainage pathway of the frontal sinus. Medical therapy is an essential component of the initial management of frontal sinusitis as well as maintenance strategies to prevent recurrence. ESS also plays an important role in relieving obstruction and facilitating the delivery of topical medications.

A thorough understanding of the anatomy of the frontal recess and the factors affecting the pathogenesis of CRS is essential to aid clinicians in managing frontal sinusitis in CRSsNP. The objective of this chapter is to review the epidemiology, pathophysiology, and management of the frontal sinus in CRSsNP.

24.2 Epidemiology

CRS affects 5 to 15% of the general population and CRSsNP comprises the majority of patients with CRS.[1,2] Frontal sinusitis in CRSsNP can be divided into primary (i.e., unoperated sinuses) or persistent (i.e., recurrent or iatrogenic following ESS). However, the incidence and prevalence of frontal sinusitis in CRSsNP have not been clearly defined. None of the literature examining the prevalence of specific sinus disease has distinguished between CRS with nasal polyposis (CRSwNP) and CRSsNP. Another barrier to determining the epidemiology of frontal sinusitis in CRSsNP is the important difference between radiological evidence of inflammation and clinical symptoms. Radiological findings do not correlate with clinical symptoms in CRSsNP, which makes it challenging to objectively quantify the incidence and prevalence of frontal sinusitis.

Some studies have examined the prevalence of radiological frontal sinus inflammation in CRS. A computed tomography (CT) anatomic study of all CRS patients found approximately 40% had radiological evidence of primary frontal sinusitis, with partial or complete opacification of the frontal sinus.[3] Other studies have examined the prevalence of frontal sinusitis in patients undergoing ESS for CRS. One suggests that over 70% of patients undergoing ESS have radiological evidence of frontal sinus involvement and another found that approximately 90% of surgical patients undergo some form of frontal sinusotomy.[4,5] These studies were examining a subset of CRS patients who elected ESS and may not represent the general cohort of CRS patients. These studies did not examine the correlation between radiological findings and clinical symptoms or severity. Further investigations are required to define the prevalence of primary frontal sinusitis associated with CRSsNP.

Persistent frontal sinusitis following ESS is not uncommon (▶ Fig. 24.1). Reported rates of recurrent frontal sinusitis vary significantly, which may be related to how persistent frontal sinusitis is defined. Many studies discuss frontal recess patency rates as the primary outcome determining operative success, which can range from 27 to 92%.[6] These patency rates often reflect the endoscopic appearance of the frontal recess and are not correlated

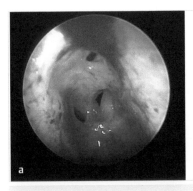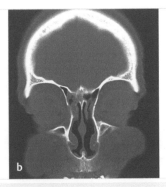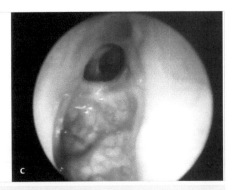

Fig. 24.1 Preoperative **(a)** endoscopic and **(b)** radiological images of persistent frontal sinusitis following ethmoidectomy. **(c)** Postoperative image following endoscopic frontal sinusotomy.

with recurrent symptoms or radiological findings.[6] Patients with stenosis are more likely to have persistent symptoms.[7] However, approximately 20% of patients with stenosis will be asymptomatic.[7]

As the length of follow-up increases, the rate of persistent frontal sinusitis also increases; approximately 30% of patients will have persistent frontal sinusitis 5 to 10 years after ESS, defined by recurrent sinonasal symptoms requiring surgical intervention.[8,9] Of note, rates of persistent frontal sinusitis following ESS have decreased over the last 10 years, with the majority of studies reporting success rates in the mid-80%.[6] This may be secondary to improved surgical techniques and the availability of mucosal sparing cutting instruments. One of the major limitations of these studies is that they do not differentiate between CRSsNP and CRSwNP.[6] In addition, success rates often reflect endoscopic ostium patency rather than symptomatic improvement.[6] Further studies with longer (5–10 years) durations of follow-up and symptomatic correlation would be helpful in determining the rate of persistent frontal sinusitis in CRSsNP.[10,11]

24.3 Pathophysiology

CRS has been well defined as an inflammatory condition of the sinonasal mucosal and much of the pathophysiology is linked to the consequences of this inflammation, such as impaired mucociliary clearance and impaired sinus drainage.[12] The cause of this inflammation varies and as such CRSsNP has a large number of potential etiologies.[12] Factors that specifically affect the frontal sinus will be discussed. These factors may contribute to the development of frontal sinusitis or to failure of medical or surgical therapy leading to persistent inflammation and obstruction.

24.3.1 Anatomic Factors

Frontoethmoidal Cells

One of the most commonly stated risk factors for developing frontal sinusitis is impaired outflow through the frontal recess. The frontal recess may be obstructed by a variety of frontoethmoidal cells such as the agger nasi, frontal cells, intersinus septal cells, and supraorbital cells.[12] It is important to note that these cells may be present in patients with no evidence of CRS.[13] Available evidence is conflicting; some studies have suggested that frontoethmoidal cells may not be associated with the presence or severity of inflammation in the paranasal sinuses, while others report an association.[4,14,15,16] This suggests that while anatomic factors may play a role, other factors such as the sinonasal inflammation underlying CRS are required to develop obstruction. Of note, Wormald et al. recently proposed a new classification system for frontoethmoidal cells (the International Frontal Sinus Anatomy Classification).[17] This system classifies cells based on their anatomic location and functional implication to the drainage of the frontal recess.[17] Incorporating a functional component into the classification may provide more insight into whether certain cells are associated with frontal sinusitis. The correlation between this classification scheme and frontal sinusitis has not yet been defined.

Osteomeatal Complex

Outflow from the frontal recess may also be obstructed distally. The osteomeatal complex may be obstructed by a variety of factors, which causes anterior ethmoid sinusitis. This can lead to obstruction of the proximal drainage of the frontal recess resulting in frontal sinusitis.[12] The attachment of the uncinate process also impacts the route of drainage from the frontal sinus. In the majority of cases, the uncinate process attaches to the lamina papyracea and the frontal recess drains directly into the middle meatus. When the uncinate process attaches to the skull base or the middle turbinate, the frontal recess drains into the ethmoid infundibulum. Identifying the location of the obstruction and the anatomic factors that may be contributing is essential to provide the most effective and least invasive treatment and prevent recurrence.

Frontal Recess Size

Narrow frontal recesses have historically been described as a potential cause of obstruction. However, current studies suggest the size of the frontal recess does not impact the prevalence of primary frontal sinusitis.[15,18] Persistent frontal sinusitis can be related to neo-ostium size, with larger openings having higher rates of postoperative patency than smaller openings.[6] The recommended size for the neo-ostium varies in the reported literature, but openings of less than 4.5 mm are reported to be at greater risk for stenosis.[6]

24.3.2 Physiological Factors

There are a variety of physiological factors that may play a role in the pathophysiology of CRSsNP. Concurrent asthma and allergy are common and subsequent treatment may improve the control of CRSsNP.[19] The role of factors such as fungal elements, microbiome disturbances, osteitis, immune deficiencies, superantigens, and biofilms are not well understood and are areas of ongoing investigation.[12] With regard to frontal sinusitis in CRSsNP, there is a paucity of literature on the impact of these factors on frontal sinusitis. The available evidence has not linked these factors to the pathophysiology of frontal sinusitis; however, further study is necessary to define what possible roles they may play.[12]

24.4 Management

An essential component of the initial and long-term management of CRSsNP consists of medical therapy, which aims to reduce underlying inflammation. Patients who have persistent symptoms despite medical therapy may benefit from ESS. Treatment considerations in the management of CRSsNP will be discussed in this section, specifically regarding their role in the treatment of frontal sinusitis.

24.4.1 Medical Management

Delivery of Topical Medications

Due to the anatomic location of the frontal recess and the variety of frontoethmoidal cells, one of the main challenges of medical therapy is delivery of medication to the frontal recess. There are a few techniques that are utilized in clinical practice to aid in the delivery of medications to the frontal recess, such as head position and delivery method. High-volume sinonasal irrigations (> 200 mL) are the most effective, especially when combined with a head down forward position (▶ Fig. 24.2).[20] Low-volume techniques, such as nasal drops, may penetrate the frontal recess when combined with a head back (i.e., nose upward) position (▶ Fig. 24.3).[20] Of note, these techniques

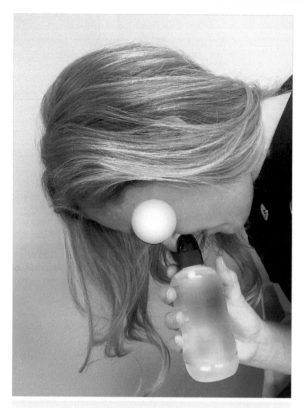

Fig. 24.2 Head down forward position, most effective for frontal sinus delivery with high-volume irrigations.

have more effective distribution to all of the paranasal sinuses following ESS.[12,21]

Appropriate Medical Therapy

Historically, medical management of patients with CRS involved the use of defined "maximal medical therapy." This referred to the process of exhausting medical treatment options before surgical interventions were offered. Recently, the concept of appropriate medical therapy (AMT) has emerged, which strives to strike a balance between trialing medical therapy, without delaying patients' access to ESS.[12] A recent study has defined AMT for both primary and recurrent CRSsNP.[22,23] The results of this study suggest that AMT should consist of high-volume sinonasal irrigations and topical intranasal corticosteroids, for a minimum of 8 weeks. In addition, patients should receive either a short course of broad-spectrum/culture-directed systemic antibiotics (2–3 weeks) or a prolonged course of systemic low-dose anti-inflammatory antibiotic (> 12 weeks).[22,23] These suggestions are in agreement with the International Consensus Statement on Allergy and Rhinology: Rhinosinusitis as well.[12] Of note, the recommendations regarding AMT do not address specific sinusitis, such as frontal sinusitis. Currently, there is no evidence to suggest that AMT for

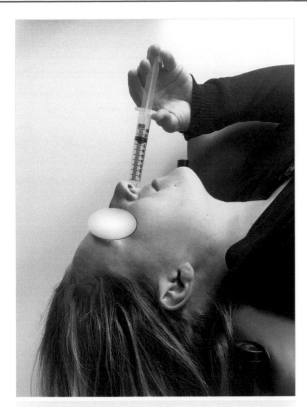

Fig. 24.3 Head back/nose upward position, most effective for frontal sinus delivery with nasal drops.

frontal sinusitis should deviate from these recommendations.[24]

Specific Medical Therapy

Currently, there are no unique recommendations for medical strategies specific to frontal sinusitis in CRSsNP.[12,22,23,24] There is some evidence supporting the use of a short course (< 3 weeks) of systemic corticosteroids in CRSsNP, which may be considered on an individual basis considering the associated therapeutic risks.[25] This may be beneficial in patients with chronic frontal sinusitis to decrease edema and inflammation in the frontal recess and decrease the resulting obstruction of the frontal recess. There is no evidence supporting the use of leukotriene receptor antagonists, systemic antihistamines, anti-immunoglobulin E or anti-interleukin 5 therapy in CRSsNP.[25] There is evidence recommending against the use of topical antibiotics and antifungals in CRSsNP.[25] Alternative medical therapies, such as intranasal xylitol, surfactants, and Manuka honey, have low levels of evidence; further study is required before recommendations regarding these treatments can be made.[12] The mainstay of therapy for frontal sinusitis in CRSsNP remains AMT, as described earlier.[22,23]

24.4.2 Surgical Management

ESS is indicated in medically refractory CRS. The goals of ESS in the frontal sinus are to improve sinonasal symptoms, relieve obstruction, and allow for natural drainage as well as facilitate the delivery of maintenance medical therapy. In unoperated sinuses, delivery to the frontal recess is limited and inconsistent, regardless of delivery method or head position.[21] Following ESS, penetration into the frontal recess is significantly improved.[21] The greater the extent of surgery, the better the penetration; for example, compared to a Draf IIa, a Draf III provides significantly better penetration of topical medications into the frontal recess (▶ Fig. 24.4).[20,26]

Identifying the location of the obstruction is important to allow surgeons to choose the most valuable surgical intervention. Some patients with mild inflammation may benefit from an anterior ethmoidectomy alone. A retrospective cohort study and a recent prospective cohort study suggest that an anterior ethmoidectomy alone may be sufficient in patients with a limited degree of sinonasal inflammation.[19,27] However, these studies were limited by a small number of patients receiving anterior ethmoidectomy compared to the group receiving frontal recess dissection and a short duration of follow-up.[19,27] In addition, undissected frontal cells are a common finding in recurrent frontal sinusitis[15] and an anterior ethmoidectomy may not improve topical medical delivery to the frontal recess.[6] Others advocate that a Draf IIa is an appropriate and effective option for most patients with refractory CRSsNP, which improves penetration of medication into the frontal recess in addition to relieving obstruction.[6,15,26] Draf III dissections are often reserved for revision or salvage cases, which are discussed in detail in another chapter.[6] Deciding the appropriate extent of surgery can be challenging, in part due to the variations in anatomy, underlying pathophysiology, and severity of disease. Additionally, the literature available to guide clinicians does not clearly define what the optimal extent of surgery involves.[6] This may contribute to significant variations in frontal sinus surgery. Physicians should participate in an open discussion about the risks, benefits, and alternative treatments with individual patients to aid in the shared decision-making process.

The frontal recess is one of the most challenging operative sites in the paranasal sinuses. Aside from the variable anatomy, narrow confines, and the proximity to vital structures, the frontal recess is unforgiving of anything short of meticulous dissection with the highest rates of postoperative stenosis and revision surgery.[6] When the drainage pathway of the frontal recess is preserved (i.e., Draf I and IIa), mucosal preservation techniques are essential to prevent stripping and exposed bone, which may be associated with circumferential scarring and postoperative stenosis.[5,28] Utilizing a variety of endoscopes

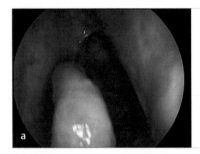
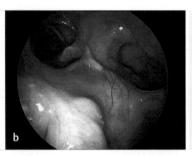

Fig. 24.4 **(a)** Right endoscopic view of a healed Draf IIb procedure/unilateral frontal floor resection and **(b)** endoscopic view of a healed Draf III procedure/bilateral frontal floor removal. Note the much widened access for topical therapy afforded by removal of the superior nasal septum and frontal intersinus septum.

(0, 30, 45, and 70 degrees) can be useful to optimize visualization, which may minimize trauma and ensure a complete dissection. Ample surgical expertise, skill, and patience are important components of successful surgery, and insight into personal surgical limitations is important to prevent iatrogenic stenosis. The use of drug-eluting stents may be of some benefit in the frontal recess and will be discussed in another chapter.

Despite these challenges, namely, the complex surgical anatomy, choosing the appropriate extent of surgery, and high recurrence and revision rates, the literature shows that ESS in frontal sinusitis is associated with improved disease-specific quality of life and long-term patency in the majority of patients.[6] Carefully matching the patient to the procedure is an important consideration to optimize the value of ESS in CRSsNP.

24.5 Conclusion

Frontal sinusitis in CRSsNP represents a unique challenge. Medical therapy is an important component of initial and maintenance therapy; however, delivery to the frontal recess is limited in unoperated sinuses. While ESS plays an important role in the management of medically refractory frontal sinusitis, it is also associated with significant risks including high rates of stenosis and revision surgery. Balancing the risks and benefits of these treatments can be difficult; however, the majority of patients receive significant symptomatic improvement with appropriate medical and surgical therapy.

References

[1] Huvenne W, van Bruaene N, Zhang N, et al. Chronic rhinosinusitis with and without nasal polyps: what is the difference? Curr Allergy Asthma Rep. 2009; 9(3):213–220

[2] Beule A. Epidemiology of chronic rhinosinusitis, selected risk factors, comorbidities, and economic burden. GMS Curr Top Otorhinolaryngol Head Neck Surg. 2015; 14:Doc11

[3] Lai WS, Yang PL, Lee CH, et al. The association of frontal recess anatomy and mucosal disease on the presence of chronic frontal sinusitis: a computed tomographic analysis. Rhinology. 2014; 52(3):208–214

[4] Eweiss AZ, Khalil HS. The prevalence of frontal cells and their relation to frontal sinusitis: a radiological study of the frontal recess area. ISRN Otolaryngol. 2013; 2013:687582

[5] Valdes CJ, Bogado M, Samaha M. Causes of failure in endoscopic frontal sinus surgery in chronic rhinosinusitis patients. Int Forum Allergy Rhinol. 2014; 4(6):502–506

[6] DeConde AS, Smith TL. Outcomes After Frontal Sinus Surgery: An Evidence-Based Review. Otolaryngol Clin North Am. 2016; 49(4):1019–1033

[7] Naidoo Y, Wen D, Bassiouni A, Keen M, Wormald PJ. Long-term results after primary frontal sinus surgery. Int Forum Allergy Rhinol. 2012; 2(3):185–190

[8] Friedman M, Bliznikas D, Vidyasagar R, Joseph NJ, Landsberg R. Long-term results after endoscopic sinus surgery involving frontal recess dissection. Laryngoscope. 2006; 116(4):573–579

[9] Ting JY, Wu A, Metson R. Frontal sinus drillout (modified Lothrop procedure): long-term results in 204 patients. Laryngoscope. 2014; 124(5):1066–1070

[10] Jacobs JB. 100 years of frontal sinus surgery. Laryngoscope. 1997; 107 (11 Pt 2):1–36

[11] Neel HB, III, McDonald TJ, Facer GW. Modified Lynch procedure for chronic frontal sinus diseases: rationale, technique, and long-term results. Laryngoscope. 1987; 97(11):1274–1279

[12] Orlandi RR, Kingdom TT, Hwang PH, et al. International Consensus Statement on Allergy and Rhinology: Rhinosinusitis. Int Forum Allergy Rhinol. 2016; 6 Suppl 1:S22–S209

[13] Lee WT, Kuhn FA, Citardi MJ. 3D computed tomographic analysis of frontal recess anatomy in patients without frontal sinusitis. Otolaryngol Head Neck Surg. 2004; 131(3):164–173

[14] Lien CF, Weng HH, Chang YC, Lin YC, Wang WH. Computed tomographic analysis of frontal recess anatomy and its effect on the development of frontal sinusitis. Laryngoscope. 2010; 120(12):2521–2527

[15] DelGaudio JM, Hudgins PA, Venkatraman G, Beningfield A. Multiplanar computed tomographic analysis of frontal recess cells: effect on frontal isthmus size and frontal sinusitis. Arch Otolaryngol Head Neck Surg. 2005; 131(3):230–235

[16] Langille M, Walters E, Dziegielewski PT, Kotylak T, Wright ED. Frontal sinus cells: identification, prevalence, and association with frontal sinus mucosal thickening. Am J Rhinol Allergy. 2012; 26(3):e107–e110

[17] Wormald PJ, Hoseman W, Callejas C, et al. The International Frontal Sinus Anatomy Classification (IFAC) and Classification of the Extent of Endoscopic Frontal Sinus Surgery (EFSS). Int Forum Allergy Rhinol. 2016; 6(7):677–696

[18] DeConde AS, Barton MD, Mace JC, Smith TL. Can sinus anatomy predict quality of life outcomes and operative times of endoscopic frontal sinus surgery? Am J Otolaryngol. 2015; 36(1):13–19

[19] Abuzeid WM, Mace JC, Costa ML, et al. Outcomes of chronic frontal sinusitis treated with ethmoidectomy: a prospective study. Int Forum Allergy Rhinol. 2016; 6(6):597–604

[20] Smith KA, Rudmik L. Delivery of topical therapies. in: Woodworth BA, Poetker DM, Reh DD, eds. Advances in Oto-Rhino-Laryngology: Rhinosinusitis with Nasal Polyposis. Basel: Karger; 2016

[21] Thomas WW, III, Harvey RJ, Rudmik L, Hwang PH, Schlosser RJ. Distribution of topical agents to the paranasal sinuses: an evidence-based review with recommendations. Int Forum Allergy Rhinol. 2013; 3 (9):691–703

[22] Rudmik L, Soler ZM, Hopkins C, et al. Defining appropriateness criteria for endoscopic sinus surgery during management of uncomplicated adult chronic rhinosinusitis: a RAND/UCLA appropriateness study. Int Forum Allergy Rhinol. 2016; 6(6):557–567

[23] Rudmik L, Soler ZM, Hopkins C, et al. Defining appropriateness criteria for endoscopic sinus surgery during management of uncomplicated adult chronic rhinosinusitis: a RAND/UCLA appropriateness study. Rhinology. 2016; 54(2):117–128

[24] Sohal M, Tessema B, Brown SM. Medical management of frontal sinusitis. Otolaryngol Clin North Am. 2016; 49(4):927–934

[25] Rudmik L, Soler ZM. Medical therapies for adult chronic sinusitis: a systematic review. JAMA. 2015; 314(9):926–939

[26] Barham HP, Ramakrishnan VR, Knisely A, et al. Frontal sinus surgery and sinus distribution of nasal irrigation. Int Forum Allergy Rhinol. 2016; 6(3):238–242

[27] Becker SS, Han JK, Nguyen TA, Gross CW. Initial surgical treatment for chronic frontal sinusitis: a pilot study. Ann Otol Rhinol Laryngol. 2007; 116(4):286–289

[28] Bradoo RA, Shah KD, Joshi AA. Factors affecting the outcome of frontal sinus surgery: a prospective study. Indian J Otolaryngol Head Neck Surg. 2013; 65 Suppl 2:260–266

25 Frontal Sinus Surgery in CRSwNP, AFRS, and ASA Triad

Nsangou Ghogomu and Robert C. Kern

Abstract

The need for revision frontal sinus surgery is significantly increased by the presence of nasal polyps, asthma, aspirin-exacerbated respiratory disease (AERD), and/or allergic fungal rhinosinusitis (AFRS). While surgery decreases the inflammatory load and opens the sinus drainage pathways in these patients, its greater goal is the creation of wide access for postoperative topical medication delivery. The endoscopic modified Lothrop procedure (EMLP, Draf III) procedure provides significantly better access for topical medications to the frontal sinus than the Draf IIa procedure. Not surprisingly, the need for revision frontal sinus surgery in patients with polyps, asthma, and AERD is significantly decreased following the Draf III compared to the Draf IIa procedure. Recent long-term clinical outcome studies suggest that for select patients with multiple risk factors for disease recurrence, Draf III may be considered the initial surgical intervention. This evolution toward earlier performance of the Draf III procedure has been made possible by significant improvement in surgical drills as well as the development of technology to allow for in-office polypectomy and placement of steroid-eluting stents to address early recurrence of otherwise inaccessible disease at or above the frontal sinus ostium. Regardless of chosen surgical approach, long-term regular follow-up in this population is critical to allow for early detection and intervention of recurrent disease or development of comorbidities.

Keywords: frontal sinus surgery, Lothrop, endoscopic modified Lothrop procedure, Draf, nasal polyps, asthma, aspirin-exacerbated respiratory disease, allergic fungal sinusitis

25.1 Epidemiology and Etiology

25.1.1 Chronic Rhinosinusitis with Nasal Polyps

At present, chronic rhinosinusitis (CRS) is divided into two phenotypes based on the presence (CRS with nasal polyps [CRSwNP]) or absence (CRS without nasal polyps [CRSsNP]) of nasal polyps.[1] CRSwNP has an estimated prevalence of 0.06%[2] and an incidence of approximately 8.3 cases per 10,000 person years.[3] While most cases of CRSwNP are idiopathic, some are part of a known underlying disease process such as cystic fibrosis (CF), aspirin-exacerbated respiratory disease (AERD), or allergic fungal sinusitis (AFRS). The majority of CRSwNP in Western countries demonstrate an eosinophilic type 2 cytokine pattern (interleukin-4 [IL-4], IL-5, and IL-13) of inflammation.[4]

Among Asian patients, Th1/Th2/Th17 neutrophilic inflammation is often associated with CRSwNP.[5]

25.1.2 Aspirin-Exacerbated Respiratory Disease

Samter's triad refers to a syndrome characterized by nasal polyps, asthma, and aspirin sensitivity.[6] The prevalence of AERD in asthmatic patients is 15% in patients with severe asthma and 10% in patients with nasal polyposis.[7] The syndrome usually begins in the third or fourth decade of life with persistent rhinitis. This is then followed by onset of asthma and finally development of aspirin intolerance.[8] It is caused by an abnormality in the arachidonic acid metabolic pathway whereby exposure to cyclooxygenase-1 (COX-1) inhibitors leads to overproduction of proinflammatory cysteinyl leukotrienes and prostaglandins, as well as underproduction of anti-inflammatory prostaglandin E2 (PGE2). This leads to a proinflammatory state in the upper and lower airways mediated by mast cells, eosinophils, and platelets.[9]

25.1.3 Allergic Fungal Sinusitis

Allergic fungal rhinosinusitis (AFRS) is a severe form of noninvasive fungal CRS caused by allergic hypersensitivity to fungal elements encountered in the sinuses of immunocompetent individuals. Approximately 5 to 10% of CRS patients have AFRS. Onset of disease is typically in late adolescence or early adulthood.[10]

25.2 Clinical Presentation and Investigations

25.2.1 Chronic Rhinosinusitis with Nasal Polyps

CRSwNP is characterized by greater than 12 weeks of nasal obstruction, loss of smell, and less frequently mucopurulent discharge and/or facial pressure. The diagnosis is confirmed by nasal endoscopy and CT scan confirming the presence of polyps in the nasal cavity and/or paranasal sinuses.[1]

25.2.2 Aspirin-Exacerbated Respiratory Disease

AERD often begins as CRSwNP without associated asthma or aspirin sensitivity. Over several years, patients develop the remaining portions of Samter's triad. Thus, diagnosis of the condition requires that all patients with CRSwNP be asked about nonsteroidal anti-inflammatory drug (NSAID) sensitivity and asthma symptoms at every follow-up visit. In patients with a history of adverse respiratory reactions to intake of aspirin or other NSAIDs, aspirin sensitivity is confirmed by provocation testing using oral aspirin or inhaled lysine-aspirin.[11] For those with new cough, wheezing, or shortness of breath, asthma can be diagnosed by demonstrating an inducible obstructive disorder on pulmonary function testing.

25.2.3 Allergic Fungal Sinusitis

The clinical presentation for patients with AFRS may be very similar to that of CRSwNP with the exception that patients complain of the presence of thicker mucus and crusting.[10] However, insidious bony erosion and expansion can be seen in 20 to 77% of AFRS patients who may remain relatively asymptomatic until intracranial or orbital complications of the disease lead them to seek medical attention.[12] Overall, the lamina papyracea is the most frequently eroded bone, but when present in the frontal sinus, erosion is most often seen in the posterior table followed by the floor overlying the orbit.[13] These patients with erosion tend to be younger, male, and African American.[14]

The Bent and Kuhn major diagnostic criteria for AFRS include presence of nasal polyposis, fungi, eo- sinophilic mucin without invasion, type 1 (immunoglobulin E [IgE] mediated) hypersensitivity to fungi, and presence of characteristic CT findings of sinus expansion or heterogeneous opacification.[15] In the presence of bony erosion of the posterior table, an MRI is more sensitive than CT at determining the extent of disease extension into the cranium.

25.3 Management Overview

25.3.1 Chronic Rhinosinusitis with Nasal Polyps

Topical and systemic steroids are the mainstay of treatment for patients with CRSwNP.[16,17] Among patients with CRSwNP, efficacy of steroids varies with inflammatory endotype, with poorer responses seen in patients who tend to have non–Th2 mediated nasal polyposis.[18,19] Early surgery is indicated for patients who fail appropriate medical management, with delays associated with worse sinonasal and pulmonary outcomes.[1,20,21]

25.3.2 Aspirin-Exacerbated Respiratory Disease

Patients with AERD typically have more extensive sinonasal disease compared to aspirin-tolerant patients. They also tend to be more recalcitrant to both medical and surgical treatments, with post functional endoscopic sinus surgery (FESS) polyp recurrence rates as high as 90% at 5 years, and revision rates as high as 90% at 10 years.[22]

Sinus surgery coupled with medical management leads to improvement in overall quality of life, asthma outcomes, and sinus-related symptoms.[23]

The initial management of AERD follows typical guidelines for CRSwNP treatment, with the addition of leukotriene-modifying agents, avoidance of NSAIDs, and use of aspirin desensitization followed by high-dose aspirin therapy. Indications for aspirin desensitization followed by high-dose aspirin therapy include failure of standard medical therapies including inhaled steroids and leukotriene-modifying agents resulting in need for frequent bursts of oral steroids and recurrent nasal polyps.[24] Contraindications include pregnancy and history of gastric ulcers. Several studies have demonstrated consistent and significant benefits of aspirin de-sensitization not just for AERD broadly, but for sinonasal disease. They have demonstrated decrease in nasal congestion, polyp size, frequency of sinusitis, need for steroids, and anosmia.[25] The evidence for leukotriene-modifying agents suggests it may have higher impact on the lower airways than the sinuses.[26]

25.3.3 Allergic Fungal Sinusitis

Unlike most forms of CRS, the primary treatment modality for AFRS is surgery. The goals of surgery include polyp removal, evacuation of eosinophilic mucin containing fungal antigen and inflammatory mediators, and provision of access for topical intranasal medication.[27]

Postoperative medical therapy following surgery is directed at decreasing inflammation, preventing allergic mucin re-accumulation, and maintaining sinus drainage. There is consistent evidence from observational studies supporting use of systemic steroids in post-op patients with AFRS. There is little direct evidence to support topical steroid use in AFRS specifically, but its benefits have been clearly demonstrated for CRSwNP and are thus considered applicable to AFRS.[28] With two-thirds of AFRS patients having a history of allergic rhinitis and 90% with elevated specific IgE to fungus, allergy treatment is recommended. Postoperative immunotherapy appears to decrease postoperative systemic steroid requirements as well as reoperation rates.[29]

While long-term systemic antifungal therapy has proven beneficial in allergic bronchopulmonary aspergillosis (ABPA), evidence is lacking to support topical or systemic antifungal therapy in AFRS. Similarly, evidence to support leukotriene modulators in AFRS is lacking with the exception of a single case report demonstrating benefit.[30]

25.4 Extent of Surgery and Outcomes

25.4.1 Goals of Surgery

Historically, FESS emphasized sinus aeration and restoration of mucociliary function by opening blocked sinus ostia. However, it is clear that this is not the full story, as 35% of patients with CRS do not have obstructed OMCs (osteomeatal complexes). The goal of surgery now focuses on decrease in inflammatory load by removal of polyps, eosinophilic and allergic mucin, and maintenance of a large enough ostium to permit not simply aeration, but rather access for irrigation and application of topical anti-inflammatory medications.[31]

25.4.2 Effect of Extent of Surgery on Outcomes for Maxillary and Ethmoid Sinuses

Patients with CRSwNP tend to have higher rates of revision surgery than patients without polyps. In the United Kingdom sinonasal audit looking at over 1,000 patients, they found that the frequency of revision surgery was 29% in CRSsNP and 55% in CRSwNP.[32,33] Among patients with polyps, disease severity and risk of recurrence are increased by the presence of more severe eosinophilic inflammation seen in asthma, AERD, and AFRS.[34,35] A study comparing outcomes for nasal polyps, asthma, and AERD showed that at 5 years after complete FESS with Draf IIa, the revision surgery rate was 40% for AERD, 20% for asthma, and 10% for CRSwNP not otherwise specified.[22]

While disease subtype and comorbidity can significantly alter disease recurrence rate, modifications to surgical extent has a significant impact on outcomes. Studies looking at recurrence rates in CRSwNP patients undergoing at least complete ethmoidectomy compared to simply anterior ethmoidectomy or similarly targeted surgeries suggest significantly higher recurrence rates in less radical surgery. Threefold differences in 5-year recurrence rates of nasal polyps (20 vs. 60%) have been demonstrated in several studies comparing incomplete to complete ethmoidectomy in patients with CRSwNP.[36,37]

These outcomes observed from more radical surgery are due to both decrease in inflammatory load and improved penetration of irrigations and topical medications after surgery.[38,39] In addition to this, the presence of larger ethmoid cavities permits placement of long-lasting bioabsorbable steroid-eluting implants as well as more

effective use of vacuum-powered microdebriders, both of which permit early intervention for recurrent polyp disease without the need for formal revision surgery.[40,41]

25.4.3 Effect of Extent of Surgery on Outcomes for the Frontal Sinus

Draf IIa versus Draf III in Patients with CRSwNP, Asthma, and AERD

Similar to findings in the ethmoids, in the frontal sinus, smaller size of frontal ostia is associated with significantly decreased penetration of saline irrigation and topical therapies. Significantly improved penetration of the frontals sinus (beyond recess) is observed in Draf III compared to Draf IIa (80 vs. 20%). Change of head position to vertex significantly improves penetration in both cases, but results in frontal lavage in 87.5% of Draf III versus 25% of Draf IIa.[42] In addition, the cavity created in patients who have undergone Draf III procedures tremendously facilitates placement of steroid-eluting stents into the ostium, and access for debridement of polyps. It would therefore come as no surprise that trends in outcomes in frontal sinus surgery for CRSwNP, AERD, and AFRS are similar to those seen for these diseases in the ethmoids.

Outcomes for frontal sinus disease vary by disease subtype as well as extent of surgery. The need for revision frontal sinus surgery following complete FESS with Draf IIa in patients with CRSwNP is approximately 17%. The presence of both asthma and polyps increases this rate to 28%; with the further addition of diffuse polyposis and frontal ostium size less than 4 mm to those factors, the failure rate is 62%.[43] This work supports the need for wider frontal sinusotomies in patients with polyp disease, especially when asthma or aspirin allergy is present.

Bassiouni and Wormald compared patients who underwent complete FESS with Draf IIa to those who had complete FESS with Draf III procedures. They found that the most common location of polyp recurrence was the frontal sinus (55%), followed by ethmoids (38%). The rate of polyp recurrence was tripled for AERD patients, and doubled in those with asthma (▶ Table 25.1). The need for revision surgery at 1 year was 37% for Draf IIa and 7% for Draf III.[44] Additional studies specifically looking at

Table 25.1 Effect of frontal surgery extent and comorbidity on polyp recurrence rates[44]

	Polyp recurrence rate by surgery type	
	FESS with Draf IIa (199 cases)	FESS with Draf III (139 cases)
CRSwNP (all)	26%	16%
With asthma	40%	16%
With AERD	55%	11%

Abbreviations: AERD, aspirin-exacerbated respiratory disease; CRSwNP, chronic rhinosinusitis with nasal polyps; FESS, functional endoscopic sinus surgery.

failure patterns in CRSwNP after Draf III found that the most common reason for failure is polyp growth obstructing the frontal ostium.[45,46] In these Draf III patients, with the bony floor of the sinus widely removed, excellent access is afforded for in-office polyp debridement and placement of steroid-eluting stents into the otherwise inaccessible upper reaches of the frontal sinus ostium.[40,41]

Use of Draf III in Allergic Fungal Sinusitis

The majority of the literature discussing the impact of AFRS on the need for revision frontal sinus surgery highlights the role of recurrent obstructing polyps as the reason for failure in this disease process and justification for a wider ostium. However, the need for early radical frontal sinus surgery in AFRS may be necessary from a practical standpoint given the extreme difficulty of removing allergic/eosinophilic mucin from the frontal sinus without a large frontal sinus opening. Postoperatively, without a Draf III cavity, it is even more challenging to displace these thick secretions with irrigations or debridements. In addition, with the significantly increased rate of bony erosion of the posterior table of the frontal sinus in AFRS, visualization

and access afforded by the Draf III procedure allow for identification and repair of cerebrospinal fluid (CSF) leaks.

25.5 Case Examples

25.5.1 Samter's Triad Successfully Managed with Draf IIa

A woman in her thirties with a long history of poorly controlled asthma was initially referred to otolaryngology for evaluation of her sinuses. The patient lacked NSAID sensitivity. Initial evaluation revealed presence of significant nasal polyps with near-complete opacification of all her sinuses. The patient opted for medical therapy. Ten years later, she returned, this time with a diagnosis of aspirin allergy, and now refractory to medical therapy. She underwent a complete FESS with Draf IIa. Two years after surgery, using budesonide irrigations, the patient has completely healthy frontal sinuses (▶ Fig. 25.1).

25.5.2 Samter's Triad Only Controlled after Draf III

A man in his twenties with poorly controlled asthma who had undergone five sinus surgeries was referred to otolaryngology for symptomatic CRSwNP refractory to medication. He underwent a sixth surgery, which included a complete FESS with Draf IIa. Within a few months, polyps and associated symptoms returned and were managed medically. Several years later, with failure of medical management (▶ Fig. 25.2), a revision FESS with Draf III was performed. Four months later, on budesonide irrigations, the patient has completely healthy frontal sinuses (▶ Fig. 25.3).

25.5.3 Nasal Polyp Recurrence in Frontal Ostium Managed in the Office

A man in his fifties with Samter's triad and a history of prior complete FESS with Draf IIa presented with medically refractory sinonasal disease. A Draf III was performed and he was maintained postoperatively on topical steroid irrigations. During a recent routine clinic follow-up, endoscopy revealed recurrence of obstructing nasal

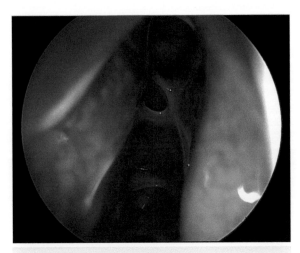

Fig. 25.1 Successful outcome following Draf IIa in a patient with aspirin-exacerbated respiratory disease.

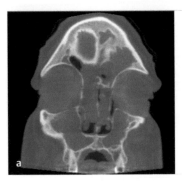
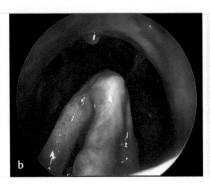

Fig. 25.2 (a, b) Preoperative CT of an asthmatic patient who had failed multiple surgeries for chronic rhinosinusitis with nasal polyps.

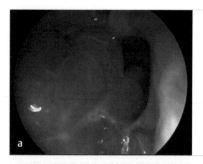
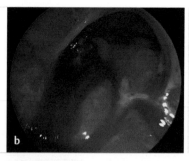

Fig. 25.3 (a, b) Postoperative outcome after complete functional endoscopic sinus surgery with Draf III in a patient with chronic rhinosinusitis with nasal polyps.

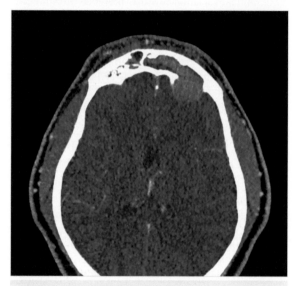

Fig. 25.4 Recurrent polyps obstructing frontal ostium in a patient with aspirin-exacerbated respiratory disease following Draf III.

polyps high in the frontal neo-ostium (▶ Fig. 25.3a). Using frontal instruments and a microdebrider, these were easily debrided, restoring thefrontal sinus patency (▶ Fig. 25.3b).

25.5.4 Allergic Fungal Sinusitis Presenting with Proptosis

A man in his twenties with allergic rhinitis and asthma presented to the emergency department complaining of vision changes. Physical examination revealed proptosis. CT scan revealed heterogeneous high-attenuation material filling the sinuses, associated with bony expansion and erosion of the posterior table and floor of the frontal sinus (▶ Fig. 25.4). An MRI of the brain revealed the presence of multiple mucoceles entering the orbit and cranium that could not be clearly distinguished on CT. He underwent a full FESS with Draf III. There was no intraoperative CSF leak.

25.6 Complications

The most significant potential complication in this class of diseases is the presence of posterior table or frontal sinus floor erosion with intracranial or orbital extension. Removal of frontal sinus disease in this situation may be associated with a CSF leak, intracranial bleed, or orbital hematoma. Details of management of these complications are discussed in depth in other chapters.

References

[1] Orlandi RR, Kingdom TT, Hwang PH, et al. International Consensus Statement on Allergy and Rhinology: Rhinosinusitis. Int Forum Allergy Rhinol. 2016; 6 Suppl 1:S22–S209

[2] Larsen K, Tos M. The estimated incidence of symptomatic nasal polyps. Acta Otolaryngol. 2002; 122(2):179–182

[3] Tan BK, Chandra RK, Pollak J, et al. Incidence and associated premorbid diagnoses of patients with chronic rhinosinusitis. J Allergy Clin Immunol. 2013; 131(5):1350–1360

[4] Lam K, Schleimer R, Kern RC. The etiology and pathogenesis of chronic rhinosinusitis: a review of current hypotheses. Curr Allergy Asthma Rep. 2015; 15(7):41

[5] Cao PP, Li HB, Wang BF, et al. Distinct immunopathologic characteristics of various types of chronic rhinosinusitis in adult Chinese. J Allergy Clin Immunol. 2009; 124(3):478–484, 484.e1–484.e2

[6] Fahrenholz JM. Natural history and clinical features of aspirin-exacerbated respiratory disease. Clin Rev Allergy Immunol. 2003; 24 (2):113–124

[7] Rajan JP, Wineinger NE, Stevenson DD, White AA. Prevalence of aspirin-exacerbated respiratory disease among asthmatic patients: a meta-analysis of the literature. J Allergy Clin Immunol. 2015; 135 (3):676–81.e1

[8] Szczeklik A, Nizankowska E, Duplaga M, AIANE Investigators. European Network on Aspirin-Induced Asthma. Natural history of aspirin-induced asthma. Eur Respir J. 2000; 16(3):432–436

[9] Morrissey DK, Bassiouni A, Psaltis AJ, Naidoo Y, Wormald PJ. Outcomes of modified endoscopic Lothrop in aspirin-exacerbated respiratory disease with nasal polyposis. Int Forum Allergy Rhinol. 2016; 6(8):820–825

[10] Luong A, Marple BF. Allergic fungal rhinosinusitis. Curr Allergy Asthma Rep. 2004; 4(6):465–470

[11] Mullol J, Picado C. Rhinosinusitis and nasal polyps in aspirin-exacerbated respiratory disease. Immunol Allergy Clin North Am. 2013; 33 (2):163–176

[12] White LC, Jang DW, Yelvertan JC, Kountakis SE. Bony erosion patterns in patients with allergic fungal sinusitis. Am J Rhinol Allergy. 2015; 29(4):243–245

[13] Nussenbaum B, Marple BF, Schwade ND. Characteristics of bony erosion in allergic fungal rhinosinusitis. Otolaryngol Head Neck Surg. 2001; 124(2):150–154

[14] Ghegan MD, Lee FS, Schlosser RJ. Incidence of skull base and orbital erosion in allergic fungal rhinosinusitis (AFRS) and non-AFRS. Otolaryngol Head Neck Surg. 2006; 134(4):592–595

[15] Bent JP, III, Kuhn FA. Diagnosis of allergic fungal sinusitis. Otolaryngol Head Neck Surg. 1994; 111(5):580–588

[16] Chong LY, Head K, Hopkins C, Philpott C, Schilder AG, Burton MJ. Intranasal steroids versus placebo or no intervention for chronic rhinosinusitis. Cochrane Database Syst Rev. 2016; 4:CD011996

[17] Kalish L, Snidvongs K, Sivasubramaniam R, Cope D, Harvey RJ. Topical steroids for nasal polyps. Cochrane Database Syst Rev. 2012; 12: CD006549

[18] Wen W, Liu W, Zhang L, et al. Nasal Health Group, China (NHGC). Increased neutrophilia in nasal polyps reduces the response to oral corticosteroid therapy. J Allergy Clin Immunol. 2012; 129(6):1522–8. e5

[19] Zhou B, He G, Liang J, et al. Mometasone furoate nasal spray in the treatment of nasal polyposis in Chinese patients: a double-blind, randomized, placebo-controlled trial. Int Forum Allergy Rhinol. 2016; 6(1):88–94

[20] Hopkins C, Rimmer J, Lund VJ. Does time to endoscopic sinus surgery impact outcomes in Chronic Rhinosinusitis? Prospective findings from the National Comparative Audit of Surgery for Nasal Polyposis and Chronic Rhinosinusitis. Rhinology. 2015; 53(1):10–17

[21] Benninger MS, Sindwani R, Holy CE, Hopkins C. Impact of medically recalcitrant chronic rhinosinusitis on incidence of asthma. Int Forum Allergy Rhinol. 2016; 6(2):124–129

[22] Mendelsohn D, Jeremic G, Wright ED, Rotenberg BW. Revision rates after endoscopic sinus surgery: a recurrence analysis. Ann Otol Rhinol Laryngol. 2011; 120(3):162–166

[23] Adelman J, McLean C, Shaigany K, Krouse JH. The role of surgery in management of Samter's triad: a systematic review. Otolaryngol Head Neck Surg. 2016; 155(2):220–237

[24] Macy E, Bernstein JA, Castells MC, et al. Aspirin Desensitization Joint Task Force. Aspirin challenge and desensitization for aspirin-exacerbated respiratory disease: a practice paper. Ann Allergy Asthma Immunol. 2007; 98(2):172–174

[25] Simon RA, Dazy KM, Waldram JD. Update on aspirin desensitization for chronic rhinosinusitis with polyps in aspirin-exacerbated respiratory disease (AERD). Curr Allergy Asthma Rep. 2015; 15(3):508

[26] Buchheit KM, Laidlaw TM. Update on the management of aspirin-exacerbated respiratory disease. Allergy Asthma Immunol Res. 2016; 8(4):298–304

[27] Marple BF. Allergic fungal rhinosinusitis: current theories and management strategies. Laryngoscope. 2001; 111(6):1006–1019

[28] Gan EC, Thamboo A, Rudmik L, Hwang PH, Ferguson BJ, Javer AR. Medical management of allergic fungal rhinosinusitis following endoscopic sinus surgery: an evidence-based review and recommendations. Int Forum Allergy Rhinol. 2014; 4(9):702–715

[29] Patadia MO, Welch KC. Role of immunotherapy in allergic fungal rhinosinusitis. Curr Opin Otolaryngol Head Neck Surg. 2015; 23(1):21–28

[30] Schubert MS. Antileukotriene therapy for allergic fungal sinusitis. J Allergy Clin Immunol. 2001; 108(3):466–467

[31] Bassiouni A, Naidoo Y, Wormald PJ. When FESS fails: the inflammatory load hypothesis in refractory chronic rhinosinusitis. Laryngoscope. 2012; 122(2):460–466

[32] Hopkins C, Browne JP, Slack R, et al. The national comparative audit of surgery for nasal polyposis and chronic rhinosinusitis. Clin Otolaryngol. 2006; 31(5):390–398

[33] Philpott C, Hopkins C, Erskine S, et al. The burden of revision sinonasal surgery in the UK-data from the Chronic Rhinosinusitis Epidemiology Study (CRES): a cross-sectional study. BMJ Open. 2015; 5 (4):e006680

[34] Van Zele T, Holtappels G, Gevaert P, Bachert C. Differences in initial immunoprofiles between recurrent and nonrecurrent chronic rhinosinusitis with nasal polyps. Am J Rhinol Allergy. 2014; 28(3):192–198

[35] Georgalas C, Cornet M, Adriaensen G, et al. Evidence-based surgery for chronic rhinosinusitis with and without nasal polyps. Curr Allergy Asthma Rep. 2014; 14(4):427

[36] Jankowski R, Pigret D, Decroocq F, Blum A, Gillet P. Comparison of radical (nasalisation) and functional ethmoidectomy in patients with severe sinonasal polyposis. A retrospective study. Rev Laryngol Otol Rhinol (Bord). 2006; 127(3):131–140

[37] Masterson L, Tanweer F, Bueser T, Leong P. Extensive endoscopic sinus surgery: does this reduce the revision rate for nasal polyposis? Eur Arch Otorhinolaryngol. 2010; 267(10):1557–1561

[38] Doellman M, Chen PG, McMains KC, Sarber KM, Weitzel EK. Sinus penetration of saline solution irrigation and atomizer in a cadaveric polyp and allergic fungal sinusitis model. Allergy Rhinol (Providence). 2015; 6(1):8–11

[39] Snidvongs K, Kalish L, Sacks R, Sivasubramaniam R, Cope D, Harvey RJ. Sinus surgery and delivery method influence the effectiveness of topical corticosteroids for chronic rhinosinusitis: systematic review and meta-analysis. Am J Rhinol Allergy. 2013; 27(3):221–233

[40] Forwith KD, Han JK, Stolovitzky JP, et al. RESOLVE: bioabsorbable steroid-eluting sinus implants for in-office treatment of recurrent sinonasal polyposis after sinus surgery: 6-month outcomes from a randomized, controlled, blinded study. Int Forum Allergy Rhinol. 2016; 6(6):573–581

[41] Gan EC, Habib AR, Hathorn I, Javer AR. The efficacy and safety of an office-based polypectomy with a vacuum-powered microdebrider. Int Forum Allergy Rhinol. 2013; 3(11):890–895

[42] Barham HP, Ramakrishnan VR, Knisely A, et al. Frontal sinus surgery and sinus distribution of nasal irrigation. Int Forum Allergy Rhinol. 2016; 6(3):238–242

[43] Naidoo Y, Bassiouni A, Keen M, Wormald PJ. Risk factors and outcomes for primary, revision, and modified Lothrop (Draf III) frontal sinus surgery. Int Forum Allergy Rhinol. 2013; 3(5):412–417

[44] Bassiouni A, Wormald PJ. Role of frontal sinus surgery in nasal polyp recurrence. Laryngoscope. 2013; 123(1):36–41

[45] Naidoo Y, Bassiouni A, Keen M, Wormald PJ. Long-term outcomes for the endoscopic modified Lothrop/Draf III procedure: a 10-year review. Laryngoscope. 2014; 124(1):43–49

[46] Morrissey DK, Bassiouni A, Psaltis AJ, Naidoo Y, Wormald PJ. Outcomes of revision endoscopic modified Lothrop procedure. Int Forum Allergy Rhinol. 2016; 6(5):518–522

26 Frontal Sinus Mucoceles

James Constable and Anshul Sama

Abstract

Paranasal sinus mucoceles are benign, epithelialized, mucus-filled sacs that commonly occur within the frontal sinus. Inflammatory and posttraumatic obstruction of normal mucociliary clearance is thought to be responsible for the majority of frontal sinus mucoceles. They most commonly present with orbital signs and/or orbital and facial discomfort. They are diagnosed radiologically; high-resolution computed tomography (CT) is most informative. Magnetic resonance imaging (MRI) is indicated if there is orbital, intracranial, or external expansion/dehiscence. Frontal mucoceles can be classified radiologically as medial, intermediate, or lateral. Management is surgical. Two important factors when planning surgery are access and sinusotomy size, whereas mucocele size and extra-frontal extension are relatively unimportant. Endoscopic approaches are generally adequate and favored. Repair of frontal sinus wall dehiscence is generally unnecessary. Osteoplastic flap may be required with lateral mucoceles and or with significant neo-osteogenesis. Special considerations, such as malignancy and revision surgery, should be made when planning a surgery.

Keywords: frontal sinus, mucocele, symptoms, investigation, classification, management, algorithm

26.1 Terminology

The term "mucocele" is a derivation of the Latin words "mucus" and "coele." Mucus is self-explanatory; "coele" translates to "cavity/chamber." Mucoceles are benign, epithelialized, mucus-filled sacs and are typically located in the cavities termed the paranasal sinuses.[1] In 1896, Rollet was the first to use the term mucocele, and in 1901, Onodi made the first attempt to describe its histology.

26.2 Epidemiology

Mucoceles are the most common benign mass lesions of the paranasal sinuses. They present equally in both genders, and are most commonly diagnosed in middle-aged patients (40–60 years).[2] Although any age of presentation is feasible, pediatric cases are extremely rare, owing at least in part to the normally protracted time delay between mucocele formation and symptom manifestation.[3] An accurate incidence/prevalence is yet to be reported; however, we can at least confirm that paranasal sinus mucoceles are relatively uncommon.[1] Of all the paranasal sinuses, they most commonly occur in the frontal sinuses (65–89%), followed by the ethmoids (8–30%), and then the maxillary sinuses (< 5%).[3,4] The rarest location is the sphenoid sinus. The remainder of this chapter will now solely focus on frontal sinus mucoceles.

26.3 Pathology

In health, the frontal sinuses (and all other paranasal sinuses) are lined with the mucosa consisting of ciliated and nonciliated columnar epithelial cells, and goblet cells. In combination, these cells produce and move mucus in a process termed "mucociliary clearance." The mucus contains protective enzymes, antibodies, and immune cells, and acts as a trap for environmental pathogens and harmful substances.[5,6] Mucociliary clearance moves mucus from within the frontal sinuses to their single points of drainage, termed the sinus ostia. Therefore, it is logical that obstruction of the frontal sinus ostium can cause disruption of mucociliary clearance, with subsequent stasis and accumulation of mucus; this obstruction explains the formation of resultant mucoceles. The causes of frontal sinus ostium obstruction are wide-ranging, and include idiopathic causes (previous surgery accounts for a third of cases), chronic rhinosinusitis, radiotherapy, maxillofacial trauma, and obstructing mass lesions (e.g., nasal polyps/neoplasms).[7,8] Causes related to inflammation (any cause) and trauma (including surgical) are the most common culprits. Regarding surgical causes, both external and endoscopic sinus surgeries are implicated.[9,10] Once formed, the epithelial lining of the mucocele continues to secrete mucus, resulting in its expansion. A mucopyocele refers to an infected mucocele. Commonly isolated bacteria include *Staphylococcus aureus*, *Haemophilus influenza*, alpha hemolytic *Streptococcus*, and gram-negative bacilli.[11] The most common anaerobic organism is *Propionibacterium acnes*.[11]

The infection itself can significantly increase the risk of local complications, and it commonly accelerates the mucocele's rate of expansion.[12] The expansion causes pressure damage to the internal walls of the frontal sinus, resulting in devitalization, bony resorption, osteolysis, and bony remodeling. Among the inflammatory cytokines that mediate this expansion are tumor necrosis factor-α (TNF-α), interleukin-1 (IL-1), IL-6, and prostaglandin E2 (PGE$_2$), with PGE$_2$ being produced in significantly elevated levels by the fibroblasts cultured from these mucoceles.[13,14] The mucocele can then extend beyond the normal anatomical limits of the frontal sinus, and compress/invade neighboring cavities and/or structures.

26.4 Clinical Presentation

There can be a significant time delay between initial mucocele formation and resultant symptoms and

Table 26.1 Examples of extra-frontal mucocele extension and associated presentations

Sites of extra-frontal extension	Associated presentations
Orbit	Diplopia, visual disturbance, orbital/ocular pain, epiphora, proptosis, ophthalmoplegia, periorbital swelling/cellulitis
Intra-cranial	Headache, meningism, focal neurology, raised intracranial pressure, intracranial sepsis
Neighboring paranasal sinuses/nasal cavity	Facial pain/pressure, rhinorrhea, hypo-/anosmia, nasal obstruction, post nasal drip
Frontal subcutaneous tissue	Frontal facial swelling/pain/cellulitis/sinocutaneous fistula

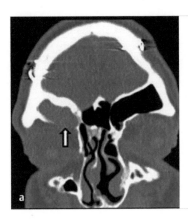 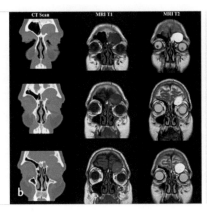

Fig. 26.1 (a) Coronal CT scan with classical expansile lesion of mucocele; (b) CT and MRI images of mucocele with intracranial and orbital expansion.

presentation. Symptoms and presentation are often dictated by mucocele extension to neighboring cavities and/or sequelae of mucocele expansion. The most common presentations are summarized in ▶ Table 26.1.

The commonest presentation is with orbital signs and symptoms, especially proptosis.[15] Facial pain/pressure, headaches, and nasal obstruction are among the other common presentations.

26.5 Investigations

Although history and examination are certainly important, frontal sinus mucocele is a radiological diagnosis. However, clinical examination may reveal concomitant abnormalities that compromise the frontal sinus ostium, and therefore warrant correction as part of its treatment (e.g., septal deviation/nasal polyposis). Plain film radiographs are capable of detecting some frontal sinus mucoceles; however, sensitivity and specificity are low, and they are of no use for surgical planning. The imaging modality of choice is high-resolution computed tomography (CT). On CT, a frontal mucocele is seen as a homogenous, well-circumscribed, expansile mass lesion within the sinus, with its contents demonstrating attenuation anywhere in the range of 10 to 40 HU (▶ Fig. 26.1).[4] Rim enhancement is demonstrated with contrast; however, the latter is indicated if there have been some intracranial or orbital complications or the diagnosis is uncertain. Bony dehiscence and frontal sinus defects are also readily demonstrated.

Magnetic resonance imaging (MRI) is indicated if there is orbital, intracranial, or external expansion or dehiscence (▶ Fig. 26.1b). On MRI, mucoceles do not show gadolinium enhancement, and variably demonstrate high T2 with low T1 signal.[4] Despite this variability, MRI can be of use when characterizing frontal sinus mucoceles, especially when other neoplastic causations for the expansion or dehiscence need to be excluded, and the extent and contents of extra-sinus expansion are to be determined. Furthermore, MRI is superior to CT for characterizing dural/brain tissue and intraorbital soft tissue that is immediately adjacent to a mucocele.[4]

26.6 Classification

A radiological classification that is often referenced for frontal sinus mucoceles is presented in ▶ Table 26.2.

This classification is based on progressive enlargement of a mucocele and associated patterns of bony erosion. The senior author has published an alternative classification (based on CT) in order to define the position of the mucocele as related to frontal sinus in a parasagittal plane ▶ Fig. 26.2.[15]

Essentially, the position of the mucocele is classified according to the mucocele's *most medial position* on a parasagittal plane. Mucoceles presenting medial to the lamina papyracea are termed "medial," those presenting medial to orbital rim's medial third are "intermediate," and all other mucoceles lateral of this are termed "lateral." The classification has been recommended to aid

Table 26.2 A radiological classification of frontal sinus muco-coeles[16]

Classification	Radiological description
I	Limited to the frontal sinus ± orbital extension
II	Frontoethmoidal mucocele ± orbital extension
IIIa	Erosion of the posterior wall of the frontal sinus, minimal or no intracranial extension
IIIb	Erosion of the posterior wall, major intracranial extension
IV	Erosion of the anterior frontal sinus wall
Va	Erosion of both anterior and posterior frontal sinus walls, minimal or no intracranial extension
Vb	Erosion of both anterior and posterior frontal sinus walls, major intracranial extension

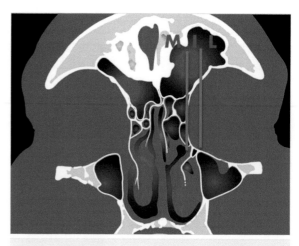

Fig. 26.2 Frontal sinus mucocele classification, based on most medial presentation in the parasagittal plane (M, medial; I, intermediate; L, lateral).

consistency in reporting of the position of frontal mucocele but in particular relevance to the management of frontal sinus mucoceles.

26.7 Management

Management of a frontal sinus mucocele is surgical. Given the potentially fatal consequences of extra-frontal extension, the surgical goals are decompression and marsupialization in the nasal cavity or paranasal sinuses. An important secondary consideration is to establish adequate drainage and prevent recurrence while minimizing associated morbidity. The agreed principle of frontal sinus mucocele surgery is to use the least destructive approach and technique possible, in order to maximize normal sinus function and therefore surgical success. In surgical management for frontal mucoceles, two factors are considered: surgical approach and size of frontal sinusotomy considered adequate for long-term drainage. Surgical approaches entail the least morbidity associated method to access the pathology or pathologies apparent in the patient's sinus and are categorized as external (transfacial or osteoplastic flap [OPF]) or endoscopic (transethmoidal, transnasal, or transseptal; ▶ Table 26.3). Having established surgical access to the pathologies, the secondary consideration in the surgical plan is determining the most adequate size of drainage pathway to maintain adequate long-term drainage.

The latter is an important consideration because we know that higher rates of frontal sinus outflow stenosis (due to scarring) and subsequent recurrence are associated with the more destructive procedures, especially the external and obliterative procedures.[7,16,17] Furthermore, the transnasal endoscopic approaches avoid inevitable facial scars, possible cosmetic deformity, and any risk to the supratrochlear and supraorbital nerves.[18,19]

Much before the advent of endoscopic surgery (around the turn of the 20th century), Riedel and other surgeons described various external procedures, with the common underlying principle of sinus mucosa obliteration. However, these ablative procedures were associated with generally unacceptable cosmetic deformity, morbidity, and recurrence rates. Despite this, Riedel's procedure is now still considered a terminal surgical option for especially difficult cases, when all other more conservative approaches (both external and endoscopic) have failed.[15] Similarly, although cranialization is another ablative procedure, it is still reserved for acute severe presentations of intracranial sepsis secondary to extra-frontal mucocele (often mucopyocele) extension.[22] Nonablative, external approaches include the Lynch–Howarth procedure and the coronal OPF. The Lynch–Howarth procedure is a frontoethmoidectomy with preservation of the sinus mucosa and stenting of the outflow tract (▶ Fig. 26.3b with stent and neo-osteogenesis). However, this approach has certain fundamental flaws as the approach entails drilling the anterior wall of the frontal drainage pathway and in turn compromises the integrity of the drainage pathway.[23] Although the OPF is also external, it offers better access to the frontal sinus while minimizing cosmetic deformity and retains the integrity of the frontal drainage pathway. Although this approach is by no means minimally invasive, it is the preferred external approach in the literature.[15,24,25]

Traditionally, the surgical approach to a frontal sinus mucocele was said to largely depend upon the mucocele's size, location within the sinus, and any associated extra-frontal extension. It would appear to be logical that large mucoceles with extra-frontal extension require an external approach. For example, cranialization has previously been strongly recommended for cases of intracranial extension.[26,27] However, this has since been disproven with various reports showing that such patients can in fact be

Table 26.3 Surgical approach and size of frontal sinusotomy

External procedures	Description
Lynch–Howarth procedure	External frontoethmoidectomy
Coronal osteoplastic flap	Osteoplastic frontal sinusotomy
Cranialization	Removal of the frontal sinus' posterior table and obliteration of its mucosa
Riedel's procedure	Removal of the frontal sinus' anterior table, floor, and obliteration of its mucosa
Others	Transverse eyebrow incision, frontal incision, modified lateral rhinotomy
Endoscopic procedures	**Description**
Draf procedures:	
1. Type I	Ethmoidectomy, including cell septa removal in frontal recess region, essentially widening the natural ostium
2. Type IIa	Frontal sinus floor resection between the lamina papyracea and the middle turbinate
3. Type IIb	Frontal sinus floor resection between the lamina and the nasal septum
4. Type III/"modified Lothrop"	Resection of both frontal sinus floors between the lamina papyracea, including resection of the upper nasal septum and frontal intersinus septum

managed with purely endoscopic techniques without the need for either anterior or posterior table reconstruction.[7,15,27,28] Similarly, endoscopic procedures have been shown to be adequate for cases of anterior table dehiscence.[15,29] Therefore, size and extra-frontal extension are relatively unimportant when choosing the surgical strategy. However, the location of the mucocele within the sinus is important, especially its most medial presenting component.[15] This is because this component considerably dictates the required endoscopic technique in order to achieve sufficient access to the mucocele. Also of high importance with reference to access and subsequent sinus drainage are the preoperative characteristics of the frontal sinus outflow tract, namely, the anteroposterior (AP) and lateromedial (LM) dimensions of the frontal sinus ostia (▶ Fig. 26.3), presence of type III/IV frontoethmoidal cells, presence and degree of osteitis or neo-osteogenesis (▶ Fig. 26.4), contralateral frontal sinus disease, and presence of concomitant sinus pathology.[15] These factors in combination with the previously described positional classification (▶ Fig. 26.2) are used as part of the editor's recommended management algorithm, which is shown in ▶ Table 26.4.[15]

Broadly speaking, this management algorithm shows that as the mucocele's most medial component lateralizes, a wider Draf procedure (i.e., more extensive endoscopic resection) is required. This is also the case for mucoceles associated with complicating variables related to the ostium (AP/LM dimensions, etc.). It also shows when a combined Draf III and OPF is indicated, higher in the surgical ladder.

Clearly, there is a wide range of influencing variables with regard to the chosen surgical strategy for frontal

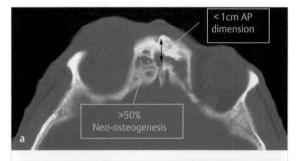
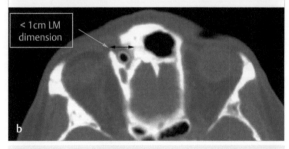

Fig. 26.3 (a) Narrow AP dimension of frontal drainage pathway with significant neo-osteogenesis; **(b)** CT scan of failed external frontoethmoidectomy procedure with stenting with limited LM dimension.

sinus mucoceles. It is therefore arguably impossible for a surgical ladder to be simple, while also including all of the preoperative characteristics to be taken into account in deciding the surgical plan. However, having used the algorithm extensively and considering the experience reported in the literature, the authors' management algorithm in ▶ Table 26.4 presents a useful aid planning surgery.[15]

Table 26.4 Management algorithm for frontal sinus mucoceles based on positional classification[15]

Complicating variables related to ostium	Position of mucocele's most medial component		
	Medial	Intermediate	Lateral
No complicating factors	Draf I/IIa	Draf IIa/IIb	Draf IIb/ III
AP/LM dimensions < 1 cm	Draf IIb	Draf III	Combined Draf III and OPF
Type III / IV FE cell			
> 50% neo-osteogenesis	Draf III	Combined Draf III and OPF	OPF

Special considerations (requiring one step up within the above algorithm)

1. Supraorbital mucocele
2. Mucocele secondary to significant pathology (osteoma/inverted papilloma/Pott's puffy tumor/Samter's triad)
3. Significant intracranial extension/involvement
4. Bilateral mucoceles/pathologies
5. Revision surgery

Indications for OPF, i.e., when an endoscopic approach may not be possible

1. Lateral mucocele with > 50% ostial neo-osteogenesis
2. In the presence of malignancy
3. Poor access to the supraorbital cell
4. Multiple (> 3) coexistent complicating variables, i.e., narrow AP/LM dimensions, etc.
5. When a concomitant pathology necessitates, e.g., grade III frontal osteoma

Abbreviations: AP/LM, anteroposterior/lateromedial; FE, frontoethmoidal; OPF, osteoplastic flap.

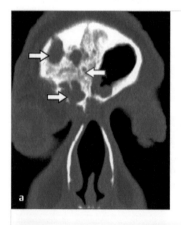
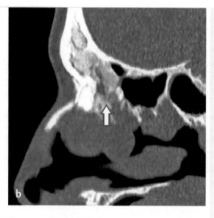
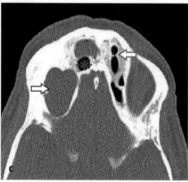
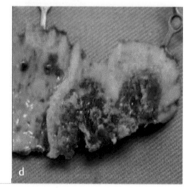

Fig. 26.4 (a–c) Coronal and sagittal CT scan examples of patients with significant neo-osteogenesis and osteitis. *Red arrow*: neo-osteogenesis and osteitis; *black arrows*: multiple mucoceles; *red asterisk*: posterior suprabulla cell. **(d)** Operative image of the frontal plate of frontal sinus in a case with osteoplastic flap demonstrating the new bone formation and osteitis.

26.8 Outcomes

Confirmed mucocele recurrence rates are inadequately reported in the literature. Various revision rates have been previously reported; however, these rates are often nonspecific as they are frequently reported as revision rates for frontal sinus surgery in general, or for all paranasal sinus mucoceles, that is, not specifically the frontal sinus. For example, Draf presented a series of 255 patients with paranasal sinus mucoceles with a revision rate of 1.6%; 51 of those 255 patients had frontal mucoceles.[20] Georgalas et al reported a series in which 122 patients underwent Draf III procedures for various pathologies; among these, paranasal sinus mucoceles had an overall revision rate of 5.6%.[21] More specific to the frontal sinus, Dhepnorrarat et al reported outcomes for 44 endoscopically treated frontoethmoidal mucoceles, with a revision rate of 5%, and a further 7% experienced stenosis with no further surgical intervention.[30] There are further examples with very similar revision rates, which include the editor's own experience. Therefore, although it is very difficult to comment on the true revision rate for frontal sinus mucoceles, it is likely to be somewhere in the range of greater than 0 to 10%.

Revision surgery is usually indicated for stenosis of the surgical neo-ostium, which is detected either through routine postoperative follow-up or more rarely due to recurrence of symptoms and mucocele. Stenosis of the neo-ostium increases the risk of mucocele recurrence, hence the necessity for revision surgery in the majority of cases. In the author's experience, risk factors for neo-ostial stenosis include all of the complicating variables highlighted in the management algorithm, hence their inclusion.[15] The algorithm also recommends that when revision surgery is required for a confirmed recurrent mucocele, a more aggressive approach is recommended.

26.9 Conclusion

A mucocele is a benign, epithelialized, mucus-filled sac. Paranasal sinus mucoceles are relatively uncommon; of these, frontal sinus mucoceles are the most common type. Presentation is often with orbital symptoms in the middle-aged. A frontal sinus mucocele is capable of expansion with subsequent bony dehiscence and extrafrontal extension. This extension can be subcutaneous, intraorbital, or intracranial; the latter is rare, but potentially dangerous. Clinical assessment includes a focused history and nasoendoscopic examination. Diagnosis of a frontal mucocele is radiological; CT is the first-line modality as it provides excellent osteological detail, relevant to surgical planning. MRI is useful in situations of diagnostic uncertainty, posterior or anterior wall dehiscence, and intraorbital/intracranial extension. The surgical aim is marsupialization and establishing adequate drainage pathway into nasal/paranasal cavity to avoid recurrence. Endoscopic techniques are considered first line and adequate for management of uncomplicated mucoceles. More extensive endoscopic and external approaches still have a place in very particular circumstances, although this is rare. Surgical escalation is required in certain situations, such as a lateral mucocele, compromised ostium dimensions, significant osteitis/neo-osteogenesis, and in revision cases. Repair of frontal sinus wall dehiscence is generally unnecessary. The surgical revision rate is approximately less than 20% and is not always representative of the true mucocele recurrence rate and also stenosis of frontal outflow tract.[20,21,30]

References

[1] Lund VJ, Milroy CM. Fronto-ethmoidal mucocoeles: a histopathological analysis. J Laryngol Otol. 1991; 105(11):921–923

[2] Arrué P, Kany MT, Serrano E, et al. Mucoceles of the paranasal sinuses: uncommon location. J Laryngol Otol. 1998; 112(9):840–844

[3] Lund V. Mucocoeles. In: Gleeson, ed. Scott-Brown's Otorhinolaryngology, Head and Neck Surgery. Vol. 2. London: Hodder Arnold; 2008:1531–1538

[4] Lloyd G, Lund VJ, Savy L, Howard D. Optimum imaging for mucoceles. J Laryngol Otol. 2000; 114(3):233–236

[5] Navarro JAC, Navarro JdL, Navarro PdL. Frontal sinus. In: The Nasal Cavity and Paranasal Sinuses. Berlin: Springer; 2001:83–91

[6] Watelet JB, Van Cauwenberge P. Applied anatomy and physiology of the nose and paranasal sinuses. Allergy. 1999; 54 Suppl 57:14–25

[7] Har-El G. Endoscopic management of 108 sinus mucoceles. Laryngoscope. 2001; 111(12):2131–2134

[8] Diaz F, Latchow R, Duvall AJ, III, Quick CA, Erickson DL. Mucoceles with intracranial and extracranial extensions. Report of two cases. J Neurosurg. 1978; 48(2):284–288

[9] Har-El G, Balwally AN, Lucente FE. Sinus mucoceles: is marsupialization enough? Otolaryngol Head Neck Surg. 1997; 117(6):633–640

[10] Busaba NY, Salman SD. Ethmoid mucocele as a late complication of endoscopic ethmoidectomy. Otolaryngol Head Neck Surg. 2003; 128 (4):517–522

[11] Brook I, Frazier EH. The microbiology of mucopyocele. Laryngoscope. 2001; 111(10):1771–1773

[12] Stiernberg CM, Bailey BJ, Calhoun KH, Quinn FB. Management of invasive frontoethmoidal sinus mucoceles. Arch Otolaryngol Head Neck Surg. 1986; 112(10):1060–1063

[13] Lund VJ, Henderson B, Song Y. Involvement of cytokines and vascular adhesion receptors in the pathology of fronto-ethmoidal mucoceles. Acta Otolaryngol. 1993; 113(4):540–546

[14] Lund VJ, Harvey W, Meghji S, Harris M. Prostaglandin synthesis in the pathogenesis of fronto-ethmoidal mucoceles. Acta Otolaryngol. 1988; 106(1-2):145–151

[15] Sama A, McClelland L, Constable J. Frontal sinus mucoceles: new algorithm for surgical management. Rhinology. 2014; 52(3):267–275

[16] Har-El G. Transnasal endoscopic management of frontal mucoceles. Otolaryngol Clin North Am. 2001; 34(1):243–251

[17] Iro H, Hosemann W. Minimally invasive surgery in otorhinolaryngology. Eur Arch Otorhinolaryngol. 1993; 250(1):1–10

[18] Kennedy DW, Josephson JS, Zinreich SJ, Mattox DE, Goldsmith MM. Endoscopic sinus surgery for mucoceles: a viable alternative. Laryngoscope. 1989; 99(9):885–895

[19] Wigand ME, Hosemann WG. Endoscopic surgery for frontal sinusitis and its complications. Am J Rhinol Allergy. 1991; 5:85–89

[20] Bockmühl U, Kratzsch B, Benda K, Draf W. Surgery for paranasal sinus mucocoeles: efficacy of endonasal micro-endoscopic management and long-term results of 185 patients. Rhinology. 2006; 44(1):62–67

[21] Georgalas C, Hansen F, Videler WJM, Fokkens WJ. Long terms results of Draf type III (modified endoscopic Lothrop) frontal sinus drainage

procedure in 122 patients: a single centre experience. Rhinology. 2011; 49(2):195–201

[22] Kamani T, Sama A. Frontal sinus mucoceles. Otorhinolarngol.. 2016; 9:65–68

[23] Rubin JS, Lund VJ, Salmon B. Frontoethmoidectomy in the treatment of mucoceles. A neglected operation. Arch Otolaryngol Head Neck Surg. 1986; 112(4):434–436

[24] Gavioli C, Grasso DL, Carinci F, Amoroso C, Pastore A. Mucoceles of the frontal sinus. Clinical and therapeutical considerations. Minerva Stomatol. 2002; 51(9):385–390

[25] Schmerber S, Cuisnier O, Delalande C, Verougstraete G, Reyt E. [Surgical strategy in paranasal sinus mucoceles]. Rev Laryngol Otol Rhinol (Bord). 2002; 123(2):93–97

[26] Delfini R, Missori P, Iannetti G, Ciappetta P, Cantore G. Mucoceles of the paranasal sinuses with intracranial and intraorbital extension:

report of 28 cases. Neurosurgery. 1993; 32(6):901–906, discussion 906

[27] Maliszewski M, Ladziński P, Kaspera W, Majchrzak K. Mucocoele and mucopyocoele of the frontal sinus penetrating to the cranial cavity and the orbit. Neurol Neurochir Pol. 2011; 45(4):342–350

[28] Hurley DB, Javer AR, Kuhn FA, Citardi MJ. The endoscopic management of chronic frontal sinusitis associated with frontal sinus posterior table erosion. Am J Rhinol. 2000; 14(2):113–120

[29] Woodworth BA, Harvey RJ, Neal JG, Palmer JN, Schlosser RJ. Endoscopic management of frontal sinus mucoeceles with anterior table erosion. Rhinology. 2008; 46(3):231–237

[30] Dhepnorrarat RC, Subramaniam S, Sethi DS. Endoscopic surgery for fronto-ethmoidal mucoceles: a 15-year experience. Otolaryngol Head Neck Surg. 2012; 147(2):345–350

27 Frontoethmoidal Osteomas

Christos Georgalas and Edward Hadjihannas

Abstract

Osteomas of the frontal and ethmoid sinuses have traditionally been surgically removed via external approaches. However, over the last 25 years, endoscopic techniques have increasingly been used for the surgical management of selected cases. Advances in visualization and instrumentation as well as the excellent access provided by Draf type III (median drainage/endoscopic modified Lothrop) procedure expanded the reach of endoscopes. Currently, the vast majority of frontal sinus osteomas can be managed endoscopically, with the exception of those with significant anterior or extreme inferolateral extension.

Keywords: frontal sinus, ethmoid sinus, osteoma, fibro-osseous tumors, ethmoid, osteoplastic flap, frontal sinusotomy

27.1 Epidemiology and Etiology

Osteomas are benign, slow-growing bone tumors with the consistency of well-differentiated mature, compact, or cancellous bone. Two CT radiological studies of 1,500[1] and 1,889[2,3] patients respectively, have demonstrated that osteomas are the most common benign tumors of the paranasal sinuses with a point prevalence of 3%.

The variable male-to-female ratio is 1.3:1[1] to 1.5:1[2,3] and their peak incidence is between the fourth and sixth decade, with an average age at presentation of 50 years.[1,2]

The majority of osteomas (58[1] to 68%[3]) are found in the frontal sinus (37% arise in the immediate vicinity of the nasofrontal duct and 21% above and lateral to the frontal ostium).[1] The second most common area are the ethmoid sinuses. The maxillary sinuses are involved in less than 20% of cases, and the sphenoid sinuses are rarely involved.[1] Gardner's syndrome or familial adenomatous polyposis is an autosomal dominant condition consisting of multiple osteomas together with soft-tissue tumors (including skin cysts and desmoid tumors) as well as large intestine polyps that have a propensity for malignant transformation.[4] Gastroenterology referral is strongly recommended because osteomas can appear an average of 17 years before the intestinal polyps[5] (see ▶ Table 27.1).

The three main pathogenetic theories surrounding the etiology of osteomas are the developmental, traumatic, and infective (▶ Fig. 27.1).[6,7] The developmental theory as proposed by Hallberg[7] states that osteomas arise from stem cells of the junctional area between the frontal and ethmoid bone. This theory is reinforced by the fact that osteomas frequently occur at the frontoethmoid suture line where the frontal sinus (membranous bone) borders the ethmoid labyrinth (endochondral ossification). Still this theory does not justify the presence of osteomas in other anatomical locations. The traumatic theory as proposed by Gerber[51] advocates that the development of osteomas occurs as a result of an abnormal proliferative response to trauma. This is supported by the fact that the incidence of osteomas is higher in men and they grow more frequently during puberty, which is the period when the rate of skeletal development is at its peak.[8] Conversely, most osteomas are detected later in life and the great majority of patients do not report any history of trauma. Also, there is no evidence to suggest an increased incidence of osteomas in patients subjected to multiple endoscopic sinus surgery procedures. The infective theory proposes that osteomas may arise due to stimulating osteoblasts within the mucoperiosteal lining of the sinus, which in turn may become secondarily calcified. Most osteomas (63%) seem to appear in healthy noninfected sinuses, even though a link between

Table 27.1 Epidemiology of sinonasal osteomas

Prevalence	Gender	Age	Location
3%	Male > female	4th–6th decade	Frontal sinus Ethmoid sinus Maxillary sinus Sphenoid sinus

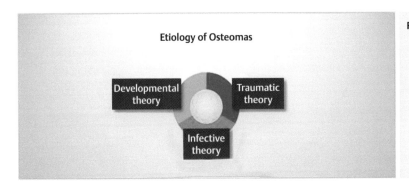

Fig. 27.1 Etiological theories of osteomas.

osteomas and sinusitis has been described.[2] There are also some other theories that suggest that osteomas may be osteodysplastic lesions, osteogenic hamartomas, embryonic bone rests, or the result of ossification of sinus polyps, but none of those have been validated[4].

27.2 Histology

Macroscopically, osteomas are round or oval, hard, ivory-white, bosselated, well-circumscribed lesions attached to the underlying bone by a broad base or occasionally by a small stalk and covered by a thin layer of fibrous periosteum.[6] Histologically, osteomas can be classified into three types: ivory or compact, mature or cancellous or spongiotic, and mixed[7]. Ivory osteomas usually have a sessile base and are characterized by hard bone with a thick matrix containing only a small amount of fibrous tissue and minimal marrow; cancellous osteomas have often a pedunculated base and are composed of cancellous bone with intertrabecular hematopoietic bone marrow or fat; mixed osteomas share characteristics from both types[6,7] (▶ Fig. 27.2).

In a study of 13 osteomas with serial radiographs, average growth rate was 1.61 mm/y, ranging from 0.44 to 6.00 mm/y.[8] According to some studies, most osteomas seem to rarely recur even if incompletely removed.[9] Nevertheless, other studies have shown that, given enough time, osteomas can recur,[10,11] even with accelerating growth following incomplete removal.[12] Malignant

transformation in osteomas is unheard of and are not to be considered neoplastic lesions.[7]

27.3 Clinical Presentation and Investigations

Osteomas are mostly asymptomatic as they grow slowly and their diagnosis is incidental. There is only a small percentage (4[1] to 10%[13]) of osteomas that present with clinical symptoms such as pressure or headache.[14,15] Such symptoms can be caused directly by the lesion itself, or indirectly by impaired drainage of the frontal sinus associated with chronic rhinosinusitis. Osteomas of the frontoethmoidal region tend to be linked with earlier symptoms. The incidence of headache in various osteoma series varies between 52[16] and 100%[14] (see ▶ Table 27.1).

Osteomas extending beyond the boundaries of the sinuses can create an external deformity[17] (▶ Fig. 27.3a, b) with occasional eyelid ptosis[18] and may result in orbital pain and proptosis, together with diplopia and chemosis if the orbital muscles are involved.[19,20,21] Also, compression or obstruction of the nasolacrimal duct can result in epiphora[22,23] (▶ Fig. 27.4). On rare occasions, compression of the optic nerve will lead to visual acuity impairment.[24,25] Complete obstruction of a sinus ostium by an osteoma may lead to secondary formation of mucocele.[26,27] Finally, intracranial extension of osteomas can cause intracranial mucoceles, meningitis, cerebral abscesses,[26,28] or tension pneumocephalus[29] (▶ Fig. 27.5a, b).

The investigation of choice for osteomas is thin-sliced computed tomography (CT), which can determine the size and location of the lesion, as well as associated sinus pathology. Characteristically on CT, osteomas appear as well-circumscribed masses of heterogeneous consistency with a high signal component when hyperostotic and a low signal component when spongiotic (▶ Fig. 27.6). The lower signal components may be confused with associated mucoceles. Magnetic resonance imaging (MRI) can be useful in cases of complications, including intracranial or intraorbital.

27.4 Management

The management of asymptomatic osteomas is controversial, in contrast with symptomatic ones, where surgical excision is universally considered to be the treatment of

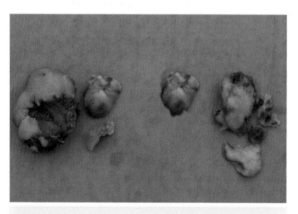

Fig. 27.2 A typical osteoma removed in pieces via an endonasal approach.

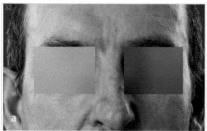
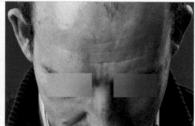
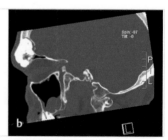

Fig. 27.3 (a, b) A frontal osteoma extending through the anterior frontal plate and displacing the orbit inferoanteriorly. This was removed via an external osteoplastic approach.

choice unless there are serious contraindications. Asymptomatic, small osteomas are usually watched and periodically monitored radiologically. Frontal sinus osteomas that appear to grow or occupy more than 50% of the sinus need surgical excision.[30] The same is suggested for osteomas that breach the boundaries of the sinus and those obstructing the nasofrontal duct. Concomitant chronic sinusitis, ethmoid sinus involvement associated complications (mucocele, orbital symptoms, neurological symptoms, external deformity), and headaches inexplicable from other etiologies are also indications for surgery[31] (see ▶ Fig. 27.7).

27.5 Approaches for Frontoethmoidal Osteomas

27.5.1 External Approaches

- *Lynch approach:* This approach, otherwise described as external frontoethmoidectomy approach (Lynch procedure), although relatively simple, does not provide adequate access, while it is usually associated with a visible scar and is not used by the authors.[32] This has

been used for small, medially and inferiorly situated frontal osteomas. Even though it is simple and fast to perform, it can be complicated by an unsightly scar, a high rate frontal recess stenosis, and does not allow access to laterally based lesions.[33]

- *Osteoplastic flap approach:* This approach, as popularized by Goodale and Montgomery, has been in use for more than 40 years[34] and has been the most widely used technique for frontal sinus osteomas (Case 2). Its main advantage is that it offers a wide access to all anatomical sides of the frontal sinus except perhaps from its inferomedial part to the nasofrontal duct and into the ethmoids. The disadvantage of this approach is its invasiveness, which can cause occasional morbidity such as hemorrhage, postoperative frontal pain, paresthesia, or anesthesia from supraorbital nerve damage, impaired cosmesis, and less commonly cerebrospinal fluid (CSF) leak and meningitis. If it is paired with obliteration of the frontal sinus it requires an abdominal incision for fat harvesting and carries the risk of late mucocele formation, which can be as high as 9% after 2 years.[35] However, in most of our cases it has proven to be a reliable approach, with minimal complications and with a scar that is practically invisible.

- *Endoscopic approach:* Endoscopic approaches to the nose and paranasal sinuses were introduced in the 1980s and by the early 1990s the first cases of endoscopic management of ethmoid osteomas were published.[36,37] The accumulating experience with endoscopic surgery improved optics and image quality as well as the design of better endoscopic instruments and high-speed drills as well as the introduction of imaging navigation expanded the indications for endoscopic approaches. Draf[38] revolutionized the management of frontal sinus pathologies including osteomas and laid the foundations of modern endoscopic frontal sinus surgery. In particular, Draf III procedure[39] (endoscopic modified Lothrope,[40] bilateral frontal sinus drillout,[41] and median drainage procedure,[42]) provides the widest possible transnasal access to the frontal sinus (Case 1).

27.5.2 Endoscopic Approaches

As with most surgical techniques, grade 1 or 2 evidence is missing; however, grade 3 evidence can be collected using case series and retrospective cohorts. The evolution

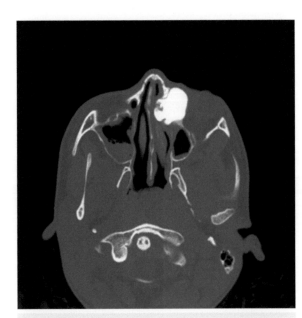

Fig. 27.4 An osteoma presenting with epiphora—the osteoma has completely obstructed the nasolacrimal duct. This was removed via a combined transconjunctival–endoscopic approach.

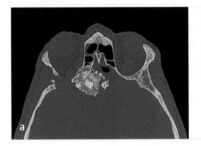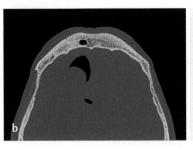

Fig. 27.5 (a, b) An intracranially extending osteoma that presented with cerebrospinal fluid rhinorrhea and pneumocephalus.

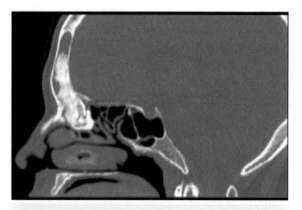

Fig. 27.6 Note the different types of bone contained in the osteoma—resulting in different appearance in the CT.

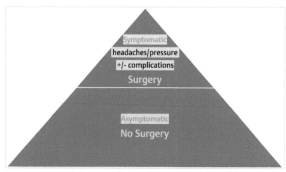

Fig. 27.7 Indications for surgery in osteomas.

Table 27.2 Frontal sinus osteoma grading system[44]

Grade I	Base of attachment is posteroinferior along the frontal recess. Tumor is medial to a virtual sagittal plane through the lamina papyracea. Anteroposterior diameter of the lesion is < 75% of the anteroposterior dimension of the frontal recess
Grade II	Base of attachment is posteroinferior along the frontal recess. Tumor is medial to a virtual sagittal plane through the lamina papyracea. Anteroposterior diameter of the lesion is > 75% of the anteroposterior dimension of the frontal recess
Grade III	Base of attachment is anterior or superiorly located within the frontal sinus AND/OR tumor extends lateral to a virtual sagittal plane through the lamina papyracea
Grade IV	Tumor fills the entire frontal sinus

of these indications testifies to the progress affected in endoscopic surgery over the last decades.

Draf in his seminal paper on the Fulda concept in 1991 suggested that any "large osteoma" was not amenable to an endoscopic approach and should be dealt with via an osteoplastic flap approach.[43]

Since then, a number of series of at least five patients with osteomas were published.

Schick et al in 2001 were the first to publish large series of sinonasal osteomata treated endoscopically (35 patients) suggesting specific exclusion criteria for endoscopic removal.[14] However, the first systematic attempt to codify the limits of endoscopic resection was by Chiu et al in 2005.[44] Drawing from their experience with nine osteomas between 1999 and 2003, they developed a grading system maintaining that only grade 1 and 2 osteomata can be removed endoscopically (see ▶ Table 27.2).

This grading system suggests that endoscopic removal of an osteoma is not feasible if:

- The base of its attachment in the frontal sinus is anteriorly or superiorly.
- There is lateral extension to a virtual sagittal plane through the lamina papyracea.
- It completely obliterates the frontal sinus.

Castelnuovo et al[16] and Bignami et al[45] suggested that the limits of endoscopic removal include orbital and intracranial extension, extension lateral to a sagittal plane through the lamina papyracea, erosion of the anterior and posterior wall, and a diameter less than 10 mm anteroposteriorly of the frontal sinus.

Endoscopic surgery has been evolving at a very fast pace, and a number of surgeons have challenged these assumptions. Just a year after the publication of the Chiu et al classification, Dubin and Kuhn[32] published their results of successful endoscopic removal of five grade III tumors—either attached superoanteriorly in the frontal sinus or extending lateral to the plane of the lamina

papyracea. In this article, an osteoplastic flap was recommended only for removal of tumors with greater than 2 cm vertical extension into the frontal sinus or occupancy of 100% of the frontal sinus.

In 2009, Seiberling et al[15] reported their results of 23 patients with varying sizes of frontal sinus osteomas treated endoscopically that included eight patients with a grade IV tumor and six patients with a grade III tumor. A Draf III procedure was used for 15 of these tumors (including all grade 3 and 4 tumors). In four out of eight grade 4 (filling the entire frontal sinus) tumors, a residual was left toward the posterior frontal plate, as it was felt that the risk of penetrating the dura was too high. In two cases, a second procedure was necessary for the complete removal of the tumor, while in one patient with extensive orbital extension, an external blepharoplasty incision was used and an extended trephine incision in another.

In 2010, Ledderose et al[46] proposed that, in carefully selected individual cases, it is possible to remove grade 3 and even grade 4 osteomas endonasally. They described the endoscopic removal of eight osteomas, three of which would have been classified nonresectable endoscopically according to the Chiu et al classification: specifically, two grade 3 tumors were removed via a Draf IIb approach and a grade 4 tumor via a Draf III approach.[44]

In 2011, Gil-Carcedo et al[47] suggested that frontal sinus osteomas are frequently diagnosed as incidental findings on CT scans and no firm criteria have been established to determine the need for surgery. They therefore proposed a revised osteoma classification based on CT appearance, together with clinical symptoms when present.

What we know now is that, while there is no number of external approaches that can prove the limits of endoscopic surgery, a small number of endoscopic approaches (replicated in more than one centers) can shatter the myth of "unresectability."

More recently in 2012 Turri-Zanoni et al[48] reported on 60 frontoethmoidal osteomas that were treated surgically. The lesion involved the far lateral portion of the frontal sinus in 23 cases and the orbital region in 6 cases. In 31 cases, a purely endoscopic approach was performed, while a combined procedure was used in 25 patients. Only in 4 patients, an exclusively external approach was required and resectability was achieved in all but 2 cases. That supports once more that the size of the osteoma, lateral extension of the tumor in the frontal sinus beyond the lamina papyracea, and intraorbital involvement are no longer absolute contraindications for an exclusively transnasal endoscopic resection.

We propose that it is not the anteroposterior diameter or the lateral extension of the osteoma that defines its resectability endoscopically, but rather the relation between the interorbital distance, the anteroposterior diameter of the frontal beak, and the lateral height of the frontal sinus. We have attempted to codify our experience with endoscopic approach to osteomas as follows (See ▶ Table 27.2[50]):

- **Lateral extent:** Using the wide access provided by a Draf III procedure and curved drills, it is possible to access the lateral supraorbital ridge, well beyond the medial orbit. We maintain that it is neither the plane of lamina papyracea nor the 2 cm lateral to it that define the lateral limits of respectability, but rather the ratio of lateral tumor extension to interorbital distance. Following the removal of the superior septum and the drilling of the nasal beak, lateral access to the frontal sinus is restricted primarily by the orbital walls. In patients with relative large intercanthal distance the lateral access that can be gained is increased, while the opposite is true for narrow nasal inlet. Lateral access to the floor of the frontal sinus (orbital roof) may, however, be limited.[49]
- **Large tumors attached to the posterior/superior frontal walls/more than 2 cm superiorly in the frontal sinus:** Similarly, tumors extending superiorly, to the posterior frontal plate—or associated with complete opacification of the frontal sinus—can also be removed endoscopically. The process of removing such tumors is generally time-consuming, and drills often fail and need replacing. The

development of more robust, higher speed curved drills in the future may further facilitate the removal of such large laterally located osteomas.
- **Orbital extension:** Orbital extension is not in itself a contraindication for endonasal approach: However, additional incisions may be required if the tumor extends anteriorly.[15] It is rather the anterior extension (anterior to the nasolacrimal duct) than the orbital extension that should determine the need for an additional external incision. In most cases, the external approach can be performed via a subconjunctival incision, with no cosmetic consequences.
- **Intracranial extension:** Limited endocranial extension does not always preclude the use of the endoscope. As one progresses to manage intracranial/intradural tumors endoscopically, the limitation of posterior wall erosion/endocranial extension sounds irrelevant, provided that the removal is done in combination with a endoscopically trained neurosurgeon.
- **Anterior extension:** The one limitation to endonasal approaches that seems to withstand the test of time is anterior extension. Extension of the tumor through the anterior frontal plate is usually physically impossible to access endoscopically, while the associated bony defect and deformity necessitate an external approach for reconstruction (▶ Table 27.3).

27.6 Summary

Advantages of the endoscopic approach include better visualization of anatomical structures, absence of scars, smaller traumatic impact along the direct approach and hence, reduction of postoperative morbidity, preservation of the physiologic mucociliary drainage, less bleeding, and a shorter hospital stay. However, the endoscopic approach can make more difficult the management of potential intraoperative complications (massive bleeding, intracranial complications, CSF leak) and requires significant time commitment (for large osteomas, significantly more than an external approach) and highly sophisticated surgical tools.

The endoscopic removal of osteomas is a procedure that should not be undertaken lightly. Significant experience in all frontal sinus approaches including Draf type III sinusotomy is required, together with great facility in the use of the drill endonasally. Although temporal bone drilling is part of the curriculum in most residency programs, the development of similar skills for drilling in the anterior skull base is not required and rarely acquired during the training. As endoscopic sinus surgery comes of age, expectantly the skills required will be more widely shared. A new generation of surgeons will be moving forward the frontiers of endoscopic surgery, and hopefully what are today the "frontiers" of endonasal surgery will be standard procedures tomorrow.

Table 27.3 Contraindications to the endoscopic approach according to different studies

Anatomic limitations	Schick et al[14]	Chiu et al[44]	Dubin and Kuhn[32]	Bignami et al[45]	Castelnuovo et al[16]	Seiberling et al[15]	Ledderose et al[46]	Turri-Zanoni et al[48]	Georgalas et al[50]
Attachment anterior frontal plate		Yes			Yes			No	Yes (when associated with large defect or very high attachment)
Attachment posterior frontal plate					Yes	No (may need to leave remnant)		No (may need to leave remnant)	No
Attachment superior frontal sinus		Yes				No	No		No
Less than 1 cm frontal sinus diameter	Yes			Yes	Yes				Relative
Extension more than 2 cm superiorly in frontal sinus			Yes			No	No		No
Lateral to lamina papyracea sagittal plane	Yes			Yes	Yes	No	No	No	No
2 cm lateral to orbit						No	No	No	No
Erosion of anterior table	Yes			Yes	Yes				Yes
Complete obstruction of frontal recess			Yes			No	No	No	No
Complete opacification of frontal sinus		Yes				No			No
Intracranial extension/erosion of posterior table	Yes			Yes	Yes				No
Extension anterior to nasolacrimal duct									Yes
(Significant) orbital extension	Yes			Yes		No (may require additional incision)		No	No

27.7 Case Examples

27.7.1 Case 1

A 69-year-old lady has been suffering from left frontal headaches and associated episodes of left orbital cellulitis for more than 10 years. She was known with a left frontoethmoidal osteoma that was occluding the left frontal recess and was associated with a concurrent left frontal mucocele. An attempt to remove it via a Lynch approach in 1995 in another institution resulted in a significant and growing residual. A CT shows an osteoma of 2.3-cm maximal diameter completely obstructing the left frontal recess (► Fig. 27.8a, b). A Draf III approach was performed and the osteoma was drilled out using a fast 70-degree rough diamond drill. Any remnants attached to the skull base

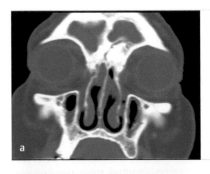
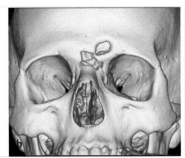

Fig. 27.8 **(a)** A coronal CT sinus of a residual frontoethmoid osteoma after a previous open approach. **(b)** A reconstruction of the anterior frontal plate, after the previous attempt elsewhere at a removal via a Lynch–Howarth approach.

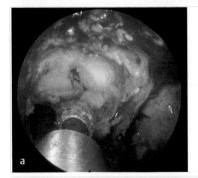
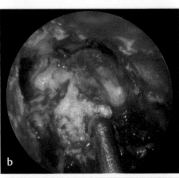
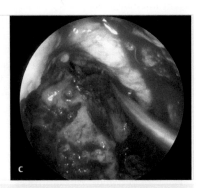

Fig. 27.9 **(a)** Drilling of the osteoma using a 70-degree rough diamond fast drill. **(b)** Removal of the final remnants of the osteoma from the anterior skull base. **(c)** Use of a laterally based flap for the Draf III neo-ostium.

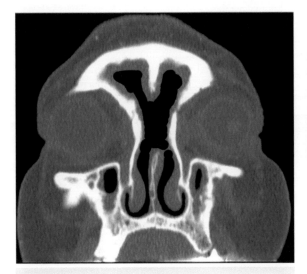

Fig. 27.10 Coronal CT sinus after removal.

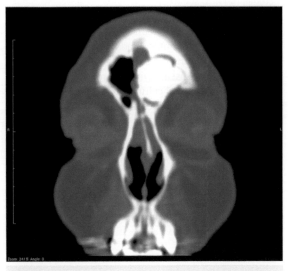

Fig. 27.11 Coronal CT sinus of a giant frontal osteoma with erosion of the posterior frontal plate and attachment to the lateral roof of the orbit.

were gently removed after mobilization. A laterally based flap was raised and then placed on the neo-ostium to prevent stenosis (▶ Fig. 27.9). A subsequent CT sinus shows a complete removal of the osteoma (▶ Fig. 27.10).

27.7.2 Case 2

A 50-year-old lady with known CRS with nasal polyps (CRSwNP) had been complaining of left frontal headaches for

the last 6 years. Subsequent CT sinus confirmed the presence of a growing osteoma of the left frontal sinus, with erosion of both the anterior and the posterior frontal table as well as the orbital roof (▶ Fig. 27.11). As the osteoma was attached to the roof of the orbit and to the posterosuperior frontal sinus, a decision was taken to remove it via an osteoplastic flap approach (▶ Fig. 27.12a, b). This was performed, and although the posterior frontal sinus plate was eroded, there was no dural tear or CSF leak. A subsequent CT sinus showed a complete removal of the osteoma (▶ Fig. 27.13).

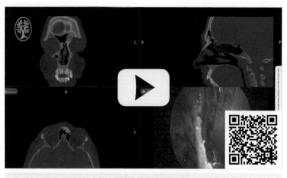

Video 27.1 Case 3 – Draf III for a frontal osteoma

27.7.3 Case 3

A 40-year-old male presented with a 2-year history of left frontal headaches and intermittent episodes of acute frontal sinusitis. On CT there was evidence of an osteoma occupying more than 50% of the left frontal sinus, with extension and attachment to the orbital roof and the posterior frontal sinus wall (▶ Fig. 27.14a). A decision was made to remove via a Draf III approach. As the left frontal ostium was obstructed by the tumor, an outside–in approach was chosen (▶ Fig. 27.14b). The wide interorbital and anteroposterior distance of the frontal neo-ostium provided adequate access for the complete removal of the osteoma (Video 27.1 and ▶ Fig. 27.14c, d).

27.7.4 Case 4

A 35-year-old male presented with a giant frontal osteoma, measuring more than 4 cm and occupying both right and left frontal sinuses, extending beyond the

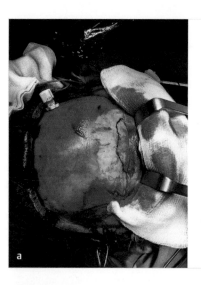
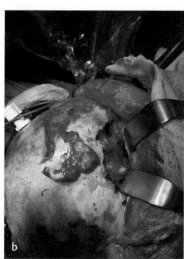

Fig. 27.12 (a) Planning of the osteoplastic flap using navigation. **(b)** Removal of the osteoma.

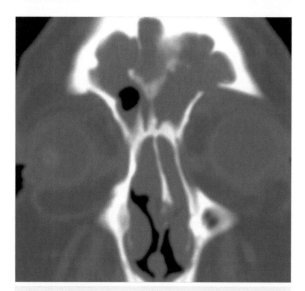

Fig. 27.13 Postoperative result: CT sinus.

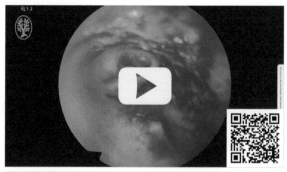

Video 27.2 Endoscopic removal of a giant frontal sinus osteoma

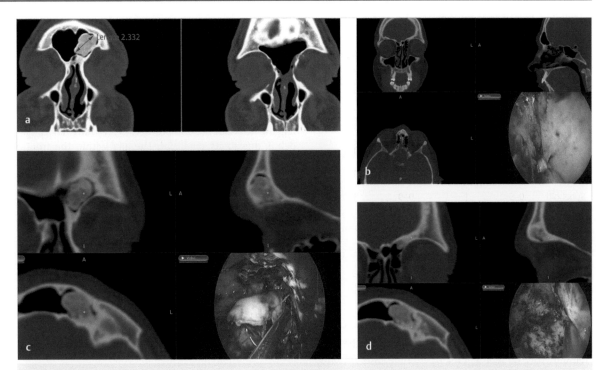

Fig. 27.14 **(a)** Pre- and postoperative CT sinus of the complete endoscopic removal of a frontal sinus osteoma attached to the posterior orbital roof and the posterior frontal plate. **(b)** Intraoperative neuronavigation image showing the neurovascular bundle of the septal branch of the anterior ethmoidal artery, the ethmoidal nerve and vessels pointing to the anterior skull base (outside – in Draf III approach). **(c)** Intraoperative neuronavigation image of the removal of the final part of the osteoma attached to the supraorbital recess. **(d)** Intraoperative neuronavigation image after complete removal – note the lateral extend of access to the frontal sinus/supraorbital recess.

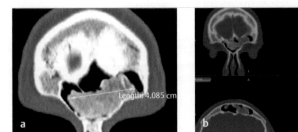 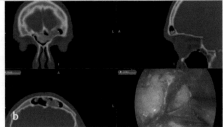 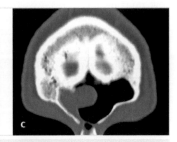

Fig. 27.15 **(a)** A preoperative CT of a giant frontal osteoma measuring 4 cm, occupying right and left frontal sinuses, extending beyond the midline of the left orbit and attached to both the posterior frontal wall and the superior wall of the orbit. **(b)** A Draf III was performed and the osteoma was drilled out and gently removed in pieces from its attachments laterly and posteriorly. **(c)** A postoperative CT confirming complete removal.

midline of the left orbit and attached to the posterior frontal plate (Fig 27.15a). The favorable frontal recess anatomy (wide interorbital and anteroposterior distance) made feasible the complete endoscopic removal via a Draf III approach (Fig. 27.15b, c; Video 27.2).

References

[1] Earwaker J. Paranasal sinus osteomas: a review of 46 cases. Skeletal Radiol. 1993; 22(6):417–423

[2] Erdogan N, Demir U, Songu M, Ozenler NK, Uluç E, Dirim B. A prospective study of paranasal sinus osteomas in 1,889 cases: changing patterns of localization. Laryngoscope. 2009; 119(12):2355–2359

[3] McHugh JB, Mukherji SK, Lucas DR. Sino-orbital osteoma: a clinicopathologic study of 45 surgically treated cases with emphasis on tumors with osteoblastoma-like features. Arch Pathol Lab Med. 2009; 133(10):1587–1593

[4] Gómez García EB, Knoers NVAM. Gardner's syndrome (familial adenomatous polyposis): a cilia-related disorder. Lancet Oncol. 2009; 10(7):727–735

[5] Alexander AAZ, Patel AA, Odland R. Paranasal sinus osteomas and Gardner's syndrome. Ann Otol Rhinol Laryngol. 2007; 116(9):658–662

[6] Eller R, Sillers M. Common fibro-osseous lesions of the paranasal sinuses. Otolaryngol Clin North Am. 2006; 39(3):585–600, x

[7] Hallberg OE, Begley JW, Jr. Origin and treatment of osteomas of the paranasal sinuses. Arch Otolaryngol. 1950; 51(5):750–760

[8] Cutilli BJ, Quinn PD. Traumatically induced peripheral osteoma. Report of a case. Oral Surg Oral Med Oral Pathol. 1992; 73(6):667–669

[9] Nielsen GP, Rosenberg AE. Update on bone forming tumors of the head and neck. Head Neck Pathol. 2007; 1(1):87–93

[10] Fu YS, Perzin KH. Non-epithelial tumors of the nasal cavity, paranasal sinuses, and nasopharynx. A clinicopathologic study. II. Osseous and fibro-osseous lesions, including osteoma, fibrous dysplasia, ossifying fibroma, osteoblastoma, giant cell tumor, and osteosarcoma. Cancer. 1974; 33(5):1289–1305

[11] Koivunen P, Löppönen H, Fors AP, Jokinen K. The growth rate of osteomas of the paranasal sinuses. Clin Otolaryngol Allied Sci. 1997; 22(2):111–114

[12] Larrea-Oyarbide N, Valmaseda-Castellón E, Berini-Aytés L, Gay-Escoda C. Osteomas of the craniofacial region. Review of 106 cases. J Oral Pathol Med. 2008; 37(1):38–42

[13] Eckel W, Palm D. Statistical and roentgenological studies on some problems of osteoma of the paranasal sinuses. Arch Ohren Nasen Kehlkopfheilkd. 1959; 174:440–457

[14] Schick B, Steigerwald C, el Rahman el Tahan A, Draf W. The role of endonasal surgery in the management of frontoethmoidal osteomas. Rhinology. 2001; 39(2):66–70

[15] Seiberling K, Floreani S, Robinson S, Wormald P-J. Endoscopic management of frontal sinus osteomas revisited. Am J Rhinol Allergy. 2009; 23(3):331–336

[16] Castelnuovo P, Valentini V, Giovannetti F, Bignami M, Cassoni A, Iannetti G. Osteomas of the maxillofacial district: endoscopic surgery versus open surgery. J Craniofac Surg. 2008; 19(6):1446–1452

[17] Baykul T, Heybeli N, Oyar O, Doğru H. Multiple huge osteomas of the mandible causing disfigurement related with Gardner's syndrome: case report. Auris Nasus Larynx. 2003; 30(4):447–451

[18] Ata N, Tezer MS, Koç E, Övet G, Erdur Ö. Large frontoorbital osteoma causing ptosis. J Craniofac Surg. 2017; 28(1):e17–e18

[19] Tsai C-J, Ho C-Y, Lin C-Z. A huge osteoma of paranasal sinuses with intraorbital extension presenting as diplopia. J Chin Med Assoc. 2003; 66(7):433–435

[20] Gerbrandy SJF, Saeed P, Fokkens WJ. Endoscopic and trans-fornix removal of a giant orbital-ethmoidal osteoma. Orbit. 2007; 26(4):299–301

[21] Rawe SE, VanGilder JC. Surgical removal of orbital osteoma; case report. J Neurosurg. 1976; 44(2):233–236

[22] Osma U, Yaldiz M, Tekin M, Topcu I. Giant ethmoid osteoma with orbital extension presenting with epiphora. Rhinology. 2003; 41 (2):122–124

[23] Lin C-J, Lin Y-S, Kang B-H. Middle turbinate osteoma presenting with ipsilateral facial pain, epiphora, and nasal obstruction. Otolaryngol Head Neck Surg. 2003; 128(2):282–283

[24] Mansour AM, Salti H, Uwaydat S, Dakroub R, Bashshour Z. Ethmoid sinus osteoma presenting as epiphora and orbital cellulitis: case report and literature review. Surv Ophthalmol. 1999; 43(5):413–426

[25] Naraghi M, Kashfi A. Endonasal endoscopic resection of ethmoido-orbital osteoma compressing the optic nerve. Am J Otolaryngol. 2003; 24(6):408–412

[26] Shady JA, Bland LI, Kazee AM, Pilcher WH. Osteoma of the frontoethmoidal sinus with secondary brain abscess and intracranial mucocele: case report. Neurosurgery. 1994; 34(5):920–923, discussion 923

[27] Nabeshima K, Marutsuka K, Shimao Y, Uehara H, Kodama T. Osteoma of the frontal sinus complicated by intracranial mucocele. Pathol Int. 2003; 53(4):227–230

[28] Summers LE, Mascott CR, Tompkins JR, Richardson DE. Frontal sinus osteoma associated with cerebral abscess formation: a case report. Surg Neurol. 2001; 55(4):235–239

[29] Park MC, Goldman MA, Donahue JE, Tung GA, Goel R, Sampath P. Endonasal ethmoidectomy and bifrontal craniotomy with craniofacial approach for resection of frontoethmoidal osteoma causing tension pneumocephalus. Skull Base. 2008; 18(1):67–72

[30] Smith ME, Calcaterra TC. Frontal sinus osteoma. Ann Otol Rhinol Laryngol. 1989; 98(11):896–900

[31] Savić DL, Djerić DR. Indications for the surgical treatment of osteomas of the frontal and ethmoid sinuses. Clin Otolaryngol Allied Sci. 1990; 15(5):397–404

[32] Dubin MG, Kuhn FA. Preservation of natural frontal sinus outflow in the management of frontal sinus osteomas. Otolaryngol Head Neck Surg. 2006; 134(1):18–24

[33] Neel HB, III, McDonald TJ, Facer GW. Modified Lynch procedure for chronic frontal sinus diseases: rationale, technique, and long-term results. Laryngoscope. 1987; 97(11):1274–1279

[34] Goodale RL, Montgomery WW. Experiences with the osteoplastic anterior wall approach to the frontal sinus; case histories and recommendations. AMA Arch Otolaryngol. 1958; 68(3):271–283

[35] Weber R, Draf W, Kratzsch B, Hosemann W, Schaefer SD. Modern concepts of frontal sinus surgery. Laryngoscope. 2001; 111(1):137–146

[36] Busch RF.. Frontal sinus osteoma: complete removal via endoscopic sinus surgery and frontal sinus trephination. Am J RhinolAllergy. 1992; 6(4):139–143

[37] Menezes CA, Davidson TM. Endoscopic resection of a sphenoethmoid osteoma: a case report. Ear Nose Throat J. 1994; 73(8):598–600

[38] Draf W, Weber R. Endonasal micro-endoscopic pansinusoperation in chronic sinusitis. I. Indications and operation technique. Am J Otolaryngol. 1993; 14(6):394–398

[39] Choudhury N, Hariri A, Saleh H. Extended applications of the endoscopic modified Lothrop procedure. J Laryngol Otol. 2016; 130 (9):827–832

[40] Gross WE, Gross CW, Becker D, Moore D, Phillips D. Modified transnasal endoscopic Lothrop procedure as an alternative to frontal sinus obliteration. Otolaryngol Head Neck Surg. 1995; 113(4):427–434

[41] Metson R, Gliklich RE. Clinical outcome of endoscopic surgery for frontal sinusitis. Arch Otolaryngol Head Neck Surg. 1998; 124 (10):1090–1096

[42] Kikawada T, Fujigaki M, Kikura M, Matsumoto M, Kikawada K. Extended endoscopic frontal sinus surgery to interrupted nasofrontal communication caused by scarring of the anterior ethmoid: long-term results. Arch Otolaryngol Head Neck Surg. 1999; 125(1):92–96

[43] Draf W. Endonasal micro-endoscopic frontal sinus surgery: the Fulda concept. Oper Tech Otolaryngol Head Neck Surg. 1991; 2:234–240

[44] Chiu AG, Schipor I, Cohen NA, Kennedy DW, Palmer JN. Surgical decisions in the management of frontal sinus osteomas. Am J Rhinol. 2005; 19(2):191–197

[45] Bignami M, Dallan I, Terranova P, Battaglia P, Miceli S, Castelnuovo P. Frontal sinus osteomas: the window of endonasal endoscopic approach. Rhinology. 2007; 45(4):315–320

[46] Ledderose GJ, Betz CS, Stelter K, Leunig A. Surgical management of osteomas of the frontal recess and sinus: extending the limits of the endoscopic approach. Eur Arch Otorhinolaryngol. 2011; 268(4):525–532

[47] Gil-Carcedo LM, Gil-Carcedo ES, Vallejo LA, de Campos JM, Herrero D. Frontal osteomas: standardising therapeutic indications. J Laryngol Otol. 2011; 125(10):1020–1027

[48] Turri-Zanoni M, Dallan I, Terranova P, et al. Frontoethmoidal and intraorbital osteomas: exploring the limits of the endoscopic approach. Arch Otolaryngol Head Neck Surg. 2012; 138(5):498–504

[49] Timperley DG, Banks C, Robinson D, Roth J, Sacks R, Harvey RJ. Lateral frontal sinus access in endoscopic skull-base surgery. Int Forum Allergy Rhinol. 2011; 1(4):290–295

[50] Georgalas C, Goudakos J, Fokkens WJ. Osteoma of the skull base and sinuses. Otolaryngol Clin North Am. 2011; 44(4):875–890, vii

[51] Gerber, P. H. : Les Osteomes du Sinus Frontal. Arch. Int. de Laryngol-Otol.-Rhin., 23:17, 1907

28 Frontal Inverted Papilloma

Paolo Battaglia, Apostolos Karligkiotis, Giacomo Pietrobon, Paolo Castelnuovo, and Mario Turri-Zanoni

Abstract

The inverted papilloma is the most frequent benign sino-nasal tumor that may involve the frontal sinus in a percentage of cases ranging from 16.6 to 19%. Although the tumor may be involving the frontal sinus, in most it vegetates within the frontal sinus with its origin from the frontal recess or ethmoid sinus. Preoperative nasal endoscopy, CT scan, and contrast-enhanced MR imaging are paramount in reaching diagnosis and planning appropriate treatment. Surgical strategies to properly manage frontal inverted papilloma must be tailored to the tumor extension and to patients' morbidity, and it may include the endoscopic endonasal approach and different kinds of external techniques such as the endoscopic frontal trephination, the osteoplastic flap, and the transorbital approach through a superior eyelid approach. The endoscopic endonasal approach is able to achieve complete resection of frontal inverted papilloma in the large majority of cases, with limited complications rate, and reduce morbidity for patients. Frontal sinusotomies according to Draf types IIa, IIb, and III are generally used. Recently the endoscopic orbital transposition has been described in order to expand the endonasal approach to the frontal sinus. Indications, contraindications, complications rates, and outcomes of each surgical technique have been analyzed in details in this chapter.

Keywords: inverted papilloma, frontal sinus, endoscopic frontal sinusotomy, osteoplastic flap

28.1 Epidemiology and Etiology

Inverted papilloma (IP) is the most common benign tumor of the sinonasal tract, accounting for approximately 0.5 to 4% of all tumors of this region. It arises from the Schneiderian mucosa of the paranasal sinuses and it typically grows with an inverted pattern into the underlying stroma. This peculiar feature differentiates it from other Schneiderian papillomas, that is oncocytic and exophytic or fungiform, though diverse patterns can coexist. The most frequent site of origin is the ethmoidal compartment (48%), followed by the maxillary sinus (28%), sphenoid (7.5%), frontal sinus (2.5%), and nasal septum (2.5%).[1]

Hence, IP of the frontal sinus represents a rare entity. The mucosa of the frontal sinus can either be the origin of the tumor or be involved later in the progression of a disease arising elsewhere, most commonly in the anterior ethmoid. Tumors can also possibly vegetate within the frontal sinus, without infiltrating its mucosal lining.

Recent case series reported an involvement of the frontal sinus ranging from 16.6 to 19% of cases (▶ Table 28.1). However, these data are distorted by the fact that different authors consider different criteria in defining the involvement of the frontal sinus by IP. In this regard, the frontal recess poses some difficulties in defining the precise origin of the lesion: some authors consider it part of the frontal sinus, though it is still strictly an ethmoidal structure; others prefer to include within the frontal IP only those tumors affecting at least one of the walls of the sinus. Theoretically, all the walls of frontal sinus can be affected by the tumor and they can possibly harbor the pedicle of the lesion. Bony modifications, such as osteitis and/or spur/osteogenesis and/or erosion, can be present, similarly to what happens in other sites. Moreover, neoplastic growth from or into the sinus can widen the frontal sinus drainage pathway, thus realizing a sort of natural sinusotomy. A massive involvement of the frontal sinus or multiple origins within it can be encountered as well. Bilateral extension of frontal IP was described in 16.3% of cases in a recent review.[2] The same study reported that squamous cell carcinoma (SCC) was associated in 4.1% of cases, thus confirming that IP of the frontal sinus is no exception to the well-known possible malignant transformation.

So far, no specific etiologic factors have been clearly defined, although there is compelling evidence of the causal role of human papillomavirus (HPV), acting as genetic modifier with a mechanism that may be similar to what happens in cervical tumors, although not precisely defined yet.[3] Another possible risk factor is represented by the cigarette smoke[4] although the current body of evidences is still limited. The recent study by Roh et al reported that a history of smoking was associated with recurrence of IP, although the total number of patients assessed was too low to infer definitive conclusions.[5] Current literature concerning etiology of IP takes into account the disease on its whole, without further considerations on the specific site. Given the paucity of cases with frontal sinus involvement, it is unlikely to obtain any new significant result in the next future.

Different staging systems have been proposed to categorize the extent of IP. Cannady et al categorized sinonasal IP into three groups as follows: group A—IP confined to the nasal cavity, ethmoid sinus, and medial maxillary sinus; group B—IP with lateral maxillary sinus, sphenoid sinus, or frontal sinus involvement; and group C—IP with extrasinus extension.[6] According to this classification system, frontal IP can be included within group B. Another staging system largely used is the one proposed by Krouse in 2000.[7] Briefly, stage I disease is

Table 28.1 Review of English literature on surgical treatment of inverted papilloma of the frontal sinus

Author	Year	Total cases	Cases with FS involvement	Type of surgery	Results	No. of relapses	Type of surgery for relapse	Status	Follow-up (mo)
Adriansen[27]	2015	20	20	EE	100% CR	2	EE	100% NED	42
Ungari[28]	2015	35	5 FS 13 FE	OPF	100% CR	2	2 OPF	100% NED	>12
Pagella[29]	2014	73	2 FS 8 FE	EE	100% CR	0	NA	100% NED	58
Sciarretta[9]	2014	110	7 FR 4 FS	EE	100% CR	1 FR 1 FS	1 EE (FR) 1 OPF (FS)	100% NED	56.7
Kim[30]	2012	578	22 as origin	10 EE 8 combined 4 external	100% CR	6	Unknown	Unknown	41
			89 as extension	59 EE 20 combined 10 external		24			
Gotlib[31]	2012	2	2	EE	100% CR	Unknown	Unknown	50% NED 50% unknown	12
Walgama[2]	2012	49	49	31 EE 13 OPF 5 EFT	100% CR	11	8 EE 1 EFT 2 OPF	100% NED	27
Lian[32]	2012	26	1	EE	100% CR	Unknown	Unknown	100% NED	28.2
Kamel[33]	2012	119	6	EE	100% CR	0	NA	100% NED	27
Bathma[34]	2011	13	4 FR	EE	100% CR	2[a]	EE	100% NED	40
Lombardi[8]	2011	212	11	EE	100% CR	2	1 EE 1 OPF	100% NED	53.8
Dragonetti[35]	2011	84	3 FS 5 FR	6 EE 2 OPF	100% CR	1 (FR)	OPF	100% NED	39.5
Gras-Cabrerizo[36]	2010	79	8 as extension	5 EE 3 external	100% CR	Unknown	Unknown	Unknown	>12
Sham[37]	2009	56	3	1 EE 2 ExFS[b]	100% CR	3	2 ExFS 1 ExFS + Lothrop	89% NED 11% DOC	84
Yoon[38]	2009	18	18	2 OPF 5 EFT	100% CR	4	3 EE 1 EFT	100% NED	36.6
Eweiss[39]	2009	4	4	EE	100% CR	1	OPF	100% NED	Unknown
Landsberg[40]	2008	30	2	EE	50% CR 50% PR	1 (persistence)	NA	50% NED 50% AWD	40

Table 28.1 (continued) Review of English literature on surgical treatment of inverted papilloma of the frontal sinus

Author	Year	Total cases	Cases with FS involvement	Type of surgery	Results	No. of relapses	Type of surgery for relapse	Status	Follow-up (mo)
Mackle[41]	2008	55	1	OPF	100% CR	Unknown	Unknown	Unknown	>36
Zhang[42]	2008	9	9c	EE	100% CR	0	NA 1 OPF	100% NED	15.1
Sautter[43]	2007	5	5	4 EE 1 EFT	100% CR	0	NA	100% NED	16.8
Mortuaire[44]	2007	65	3	Unknown	100% CR	1	External (lateral rhinotomy)	Unknown	28
Woodworth[11]	2007	110	10 FR 9 FS	10 EE 5 OPF 2 EFT 2 EE + Lynch	100% CR	8	5 EE 1 EFT 1 EE + OPF 1 EE + Lynch	100% NED	40
Minovi[45]	2006	87	13	4 EE 9 OPF	100% CR	Unknown	Unknown	100% NED	74
Katori[46]	2005	39	2 as origin 8 as extension	Both EE and external	100% CR	5d	Both EE and external	Unknown	35
Dubin[17]	2005	18	6	2 EE 1 OPF 3 EE + staged OPF	67% CR 33% PR	3e	2 EE 1 OPF	83% NED 17% DOC	13.3
Jameson[47]	2005	18	1 FS 1 FR	1 OPF 1 EE	100% CR	0	NA	100% NED	29
Wolfe[48]	2004	50	3 FS 2 FR	3 EE 1 OPF 1 Lynch	100% CR	0	NA	100% NED	31.1

Abbreviations: AWD, alive with disease; CR, complete resection; DOC, dead of other causes; EE, endoscopic endonasal; EFT, endoscopic frontal trephination; ExFs, external frontal sinusotomy; FE, frontoethmoidal; FR, frontal recess; FS, frontal sinus; Lynch, external approach through Lynch incision; NED, no evidence of disease; OPF, osteoplastic flap; PR, partial resection; NA, non applicable.
aThe 2 relapses occurred in the same patient.
bThe external frontal sinusotomy was realized via an eyebrow incision.
cFrontal sinus and frontal recess are considered altogether.
dOne relapse in frontal sinus originally involved only the ethmoid. 2 patients recurred twice each after endoscopic and external approach (not further specified).
eTwo out of 3 cases were in fact persistence: a staged OPF was performed because of suspicious partial resection after endoscopic approach, confirmed by pathology.

limited to the nasal cavity alone, stage II includes involvement of the ethmoid and the medial or superior portion of the maxillary sinus, stage III indicates extension to the lateral or inferior aspect of the maxillary sinus or into the frontal and sphenoid sinuses, and stage IV is reserved for malignant transformation or tumor spread outside of the paranasal sinuses. According to Krouse, IP of the frontal sinus is generally considered stage T3, unless it presents with associated malignancy, which conveys a higher stage (T4).

28.2 Clinical Presentation and Investigations

IP can present itself in several different clinical ways, similarly to other sinonasal tumors, albeit it can be diagnosed incidentally even in completely asymptomatic patients. The most common symptom reported is nasal obstruction (45–94%), generally unilateral, followed by hyposmia (3–18.7%), rhinorrhea (12.3–18.2%), headache or generic facial pain (1.8–17%), epistaxis (5–11%), and epiphora (1–

6%), in a variable percentage of cases.[8,9,10,11] In the case of papilloma involving the frontal sinus, nasal obstruction remains the most frequent complaint (69%), with headache being the second most common symptom (7–31%). More severe symptoms, such as impairment of vision or ocular motility and intense pain or even neurologic signs, must be carefully investigated since they might be indicative of a malignant transformation. Nonetheless, occasional discovery of the lesion is possible in a small percentage of cases.

As a general rule, a detailed inspection of nasal fossae, eyes, oral cavity, and facial profile is mandatory in these patients. Nasal endoscopy is currently considered the first mandatory diagnostic step for the assessment of sinonasal and skull base pathologies. Endoscopic exploration of the nasal fossa, nasopharynx, and skull base allows detection of any tissue abnormality or lesions in these compartments. In several cases, lesion obstructing the middle meatus and possibly prolapsing into the nasal cavity is well evident. In other cases, unless the ethmoidal compartment and the frontal sinus are massively involved by IP, the endoscopic endonasal evaluation shows no evidence of the disease. Hence, imaging is essential in every case and it must include both CT scan and contrast-enhanced magnetic resonance (MR). Complementary information provided by these two examinations must be integrated in order to allow the precise evaluation of the site, size, and extent of the lesions as well as to have information on anatomical details (e.g., septal spur, concha bullosa, shape of the frontal recess, pneumatization of the frontal sinus, and presence of intrafrontal cells) that can influence surgery. Although definitive diagnosis requires biopsy and histological examination to confirm the nature of the lesion, IP exhibits peculiar features on both CT scan and MR. Osteitic

changes of the bone underlying IP, especially the area of the pedicle, are common.[12] A focal hyperostosis/neo-osteogenesis, creating a cone-shaped thickening, predicts the site of attachment in a high percentage of cases[13] (▶ Fig. 28.1). On the contrary, bony whole-thickness erosion or destruction is not typical of IP and is likely due to a synchronous carcinoma.

The MR is necessary to complement CT scan, which is not able to distinguish between disease and inflammation or fluid retention. In both T1- and T2-weighted sequences, the IP displays a typical columnar or convoluted cerebriform pattern that is not shown by malignant tumors and thus allows differential diagnosis[14] (▶ Fig. 28.2).

Imaging should always precede biopsy of the sinonasal tumor since it is mandatory to rule out the presence of meningoencephaloceles or highly vascularized lesions before approaching it surgically. After proper radiological assessment, generally the biopsy is taken under endoscopic endonasal control in local anesthesia. In case the tumor is not easily accessible but is highly suggestive for IP from a radiological viewpoint, the patient is scheduled for surgery under general anesthesia and a biopsy is sent for frozen section once the tumor is reached.

28.3 Management

Surgery is the treatment of choice for IP. Resection needs to be radical because of both the well-known tendency to relapse locally and the possibility of associated malignancy, namely, squamous cellular carcinoma, either synchronous or metachronous.[1]

Removal of the lesion is accomplished with a progressive multilayer resection, according to the "disassembling"

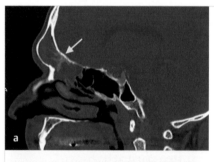
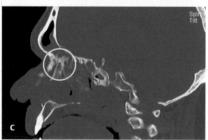
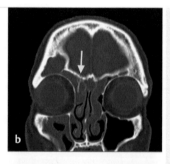
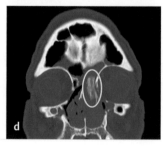

Fig. 28.1 (a–d) CT scan imaging of inverted papilloma of the frontal sinus in coronal and sagittal views. Focal hyperostosis is located in the insertion area of the tumor pedicle, for example, in the posterior wall of the frontal sinus (**a,b**; *yellow arrows*) or in the frontal recess (**c,d**; *yellow rings*).

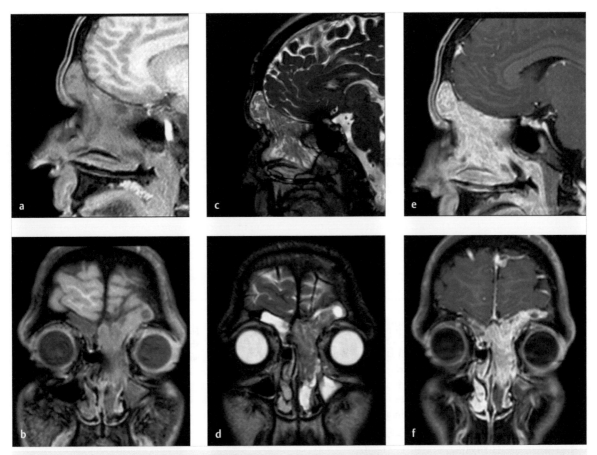

Fig. 28.2 MR imaging of inverted papilloma of the frontal sinus in coronal and sagittal views. Diffuse frontoethmoidal involvement is evident in **(a,b)** T1-weighted scans and a typical columnar/cerebriform pattern can be appreciated in both **(c,d)** T2-weighted scans and **(e,f)** T1-weighted scans after gadolinium enhancement.

technique.[8] This consists of an initial tumor debulking, followed by a subperiosteal dissection and a final drilling of the underlying bone in order to eliminate any possible residual tumoral cell grown inside bony crevices.[12]

Nowadays, the endoscopic resection is considered the standard surgical treatment for sinonasal IP. In a relatively recent review, Busquets and Hwang proved endoscopic resection to be at least as successful as craniofacial resection in terms of oncological radicality and recurrence rate.[15] Nonetheless, what is crucial is complete resection of the tumor: endoscopy is simply a tool and it is inadequate or insufficient if it does not allow a thorough access to the lesion. In this regard, the frontal sinus involvement poses a unique challenge. Whenever IP involves the frontal sinus, both endoscopic resection and external procedures may be contemplated, and possibly integrated, depending on the following aspects:
- Extension of the tumor to the surrounding structures.
- Size of the lesion.
- Site of the tumor inside the frontal sinus and number of attachments.

- Anatomy and pneumatization of the frontal sinus (anteroposterior diameter of the sinus, interorbital distance, intrafrontal cells, frontal beak projection).

Of course, surgeon's experience and available instrumentations play a major role in choosing the most convenient approach. Nevertheless, some general indications can be outlined.

Endoscopic resection spans from a simple clearance of frontal drainage pathway (Draf type I) to a wider access realized through a frontal sinusotomy (Draf type IIa/IIb) or a modified endoscopic Lothrop procedure, also known as Draf type III (▶ Fig. 28.3). External procedures include endoscopic frontal trephination (EFT) and osteoplastic flap (OPF) with or without obliteration of the frontal sinus. In selected cases, endoscopic endonasal and traditional external approaches can be combined to obtain more satisfying results.

When the IP originates somewhere else (e.g., frontal recess or anterior ethmoid) and simply vegetates in the frontal sinus, endoscopic resection is undoubtedly the

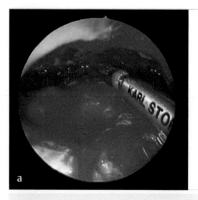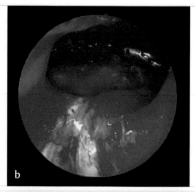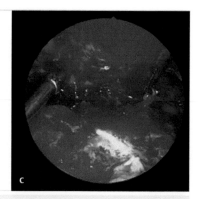

Fig. 28.3 Endoscopic intraoperative view of Draf type III frontal sinusotomy. The removal of intersinus septum and cranial portion of the anterior third of the nasal septum allows wider access for **(a)** curved drill or **(b)** curved forceps, while controlling instruments from the contralateral side. **(c)** Use of multiple instruments, for example, forceps and suction, is also made possible.

most appropriate solution. Furthermore, the attachment of the tumor to the posterior or medial frontal wall in patients with a well-pneumatized sinus is considered a favorable condition for an endoscopic endonasal approach. Conversely, involvement of the anterior wall and/or the lateral or superior aspect of the frontal sinus, particularly in a well-pneumatized frontal sinus, represents a challenge to the exclusive endonasal approach and the proper surgical approach should be chosen case by case in a patient-tailored fashion. Finally, the massive extension of the IP into the sinus, with involvement and/or erosion of all the bony frontal walls, represents a contraindication for the endoscopic endonasal procedure, requiring at least a combined transnasal–transcranial approach.[16,17]

In a recent publication, the authors outlined a series of absolute contraindications to a purely endoscopic approach to the frontal sinus' disease.[18] These can be summarized as follows:

- Small anteroposterior diameter of the frontal sinus (< 1 cm) and small interorbital distance.
- Erosion of the posterior wall of the frontal sinus with intracranial extension.
- Extension of the lesion through the anterior frontal bony plate.
- Massive lateral supraorbital attachment of the lesion in laterally pneumatized frontal sinus.
- Massive involvement of the mucosa of the frontal sinus and/or of supraorbital cell.
- Histological evidence of SCC in IP at frozen sections.
- Presence of abundant scar tissue from previous surgery or relevant posttraumatic anatomic changes of the frontal bone.

The preoperative planning based on imaging (CT and MR scans) is usually able to predict the surgical approach required to remove radically the IP involving the frontal sinus. When the surgical removal is planned through an exclusive endoscopic endonasal approach, the patient should always be informed prior to surgery that a conversion/switching of operative technique to a traditional external procedure might be necessary. Even if an external procedure is planned from the very beginning in order to fully approach the lesion, a combined endoscopic endonasal surgery should always be performed in order to clean the frontal recess and ensure the patency of the natural ostium of the sinus, preventing postoperative scar tissue formation or fluid retention.

The most recent literature shows a prevalence of endoscopic endonasal procedures for treatment of IP originating or extending into the frontal sinus. Good results can be achieved in terms of complete resection of the lesions. Rates of relapse or persistence are variable. Surgery for recurrences still includes endoscopic endonasal procedures, whenever feasible, though an external approach is likely to be necessary in a higher percentage of cases (see ▶ Table 28.1).

The EFT is used by some authors because it allows positioning of both scopes and instrumentations in an otherwise inaccessible portion of the frontal sinus. Before performing the trephination, radiological imaging of the frontal sinus is necessary (e.g., skull x-ray or CT scan) to assess the size of the sinuses and the location of the intersinus septum. A 1- to 2-cm skin incision is carried 1 cm lateral to the midline of a line connecting the supraorbital rims. Once the bone is reached, a 4-mm drill is used to realize the frontal trephine. The trephine may be enlarged using Kerrison rongeurs to gain better accommodation of instruments. It is also possible to insert a catheter to irrigate the sinus and check for the frontal outflow tract endonasally.[19] ▶ Table 28.1 summarizes the outcomes of EFT in treatment of IP of the frontal sinus in the last 10 years. A combination of EFT and endoscopic endonasal approach is always necessary.

OPF provides a wider external exposition of the surgical field, though it is undoubtedly more invasive. When performing this approach, it is mandatory not to exceed the borders of the frontal sinus. Usually a sterile template is realized preoperatively, based on a skull X-ray with occipitofrontal view (so-called Caldwell's view). Alternatively, intraoperative magnetic navigation system can be used for a precise delineation of the frontal sinus' contour, as recently described.[20] At the end of the procedure, obliteration of the frontal sinus with fat has been proposed in the past by several authors.[21,22,23] However, refinements in endoscopic endonasal surgery as well as better understandings of the frontal sinus drainage pathways strongly suggest avoiding such procedure because of both the impossibility of an efficient endoscopic follow-up for recurrences and the risk of mucocele formation in case of even minimal mucosal residues.[11,19,24]

It is noteworthy that a recent review of the literature was unable to demonstrate superiority of one surgical approach over others for successful removal of IP of frontal sinus.[2] Those authors concluded that surgeons should handle all different types of surgical techniques and be ready to convert from endoscopic to external approaches whenever dictated by intraoperative findings, possibly with a single-staged operation.

Recently, new endoscopic techniques have been developed to expand the approach to the frontal sinus' pathology, including IP. The so-called orbital transposition allows access to the far lateral portion of the frontal sinus through removal of lamina papyracea, cauterization of ethmoidal arteries, and lateralization of the orbital content.[18] Other solutions proposed to access the far lateral portion of the frontal sinus include the transorbital route via a superior eyebrow incision that gives access to the orbital roof and to the anterolateral aspect of the frontal sinus.[25] Surgical outcomes obtained with these techniques are encouraging, with limited rates of complications and recurrences (▶ Table 28.1). Such techniques, however, are used only for well-selected cases and in centers with large experience in endoscopic and external procedures. Surgical tips and tricks to overcome technical problems and avoid possible complications are provided in ▶ Table 28.2.

28.4 Case Examples

28.4.1 Case 1

A 48-year-old man was referred to our attention because of persistent left respiratory nasal obstruction and epistaxis. Endoscopic examination and imaging revealed a papillomatous lesion occupying the maxillary sinus and the ethmoidal compartment, including the frontal recess and, possibly, the lower part of the frontal sinus. The patient underwent an endoscopic endonasal approach with Draf type IIa frontal sinusotomy and a complete removal of the lesion was achieved. The tumor appeared to simply vegetate in the frontal sinus, as shown in ▶ Fig. 28.4a–c. No complications occurred during surgery and postoperatively. The patient is free of disease after a 10-year follow-up (▶ Fig. 28.4d).

Table 28.2 Surgical tips and tricks in the treatment of inverted papilloma involving the frontal sinus

Point of difficulty	Technical solution
Presence of intra-frontal cells	Pre-op evaluation with multiplanar CT scan, in order to disassemble the cells of the frontal recess and sinus
Involvement of the lateral aspect of the frontal sinus	• Draf type IIB or III • Use the contralateral nasal fossa to increase the angulation of instruments • Curved and double-curved instruments • Orbital transposition technique
Inverted papilloma attachment to the anterior or posterior frontal wall	• Consider preoperatively the interorbital distance and the anteroposterior diameter of the frontal sinus in order to select the best surgical approach
Orbital involvement	• Preoperative evaluation with MRI (fat-suppressed images) • Preserve the periorbital layer in order to prevent diplopia and enophthalmos • Rule out malignant transformation (frozen sections)
Intracranial involvement	• Preoperative evaluation with MRI (T2-FLAIR sequences) • Consider external approaches (OPF vs. cranioendoscopic approach) • Rule out malignant transformation (frozen sections)

Abbreviations: CT, computed tomography; FLAIR, fluid-attenuated inversion recovery; MRI, magnetic resonance imaging; OPF, osteoplastic flap.

28.4.2 Case 2

A 58-year-old man was referred to our department for a recurrent left frontoethmoidal IP. He had previously undergone two endoscopic resections for the same disease. He complained of headache. He was a former smoker. Preoperative MR scan showed a lesion of the left ethmoidal recess, extending into the frontal sinus (▶ Fig. 28.5a, b). An endoscopic endonasal resection was achieved through a complete ethmoidectomy and a Draf type IIb frontal sinusotomy. No complications occurred intraoperatively and postoperatively. At the last follow-up performed 5 years after surgery, the patient is free of disease (▶ Fig. 28.5c, d).

28.4.3 Case 3

A 59-year-old man was referred to our department after an excisional biopsy of IP of the left frontal sinus. The patient complained of headache, unilateral left nasal respiratory obstruction, rhinorrhea, and episodic epistaxis. He was a former smoker (stopped 12 years earlier). The CT scan and MRI showed a lesion occupying the frontal sinus bilaterally and extending to the ethmoidal compartment

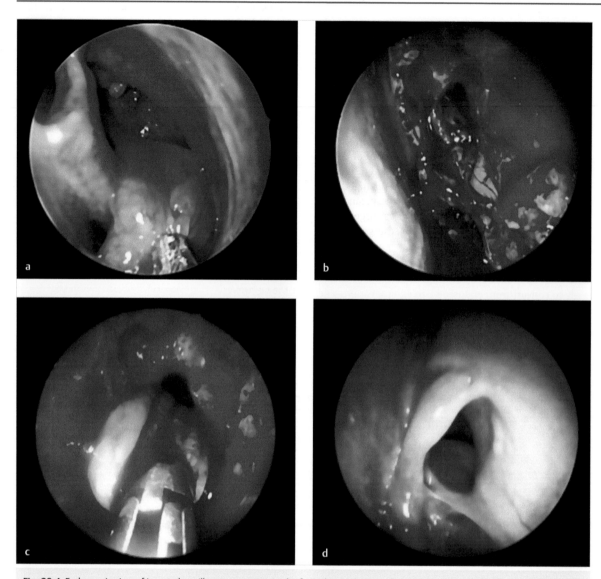

Fig. 28.4 Endoscopic view of inverted papilloma vegetating in the frontal sinus (patient described in Case 1). **(a)** The tumor obliterates the left middle meatus and originates in the frontal recess. **(b)** After completion of anterior ethmoidectomy, vegetation of the lesion into the frontal sinus can be appreciated. **(c)** Removal of the papilloma is achieved by simple stripping the tumor with Blakesley nasal forceps. **(d)** Postoperative endoscopic control during follow-up shows open and explorable frontal sinusotomy, without any sign of recurrent disease.

and nasal fossa bilaterally (▶ Fig. 28.6). Because of the extension of the disease, a combined endoscopic–external approach was planned. An OPF was realized accordingly to the technique previously described, while a Draf type III frontal sinusotomy was performed endonasally. During the follow-up, the patient underwent a revision surgery for frontal stenosis and mucocele's formation. The last clinical and radiological follow-up performed 5 years after surgery is negative for relapse of disease (▶ Fig. 28.7).

28.5 Complications: Management

Complications related to surgical treatment of IP involving the frontal sinus are similar to those associated with any other sinonasal surgery and so is their management. Major complications of both endoscopic surgery and craniofacial resection may be divided into intraoperative and postoperative. The latter may be further subdivided into early and late. ▶ Table 28.3 and ▶ Table 28.4 summarize the most frequent complications that may occur in such a surgery.

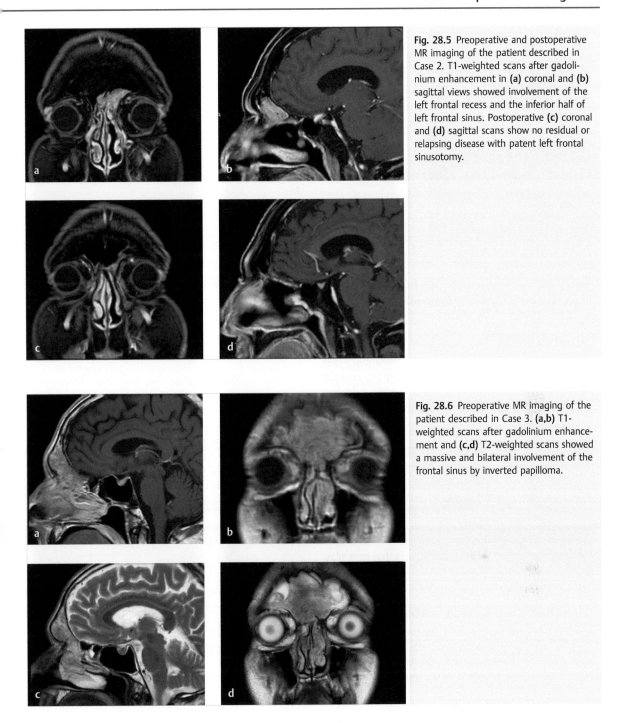

Fig. 28.5 Preoperative and postoperative MR imaging of the patient described in Case 2. T1-weighted scans after gadolinium enhancement in (a) coronal and (b) sagittal views showed involvement of the left frontal recess and the inferior half of left frontal sinus. Postoperative (c) coronal and (d) sagittal scans show no residual or relapsing disease with patent left frontal sinusotomy.

Fig. 28.6 Preoperative MR imaging of the patient described in Case 3. (a,b) T1-weighted scans after gadolinium enhancement and (c,d) T2-weighted scans showed a massive and bilateral involvement of the frontal sinus by inverted papilloma.

Complete resection of IP requires drilling of the bone underlying the lesion; thus, the surgeon may face a few complications caused by excessive or inappropriate use of the bur. In this regard, the use of a diamond bur is recommended, while the use of aggressive and sharp bur has to be reserved only for selected cases and in expert hands.

Possible site of iatrogenic cerebrospinal fluid (CSF) leakage differs between the two approaches. During endoscopic surgery, it is more likely to damage either the inferior part of the posterior wall of the frontal sinus or the ethmoidal roof (e.g., olfactory cleft). Conversely, during external procedure, the whole posterior wall may be injured, as well as other portions of the frontal bone, in case the osteotomies are mistakenly realized outside the borders of the sinus. CSF leakage mandates an immediate skull base reconstruction. The type of sealing depends on the site and extent of exposure. A small defect, localized either on the posterior frontal wall or on the ethmoidal

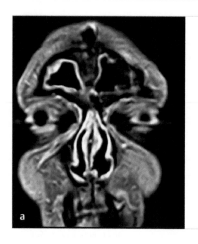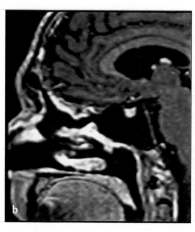

Fig. 28.7 Postoperative MR imaging of the patient described in Case 3. T1-weighted scan after gadolinium enhancement in **(a)** coronal view shows mild inflammatory retention on the right side of the frontal sinus, while a patent left side is seen in the **(b)** sagittal view.

Table 28.3 Complications associated with endoscopic endonasal approaches to frontal sinus inverted papilloma

Intraoperative	Postoperative	
	Early	Late
Bleeding from AEA	CSF leakage	Frontal ostium stenosis
CSF leakage	Sinonasal infection	Mucocele
Damage to orbital content (muscles and nerve) and/or lacrimal pathway	Periorbital hematoma and/or swelling	Chronic rhinosinusitis
Collapse of nasion due to excessive drilling (Draf type III)	Meningitis	

Abbreviations: AEA, anterior ethmoidal artery; CSF, cerebrospinal fluid.

Table 28.4 Complications associated with external approaches to frontal sinus inverted papilloma

Intraoperative	Postoperative	
	Early	Late
CSF leakage	Infection of skin wound	Frontal ostium stenosis
Fracture of bony flap	Frontal subcutaneous hematoma	Mucocele
Bleeding from supraorbital and/or supratrochlear vessels	CSF leakage	Frontal bone osteitis
Damage of frontal nerve branches (SON or STN)	Meningitis	Frontal cutaneous anesthesia
	Sinonasal infection	Frontal/supraorbital aesthetic impairment

Abbreviations: CSF, cerebrospinal fluid; SON, supraorbital nerve; STN, supratrochlear nerve.

roof, may be repaired with a simple mucoperiosteum graft, harvested from the middle turbinate, from the septum or from the floor of the nasal fossa. A larger bony defect with dural tear can be repaired with a multilayer technique using fascia lata harvested from the patient's thigh and possibly cartilaginous or bony grafts, performing a so-called Gasket seal procedure.[26] The resurfacing of the skull base reconstruction using pedicled septal flap or even with free graft of the nasal mucosa is able to promote the healing of the surgical site and to prevent scar tissue formation while reducing postoperative nasal crusting. Attention needs to be paid when drilling the frontal beak to realize a Draf type III frontal sinusotomy. Excessive resection of bone, as far as the subcutaneous plane, may cause collapse of the nasion area with ensuing aesthetic deficit. In case of orbital hematoma caused by bleeding of the anterior ethmoidal artery, a lateral canthotomy is realized in order to reduce intraorbital pressure and to preserve optic nerve function.

When harvesting an OPF, it is important to realize osteotomies along a single line in order to avoid loss of bony resistance and possible fracture of the bone flap. In case the flap gets damaged, it can be rearranged with plates and screws or even be replaced by a titanium mesh, shaped accordingly to the frontal defect and fixed with screws. During harvesting of the OPF, it is also recommended to spare part of the bone of the supraorbital ridge, so that space for inferiorly fixing screws is made. This is important considering that it is difficult to correct an aesthetic impairment derived from improper inferior osteotomies of the OPF. Another possible complication related to external surgical procedures to address the frontal sinus is the injury of the frontal nerve branches. The frontal nerve gives off a larger lateral branch, the supraorbital nerve (SON), and a smaller medial branch, the supratrochlear nerve (STN). Both exit the orbit anteriorly. The SON exits from the supraorbital foramen or notch along the superior rim of the frontal bone, accompanied by the supraorbital artery. In the supraorbital notch, the SON gives off small filaments that supply the mucosal membrane of the frontal sinus and filaments that supply the upper eyelid. The SON is usually located 2.7 cm from the midline and it sends fibers all the way to the vertex of the scalp, providing sensory innervation to the forehead, upper eyelid, and anterior scalp. The STN instead is usually located 1.7 cm from the midline and it supplies sensory innervations to the bridge of the nose, the medial part of the upper eyelid, and the medial forehead. Intraoperative identification and preservation of such nerves is always mandatory.

References

[1] Lund VJ, Stammberger H, Nicolai P, et al. European Rhinologic Society Advisory Board on Endoscopic Techniques in the Management of Nose, Paranasal Sinus and Skull Base Tumours. European position paper on endoscopic management of tumours of the nose, paranasal sinuses and skull base. Rhinol Suppl. 2010; 22(22):1–143

[2] Walgama E, Ahn C, Batra PS. Surgical management of frontal sinus inverted papilloma: a systematic review. Laryngoscope. 2012; 122 (6):1205–1209

[3] Altavilla G, Staffieri A, Busatto G, Canesso A, Giacomelli L, Marioni G. Expression of p53, p16INK4A, pRb, p21WAF1/CIP1, p27KIP1, cyclin D1, Ki-67 and HPV DNA in sinonasal endophytic Schneiderian (inverted) papilloma. Acta Otolaryngol. 2009; 129(11):1242–1249

[4] Buchwald C, Franzmann MB, Tos M. Sinonasal papillomas: a report of 82 cases in Copenhagen County, including a longitudinal epidemiological and clinical study. Laryngoscope. 1995; 105(1):72–79

[5] Roh HJ, Mun SJ, Cho KS, Hong SL. Smoking, not human papilloma virus infection, is a risk factor for recurrence of sinonasal inverted papilloma. Am J Rhinol Allergy. 2016; 30(2):79–82

[6] Cannady SB, Batra PS, Sautter NB, Roh HJ, Citardi MJ. New staging system for sinonasal inverted papilloma in the endoscopic era. Laryngoscope. 2007; 117(7):1283–1287

[7] Krouse JH. Development of a staging system for inverted papilloma. Laryngoscope. 2000; 110(6):965–968

[8] Lombardi D, Tomenzoli D, Buttà L, et al. Limitations and complications of endoscopic surgery for treatment for sinonasal inverted papilloma: a reassessment after 212 cases. Head Neck. 2011; 33 (8):1154–1161

[9] Sciarretta V, Fernandez IJ, Farneti P, Pasquini E. Endoscopic and combined external-transnasal endoscopic approach for the treatment of inverted papilloma: analysis of 110 cases. Eur Arch Otorhinolaryngol. 2014; 271(7):1953–1959

[10] Kim WS, Hyun DW, Kim CH, Yoon JH. Treatment outcomes of sinonasal inverted papillomas according to surgical approaches. Acta Otolaryngol. 2010; 130(4):493–497

[11] Woodworth BA, Bhargave GA, Palmer JN, et al. Clinical outcomes of endoscopic and endoscopic-assisted resection of inverted papillomas: a 15-year experience. Am J Rhinol. 2007; 21(5):591–600

[12] Chiu AG, Jackman AH, Antunes MB, Feldman MD, Palmer JN. Radiographic and histologic analysis of the bone underlying inverted papillomas. Laryngoscope. 2006; 116(9):1617–1620

[13] Bhalla RK, Wright ED. Predicting the site of attachment of sinonasal inverted papilloma. Rhinology. 2009; 47(4):345–348

[14] Maroldi R, Farina D, Palvarini L, Lombardi D, Tomenzoli D, Nicolai P. Magnetic resonance imaging findings of inverted papilloma: differential diagnosis with malignant sinonasal tumors. Am J Rhinol. 2004; 18(5):305–310

[15] Busquets JM, Hwang PH. Endoscopic resection of sinonasal inverted papilloma: a meta-analysis. Otolaryngol Head Neck Surg. 2006; 134 (3):476–482

[16] Yoon BN, Batra PS, Citardi MJ, Roh HJ. Frontal sinus inverted papilloma: surgical strategy based on the site of attachment. Am J Rhinol Allergy. 2009; 23(3):337–341

[17] Dubin MG, Sonnenburg RE, Melroy CT, Ebert CS, Coffey CS, Senior BA. Staged endoscopic and combined open/endoscopic approach in the management of inverted papilloma of the frontal sinus. Am J Rhinol. 2005; 19(5):442–445

[18] Karligkiotis A, Pistochini A, Turri-Zanoni M, et al. Endoscopic endonasal orbital transposition to expand the frontal sinus approaches. Am J Rhinol Allergy. 2015; 29(6):449–456

[19] Kountakis SE, Senior BA, Draf W. The Frontal Sinus. Berlin: Springer; 2005

[20] Volpi L, Pistochini A, Bignami M, Meloni F, Turri Zanoni M, Castelnuovo P. A novel technique for tailoring frontal osteoplastic flaps using the ENT magnetic navigation system. Acta Otolaryngol. 2012; 132(6):645–650

[21] Hardy JM, Montgomery WW. Osteoplastic frontal sinusotomy: an analysis of 250 operations. Ann Otol Rhinol Laryngol. 1976; 85(4, Pt 1):523–532

[22] Donald PJ, Ettin M. The safety of frontal sinus fat obliteration when sinus walls are missing. Laryngoscope. 1986; 96(2):190–193

[23] Weber R, Draf W, Kahle G, Kind M. Obliteration of the frontal sinus: state of the art and reflections on new materials. Rhinology. 1999; 37 (1):1–15

[24] DeConde AS, Smith TL. Outcomes after frontal sinus surgery: an evidence-based review. Otolaryngol Clin North Am. 2016; 49(4):1019–1033

[25] Dallan I, Castelnuovo P, Sellari-Franceschini S, Locatelli D. Endoscopic orbital and Transorbital Approaches. Tuttlingen, Germany: Endo Press GmbH; 2016

[26] Leng LZ, Brown S, Anand VK, Schwartz TH. "Gasket-seal" watertight closure in minimal-access endoscopic cranial base surgery. Neurosurgery. 2008; 62(5) Suppl 2:E342–E343, discussion E343

[27] Adriaensen GF, van der Hout MW, Reinartz SM, Georgalas C, Fokkens WJ. Endoscopic treatment of inverted papilloma attached in the frontal sinus/recess. Rhinology. 2015;53(4):317–324.

[28] Ungari C, Riccardi E, Reale G, et al. Management and treatment of sinonasal inverted papilloma. Ann Stomatol (Roma). 2015;6(3–4):87–90.

[29] Pagella F, Pusateri A, Giourgos G, Tinelli C, Matti E. Evolution in the treatment of sinonasal inverted papilloma: pedicle-oriented endoscopic surgery. Am J Rhinol Allergy. 2014;28(1):75–81.

[30] Kim DY, Hong SL, Lee CH, et al. Inverted papilloma of the nasal cavity and paranasal sinuses: a Korean multicenter study. Laryngoscope. 2012;122(3):487–494.

[31] Gotlib T, Krzeski A, Held-Ziółkowska M, Niemczyk K. Endoscopic transnasal management of inverted papilloma involving frontal sinuses. Wideochir Inne Tech Maloinwazyjne. 2012;7(4):299–303.

[32] Lian F, Juan H. Different endoscopic strategies in the management of recurrent sinonasal inverted papilloma. J Craniofac Surg. 2012;23(1): e44–48.

[33] Kamel RH, Abdel Fattah AF, Awad AG. Origin oriented management of inverted papilloma of the frontal sinus. Rhinology. 2012;50(3):262–268.

[34] Bathma S, Harvinder S, Philip R, Rosalind S, Gurdeep S. Endoscopic management of sinonasal inverted papilloma. Med J Malaysia. 2011;66(1):15–18.

[35] Dragonetti A, Gera R, Sciuto A, et al. Sinonasal inverted papilloma: 84 patients treated by endoscopy and proposal for a new classification. Rhinology. 2011;49(2):207–213.

[36] Gras-Cabrerizo JR, Massegur-Solench H, Pujol-Olmo A, Montserrat-Gili JR, Ademá-Alcover JM, Zarraonandia-Andraca I. Endoscopic medial maxillectomy with preservation of inferior turbinate: how do we do it? Eur Arch Otorhinolaryngol. 2011;268(3):389–392.

[37] Sham CL, Woo JK, van Hasselt CA, Tong MC. Treatment results of sinonasal inverted papilloma: an 18-year study. Am J Rhinol Allergy. 2009;23(2):203–211.

[38] Yoon BN, Batra PS, Citardi MJ, Roh HJ. Frontal sinus inverted papilloma: surgical strategy based on the site of attachment. Am J Rhinol Allergy. 2009;23(3):337–341.

[39] Eweiss A, Al Ansari A, Hassab M. Inverted papilloma involving the frontal sinus: a management plan. Eur Arch Otorhinolaryngol. 2009;266(12):1895–1901.

[40] Landsberg R, Cavel O, Segev Y, Khafif A, Fliss DM. Attachment-oriented endoscopic surgical strategy for sinonasal inverted papilloma. Am J Rhinol. 2008;22(6):629–634.

[41] Mackle T, Chambon G, Garrel R, Meieff M, Crampette L. Endoscopic treatment of sinonasal papilloma: a 12 year review. Acta Otolaryngol. 2008;128(6):670–674.

[42] Zhang L, Han D, Wang C, Ge W, Zhou B. Endoscopic management of the inverted papilloma with attachment to the frontal sinus drainage pathway. *Acta Otolaryngol.* 2008;128(5):561–568.

[43] Sautter NB, Citardi MJ, Batra PS. Minimally invasive resection of frontal recess/sinus inverted papilloma. Am J Otolaryngol. 2007;28(4):221–224.

[44] Mortuaire G, Arzul E, Darras JA, Chevalier D. Surgical management of sinonasal inverted papillomas through endoscopic approach. Eur Arch Otorhinolaryngol. 2007;264(12):1419–1424.

[45] Minovi A, Kollert M, Draf W, Bockmühl U. Inverted papilloma: feasibility of endonasal surgery and long-term results of 87 cases. Rhinology. 2006;44(3):205–210.

[46] Katori H, Tsukuda M. Staging of surgical approach of sinonasal inverted papilloma. *Auris Nasus Larynx.* 2005;32(3):257–263.

[47] Jameson MJ, Kountakis SE. Endoscopic management of extensive inverted papilloma. Am J Rhinol. 2005;19(5):446–451.

[48] Wolfe SG, Schlosser RJ, Bolger WE, Lanza DC, Kennedy DW. Endoscopic and endoscope-assisted resections of inverted sinonasal papillomas. Otolaryngol Head Neck Surg. 2004;131(3):174–179.

29 The Frontal Sinus: Fibro-Osseous Lesions

Catherine Banks and Raymond Sacks

Abstract

The frontal sinus remains a challenging area in endoscopic sinus surgery. The tight anatomical confinement results in limited visibility and a reliance on angulated instruments. The anatomy can be variable and range from simple to complex. A greater understanding of the anatomy and advances in technology, combined with increasing expertise in endoscopic sinus surgery has redefined former surgical limitations. Despite this, external procedures and combined procedures will continue to play a role in select cases. This chapter will discuss fibro-osseous lesions, a heterogeneous group of benign tumors characterized by the replacement of normal bone with a fibrous cellular stroma, containing various amounts of foci of mineralization or ossification. The focus will be on 2 distinct entities, fibrous dysplasia, and ossifying fibroma of the frontal sinus. Epidemiology and etiology will be reviewed, along with clinical presentations and investigations, including features of the radiology, anatomical pathology and the potential for malignancy. Conservative and surgical management will be detailed and case examples and complications highlighting key considerations will be outlined. Osteomas are dealt with in a separate chapter in this text. A benign lesion mandates a planned surgical approach, with justification of decisions and balancing complete resection versus an acceptable subtotal resection to minimize morbidity. Our key surgical considerations are outlined at the end of this chapter.

Keywords: frontal sinus, fibro-osseous lesions, fibrous dysplasia, polystotic fibrous dysplasia, monostotic fibrous dysplasia, ossifying fibroma, cementifying fibroma or cemento-ossifying fibroma, psammomatoid ossifying fibroma

The frontal sinus remains a challenging area in endoscopic sinus surgery. The tight anatomical confinement results in limited visibility and a reliance on angulated instruments. The anatomy can be variable and range from simple to complex. A greater understanding of the anatomy and advances in technology, combined with increasing expertise in endoscopic sinus surgery, have redefined former surgical limitations. Despite this, external procedures and combined procedures will continue to play a role in select cases.

Fibro-osseous lesions are a heterogeneous group of benign tumors characterized by the replacement of normal bone with a fibrous cellular stroma, containing various amounts of foci of mineralization or ossification.[1] This chapter will focus on the two distinct entities: fibrous dysplasia (FD) and ossifying fibroma (OF) of the frontal sinus. Osteomas are dealt with in a separate chapter in this book. A benign lesion mandates a planned surgical approach, with justification of decisions and balancing complete resection versus an acceptable subtotal resection to minimize morbidity. Each of the bony conditions have unique considerations that will be addressed (▶ Table 29.1). Our key surgical considerations are outlined at the end of this chapter.

29.1 Fibrous Dysplasia

FD is a dysplastic skeletal anomaly in which normal bone is distorted and replaced by poorly organized and inadequately mineralized immature bone and fibrous tissue.[2]

There are two forms:
- Polyostotic (25%), involving more than one bone, and is typically unilateral.
- Monostotic (75%), involving only one bone.[1]

Polyostotic FD is associated with McCune–Albright syndrome, endocrine abnormalities, precocious puberty, and cutaneous hyperpigmentation. It is rare and more common in female patients.[1]

Monostotic FD is not always strictly limited to one bone, but may extend across suture lines to involve adjacent bones; thus, the commonly used notation "monostotic" in these cases is not always accurate, and the term craniofacial FD is preferred.[3]

29.1.1 Epidemiology and Etiology

The true incidence of FD involving the sinonasal system is not known.[1] Males and females are equally affected.[1] FD is a disease of growing bones, with most cases presenting in early childhood and adolescents. More than 80% of craniofacial FD cases are diagnosed within the first two decades of life.[2] The natural history of FD is difficult to predict, but a study of 109 patients over 32 years found that in the craniofacial region, 90% of craniofacial lesions were present by 3.4 years.[4] The growth rate is variable, and although it typically becomes quiescent after puberty,[1] it can remain active well beyond these years.[4,5] It can also become reactivated during periods of estrogen excess, such as pregnancy.[6] If rapid change does occur, malignant transformation or bone aneurysmal cyst needs to be considered.

FD is a nonhereditary postzygotic condition caused by a set of mutations in the *GNAS1* gene, located on chromosome 20q13.2.[1,2] This affects the activation of a G protein subunit alpha (GS alpha) early in the course of development. Ultimately, increased cell proliferation and inappropriate differentiation of cells in the osteoblastic lineage result in overproduction of disorganized

Table 29.1 Summary characteristics of fibro-osseous lesions

Incidence	Osteoma	Fibrous dysplasia	Ossifying fibroma
	~0.5%	Unknown	Unknown
Demographics	Male > female 5th–6th decade	Males = females 1st–2nd decade	Males < females 3rd–4th decade
Assoc. conditions	Gardner's syndrome	McCune–Albright syndrome	
Etiology	Unknown	Mutation GNAS1 gene	Unknown
Location	Frontal or ethmoid > maxillary > sphenoid sinuses	Maxillary > mandibular > ethmoid > sphenoid sinuses	Mandibular > maxillary > ethmoid sinuses
Most common presentation	Incidental finding Headache Sinusitis	Facial asymmetry Nasal obstruction Headache	Facial swelling Nasal obstruction Proptosis
Natural history	Slow growing	Slow indolent growth can undergo rapid growth during puberty and pregnancy	Slow growing but locally aggressive
Imaging	Well-marginated bone density Lesion arising from the wall of the sinus	"Ground glass" density on bone CT: varies with amount of fibrous tissue	Classically a thick bony rim surrounding low attenua- tion fibrous area
Histopathology	Ivory: solid compact bone with few to no haversian systems Mature: fibrous tissue with numerous trabecula and haversian systems	Immature woven disorganized cellu- lar fibroblastic stroma containing variable amounts of bone trabeculae	Peripherally lamellar bone element, central, woven. Fibrous stroma: fibroblasts and collagen
Management	Observe Surgery if symptoms/complication	Observe Surgery if symptoms/complication	Complete resection
Malignancy potential	No	< 1%	No

immature fibrotic bone. This mutation is seen in McCune–Albrights syndrome, and both polyostotic and monostotic FD.[2,4]

Anatomical Locations

Twenty-five percent of monostotic cases arise in the facial skeleton. The maxilla and mandible are the most common sites in the head and neck. It can arise in various sites of the maxillofacial skeleton. It is suggested that FD of the paranasal sinus and skull base at the intracranial and orbital interface can behave more aggressively.[5]

The most common location in monostotic FD is the zygomatic–maxillary complex. The paranasal sinus involvement include, in decreasing frequency, the sphenoid, ethmoid, and maxillary sinuses. It is rare, but reported in the frontal sinus[7] (▶ Fig. 29.1).

29.1.2 Clinical Presentation and Investigations

Painless swelling of the facial bones leading to facial asymmetry is the most common clinical sign of FD in the head and neck, followed by pain, ocular symptoms, and neurological changes, due to diffuse thickening of the bones involving the paranasal sinus, orbits, and foramina of the skull base.[2] FD can be an incidental finding on imaging obtained for other reasons, such as evaluation of hearing loss. Complete obliteration of the paranasal sinus can occur.

Radiological Features

Radiographic appearance of the lesions depends on the stage of the disease. One study has concluded that radiological appearance is dependent on age. Early lesions can be radiolucent and as it undergoes calcification become more opaque. Craniofacial FD typically have a "ground glass" appearance on bone window CT scans; other patterns include cystic or pagetoid features. The affected bone has an expansible appearance with ill-defined borders that blend with the surrounding bone.[2,5]

Pathology

Normal bone is replaced with a cellular fibroblastic stroma containing variable amounts of bone trabeculae. The bone trabeculae are described as resembling Chinese script letters. They are composed of immature woven

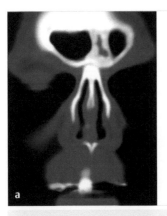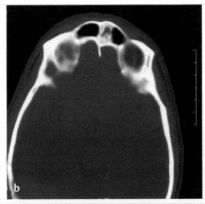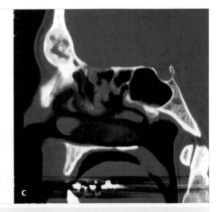

Fig. 29.1 CT scan demonstrating monostotic fibrous dysplasia confined to the frontal sinus. **(a)** Coronal CT scan demonstrating fibrous dysplasia confined to the frontal sinus. **(b)** Axial CT scan demonstrating fibrous dysplasia confined to the frontal sinus. **(c)** Sagittal CT scan demonstrating fibrous dysplasia confined to the frontal sinus.

bone, rich in osteoid, and not rimmed with osteoblast. It has been suggested that the bone of craniofacial FD, unlike that of long bones, may undergo a process of maturation leading to lamellar bone formation. The lamellar bone formation seen in craniofacial FD, but not in FD of the long bones, may be related to a maturation process of the bone.[2]

Malignancy

Radiation is contraindicated in FD and is associated with malignant transformation of FD to an osteosarcoma or less frequently fibrosarcoma, or chondrosarcoma. The rate is low at 0.5%. Spontaneous transformation is very rare. McCune–Albright syndrome has a 4% rate of malignant transformation.[1] Malignant transformation needs to be considered in any patient with a rapid increase in size or pain, with clinical or radiographic evidence of change. They need a biopsy to rule out sarcomatous transformation.[8]

29.1.3 Management

Conservative

Patients who are asymptomatic, or have minimal symptoms or cosmetic deformity, should be observed with serial imaging.[1,8]

Bisphosphonates are a controversial treatment option. Although they have been shown to decrease the incidence of fractures and bony pain in noncraniofacial FD,[1,4] craniofacial FD treated with bisphosphonates has variable results in terms of both rate of growth and pain reduction. Bisphosphonate-induced osteoradionecrosis is a key concern, particularly as patients are so young. Further studies are imperative before these medications can be recommended.

Surgical Indications

The surgical treatment of choice depends on the patient's symptoms, extent of the disease, and age. FD of the frontal sinus is rare. No general recommendation or large series exist in the literature. Therefore, indications, recommended techniques, and timing remain controversial. Endonasal endoscopic treatment of FD, especially for the relief of ocular symptoms (optic nerve decompression) or complications such as chronic rhinosinusitis, mucocele, or pneumocephaly, is commonly performed. The general consensus is that the degree of surgical resection should be based on the location and the severity of the symptoms. Treatment approaches include those discussed earlier. Localized resection in the frontal sinus is possible in select cases, utilizing a Draf III approach.[7]

Endoscopic approaches include Draf IIa, Draf IIb, and Draf III (endoscopic modified Lothrop procedure [EMLP]). The authors commonly employ a Draf IIb technique for smaller localized lesions (▶ Fig. 29.2) and a Draf III technique for larger lesions (▶ Fig. 29.3). The Draf III approach is almost always utilized via the outside-in technique as described by Harvey. This technique has been previously described in the literature[9] and involves identification of the medial orbital wall and bilateral removal of the overlying mucosa over the frontal process of the maxilla extending to involve the septal mucosa in preparation for the septal window. The septal window is created 1.5 cm anterior to the middle turbinate root and extends posteriorly to the first olfactory neuron. The septal window can be individualized based on the size and extent of access needed. Drilling begins with a 0-degree 5-mm 15-degree diamond bur. Initial removal begins with the midline crest of the septal bone. Attention is then directed to identifying the periosteum, the lateral limits of the dissection. Bone is then removed between the identified

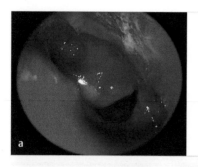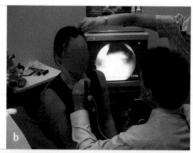

Fig. 29.2 (a, b) Draf IIb approach and result.

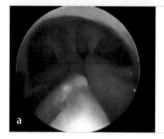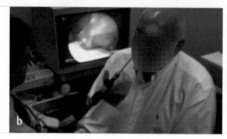

Fig. 29.3 (a, b) Postoperative view of Draf III.

lateral limits and the previously identified first olfactory neuron. These landmarks serve as a guide to remove the intervening bone laterally and anteriorly toward the nasal beak and posterior to the first olfactory neuron. The mucosa of the floor of the frontal sinus is identified and the frontal sinus is entered. It is ideal for large osteomata occluding the frontal recess, as the technique does not rely on identification of the frontal recess in the first instance as this is typically obliterated by tumor. The other major advantage is that the entire procedure is performed with a 0-degree endoscope and a 5-mm diamond high-speed bur, which allows rapid removal of both the frontal beak and the lesion, a procedure that traditionally took a prolonged period of time with angulated endoscopes and angulated instruments. Endoscopic techniques can be technically difficult and complications, such as frontal stenosis, incomplete resection, or prolonged operational time, need to be weighed carefully against ease of access and reduced surgical time.

Complete resection of extensive FD lesions in the paranasal sinuses is difficult. Unacceptable morbidity from surgery is possible. Recurrence remains a valid concern as the FD bone blends with surrounding normal bone. It is therefore essential to balance the morbidity from the surgery with the patient's symptoms and concerns. Radical resection is not warranted for this benign condition.

29.2 Ossifying Fibroma

OF is a benign tumor composed of bone, fibrous tissue, and mineralized material of varying appearances.[1] The nomenclature surrounding OF remains obscure. Variants of OF have been described. These include cemento-ossifying fibroma (COF), juvenile active OF (JAOF), and aggressive psammomatoid OF (APOF). For the purpose of this chapter, OF is considered synonymous with COF and psammomatoid OF (POF).

29.2.1 Epidemiology and Etiology

The precise incidence of OF, however, remains unknown.[10] The lesion can occur at any age and in both sexes, but it has been reported to most frequently occur in the third to fourth decade with a female predominance,[11] with a male-to-female ratio of 1:5.[1]

Anatomical Locations

OF is most frequently located in the facial skeleton, usually involving the mandible. It is rare for OF to arise in paranasal sinuses and nasal cavity.[12] The maxillary and ethmoidal sinuses are the more commonly involved sites of sinonasal OF, but it can develop in any site within the paranasal sinuses. It is thought that sinonasal OF behave more aggressively,[1,11] but this is controversial.[12] In one of the largest studies to date, the ethmoid sinus was the most commonly involved site, followed by the sphenoid sinus, nasal cavity, orbit, maxillary sinus, and frontal sinus.[11]

The etiology of OF has so far not been clarified. The tumor located in the paranasal sinus is believed to originate from ectopic periodontal membrane because of the cementum and osteoid substance from the mesenchymal blast cells, which exist in the periodontal membrane. Other theories include trauma and developmental causes.[1,11]

Characteristics and Growth or Variants

Juvenile trabecular OF (JTOF) and juvenile psammomatoid OF (JPOF) are two histological variants of JAOF. Some controversy exists regarding the nomenclature.[12] The term "juvenile" can be misleading as not all JOF are diagnosed in juveniles, not all JAOF exhibit locally aggressive behavior, and not all lesions classified as JAOF have the same histopathological features.[12] As a result of the inconsistent nomenclature, our understanding of these uncommon lesions is incomplete.

Recently, Manes et al[12] performed a systematic review of literature (137 cases involving the paranasal sinuses) to identify clinical differences between the different variants of OF. Variants were divided into three categories:

- OF.
- Cementifying fibroma or COF.
- APOF, POF, or JAOF.

This study identified no differences in the clinical behavior of the variants,[12] unlike other studies where juvenile OF has an onset at an earlier age and is clinically more aggressive with extension of the tumor to the paranasal sinuses and orbit.[1,10,11,13]

29.2.2 Clinical Presentation and Investigations

Clinical presentation depends on its location and extent. OF of the mandible is usually asymptomatic; in other locations, it can lead to facial pain, swelling, nasal obstruction, rhinosinusitis, and ocular symptoms.

Radiological Features

CT images show a characteristic sharp-demarcated expansile mass covered by a bony rim with a multiloculated low attenuation fibrous area of varying density internally[1] (▶ Fig. 29.4).

Cortical disruption and involvement of adjacent structures can occur. Diagnosis of OF by radiology alone is inaccurate and histological confirmation is recommended.

Radiological–histopathological correlation is high for osteoma and FD and low for OF.[5] Preoperative diagnosis of OF, OF versus FD, or indeterminate lesions warrants a

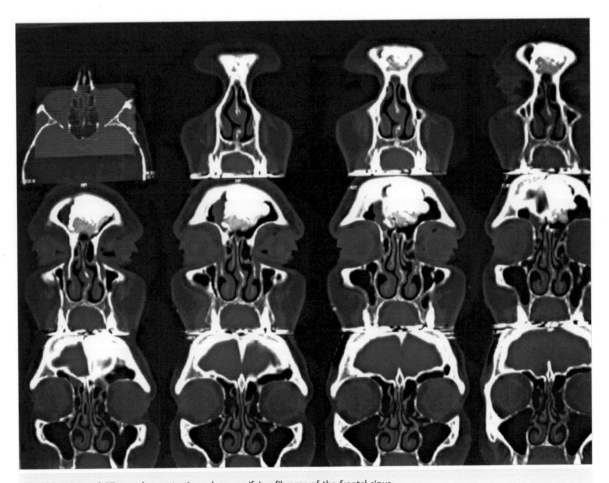

Fig. 29.4 Coronal CT scan demonstrating a large ossifying fibroma of the frontal sinus.

biopsy to establish diagnosis to guide definitive management, especially if preoperative CT imaging is concerning for an aggressive fibrosseousneoplasm.[5] The OF variants demonstrate overlapping radiological characteristics. Both magnetic resonance imaging (MRI) and CT cannot reliably differentiate the three subtypes.[5]

Histology

Macroscopically OF is often oval or circular, gray or white, with a firm shell. Histologically, the lesion consists of two main components: (1) fibrous stroma and (2) bone element. The fibrous stroma generally consists of fibroblasts and collagenous fibers. Bone elements include mineralized bodies, woven bone, and lamellar bone. Tumors in which the main mineralized component is bone are known as OFs. This is in contrast to tumors in which the main mineralized component is cementum, which are known as cementifying fibromas. Histologically, COF may have overlapping features with APOF, and the two lesions may be confused. These lesions are not thought to have malignant tendencies.

29.2.3 Management

OFs are benign tumors with possible local aggressive variants with a high rate of recurrence of 13.5% if incompletely resected.[12] The treatment of choice is dependent on the patients' symptoms, location of the tumor, and growth behavior. Options include a "wait-and-scan" policy, conservative surgical therapy, and radical surgery.[11] It is generally accepted that, if possible, a radical resection is warranted because of the slowly progressive and invasive nature of growth with the risk of local recurrence in the paranasal sinuses.[1,11]

Approaches

There are limited small case series demonstrating complete surgical resection of frontal sinus OF by a transnasal endoscopic approach.[1,11] Endoscopic resection can be technically challenging as OF can be vascular and adherence to the dura and periorbital can make dissection challenging.[10] Wang et al[11] demonstrated the need to drill the outer lamellar of the tumor and to remove all pathological bone until healthy smooth bone is seen in order to prevent recurrence.

Combined approaches may be to access the frontal sinus as discussed earlier.

29.2.4 Surgical Steps

Approach to fibro-osseous lesion in paranasal sinus (see ▶ Table 29.2–▶ Table 29.5).

29.2.5 Consent

State the planned approach, if transnasal endoscopic always consent for external approach. Risks and advantages and disadvantages of each approach are discussed.

Are the patients symptomatic or do they have pending or current complications?

If so:
1. **Secure diagnosis:**
   a) CT scan of paranasal sinus ± MRI to delineate lesion from retained secretions or, if any, intracranial or intraorbital extension.
   b) Perform a biopsy unless it is obvious that it is osteoma. Ensure that good representative specimen is obtained.
2. **Correlation of radiology and histology at multidisciplinary meeting.**
3. **Formulation of approach:**
   a) Examine the patient's anatomy on CT scan. Limiting factors for endoscopic approach include the following:
      1. Is the anteroposterior (AP) diameter of the frontal sinus on sagittal view < 1 cm?

Table 29.2 Preparation: outline of a systematic approach applied to all frontal sinus procedures

Surgical steps: preparation	Key highlights
Anesthetic Endotracheal tube (ETT) to the right side Total intravenous anaesthesia (TIVA)	Clear communication with anesthetist vital prior to case. aims: • Systolic: 90 mm Hg • Mean arterial pressure (MAP): 60 mm Hg • Heart rate (HR): 60 beats per minute
Nasal cavity preparation Cotton pledgets: 2 mL adrenaline 1:1,000 with 4 mL Naropin	
Patient position Head extension 30–40 degrees Reverse Trendelenburg 15–25 degrees	
Image guidance registration If required	
Infiltration of nasal cavity Placement: denoted by X: • Middle turbinate • Lateral wall anterior to the middle turbinate • Septum near the swell body	

Table 29.3 Draf IIb

Surgical steps	Key highlights
1. Exposure of the medial orbital wall: a sphenoethmoidectomy or at least an anterior ethmoidectomy to expose the medial orbital wall	An adrenaline soaked cotton pledget is placed posterior to agger nasi and anterior to ethmoidal bulla on removal of the uncinate.
2. Axilla of MT to be dissected superiorly until bone can no longer be removed with Kerrison rongeur or handheld instrumentation	
3. Complete resection of the remaining agger cell to ensure exposure of the frontal recess. Landmarks: Posterior: anterior wall of the ethmoid bulla Medial: vertical portion of the middle turbinate Lateral: orbital wall Anterior: nasal beak	
4. Ensure no violation of the mucosa over the anterior skull base is caused, this being the posterior boundary of the dissection	
5. Progress in anteromedial direction from Draf IIa, Draf IIb	If unable to get adequate exposure for surgical resection or the need for machine held instruments then convert to Draf III

Note: The Draf IIb technique is commonly employed for smaller more localized lesions. It is performed entirely with handheld instruments. If it is not possible to get adequate exposure of the frontal recess with handheld instruments, then conversion to Draf III is required. The risk of mucosal trauma and bone exposure with machine instruments are associated with cicatrization of the frontal sinus. The fundamental concept in any frontal sinus procedure is exposure of the key landmarks. A great deal of time is spent decongesting the nose with adrenaline-soaked cotton pledgets at the start of the case; however, we would advocate careful placement of a cotton pledget following removal of the uncinate process. This pledget is placed gently in the frontal recess, anterior to the bulla ethmoidalis and posterior to the posterior wall of the agger nasi. This decongests this area further permitting superior visualization during resection of the cells of the frontal recess and frontal os. The use of a 70-degree scope is essential for Draf IIb.

2. What is the pneumatization of the FS?
An extensive pneumatization will limit access superiorly and laterally.
    3. What is the interorbital distance? Will equipment be easily maneuvered?
4. **Consider disease:**
  a) Site of involvement:
    1. endoscopic limitation.
  b) Site of attachment (if any):
    1. Sessile.
    2. Pedunculated.
    3. Impervious.
  c) Size of lesion.
  d) Extension intraorbital or intracranial:
    1. Intraorbital—with anterior extension and anterior to nasolacrimal duct.
    2. Intracranial—extensive involvement will require neurosurgical team.
  e) Disease process surgical considerations:
    1. Osteoma: If dense, it may require excessive drilling especially if large and lateral; angulated drills have decreased rotation per minute, which results in prolonged operation time.

2. FD: Symptomatic relief rather than cure if there is extensive bony involvement.
3. OF: Locally aggressive with high recurrence rate if incompletely resected. It can be vascular, resulting in limited view endoscopically.
5. **Patient:**
  a) Age:
    1. Young—resect small asymptomatic osteoma, a simplified procedure that results in cure.
  b) Comorbidities:
    1. Safe for general anesthetic.
    2. Able to comply and tolerate postoperative follow-up.

29.3 Summary

FD and OF of the frontal sinus can represent a challenge to the surgeon. Understanding the nature of these lesions assists with a methodical approach and plan on if and when to operate. The benign lesion mandates a planned surgical approach, with justification of decisions and balancing complete resection versus an acceptable subtotal resection to minimize morbidity.

Table 29.4 Draf III

Surgical steps	Key highlights
1. Identify key initial landmarks Identify the medial orbital wall by either a sphenoethmoidectomy or at least an anterior ethmoidectomy	
2. Mucosa removal Continuous incision extending over the frontal process of the maxillary bone extending on to the roof and anteroinferiorly on to the septum	
3. Septal window Located 1.5 cm anterior to the middle turbinate root Include any swell body and is posterior to first olfactory neuron Raise as a single flap toward the olfactory cleft, starting in the apex The olfactory neuron is identified as a single neuron orientated medially	Septal bone removal is aided using a 2-mm 40-degree Kerrison rongeur and Heavy Mayo scissors superiorly and inferiorly
4. Drilling 0-degree endoscope 5-mm 15-degree diamond bur Removal • Midline crest of the septal bone inferior to the frontal sinus • Lateral limits defined by identifying the periosteum • Bone is uniformly removed anterior to the first olfactory cleft neuron	Do not enter the frontal sinus mucosa prematurely to prevent bleeding
5. Connect the frontal recess to the frontal sinus Use a Kerrison rongeur to assist with this procedure	
6. Square off the cavity Drill remaining cavity to create widest possible. • Medial orbital wall to orbital roof • Bone drilled back to the first olfactory neuron	
7. Silastic sheet Placement of the silastic sheet	 This image is provided courtesy of Richard Harvey

Note: The outside-in technique has been well documented by Richard Harvey.[9,14] This technique removes the complexity of the procedure by permitting less reliance on angulated scopes and curved instruments but also reduces operating time. The table 29.4 provides an outline of the steps involved in a Draf III approach adopting the Harvey technique.

Table 29.5 Post-operative care

Postoperative care	Key highlights
Nasopore is placed in the frontal recess—this is carefully suctioned at 7–10 d	
Nasal irrigation to commence day 1 postoperatively	200–240 mL wash bottle is used
Oral antibiotics with adequate *Staphylococcus aureus* coverage are commenced postoperatively for 1 wk	
Systemic steroids 25 mg orally daily are used for 2 wk	
Nasal steroid irrigation Budesonide 1 mg/2 mL to commence day 7 postoperatively	200–240 mL wash bottle is used
Follow-up (F/U) 1 wk: complete but nontraumatic clearance of Nasopore 6 wk 3 mo	Meticulous postoperative care is needed to prevent cicatricial stenosis Avoid too much manipulation during this phase

References

[1] Lund VJ, Stammberger H, Nicolai P, et al. European Rhinologic Society Advisory Board on Endoscopic Techniques in the Management of Nose, Paranasal Sinus and Skull Base Tumours. European position paper on endoscopic management of tumours of the nose, paranasal sinuses and skull base. Rhinol Suppl. 2010; 22(22):1–143

[2] El-Mofty SK. Fibro-osseous lesions of the craniofacial skeleton: an update. Head Neck Pathol. 2014; 8(4):432–444

[3] El-Mofty S. Bone lesions in Diagnostic Surgical Pathology of the head and neck. 2nd ed. Philadelphia, PA: Saunders, Elsevier; 2009

[4] Ricalde P, Magliocca KR, Lee JS. Craniofacial fibrous dysplasia. Oral Maxillofac Surg Clin North Am. 2012; 24(3):427–441

[5] Efune G, Perez CL, Tong L, Rihani J, Batra PS. Paranasal sinus and skull base fibro-osseous lesions: when is biopsy indicated for diagnosis? Int Forum Allergy Rhinol. 2012; 2(2):160–165

[6] Bowers CA, Altay T, Shah L, Couldwell WT. Pregnancy-induced cystic degeneration of fibrous dysplasia. Can J Neurol Sci. 2012; 39(6):828–829

[7] Charlett SD, Mackay SG, Sacks R. Endoscopic treatment of fibrous dysplasia confined to the frontal sinus. Otolaryngol Head Neck Surg. 2007; 136(4) Suppl:S59–S61

[8] Ooi EH, Glicksman JT, Vescan AD, Witterick IJ. An alternative management approach to paranasal sinus fibro-osseous lesions. Int Forum Allergy Rhinol. 2011; 1(1):55–63

[9] Knisely A, Barham HP, Harvey RJ, Sacks R. Outside-in frontal drill-out: how i do it. Am J Rhinol Allergy. 2015; 29(5):397–400

[10] Ciniglio Appiani M, Verillaud B, Bresson D, et al. Ossifying fibromas of the paranasal sinuses: diagnosis and management. Acta Otorhinolaryngol Ital. 2015; 35(5):355–361

[11] Wang H, Sun X, Liu Q, Wang J, Wang D. Endoscopic resection of sinonasal ossifying fibroma: 31 cases report at an institution. Eur Arch Otorhinolaryngol. 2014; 271(11):2975–2982

[12] Manes RP, Ryan MW, Batra PS, Mendelsohn D, Fang YV, Marple BF. Ossifying fibroma of the nose and paranasal sinuses. Int Forum Allergy Rhinol. 2013; 3(2):161–168

[13] Ledderose GJ, Stelter K, Becker S, Leunig A. Paranasal ossifying fibroma: endoscopic resection or wait and scan? Eur Arch Otorhinolaryngol. 2011; 268(7):999–1004

[14] Chin D, Snidvongs K, Kalish L, Sacks R, Harvey RJ. The outside-in approach to the modified endoscopic Lothrop procedure. Laryngoscope. 2012; 122(8):1661–1669

30 Malignant Disease Involving the Frontal Sinus

Dennis Tang, Christopher Roxbury, Kelsey McHugh, Deborah Chute, and Raj Sindwani

Abstract

Primary malignant neoplasms of the frontal sinuses are rare entities. They can be divided into epithelial malignancies (including squamous cell carcinoma, sinonasal undifferentiated carcinoma, small cell neuroendocrine carcinomas, adenocarcinoma, esthesioneuroblastoma) and nonepithelial malignancies (including non-Hodgkin's lymphoma and malignant melanoma). Patients commonly present with sequelae of nasal obstruction, epistaxis, and orbital complaints. Imaging is critical for staging and treatment planning. The staging system developed by the University of Florida is the most commonly cited system, although no staging system has been universally accepted. Treatment options include surgery, chemotherapy, and radiation. Surgical treatment can be performed via endoscopic, open, or combined approaches. Endoscopic approaches are ideal for small, low-grade malignancies with favorable anatomy. Open or combined approaches are required for larger tumors especially those with orbital and cranial involvement. Reconstruction depends on the size of the defect and range from mucosal grafts to free flaps.

Keywords: sinonasal malignancies, squamous cell carcinoma, sinonasal undifferentiated carcinoma, melanoma, adenocarcinoma, non-Hodgkin's lymphoma, small cell neuroendocrine carcinoma, esthesioneuroblastoma

30.1 Epidemiology and Etiology

Malignant diseases involving the frontal sinuses can be broadly categorized into epithelial malignancies and nonepithelial malignancies. Epithelial malignancies include squamous cell carcinoma, sinonasal undifferentiated carcinoma (SNUC), small-cell neuroendocrine carcinoma (SNEC), adenocarcinoma, and esthesioneuroblastoma. Nonepithelial malignancies that may affect the frontal sinuses include melanoma and sinonasal non-Hodgkin's lymphoma (NHL). Other forms of frontal sinus malignancies including rhabdomyosarcoma, fibrosarcoma, or sinonasal teratocarcinosarcoma are exceedingly rare and beyond the scope of this chapter.

Squamous cell carcinoma is the most common primary malignancy of the frontal sinus.[1] Initially, cancers of the frontal sinuses have nonspecific symptoms. Many patients present at advanced stages, resulting in poor overall prognosis. Risk factors for developing squamous cell carcinoma of the paranasal sinuses include exposure to wood dust, formaldehyde, and nickel.[2] These irritants are thought to cause chronic inflammation leading to development of cancer. Squamous cell carcinomas of the paranasal sinuses are histopathologically similar to squamous cell carcinoma in other regions of the head and neck (▶ Fig. 30.1). Surgical resection is the preferred primary treatment of choice with postoperative adjuvant therapy for advanced disease.

SNUC is a rare and highly aggressive malignancy that was first described by Frierson et al in 1986.[3] The underlying etiology of SNUC remains unknown. Typical presenting symptoms include nasal obstruction, epistaxis, vision changes, and headaches.[4] Nearly 60% of patients diagnosed with SNUC have extension beyond the paranasal sinuses. Median survival is 22.1 months.[5] These tumors show poor differentiation on histology, and immunohistochemistry is key in differentiating SNUC from other tumors (▶ Fig. 30.2). Multimodal therapy is recommended, including aggressive surgical resection when possible and adjuvant chemoradiation therapy.

Mucosal melanoma is another aggressive tumor of the paranasal sinuses. Unlike cutaneous melanoma, mucosal melanoma tends to present in older patients and sun exposure is not a risk factor. Although more commonly found in the nasal cavity and maxillary sinuses, mucosal melanoma is known to occur in the frontal sinus as well.[6] Complete surgical resection with clear margins is recommended where possible. Elective neck dissection without clinical evidence of locoregional metastasis is controversial due to low rate of regional metastasis.[7] Although there is an abundance of literature regarding sentinel node biopsy in cutaneous melanoma, the utility of sentinel node biopsy in mucosal melanoma still needs to be elucidated. Oldenburg and Price describe two cases of sinonasal mucosal melanoma that were found to have positive sentinel nodes on biopsy leading to cervical lymphadenectomy in both patients.[8] Pathological features of the tumor may guide decision-making with respect to cervical lymph node dissection, with lower risk of metastasis noted in macular mucosal melanoma and in those tumors with less than 5- to 7-mm tumor depth.[9] Postoperative radiation therapy is recommended in advanced disease. Systemic therapy is never used as monotherapy for mucosal melanoma but may have utility in combination with another modality of treatment.[7] Overall prognosis remains poor with 50% of patients developing distant metastases after treatment.[9] Despite advances in technology, average survival is approximately 2 years.[7]

Adenocarcinoma of the paranasal sinuses primarily occurs in the maxillary sinus. Primary tumors of the frontal sinus are rare. The World Health Organization classifies sinonasal adenocarcinoma into intestinal-type adenocarcinomas (ITACs) and nonintestinal sinonasal adenocarcinomas (non-ITACs). ITACs are known to have very strong association with wood and other dust exposures,[10] and are

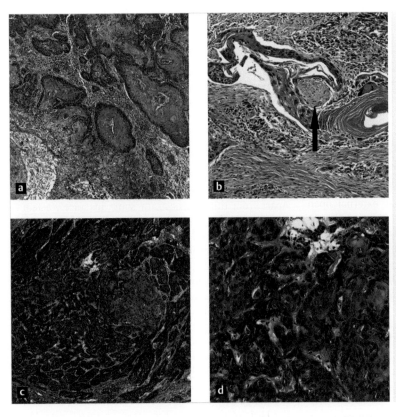

Fig. 30.1 Squamous cell carcinoma. **(a)** Low-power magnification shows invasive nests of well-differentiated to moderately differentiated keratinizing squamous cell carcinoma with tumor cells violating their basement membrane, invading the lamina propria both singly and in small clusters, groups, or nests (hematoxylin and eosin [H&E] × 40). **(b)** High-power magnification shows a nest of moderately differentiated, keratinizing squamous cell carcinoma wrapping around a nerve (*arrow*), forming a focus of perineural invasion with an adjacent keratin pearl (H&E × 100). **(c)** Low-power magnification shows nests and interanastomosing cords of poorly differentiated squamous cell carcinoma with an associated inflammatory and desmoplastic stromal response at its periphery (H&E × 40). **(d)** High-power magnification highlights hyperchromatic, pleomorphic tumor cells with irregular nuclear contours, variably conspicuous nucleoli, occasional mitoses, and apoptosis (H&E × 100).

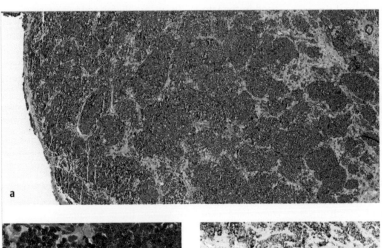

Fig. 30.2 Sinonasal undifferentiated carcinoma. **(a)** Intermediate-power magnification demonstrates a hypercellular proliferation of cells arranged in lobules and trabecularlike cords (hematoxylin and eosin [H&E] × 40). **(b)** High-power magnification shows sheets of pleomorphic cells with high nuclear-to-cytoplasm ratios, prominent central nucleoli, irregular nuclear contours, high mitotic activity (*circle*), and prominent individual cell apoptosis (*arrows*; H&E × 300). **(c)** Though these tumors lack morphological evidence of glandular or squamous differentiation, they are consistently immunoreactive with epithelial markers such as the cytokeratin CAM5.2, which highlights positive tumor cells via its brown cytoplasmic staining (CAM5.2 × 100).

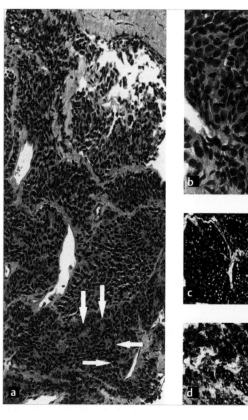
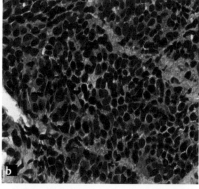
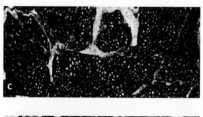
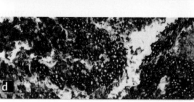

Fig. 30.3 Small cell neuroendocrine carcinoma. **(a)** Low-power magnification demonstrates a tumor composed of nests and sheets of cells with high nuclear-to-cytoplasmic ratios, indistinct cell borders, and occasional neural-type rosette formations (*arrows*; hematoxylin and eosin [H&E] × 100). **(b)** High-power magnification shows sheets of malignant cells with finely stippled nuclear chromatin (salt and pepper chromatin) and nuclear molding (H&E × 400). **(c)** Immunohistochemical staining for neuroendocrine markers such as synaptophysin or chromogranin highlights positive tumor cells via their brown cytoplasmic staining (synaptophysin × 100). **(d)** Immunohistochemical staining for cytokeratin positively stains the cytoplasm of tumor cells brown (CAM5.2 × 100).

aggressive neoplasms, as over 60% of patients will die of their disease, particularly those with a higher grade tumor,[11] and complete resection is the treatment of choice, with postoperative radiation therapy in advanced disease. Non-ITACs are divided into low and high grades, which have distinctly different morphologies and associated outcomes. Low-grade non-ITACs typically appear papillary or tubular with monomorphic cuboidal cells, a subset of which are believed to have seromucinous differentiation.[12] Treatment is complete surgical removal with negative margins if possible, and postoperative radiotherapy in advanced cases. Approximately 25% of patients with a low-grade non-ITAC will recur, but less than 10% will succumb to disease, usually due to loss of local control.[13] High-grade non-ITACs have a variety of histological features but show at least focal glandular differentiation.[14] This likely represents a heterogeneous group of tumors currently not well understood. Survival is generally poor, with most patients succumbing to disease within 5 years of diagnosis.[13]

SNEC, also known as oat-cell carcinoma, typically affects the lung. In rare instances, it is known to develop within the paranasal sinuses. Histologically, these tumors can be difficult to differentiate from SNUC and esthesioneuroblastoma. SNEC appears as small cells with a distinct staining pattern (▸ Fig. 30.3). Similar to other tumors in the sinonasal cavity, SNEC presents with nonspecific symptoms including nasal obstruction, epistaxis,

and discharge. Chemoradiation is a reasonable primary treatment modality with surgery reserved for nonresponders.[15]

Esthesioneuroblastoma originates from the olfactory neuroepithelium of the nasal cavity. Histology is key to differentiate this tumor from other small round blue cell tumors (▸ Fig. 30.4). Esthesioneuroblastoma cells are often in syncytial arrangement with a web of neuronal processes (neuropil) forming the background stroma. Homer Wright pseudorosettes and Flexner–Wintersteiner rosettes are classically seen. Homer Wright pseudorosettes are formed from palisading cells surrounding neuropil, while Flexner–Wintersteiner rosettes are true rosettes comprising glandlike spaces lined by ciliated columnar cells. The current histological grading system was proposed by Hyams in 1982, which categorizes cases of esthesioneuroblastoma into four grades ranging from well-differentiated to poorly differentiated (▸ Table 30.1).[16] In the past, anterior craniofacial resection was considered standard of care. However, with the advancement of endoscopic techniques, an endoscopic resection is possible when the anatomy is favorable. A meta-analysis has shown no difference in survival rates between open and endoscopic resections.[17] Esthesioneuroblastoma has a propensity for prolonged time before local recurrence and distant metastasis. Therefore, long-term follow-up for up to 10 years is recommended.[18]

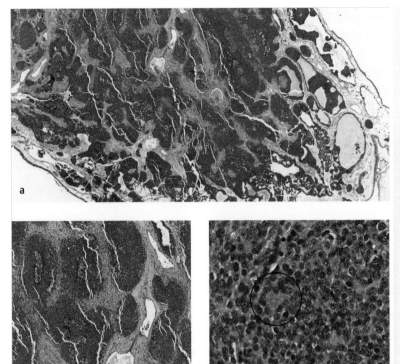

Fig. 30.4 Esthesioneuroblastoma (olfactory neuroblastoma). **(a)** Low-power magnification demonstrates a tumor composed of well-developed nests of small round blue cells arranged in a lobular architecture and undermining a respiratory mucosa uninvolved by neoplasm (hematoxylin and eosin [H&E] × 10). **(b)** Intermediate-power magnification shows nests of small round blue cells percolating through a finely fibrillary neural matrix (H&E × 40). **(c)** High-power magnification highlights small round blue cells with uniform nuclei and delicate salt and pepper chromatin arranged in sheets with occasional pseudorosette formation (Homer–Wright pseudorosette; *circled*; H&E × 400).

Table 30.1 Hyams' grading scale for esthesioneuroblastoma

Histological Feature	Grade 1	Grade 2	Grade 3	Grade 4
Architecture	Lobar	Lobar	±	±
Mitotic activity	Absent	Present	Prominent	Marked
Nuclear pleomorphism	Absent	Moderate	Prominent	Marked
Fibrillary matrix	Prominent	Present	Minimal	Absent
Rosette	HW	HW	FW	FW
Necrosis	Absent	Absent	±	Common

Abbreviations: FW, Flexner–Wintersteiner; HW, Homer Wright.

NHL is the second most common malignancy affecting the paranasal sinuses after SCC. These malignancies have similar clinical presentations compared to other tumors of this region. Surgery seldom has a role in treatment of NHL and chemotherapy and/or radiation remains the mainstay of treatment.

30.2 Clinical Presentation and Investigation

A thorough history and physical examination should be performed on all patients with concern for primary tumor of the frontal sinuses. Symptoms of nasal obstruction, epistaxis, or dysosmia should be evaluated. Clear rhinorrhea, especially with changes in position, may be concerning for cerebrospinal fluid (CSF) leak and dural involvement. Orbital symptoms such as pain, diplopia, or visual disturbances may indicate orbital involvement. All patients with suspicion for frontal sinus malignancy should be evaluated with nasal endoscopy. The nasal cavity should be examined for extension of the mass from the frontal sinuses. Initial evaluation with high-resolution computed tomography with slices less than 1.0 mm is recommended. This can evaluate for osseous erosion or invasion. Magnetic resonance imaging (MRI) should be used to further characterize the tumor. Specifically, dural or intradural extension can be viewed on MRI. Previous studies have shown a specificity of 97.9% for dural enhancement on MRI and tumor extension.[19] In patients with suspicion of dural involvement, thorough discussion with neurosurgery is required to determine resectability and preoperative planning. These images can also be used for intraoperative neuronavigation.

30.3 Staging

Due to the rarity of primary malignancies of the frontal sinus, no staging system has been universally established. The American Joint Committee on Cancer staging system for paranasal sinus tumors exclude those in the frontal sinus. A staging system was developed at the University of Florida for evaluating tumors of the nasal cavity, sphenoid, and frontal sinuses.[20] Stage I tumors are limited to the site of origin. Stage II involves extension into adjacent sites (orbit, skin, nasopharynx, pterygomaxillary fossa). Stage III involves base of skull or pterygoid plate destruction and/or intracranial extension. However, no staging system has garnered widespread use.

30.4 Management

Approaches to surgical resection of frontal sinus malignancies can be divided into three categories: endoscopic, open, or combined.

Endoscopic approaches can be appropriate for small, low-grade malignancies. The patient's anatomy must be taken into consideration prior to attempting an endoscopic approach. According to Draf, the Draf III procedure requires an anterior to posterior dimension of at least 0.8 cm to be technically feasible.[21] Furthermore, a pronounced convexity of the posterior wall can impede the ability of endoscopic instruments from reaching the full extent of a tumor. Tumors in the lateral portion or with lateral spread are considered by some clinicians to be a contraindication to endoscopic approaches.[22] Frontal sinus trephination (or osteoplastic flap approaches) may be used to assist with exposure of tumors that are difficult to reach transnasally.

The resection of most malignant tumors involving the frontal sinus necessitates an open approach to sufficiently achieve total resection of the tumor. The open frontoethmoidectomy was first described by Knapp in 1908 as a transorbital approach to the frontal sinus. An incision is made beneath the medial aspect of the eyebrow along a curvilinear path midway between the nasal dorsum and medial canthus. The dissection is carried through the soft tissue to the periosteum of the frontal process of the maxilla. The periosteum is elevated along the medial orbital wall exposing the frontoethmoidal suture line. Identification of the anterior ethmoid artery along the frontoethmoidal suture approximately 24 mm posterior to the lacrimal crest marks the floor of the anterior

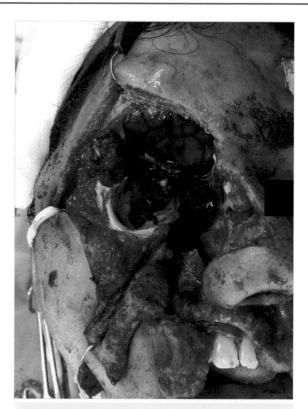

Fig. 30.5 Intraoperative exposure using a brow incision extend along a lateral rhinotomy. A supraorbital craniotomy was performed exposing the frontal lobe. The patient had tumor invading into the orbit and an orbital exenteration was also performed.

cranial fossa. The floor of the frontal sinus can be opened at this point to expose the mass. If necessary, the incision can be extended along the superior orbital rim to expose the lateral portion of the frontal sinus. The incision can be extended inferiorly along a lateral rhinotomy incision to expose the nasal cavity, which may be necessary for larger tumors. For tumors that extend intracranially, a supraorbital craniotomy may be performed (▶ Fig. 30.5). This allows access to the anterior cranial fossa with exposure posteriorly to the pituitary gland. For masses that invade extensively into the cranial vault, a bifrontal craniotomy may be necessary. This should be considered to safely control the neurovascular structure in patients undergoing orbital exenteration with significant intracranial involvement.

Depending on the pathology, adjuvant chemotherapy or radiation therapy may be necessary. Since the majority of these tumors present at advanced stage, a multidisciplinary approach involving radiation and medical oncology is often necessary.

Reconstruction depends on the size of the defect. Small defects can be closed using local rotational flaps. Most often, these can be performed via advancement of the scalp. Larger defects may necessitate a free flap especially

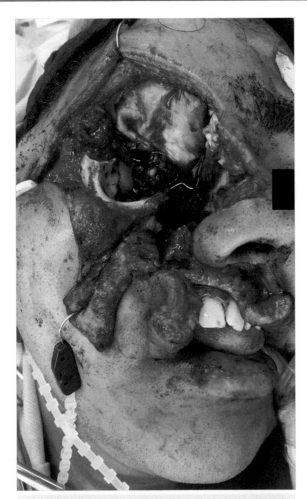

Fig. 30.6 Defect closed using fascia lata graft to reconstruct the dural defect.

30.5 Case Example

A 32-year-old gentleman presented with diplopia, right eye swelling, headache, and right facial numbness. He had a 50-lb weight loss over the course of 8 months. On examination, he was noted to have proptosis of his right eye, diplopia with upward gaze, and right-sided upper trigeminal anesthesia. MRI revealed an enhancing soft-tissue mass involving the right frontal and right ethmoidal air cells with destruction of the right lamina papyracea, postseptal orbital involvement, and intracranial involvement. The mass measured 3.5 cm × 3.5 cm in size. The patient was taken to the operating room for a transnasal biopsy, which was consistent with SNUC. His case was discussed at a multidisciplinary tumor board and the decision was made to proceed with surgical resection and adjuvant chemoradiation therapy. His resection was performed via a right craniofacial approach including a lateral rhinotomy, orbital exenteration, ethmoidectomy, and partial maxillectomy. An orbitofrontal craniotomy was performed to resect the intracranial component of the tumor. A fascia lata onlay graft was placed in the subdural space to close the dura. A large anterolateral thigh free flap was used to reconstruct the defect. The inferior orbital rim was preserved and used to suspend the free flap. A subarachnoid drain was placed and CSF was drained until postoperative day 5. His postoperative course was uncomplicated. He received 64 Gy of radiation in 32 fractions with concurrent cisplatin and etoposide.

30.6 Complications: Management

Complications of resection of frontal sinus malignancies include CSF leak, pneumocephalus, meningitis, intracranial abscess, and/or stroke. Pneumocephalus can occur from air egressing from the sinonasal tract into the cranial cavity caused by defects in the dura. Presenting symptoms include changes in mental status and headache. This should be evaluated immediately with a CT scan. Small amounts of air can be managed with observation; however, larger amounts of air should be evacuated. CSF leak is another common complication, typically presenting with clear rhinorrhea. A small leak can be managed by placement of a subarachnoid drain. If drainage continues, operative repair may be indicated. Infections of the central nervous system are a major source of morbidity and mortality after open frontal sinus surgery. Appropriate perioperative prophylactic antibiotics and separation of the sinonasal mucosa from the intracranial compartment are key in reducing infection risks.

in the cases requiring orbital exenteration or in the cases with large dural defects (▶ Fig. 30.6). The anterolateral thigh free flap offers the necessary bulk to fill the orbital exenteration cavity. A critical aspect of reconstruction is abutment of the free flap to the cranial vault to facilitate healing. If the orbital rim or orbital floor is left intact, these allow for a reliable shelf to support the free flap. A 30-mL Foley balloon can be placed intranasally to suspend the reconstruction. Large dural defects should be repaired with a multilayered approach. Multiple methods can be used to repair the dura including acellular dermal matrix, collagen matrix, fat grafts, fascia lata grafts, the temporoparietal fascia flap, or the pericranial flap.

30.7 Tips and Tricks

Point of difficulty	Technical solution
1. Is an endoscopic approach possible?	1. Tumor should not extend past the midpupillary line due to decreased access. A narrow frontal outflow tract in the anteroposterior direction limits ability for endoscopic instrumentation
2. Should an orbital exenteration be performed?	2. Preoperative imaging should be obtained. Bowing of an intact periorbita from mass effect should be distinguished from invasion

References

[1] Dutta R, Dubal PM, Svider PF, Liu JK, Baredes S, Eloy JA. Sinonasal malignancies: A population-based analysis of site-specific incidence and survival. Laryngoscope. 2015; 125(11):2491–2497

[2] Siew SS, Kauppinen T, Kyyronen P, Heikkila P, Pukkala E. Occupational exposure to wood dust and formaldehyde and risk of nasal, nasopharyngeal and lung cancer among finnish men: a whole-population-based retrospective cohort study. Epidemiol Prev. 2010; 34:158

[3] Frierson HF, Jr, Mills SE, Fechner RE, Taxy JB, Levine PA. Sinonasal undifferentiated carcinoma. An aggressive neoplasm derived from schneiderian epithelium and distinct from olfactory neuroblastoma. Am J Surg Pathol. 1986; 10(11):771–779

[4] Xu CC, Dziegielewski PT, McGaw WT, Seikaly H. Sinonasal undifferentiated carcinoma (SNUC): the Alberta experience and literature review. J Otolaryngol Head Neck Surg. 2013; 42:2

[5] Chambers KJ, Lehmann AE, Remenschneider A, et al. Incidence and survival patterns of sinonasal undifferentiated carcinoma in the United States. J Neurol Surg B Skull Base. 2015; 76(2):94–100

[6] Narasimhan K, Kucuk O, Lin HS, et al. Sinonasal mucosal melanoma: a 13-year experience at a single institution. Skull Base. 2009; 19 (4):255–262

[7] Gore MR, Zanation AM. Survival in sinonasal melanoma: a meta-analysis. J Neurol Surg B Skull Base. 2012; 73(3):157–162

[8] Oldenburg MS, Price DL. The utility of sentinel node biopsy for sinonasal melanoma. J Neurol Surg B Skull Base. 2017; 78(5):425–429

[9] Manolidis S, Donald PJ. Malignant mucosal melanoma of the head and neck: review of the literature and report of 14 patients. Cancer. 1997; 80(8):1373–1386

[10] Michel J, Radulesco T, Penicaud M, Mancini J, Dessi P. Sinonasal adenocarcinoma: clinical outcomes and predictive factors. Int J Oral Maxillofac Surg. 2017; 46(4):422–427

[11] Barnes L. Intestinal-type adenocarcinoma of the nasal cavity and paranasal sinuses. Am J Surg Pathol. 1986; 10(3):192–202

[12] Purgina B, Bastaki JM, Duvvuri U, Seethala RR. A subset of sinonasal non-intestinal type adenocarcinomas are truly seromucinous adenocarcinomas: a morphologic and immunophenotypic assessment and description of a novel pitfall. Head Neck Pathol. 2015; 9(4):436–446

[13] Stelow EB, Brandwein-Gensler M, Frachi A, Nicolai P, Wenig B. Non-intestinal-type adenocarcinoma. In: El-Naggar AK, Chan JK, Rubin Grandis J, Takata T, Slootweg PJ, eds. WHO Classification of Head and Neck Tumors. Lyon: International Agency for Research on Cancer; 2017:24–25

[14] Stelow EB, Jo VY, Mills SE, Carlson DL. A histologic and immunohistochemical study describing the diversity of tumors classified as sinonasal high-grade nonintestinal adenocarcinomas. Am J Surg Pathol. 2011; 35(7):971–980

[15] Babin E, Rouleau V, Vedrine PO, et al. Small cell neuroendocrine carcinoma of the nasal cavity and paranasal sinuses. J Laryngol Otol. 2006; 120(4):289–297

[16] Hyams VJ. Olfactory neuroblastoma (case 6). In: Batasakis J, Hyams VJ, Morales A, eds. Special Tumors of the Head and Neck. Chicago, IL: ASCP Press; 1982:24–29

[17] Devaiah AK, Andreoli MT. Treatment of esthesioneuroblastoma: a 16-year meta-analysis of 361 patients. Laryngoscope. 2009; 119 (7):1412–1416

[18] Gore MR, Zanation AM. Salvage treatment of local recurrence in esthesioneuroblastoma: A meta-analysis. Skull Base. 2011; 21(1):1–6

[19] Moiyadi AV, Pai P, Nair D, Pal P, Shetty P. Dural involvement in skull base tumors-accuracy of preoperative radiological evaluation and intraoperative assessment. J Craniofac Surg. 2013; 24(2):526–530

[20] Katz TS, Mendenhall WM, Morris CG, Amdur RJ, Hinerman RW, Villaret DB. Malignant tumors of the nasal cavity and paranasal sinuses. Head Neck. 2002; 24(9):821–829

[21] Draf W. Endonasal frontal sinus drainage type I–III according to Draf. In: Kountakis S, Senior B, Draf W, eds. The Frontal Sinus. Berlin, Germany: Springer; 2005:219–232

[22] Sieśkiewicz A, Lyson T, Piszczatowski B, Rogowski M. Endoscopic treatment of adversely located osteomas of the frontal sinus. Ann Otol Rhinol Laryngol. 2012; 121(8):503–509

31 Acute Frontal Osteomyelitis: Intracranial and Orbital Complications

Ashok Rokade and Dimitris Ioannidis

Abstract

Acute frontal sinusitis can be associated with a range of serious orbital, intracranial, and osseous complications with unique challenges in diagnosis and management. These entities have a variable clinical presentation and can frequently be concurrent and overlapping. Contrast-enhanced sinus CT is the standard initial, and often definitive, imaging modality for diagnosis and surgical planning, whereas MRI may offer superior soft-tissue resolution and is most appropriate in the context of suspected intracranial complications. Management requires a multidisciplinary approach by ENT (ear, nose, and throat), ophthalmology, neurosurgery, infectious diseases, and microbiology. In early stages, conservative management with antibiotics may be sufficient. However, surgical intervention to drain a formed collection of infectious material along with drainage of the affected sinus may be necessary in many cases and may require endoscopic or external approaches or their combination. Most commonly in the acute setting drainage of the frontal sinus via limited functional endoscopic sinus surgery and mini-trephination/trephination in combination with drainage of a potential collection via a Lynch–Howarth or transblepharoplasty approach for orbital collections, skull trephination/craniotomy for intracranial collections and surgical debridement of sequestered bone in case osteomyelitis is performed. Extended drainage of the sinus in order to prevent disease recurrence and/or surgical reconstruction of a potential cosmetic osseous defect is usually scheduled at a later time when the acute infection has settled. This definite treatment may vary from an endoscopic endonasal Draf IIa, IIb, and III (modified endoscopic Lothrop) procedure or even external frontoethmoidectomy to osteoplastic flap or cranialization of the sinus depending on the individual circumstances.

Keywords: frontal sinusitis, complications, orbital, intracranial, osseous, abscess, subdural, epidural, subperiosteal, cerebritis, cellulitis, Pott's puffy tumor

31.1 Epidemiology and Etiology

31.1.1 Epidemiology

The incidence of complications of acute rhinosinusitis (ARS) is estimated to be 2.5 to 4.3 per million population.[1,2,3,4] Acute frontal sinusitis (AFS) can be associated with orbital, intracranial, and osseous complications. Although the occurrence of each individual type is variable in the literature, the orbital complications are the commonest ones and twice as frequent as the intracranial, and the osseous complications are the least common.[3,5,6]

AFS and its complications present a higher prevalence in males (2.6–3.3:1) in their second to third decades of life,[6,7,8] likely due to frontal sinus development and vascularity peaking in this age group.[9] A higher prevalence during the winter months, probably due to the seasonal variation of upper respiratory tract infections (URTI), is also noted.[2]

Orbital complications consist of preseptal cellulitis, orbital cellulitis, subperiosteal abscess, orbital abscess, and cavernous sinus thrombosis according to the most commonly used Chandler's classification (▶ Table 31.1). Eighty-five percent of orbital complications of ARS are seen in the pediatric population. They are associated, in order of decreasing frequency, with the ethmoid, maxillary, and frontal sinusitis.[1,3,4,5] However, in frontal sinusitis in particular, the spread to the orbit can be more rapid, have worse outcomes, and have a higher rate of requiring surgical intervention.[3,9]

Intracranial complications of ARS include epidural or subdural abscess formation, intraparenchymal brain abscess, meningitis, cerebritis, and superior sagittal or cavernous sinus thrombosis. Intracranial complications can occur at any age. Frontal sinusitis is their most common source among all other sinuses.[9,10]

Osseous complications rarely result from vascular necrosis and osteomyelitis of the anterior and posterior table of the frontal sinus. Osteomyelitis of the anterior table may result in subperiosteal abscess formation that may be confused with a neoplasm (hence the term Pott's puffy tumor). Osteomyelitis of the posterior table may be linked to intracranial complications.[1,9]

Table 31.1 Classification of ARS complications

Orbital complications	Intracranial complications	Osseous complications
Preseptal cellulitis	Epidural	Putt's puffy tumor
Orbital cellulitis	Subdural abscess	
Subperiosteal abscess	Intraparenchymal brain abscess	
Orbital abscess	Meningitis/cerebritis	
Cavernous sinus thrombosis	Cavernous/superior sagittal sinus thrombosis	

233

Table 31.2 Anatomical and pathological causes of acute frontal sinusitis

Complex frontal recess cell anatomy	Anatomical variations narrowing the outflow tract	Nasal pathology causing obstruction
Prominent agger nasi	Large concha bullosa	Nasal polyps/tumor
Type I–IV Kuhn's cells	Medially rotated uncinate process that contacts the middle turbinate	Trauma
Supraorbital ethmoid cell	Laterally convex middle turbinate that contacts the lateral nasal wall	Chronic mucosal inflammation
Bulla frontalis	Severe septal deviation	Scaring and stenosis due to previous surgery

31.1.2 Etiology

Anatomic variations and nasal pathology favoring obstruction of the nasofrontal outflow tract may facilitate the development of AFS and its complications (► Table 31.2).

Anatomic relationships play a pivotal role in the spread of the infection and the development of complications in the context of AFS. These may develop either by direct spread of the infection from the frontal sinus to the orbits through bony dehiscences, neurovascular foramina, and open suture lines or by means of retrograde thrombophlebitis via the valveless diploic veins.[8,11]

The horizontal orbital plate of the frontal bone that forms the roof of the orbit is the thinnest wall of the frontal sinus. It also joins with the ethmoid bone to form both the roof of the nasal cavity and the floor of the anterior cranial fossa. The periorbita while attached firmly to the underlying bone at the orbital rims, suture lines, orbital fissures, and lacrimal crest is loosely adherent elsewhere. This allows infection to spread and form a subperiosteal abscess.[9,12] The periorbita unites at the orbital rim with the periosteum of the frontal and maxillary bones and forms the orbital septum of the upper and lower eyelids. This forms an anatomic barrier to infection that defines the preseptal and postseptal spaces.[12] The relation of the infection to the orbital septum is the basis of the classification of orbital infections. A subperiosteal abscess forms between the periorbita and the sinus bone and is extraconal (i.e., located outside the ocular muscles), while the orbital abscess is intraconal (contained within the space defined by the ocular muscles).

The valveless diploic veins of the orbit allow free communication between the facial, sinus, orbital, and intracranial venous network facilitating the spread of the infection. These join to form two main veins: (1) the superior ophthalmic vein, which is formed by the union of the angular and supraorbital veins, travels posterolaterally through the orbit, and exits through the superior orbital fissure to enter the cavernous sinus[9,13] and (2) the inferior ophthalmic vein, that originates near the anterior orbital floor and terminates by sending one branch to the pterygoid plexus through the inferior orbital fissure and a second, larger branch to the superior ophthalmic vein. Both branches drain ultimately into the cavernous sinus providing the route for the spread of the infection.[12]

Differences have been reported in the microbial flora isolated in adult and pediatric patients with orbital complications. In adults, the isolates consist of polymicrobial, anaerobic, and odontogenic microorganisms, in contrast to the *Staphylococcus pneumoniae,* nontypeable *Haemophilus influenzae,* and *Moraxella catarrhalis* that are prevalent in the pediatric population. Single aerobic pathogens are more common in infection within the first decade of life as compared with polymicrobial infection and more severe presentation of postseptal infections in the older groups.[14]

Intracranial spread may result from erosion of the sinus bone, but most commonly occurs by hematogenous spread through the valveless diploic veins that extend through the posterior table of the sinus and directly communicate with the venous plexus of the dura and periosteum.[15] Bacterial thrombi can travel through this network and spread to distant intracranial sites, leading to epidural, subdural, or intracerebral abscesses, meningitis, or even cavernous or superior sagittal sinus thrombosis via a retrograde thrombophlebitis.[9,16]

Abscesses tend to form in the white matter rather than in the gray matter due to its poorer blood supply. All cerebral complications start as encephalitis, but as necrosis and liquefaction of brain tissue progresses, a capsule develops, resulting in brain abscess over a period of weeks. Studies show a high incidence of anaerobic or mixed aerobic–anaerobic organisms in patients with intracranial complications.[1]

Spread of frontal sinusitis to the frontal bone leads to osteomyelitis.[17] This may result from direct extension of frontal sinusitis to the bone, hematogenous spread, or retrograde thrombophlebitis via the diploic veins of Galen. Osteomyelitis of the anterior table can result in a subperiosteal abscess formation that clinically manifests as a fluctuant swelling of the skin over the frontal bone. This is known as Pott's puffy tumor. Osteomyelitis of the posterior table may lead to intracranial complications, as described earlier.[1,18]

31.2 Clinical Presentation and Investigations

31.2.1 Orbital Complications

Patients with orbital complications typically present with a history of a recent upper respiratory infection and

Table 31.3 Chandler's classification of orbital complications of acute sinusitis

Preseptal cellulitis	Nontender inflammatory edema of the eyelids and conjunctiva. This is located anterior to the orbital septum and considered secondary to restricted venous drainage	
Orbital cellulitis	Pronounced inflammation and edema of the orbital soft tissues without abscess formation. Characteristic signs consist of proptosis, chemosis, and decreased extraocular motility	
Subperiosteal abscess	Abscess formation in the potential space between periorbita and bone. This causes mass effect, displacing the orbital contents. Chemosis and proptosis are always present, while reduced ocular mobility and vision loss may develop over time	
Orbital abscess	Pus and necrotic material collection within the orbital tissue. Severe proptosis and near complete ophthalmoplegia are noted with visual loss in the majority of cases	
Cavernous sinus thrombosis	Characterized by proptosis, chemosis, ophthalmoplegia, and decreased visual acuity along with nonspecific signs and symptoms as fever, headache, periorbital edema, and photophobia. The development of bilateral ocular symptoms is the classic finding in this condition. Meningitic symptoms or cranial nerve III, IV, V1, V2, VI palsies in the presence of a unilateral orbital infection are also indicative of cavernous sinus thrombosis	

symptoms of acute bacterial rhinosinusitis accompanied with fever, eyelid edema, and conjunctival injection. The classic Chandler classification suggests progression of the spread of the infection in stages with characteristic clinical manifestations (▶ Table 31.3).[1,9,14]

Despite this being the most commonly used classification, it has been debated that preseptal cellulitis should be classified as an eyelid, rather than as an orbital infection,[11,19] due to its different clinical presentation, treatment, and prognosis and that cavernous sinus thrombosis should more appropriately be considered an intracranial complication rather than the end stage of orbital infection.[7]

Preseptal cellulitis is by far the most common complication accounting for nearly 80% of the orbital complications reported in the literature.[8] It involves the infection of the soft tissue anterior to the orbital septum. Typically, there is no associated proptosis and no restriction of eye movement, although this may be difficult to assess, especially in young children.[20] Diagnosis is clinical and does not require imaging.[8,22]

> **Box 31.1 Signs indicating postseptal involvement[12,14]**
>
> Proptosis
> Restricted ocular movement
> Changes in red/green color discrimination
> Decreased visual acuity
> Afferent pupillary defect

Orbital cellulitis, orbital abscess, and subperiosteal abscess may all manifest with proptosis, restricted and painful ocular movement, conjunctival edema (chemosis), ocular pain, and tenderness (Box 31.1).[6] In the cases of abscess formation, ophthalmoplegia is more prominent and the risk for visual loss is higher. In most series, fever and raised leucocytes—and increased inflammatory markers are noted.[22]

In the absence of prompt intervention, the infection may result in central retinal artery occlusion, optic neuritis, corneal ulceration, or panophthalmitis leading to blindness. It can also spread intracranially, causing intracranial complications.[23]

31.2.2 Intracranial Complications

Intracranial complications may present with nonspecific symptoms and signs, like acute or progressive headache, high fever, lethargy, reduced consciousness, or with focal neurological signs or sign of increased intracranial pressure depending mainly on the location of the infection (▶ Table 31.4).[2,24,25]

A recent history of sinusitis symptoms and/or a localized forehead pressure/discomfort is preceding in most cases, even if nasal symptoms are absent at the time of presentation.[9]

Epidural abscesses are most commonly formed directly behind an intact posterior table of the frontal sinus due to the dura being loosely attached in this region. Symptoms may be very mild until the collection becomes large enough to cause increase of the intracranial pressure. Due

Table 31.4 Warning signs for intracranial complication

Severe frontal headache	Cranial nerve palsy
Fever > 39 °C	Focal neurological signs
Altered mental status	Hemiparesis
Photophobia	Seizures
Nuchal rigidity	Nausea, vomiting

to the proximity to the orbit, edema and tenderness of the forehead along with orbital swelling may be common. Subdural abscess formation may allow spread of the inflammation to the underlying cortex[21] and induce vasculitis and septic venous thrombosis. This leads to increasing inflammatory edema, further aggravating intracranial hypertension. The infection may spread posteriorly over the cerebral hemisphere and inferiorly into the interhemispheric fissure and subsequently to the contralateral side of the brain under or through the falx cerebri. It can also lead to superior sagittal sinus thrombosis. Both epidural and subdural abscess formation can be associated with meningitis.[10]

The intracerebral abscess mainly occurs in the frontal lobe.[26] Although an intracranial abscess can be relatively asymptomatic, subtle behavioral changes may be indicative of altered neurological function, altered consciousness, gait instability, and severe, progressive headache.[27]

Typical symptoms of spread of infection to the cortex may include hemiparesis, hemiplegia, cranial neuropathies, and seizures. Increase of intracranial pressure can cause nausea, vomiting, bradycardia, hypertension, and decreased level of consciousness; it can even lead to death from transtentorial herniation. This can be precipitated by lumbar puncture in cases of markedly elevated intracranial pressure.[9]

In cases of cavernous and superior sagittal sinus thrombosis, meningeal signs and focal neurological deficits are almost always present, while chemosis, proptosis, ophthalmoplegia, cranial nerves II and III palsies, and visual loss may progressively develop.[10] Contralateral symptoms are pathognomic of dural sinus thrombosis. Early clinical recognition of cavernous and superior sagittal sinus thrombosis is important, as mortality can be as high as 30 and 80%, respectively.[10]

31.2.3 Osseous Complications

In case of anterior frontal sinus table osteomyelitis, a "doughy" edema and a tender, fluctuant swelling of the forehead due to subperiosteal abscess (Pott's puffy tumor) may appear[1,20] along with headache, fever, and bilateral eyelid edema.[17] Increased leukocytes with neutrophilia

and raised inflammatory markers may be noted. The organisms most frequently isolated in osteomyelitis of the skull are *Streptococcus milleri*, viridians, or *S. aureus*.[14]

31.2.4 Investigations

The diagnostic evaluation of AFS complications necessitates multidisciplinary approach with otolaryngology, neurosurgery, ophthalmology, and infectious diseases input as these entities can be frequently concurrent and overlapping.[28]

A thorough clinical examination is necessary. This includes nasal endoscopy to assess for the presence of pus in the middle meatus and collection of swabs for gram stain and culture along with blood cultures, which can be crucial in guiding antibiotic therapy. White blood count (WBC) count, although not specific, can be useful as, when elevated, it is highly suggestive of a complication in the cases of ARS unresponsive to treatment.[14]

In particular in suspected orbital complications, it is vital to objectively assess the degree of proptosis (exophthalmometer), orbital pressure (tonometer), visual acuity, color vision, and ocular movements and these should always be clearly documented.

Contrast-enhanced CT scan of the sinuses is the standard initial, and often definitive, imaging modality[6,8,25] for diagnosis and surgical planning. It allows delineation of bony erosions of the frontal sinus, phlegmons, and rim-enhancing fluid collections in the orbital and intracranial soft tissue.[21] In the case of a subperiosteal abscess (▶ Fig. 31.1), CT scans usually reveal edema of the medial rectus muscle, lateralization of the periorbita, and displacement of the globe downward and laterally, whereas when an orbital abscess (▶ Fig. 31.2) is formed, the detail of the extraocular muscle and the optic nerve is obliterated by a confluent mass. Air due to anaerobic bacteria can be present in such cases.[1]

MRI offers superior soft-tissue resolution and is most appropriate in the context of suspected intracranial complications and negative or inconclusive CT (▶ Fig. 31.3a, b).[24,26,29] High-resolution CT with contrast is, however, essential for diagnosis and allows accurate definition of bone involvement (▶ Fig. 31.4, ▶ Fig. 31.5).

Cavernous sinus thrombosis causes superior ophthalmic vein engorgement, which can be diagnosed by the presence of filling defects on contrast CT. The cornerstone of diagnosis is, however, MR venogram, demonstrating absence of venous flow in the affected cavernous sinus.[1,24,26]

Lumbar puncture can be useful in ruling out meningitis, but should only be considered taking into account imaging, signs of increased intracranial pressure, and the risk of brain herniation.[10]

In the cases of Pott's puffy tumor, contrast-enhanced sinus and head CT should be obtained (▶ Fig. 31.6).

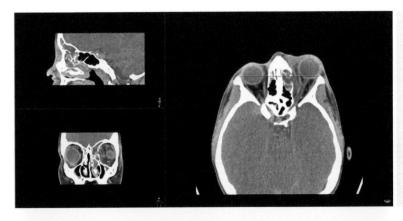

Fig. 31.1 Subperiosteal abscess (CT with contrast).

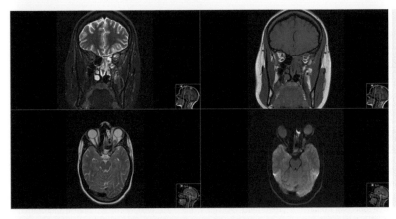

Fig. 31.2 Orbital abscess (MRI).

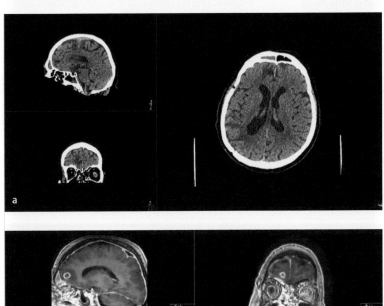

Fig. 31.3 Cerebral abscess **(a)** CT and **(b)** MRI.

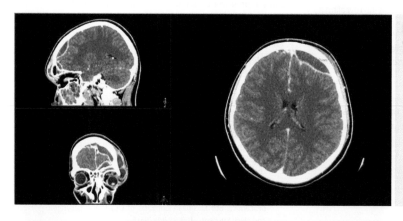

Fig. 31.4 Epidural abscess (CT with contrast).

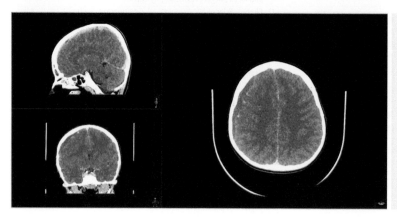

Fig. 31.5 Subdural abscess (CT with contrast).

Typically, a subperiosteal abscess in the frontal region is noted on soft-tissue windows and bony erosion related to osteomyelitis is better defined in bony windows. The extent of the concomitant sinusitis and potentially coexisting intracranial abscess is also demonstrated, allowing differentiation for other conditions with similar presentation.[14,17] MRI may be useful in case of concurrent intracranial complications.[14]

31.3 Management

Management of complications of ARS requires a multidisciplinary approach involving ENT (ear, nose, and throat), ophthalmology, neurosurgical and infectious diseases, and microbiology input. In early stages of suspected complications, a conservative management with antibiotics and topical nasal therapy including regular nasal douching and decongestants may be sufficient. However, surgical intervention to drain a formed collection of infectious material along with drainage of the affected sinus may be required.

It is important to note that AFS complications may be concurrent and overlapping (e.g., Pott's puffy tumor and intracranial extension, orbital and intracranial complications) and that even after its successful management, long-term follow-up for a minimum of 6 months is necessary to ensure complete resolution and exclude disease recurrence or any complication of treatment.

31.3.1 Frontal Sinus Drainage Techniques

Surgical drainage of the affected frontal sinus in the context of AFS complications may include endoscopic or external approaches or the combination of both.

Functional endoscopic sinus surgery (FESS) aims to re-establish sinus drainage and remove inflammatory material. Care is taken to preserve normal sinus physiology and function. It is more technically challenging in comparison to external approaches, but it achieves better cosmetic outcome, avoiding scars and deformities, and allows the surgeon to address potentially concurrent disease in other sinuses at the same time. On occasion, opening the lower anterior ethmoids and Agger nasi region may be sufficient to relieve the obstruction of frontal sinus outflow tract (Draf I). There are times, however, that the frontal recess needs to be surgically addressed (Draf IIa and IIb) while trying to preserve as much mucosa as possible to prevent scarring and stenosis. This can be challenging in the acute setting due to active infection

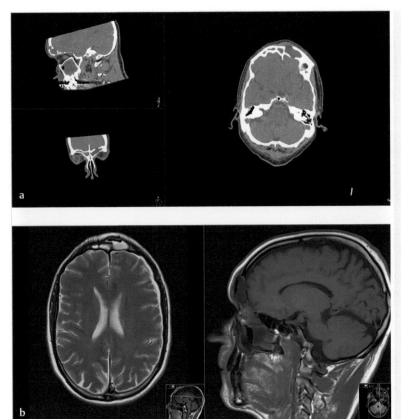

Fig. 31.6 Pott's Puffy tumour **(a)** CT and **(b)** MRI.

and higher bleeding risk.[30] The use of balloon sinuplasty in the setting of AFS has been reported, but its effectiveness is not universally accepted.[31]

FESS can be used in combination with trephination in the presence of thick septations, high frontal cells within the sinus, and lateralized frontal sinus disease. Extended drainage of the sinus in order to prevent disease recurrence is usually scheduled at a later time when the acute infection has settled. This definite treatment may vary from an endoscopic endonasal Draf IIa, IIb, and III (modified endoscopic Lothrop) procedure, to osteoplastic flap or even cranialization of the sinus depending on the individual circumstances.

In particular, trephination is a technique commonly used to drain the inflammatory material from the frontal sinus in the acute setting in conjunction to endoscopic endonasal approach. It involves a small (usually 1-cm long) incision below the medial supraorbital rim skin down to the periosteum, elevation of the periosteum, and drilling through the floor of the frontal sinus. Alternatively, a similar incision can be made within a skin crease of the forehead skin, which allows drilling through the anterior table of the frontal sinus using the mini-trephine technique.[32] This allows drainage of the infectious material from the frontal sinus. Catheter insertion may be useful for postoperative irrigation and drainage (usually for a 7- to 10-day period). It may allow inspection of the frontal sinus cavity and the nasofrontal duct using a 4-mm 0- and 30-degree telescopes.

Alternatively, a Lynch–Howarth approach can be used to drain the frontal sinus as well as medially located periorbital collections. It involves a curvilinear or Z-incision above the caudal margin of the lateral nasal bone halfway between the nasal dorsum and the medial canthus through the periosteum. The periosteum is then elevated off the lacrimal fossa, lamina papyracea, and floor of the frontal sinus, and the anterior ethmoidal artery found in the frontoethmoidal suture line is clipped or cauterized and the frontal sinus is then drilled open medially. This approach is technically simple, but may cause some disfigurement with resultant scarring, and is related to higher risk of recurrence and of mucocele formation.

The transblepharoplasty approach may be useful in the cases with lateral frontal sinus disease eroding into the orbit, either alone or in combination with FESS.[33] An incision is placed within a skin fold above the tarsal plate at least 8 mm above the lid. The orbital portion of the orbicularis oculi is located, the muscle is incised, and a plane is developed between this muscle and the levator aponeurosis toward the orbital rim while keeping the orbital septum intact.[30] A periosteal incision is made anterior to the orbital septum at the superior orbital rim and a subperiosteal dissection is completed in all directions, with the medial limit defined by the supraorbital notch and neurovascular bundle and the lateral and posterior limits defined by the extent of frontal sinus pneumatization. The frontal sinus floor is directly accessible and the area of dehiscence (in case of mucocele) is easily identified and treated. The flap is redraped in place once the patency of the outflow tract is achieved endoscopically.[30]

External frontoethmoidectomy, less frequently used over the years, can be used for the treatment in cases of mucoceles, pyoceles, and sinocutaneous fistulas, as well as for the treatment of various intracranial complications of frontal sinusitis.

31.3.2 Management of Orbital Complications

The first-line treatment for preseptal and orbital cellulitis consists of topical decongestants and intravenous (IV) antibiotics. These should cover both aerobic and anaerobic microbes.[1] In case of clinical improvement with the patient being afebrile for 48 hours, a switch to oral antibiotics can be considered.[25] If, however, no clinical improvement is noted in 24 to 48 hours or imaging indicates abscess formation, then surgical exploration and drainage along with concurrent drainage of the affected sinuses is the next appropriate step (Box 31.2).[22,34]

Drainage can be performed endoscopically through the ethmoids and the lamina papyracea or with external approach (Lynch–Howarth, transblepharoplasty approach), depending on the location of the abscess and the surgeon's expertise.

In the case of children younger than 4 years, with no decrease in visual acuity and no systemic involvement, who present small medially located subperiosteal abscess on imaging (volume < 0.5–1 mL), conservative management with IV antibiotics without surgical intervention has been argued, if close observation is feasible and clear signs of clinical improvement within 24 to 48 hours are noted.[25,35]

Prompt treatment of orbital complications is crucial as progression can be rapid and cause corneal ulceration, panophthalmitis, optic neuritis, blindness from central retinal artery occlusion, or intracranial spread and sequelae.[23]

Box 31.2 Indications for surgical intervention in orbital complications of ARS[1]

1. Evidence of subperiosteal or intraorbital abscess in CT or MRI
2. Reduced visual acuity/reduced color vision/affected afferent pupillary reflex, or inability to assess vision
3. Progressing or not improving orbital signs (diplopia, ophthalmoplegia, proptosis, swelling, chemosis) after 48-h intravenous antibiotics
4. Progressing or not improving general condition (fever, infection parameters) after 48 h of intravenous antibiotics

---

31.3.3 Management of Intracranial Complications

Most intracranial complications at early stages are managed with broad-spectrum IV antibiotics to reduce local spread of the infection and enable abscess organization.[35] Early treatment is crucial and recent studies illustrate that antimicrobial therapy at the early phase of cerebritis may prevent abscess formation. If an abscess is formed, surgical treatment may be necessary to ensure adequate therapy and complete resolution of infection.[35,36,37] Concurrent drainage of the frontal sinus and other affected sinuses can be useful, but does not substitute intracranial abscess drainage.[38]

Emergency surgery is needed if neurological signs related to a mass effect progress as in the cases of subdural empyema that requires prompt surgical evacuation as a delay in surgical drainage and decompression can be associated with high morbidity and mortality.

Abscesses smaller than 2.5 cm generally respond to antibiotics, whereas a single abscess larger than 2.5 cm requires excision or aspiration. In the cases of multiple abscesses or abscesses in vital or inaccessible brain areas (i.e., brainstem), repeated aspirations are preferred to complete excision. High-dose antibiotics for an extended period may be an alternative approach in this group of patients.[37]

The duration of therapy depends on the patient's condition, causative organisms, number and size of abscesses, and response to treatment. A 4- to 6-week course may be adequate for cerebritis and in patients who underwent surgical drainage, but in the case of encapsulated abscesses, multiloculated abscesses, abscesses in vital intracranial locations, or immunocompromised patients, a longer course of 6 to 8 weeks may become necessary.[35,37]

The length of therapy is guided by continuous clinical assessment and follow-up imaging studies at least once per week to assess treatment response.[37]

Initial empiric treatment should cover oral *Streptococci* (including *milleri* group), methicillin-susceptible *Staphylococci*, anaerobes, and *Enterobacteriaceae* until microbiology and sensitivities are available.[39] A combination of third-generation cephalosporin and metronidazole is adequate in most cases of community-acquired brain abscess in immunocompetent patients.

The use of corticosteroid is controversial and can be advocated when a significant mass effect is visible on imaging and the patient's mental status is depressed.[37]

Surgical drainage of the brain abscess can be achieved with aspiration through a burr hole or complete excision after craniotomy. Needle aspiration under CT guidance is most commonly used and preferred especially if the speech, motor, or sensory cortex areas are involved or the patient is comatose. Craniotomy is generally performed in patients with multiloculated abscesses and in the cases that do not resolve with repeated aspirations but are associated with higher morbidity.[40,41] Excision is also indicated even after initial aspiration or drainage in patients with depressed sensorium, increased intracranial pressure, no clinical improvement within 7 days, and/or a progressively growing abscess.[40,41]

In case of cavernous sinus thrombosis, the mortality and morbidity rates remain as high as 30 and 60%, respectively, in the adult population. Management mainly consists of IV antibiotics and drainage of the affected sinuses. Steroids may be helpful in reducing inflammation. The use of anticoagulants in these patients remains controversial but is probably indicated on condition of negative imaging for intracerebral hemorrhagic changes.[42]

31.3.4 Management of Osseous Complications

Management of osseous complications in the acute setting includes drainage of the affected sinus either by endoscopic and/or external trephination and surgical debridement of sequestered bone along with broad-spectrum IV antibiotics.[43] Further surgical reconstruction of the cosmetic osseous defect and definitive drainage procedure of the persistent frontal sinus disease can be scheduled at a later time if necessary.[14]

31.4 Case Examples

31.4.1 Case 1: Subperiosteal Abscess (Contrast-Enhanced CT)

A 13-year-old adolescent girl with a previous history of orbital cellulitis was admitted with new-onset periorbital cellulitis after a few days with ARS symptoms. Imaging with a contrast-enhanced CT revealed a subperiosteal abscess on the ground of ARS (▶ Fig. 31.1). The abscess was drained with a combination of external approach via a Lynch–Howarth incision and FESS.

31.4.2 Case 2: Orbital Abscess (Magnetic Resonance Imaging)

A 23-year-old woman presented with a week's history of spiking temperature, headaches, and left ptosis. Imaging with CT and MRI revealed abscess of the superior rectus/levator complex abscess along with a small epidural abscess and cerebritis (▶ Fig. 31.2). The orbital collection was drained by the maxillofacial team with a transblepharoplasty approach, while ENT drained the sinuses with FESS. The central nervous system involvement was managed conservatively with IV antibiotics.

31.4.3 Case 3: Cerebral Abscess (Magnetic Resonance Imaging)

A 73-year-old man with a history of two episodes of seizure/confusion and left-sided weakness was originally scanned with a CT scan. The scan reported a hypodense area at the medial frontal lobe with no associated enhancement potentially suggestive of a frontal lobe infarct at the ACA territory. A right-sided extra-axial collection with density just above that of cerebrospinal fluid and a maximum depth of 3 mm was also noted (▶ Fig. 31.3a).

Subsequent MRI (▶ Fig. 31.3b) raised the suspicion of a frontal lobe abscess in the context of frontal sinusitis (restricted diffusion centrally).

This was confirmed intraoperatively—burr hole craniotomy and aspiration along with frontal sinus minitrephine and limited FESS.

31.4.4 Case 4: Epidural Abscess (Contrast-Enhanced CT)

A 21-year-old man with a history of CRSwNP (chronic rhinosinusitis without nasal polyp) presented with ARS and periorbital cellulitis, headache, and fever. Imaging with a contrast-enhanced CT revealed pansinusitis, a large extradural collection (▶ Fig. 31.4), and eyelid abscess. The patient was managed jointly by neurosurgery, ENT, and ophthalmology with burr hole drainage of the collection, frontal trephine, and FESS, and drainage of the eyelid abscess. This was followed by long-term IV antibiotics.

31.4.5 Case 5: Subdural Abscess (Contrast-Enhanced CT)

An 11-year-old boy presented on treatment by GP (general practitioner) for ARS presented with right-sided headache, photophobia, drowsiness, and left-sided weakness. Contrast-enhanced CT revealed the presence of a subdural abscess at the frontal parietal convexity, 1 cm in depth toward the vertex (▶ Fig. 31.5). Some peripheral enhancement is noted. Mass effect with midline shift left and effacement of the right lateral ventricle are also noted.

The child was treated with emergency craniotomy for drainage of the subdural abscess along with FESS to address the sinus infection followed by 6 weeks of IV antibiotics. Subsequent MRI confirmed the presence of a cerebrovascular accident (CVA) and the patient was put on aspirin and FU by neurology.

31.4.6 Case 6: Pott's Puffy Tumor

A 50-year-old man presented a history of ARS and left forehead swelling on the grounds of known CRS scanned with a sinus CT (▶ Fig. 31.6a). The scan revealed Pott's puffy tumor (CT bone window) with erosion of the anterior and posterior frontal sinus table as well as the orbital roof in the context of pansinusitis. MRI (▶ Fig. 31.6b) revealed the presence of a 3-mm left subdural collection. No intraorbital extension was noted.

The patient was managed with a combination of external drainage and limited FESS, followed by long-term antibiotics.

References

[1] Fokkens WJ, Lund VJ, Mullol J, et al. EPOS 2012: European position paper on rhinosinusitis and nasal polyps 2012. A summary for otorhinolaryngologists. Rhinology. 2012; 50(1):1–12

[2] Piatt JH, Jr. Intracranial suppuration complicating sinusitis among children: an epidemiological and clinical study. J Neurosurg Pediatr. 2011; 7(6):567–574

[3] Hansen FS, Hoffmans R, Georgalas C, Fokkens WJ. Complications of acute rhinosinusitis in The Netherlands. Fam Pract. 2012; 29(2):147–153

[4] Stoll D, Klossek JM, Barbaza MO, Groupe ORLI. Prospective study of 43 severe complications of acute rhinosinusitis. Rev Laryngol Otol Rhinol (Bord). 2006; 127(4):195–201

[5] Eufinger H, Machtens E. Purulent pansinusitis, orbital cellulitis and rhinogenic intracranial complications. J Craniomaxillofac Surg. 2001; 29(2):111–117

[6] Mortimore S, Wormald PJ. The Groote Schuur hospital classification of the orbital complications of sinusitis. J Laryngol Otol. 1997; 111(8):719–723

[7] Mortimore S, Wormald PJ. Management of acute complicated sinusitis: a 5-year review. Otolaryngol Head Neck Surg. 1999; 121(5):639–642

[8] Younis RT, Lazar RH, Bustillo A, Anand VK. Orbital infection as a complication of sinusitis: are diagnostic and treatment trends changing? Ear Nose Throat J. 2002; 81(11):771–775

[9] Kountakis SE, Senior B, Draf W. The frontal Sinus. Heidelberg: Springer; 2005

[10] Goldberg AN, Oroszlan G, Anderson TD. Complications of frontal sinusitis and their management. Otolaryngol Clin North Am. 2001; 34(1):211–225

[11] Voegels RL, Pinna FdeR. Sinusitis orbitary complications classification: simple and practical answers. Rev Bras Otorrinolaringol (Engl Ed). 2007; 73(5):578

[12] Bedrossian EH. Surgical anatomy of the orbit. In: Della Rocca RC, Bedrossian EH, Arthurs BP, eds. Ophthalmic plastic surgery: Decision making and techniques. New York, NY: McGraw-Hill; 2002:207–227

[13] Healy GB. Chandler et al.: "The pathogenesis of orbital complications in acute sinusitis." (Laryngoscope 1970;80:1414–1428). Laryngoscope. 1997; 107(4):441–446

[14] Gore RG, Herman P, Senior B, Fokkens F. Complications of acute rhinosinusitis. In: Georgalas C, Fokkens WJ, eds. Rhinology and Skull Base Surgery: from the lab to the Operating Room—An Evidence-Based Approach. New York, NY: Thieme; 2013

[15] Gallagher RM, Gross CW, Phillips CD. Suppurative intracranial complications of sinusitis. Laryngoscope. 1998; 108(11, Pt 1):1635–1642

[16] Osborn MK, Steinberg JP. Subdural empyema and other suppurative complications of paranasal sinusitis. Lancet Infect Dis. 2007; 7(1):62–67

[17] Collet S, Grulois V, Eloy P, Rombaux P, Bertrand B. A Pott's puffy tumour as a late complication of a frontal sinus reconstruction: case report and literature review. Rhinology. 2009; 47(4):470–475

[18] Parida PK, Surianarayanan G, Ganeshan S, Saxena SK. Pott's puffy tumor in pediatric age group: a retrospective study. Int J Pediatr Otorhinolaryngol. 2012; 76(9):1274–1277

[19] Velasco e Cruz AA, Demarco RC, Valera FC, Anselmo-Lima WT, Marquezini RM. Orbital complications of acute rhinosinusitis: a new classification. Rev Bras Otorrinolaringol (Engl Ed). 2007; 73(5):684–688

[20] Ho CF, Huang YC, Wang CJ, Chiu CH, Lin TY. Clinical analysis of computed tomography-staged orbital cellulitis in children. J Microbiol Immunol Infect. 2007; 40(6):518–524

[21] Choi SS, Grundfast KM. Complications in sinus disease. In: Kennedy DW, Bolger WE, Zinreich SJ, eds. Diseases of the sinuses: Diagnosis and management. Ontario, ON: B.C. Decker; 2001:169–177

[22] Coenraad S, Buwalda J. Surgical or medical management of subperiosteal orbital abscess in children: a critical appraisal of the literature. Rhinology. 2009; 47(1):18–23

[23] Hicks CW, Weber JG, Reid JR, Moodley M. Identifying and managing intracranial complications of sinusitis in children: a retrospective series. Pediatr Infect Dis J. 2011; 30(3):222–226

[24] Bayonne E, Kania R, Tran P, Huy B, Herman P. Intracranial complications of rhinosinusitis. A review, typical imaging data and algorithm of management. Rhinology. 2009; 47(1):59–65

[25] Hoxworth JM, Glastonbury CM. Orbital and intracranial complications of acute sinusitis. Neuroimaging Clin N Am. 2010; 20(4):511–526

[26] Eweiss A, Mukonoweshuro W, Khalil HS. Cavernous sinus thrombosis secondary to contralateral sphenoid sinusitis: a diagnostic challenge. J Laryngol Otol. 2010; 124(8):928–930

[27] Eviatar E, Gavriel H, Pitaro K, Vaiman M, Goldman M, Kessler A. Conservative treatment in rhinosinusitis orbital complications in children aged 2 years and younger. Rhinology. 2008; 46(4):334–337

[28] Lang EE, Curran AJ, Patil N, Walsh RM, Rawluk D, Walsh MA. Intracranial complications of acute frontal sinusitis. Clin Otolaryngol Allied Sci. 2001; 26(6):452–457

[29] Blumfield E, Misra M. Pott's puffy tumor, intracranial, and orbital complications as the initial presentation of sinusitis in healthy adolescents, a case series. Emerg Radiol. 2011; 18(3):203–210

[30] Medscape. Acute Frontal Sinusitis Surgery. Accessed September 26, 2017. Available at: https://emedicine.medscape.com/article/862292-overview

[31] Hopkins C, Noon E, Roberts D. Balloon sinuplasty in acute frontal sinusitis. Rhinology. 2009; 47(4):375–378

[32] Seiberling K, Jardeleza C, Wormald PJ. Minitrephination of the frontal sinus: indications and uses in today's era of sinus surgery. Am J Rhinol Allergy. 2009; 23(2):229–231

[33] Knipe TA, Gandhi PD, Fleming JC, Chandra RK. Transblepharoplasty approach to sequestered disease of the lateral frontal sinus with ophthalmologic manifestations. Am J Rhinol. 2007; 21(1):100–104

[34] Todman MS, Enzer YR. Medical management versus surgical intervention of pediatric orbital cellulitis: the importance of subperiosteal abscess volume as a new criterion. Ophthal Plast Reconstr Surg. 2011; 27(4):255–259

[35] Kombogiorgas D, Seth R, Athwal R, Modha J, Singh J. Suppurative intracranial complications of sinusitis in adolescence. Single institute experience and review of literature. Br J Neurosurg. 2007; 21(6):603–609

[36] Honda H, Warren DK. Central nervous system infections: meningitis and brain abscess. Infect Dis Clin North Am. 2009; 23(3):609–623

[37] Medscape. Brain abscess treatment and management. Accessed November 2, 2017. Available at: https://reference.medscape.com/article/212946-treatment

[38] DelGaudio JM, Evans SH, Sobol SE, Parikh SL. Intracranial complications of sinusitis: what is the role of endoscopic sinus surgery in the acute setting. Am J Otolaryngol. 2010; 31(1):25–28

[39] Sonneville R, Ruimy R, Benzonana N, et al. ESCMID Study Group for Infectious Diseases of the Brain (ESGIB). An update on bacterial brain

abscess in immunocompetent patients. Clin Microbiol Infect. 2017; 23(9):614–620

[40] Kocherry XG, Hegde T, Sastry KV, Mohanty A. Efficacy of stereotactic aspiration in deep-seated and eloquent-region intracranial pyogenic abscesses. Neurosurg Focus. 2008; 24(6):E13

[41] Ratnaike TE, Das S, Gregson BA, Mendelow AD. A review of brain abscess surgical treatment: 78 years: aspiration versus excision. World Neurosurg. 2011; 76(5):431–436

[42] Bhatia K, Jones NS. Septic cavernous sinus thrombosis secondary to sinusitis: are anticoagulants indicated? A review of the literature. J Laryngol Otol. 2002; 116(9):667–676

[43] Josephson JS, Rosenberg SI. Sinusitis. Clin Symp. 1994; 46(2):1–32

32 Fungal Frontal Sinusitis: Allergic and Nonallergic

Fahad Alasousi, Anali Dadgostar, Amin Javer, and Carl M. Philpott

Abstract

The frontal sinus is affected less commonly with fungal infection or affectation. This is due to its location and relatively narrow access to its natural ostium, which give the frontal sinus its special characteristics. These characteristics also influence the surgical and medical management of fungal frontal sinusitis in its various forms. This chapter will consider the various fungal etiologies, including invasive and noninvasive forms that can occur and will provide the reader with guidance on the typical clinical presentation as well as to the recommended management of such cases. Some case examples are used to illustrate the key points. It is notable that surgical management is almost invariably needed, but the medical management will vary depending on the etiology.

Keywords: frontal sinus, fungal, sinusitis, allergic, nonallergic, invasive

32.1 Introduction

Fungal sinusitis can be a significant disorder in any of the sinuses and may prove especially problematic in the frontal sinus when severe. This chapter will delineate the different forms of fungal sinusitis and their discerning features as well as consider how the management of these conditions in the frontal sinus specifically may require additional challenges. To help illustrate this, a specific case example is included that highlights these challenges. Based on the clinical picture, imaging, and histology, fungal sinusitis can be broadly classified into invasive and noninvasive fungal rhinosinusitis.

32.2 Epidemiology and Etiology

32.2.1 Invasive

Acute Invasive Fungal Rhinosinusitis

Acute fulminant invasive fungal rhinosinusitis is a potentially lethal disease entity with low survival rate (49.7%).[1] It primarily affects patients with conditions associated with severe neutropenia (absolute neutrophil count [ANC] < 500/µL)[2] and/or impaired neutrophil function, that is, patients undergoing transplantation, leukemia, and uncontrolled diabetic ketoacidosis, patients receiving chemotherapy and hemochromatosis,[3,4] and especially those in receipt of bone marrow transplantation.[5,6] The genera of Aspergillus and Mucor are the most common organisms that have been associated with acute invasive fungal rhinosinusitis (AIFRS),[2,7] hence why the condition is also sometimes referred to as mucormycosis.

Chronic Invasive Fungal Rhinosinusitis

Chronic invasive fungal rhinosinusitis (CIFRS) is encountered in patients who are not immunocompromised or have a limited immunocompromised status, such as diabetics or patients on long-term corticosteroids.[8] It is a slowly destructive disease over a time course of more than 12 weeks and can reach up to 12 months' duration. Granulomatous invasive fungal rhinosinusitis (GIFRS) is a subtype of CIFRS that is more commonly encountered in healthy and immune competent patients in the Middle East, North Africa, and India.[3]

Granulomatous Invasive Fungal Sinusitis

This form of invasive fungal sinusitis is attributed to infection with *Aspergillus flavus* and is principally seen in North Africa, India, and Pakistan. The infection manifests as a locally invasive disease over at least 3 months' duration but usually occurs in immunocompetent individuals.

32.2.2 Noninvasive

Eosinophilic Fungal Sinus Disease

Eosinophilic fungal sinus disease, secondary to an over-responsiveness to fungus with or without fungal hypersensitivity, can be subdivided into the following:
- Allergic fungal rhinosinusitis (AFRS).
- Eosinophilic mucinous rhinosinusitis (EMRS)/eosinophilic mucinous fungal rhinosinusitis (EFRS).

Allergic Fungal Rhinosinusitis and Its Derivatives

AFRS may be considered a form of chronic rhinosinusitis (CRS) and accounts for 7 to 10% of CRS. In the late 1970s, AFRS was recognized as an upper airway manifestation of allergic bronchopulmonary aspergillosis (ABPA).[9,10] It was in 1994 that Bent and Kuhn defined the five diagnostic criteria for AFRS (► Table 32.1).[11,12] The EFRS and EMRS derivatives show similar traits and may overlap with aspirin exacerbated respiratory disease.[13]

Sinus Mycelia

Sinus mycelia, also known as fungal balls, represent an accumulation of fungal material in which the immune system is neither over-responsive nor under-responsive. They are mainly caused by the *Aspergillus* species (e.g., *A. fumigatus*) in immunocompetent patients. Demographics include being more common in middle-aged and elderly women, in contrast to all forms of invasive and chronic aspergillosis, which are more common in males.

Table 32.1 Diagnostic criteria for allergic fungal rhinosinusitis

Major	Minor
Type 1 hypersensitivity[a]/immunocompetence[b]	Asthma
Nasal polyposis	Unilateral disease
Characteristic CT findings	Bone erosion
Eosinophilic mucin without invasion	Fungal cultures
Positive fungal stain	Charcot–Leyden crystals
	Serum eosinophilia

[a]Bent and Kuhn.[11]
[b]Vancouver.

32.3 Clinical Presentation and Investigations

32.3.1 Invasive

Acute Invasive Fungal Rhinosinusitis

Although nonspecific, red flags for AIFRS include pyrexia and symptoms of localization to the paranasal sinus area (e.g., facial pain and pressure, nasal congestion, orbital swelling). Symptoms of greater concern include visual disturbances, paresthesia, and cranial neuropathy, indicating late presentation and more advanced disease. On endoscopic examination, the findings can range from edema to dry or pale mucosa in the early stages to Frank necrosis in the advance stages. The middle turbinate (67%) and the nasal septum (24%) are the most common sites to show clinical findings.[4]

Histopathological features include fungi invading the mucosal barriers and tissue necrosis.[8,14] Management requires an attempt at reversal of the underlying immunocompromised state with the need for a multidisciplinary approach including both medical and surgical interventions. It is therefore important to have a high index of suspicion in patients who are considered high-risk populations. This is accomplished by taking prompt biopsies and pathological evaluation in such patients. High-resolution, noncontrasted CT scan is a crucial part for the workup, while MRI is recommended in patients who present with signs or symptoms of orbital or intracranial involvement. Thickening of the periantral fat plane has been reported as an early indicator of AIFRS.[15]

Chronic Invasive Fungal Rhinosinusitis

Orbital and CNS involvement is less common than in AIFRS, although orbital apex syndrome is possible. Radiological findings include hyperdense soft tissue and bony involvement on CT scan with a very hypointense T2 signal on MRI with possible evidence of intracranial involvement. CIFRS is distinguished histologically by the formation of noncaseating granulomas in which giant cells contain the residing hyphae.[16] *A. flavus, A. fumigatus, Alternaria, Pseudallescheria boydii,* and *Sporothrix schenckii* have been reported to be the organisms associated with CIFRS. The presentation does not differ from AIFRS, but it is suspected when the symptoms of CRS are refractory to medical management and progressing in severity, especially persistent headache, visual disturbance, or development of cranial nerve deficits. Tissue biopsy is the only definitive tool to diagnose CIFRS,[17] but radiological imaging can be helpful and is important for surgical planning. Fungal invasion of the mucosa is found on pathological analysis.

Granulomatous Invasive Fungal Sinusitis

Typical presenting symptoms include those of CRS and possibly of proptosis or an enlarging mass in the affected sinus. Histological examination of material will show a pattern of noncaseating granulomas and of foreign body/Langhans giant cells with central necrosis. These cases need surgical debridement, followed by systemic antifungal medication. Disease recurrence is uncommon, and granulomatous invasive fungal sinusitis generally has a good prognosis.

32.3.2 Noninvasive

Allergic Fungal Rhinosinusitis

As aforementioned, Bent and Kuhn defined five diagnostic criteria for AFRS (▶ Table 32.1).[11,12] The name itself may indeed be a misnomer as a type I hypersensitivity reaction is not always proven despite the evidence of the other key clinical features, and a modified version has been proposed whereby immunocompetence replaces type I hypersensitivity, reflecting the group of characteristic patients seen in rhinological practice.[18] The constant features in these patients are a distinct clinical pattern of recurrent nasal polyposis and accumulation of fungal mucin. AFRS classically involves all sinus cavities with impacted thick mucin, polyps, and chronic inflammation with pushing bony margins. Characteristic radiological signs on CT include double densities with a rail track pattern in the sinus, sinus expansion, remodeling of the sinus wall, and bony erosion. MRI findings are usually consistent with hypointense areas on T1 and signal voids on T2.[19]

Eosinophilic Mucinous Rhinosinusitis

In a study conducted by Ponikau et al on CRS patients, 93% of the patients undergoing sinus surgery had both eosinophilic mucin and fungus.[20] However, less than half of the almost 100 patients in whom eosinophilic mucin

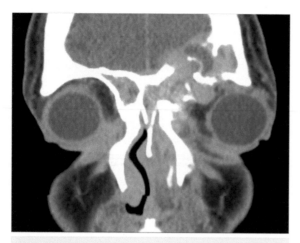

Fig. 32.1 Bony expansion around left frontal sinus.

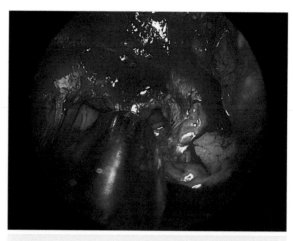

Fig. 32.2 Frontal sinus filled with dense fungal mucin.

and fungus were present were allergic. They demonstrated the movement of eosinophils out of blood vessels and into the sinus cavity to engulf fungal hyphae. They proposed that a cell-mediated response provoked by fungi in susceptible hosts was responsible and coined the term EMRS. Some studies attempted to differentiate EMRS and AFRS patients based on demographics. They suggested EMRS patients to be relatively younger, less likely to have asthma and aspirin sensitivity, and more likely to have bilateral disease when compared with AFRS patients.[21] However, in reality, there is significant overlap in the clinical pictures between EMRS and ARFS.[22] Orbital involvement and higher immunoglobulin E (IgE) levels have been found to be more common in AFRS patients. This may be due to variations in climate, genetic susceptibility, and socioeconomic factors. Orlandi et al carried out a microarray gene analysis between these two subgroups.[23] They showed 38 genes or potential genes were differentially expressed in AFRS patients, while 10 genes were differentially expressed in EMRS patients.

Sinus Mycelia

Typical presentation is with symptoms relating to chronic sinusitis of one sinus, which is usually the maxillary and less commonly the sphenoid sinus, but they can also be incidental findings on CT scans requested for nonsinugenic causes/symptoms. Typical symptoms, if present, include nasal discharge, nasal obstruction, headache, facial pain, and cacosmia, the latter of which may be a predominant symptom. Occasionally, they can be associated with unilateral proptosis and facial hypoesthesia.

Radiological imaging (CT scan) will demonstrate a unilateral, single sinus disease with heterogeneous opacification (▶ Fig. 32.1). Fungal cultures are positive in less than one-third of patients despite fungal elements on

histopathology in more than 90% of those affected. There is no predominance of eosinophils or granulomata or allergic mucin, and no histopathological evidence of fungal invasion of mucosa is seen. Treatment is surgical, invariably an endoscopic approach to remove the fungal ball and open the affected sinus; however, in an asymptomatic patient, a discussion about watchful waiting may be needed depending on the age and comorbidities of the patient. At surgery, the sinus is usually found to be full of dense brown/green material, which often requires irrigation to help dislodge (▶ Fig. 32.2). Following removal of the fungal ball, no antifungal treatment is required and no long-term follow-up is required once patency and healing of the sinus are confirmed endoscopically.

32.3.3 Special Considerations in Frontal Sinus Fungal Disease

The frontal sinus is the least susceptible to fungal *infection* due to the location of the ostium. Acute fulminant and chronic invasive fungal sinusitis therefore rarely involve the frontal sinus with only 14.8% of cases being reported to involve the frontal sinus in a large case series[24]; other series have reported slightly higher levels of involvement (17–21%).[25,26] Fungal ball involvement of the frontal sinus is also rare.[27,28] There are few case reports in the English literature describing primary sinus mycelia in the frontal sinus.[27,29,30]

In contrast, it is estimated that 71% of AFRS cases have frontal sinus involvement,[31] highlighting the difference between an infective and an inflammatory and reactive process. The relatively thin bones that are in close proximity to the frontal sinus (lamina papyracea, cribriform plate) are more susceptible to changes in a manner equivalent to pressure necrosis secondary of the accumulation of dense eosinophilic fungal mucin. This may result in erosion and extension of the disease to the orbit and intracranial space,[32] but is a more indolent process than is seen in the invasive forms of fungal disease.

32.4 Management

32.4.1 Medical Management

AIFRS is routinely managed medically with systematic antifungal therapy in conjunction with surgical intervention. Amphotericin B in liposomal formulation has been the mainstay therapy for the past 50 years.[4,33] Adverse effects with the use of systemic antifungal therapy are common, with nephrotoxicity being the most serious, occurring early in the course of treatment, and usually being reversible in most patients. Tubular damage is a well-known problem associated with amphotericin B therapy, but acute renal failure is the most serious complication.[4] Topical antifungal therapy should be considered as well.[34] A patient who recovers their neutrophil count and function has a better prognosis.[35]

32.4.2 Surgical and Postoperative Management in the Frontal Sinus

AIFRS requires an approach consistent with aggressive surgical debridement. Resection of gross necrotic tissue is necessary and sometimes requires a staged approach. Aggressive debridement and early diagnosis are associated with positive prognostic factors.[36] Urgent endoscopic sinus surgery to debride the affected areas is needed along with systemic antifungals, and once controlled the patients should continue on itraconazole for up to 1 year. Recurrence is common and thus long-term follow-up is needed to ensure the disease remains controlled. The surgical management of CIFRS does not differ from that of AIFRS and radical surgical resection and intravenous amphotericin B are recommended.[37,38,39,40]

Sinus mycelia can usually be addressed endoscopically, although several authors advocate an external approach for its management.[27,29,30] However, with the advancement in surgical techniques and instrumentation, endoscopic eradication is achievable with or without external trephination in an "above-and-below" fashion.[41] A complete endoscopic frontal sinusotomy is necessary with extension to a frontal sinus rescue (modified IIb) or a traditional Draf IIb approach often being a necessity to get proper access for removal of the fungal debris.

Isolated fungal frontal sinusitis is rare and only few case reports are available in the literature.[27] Their consistent clinical pattern is the key factor in their management as, unlike the management of classical CRS, the cornerstone for treatment of AFRS is surgery followed by close long-term endoscopic follow-up. AFRS patients require meticulous and complete endoscopic sinus surgery, along with careful and regular follow-up in the outpatient clinic

in order to try and prevent polyp reformation and accumulation of mucin; a comprehensive postoperative medical regimen is almost always a necessity for long-term control.[42]

In AFRS, surgery aims to eradicate all eosinophilic mucin and fungal debris, provide adequate ventilation and drainage to the sinus, and facilitate postoperative access for topical medication, debridement, and monitoring of disease.[32] In the cases with extensive fungal disease that is difficult to control postoperatively in the clinic, revision surgery with Draf IIb or III may be required. Frontal sinus obliteration must not be used if frontal osteoplastic flap is considered, as it is almost impossible to eradicate all mucosal disease and recurrence is high.[43] Monitoring of disease status requires a combination of symptom reporting with patient-reported outcome measures such as the SNOT-22 (Sinonasal Outcome Test 22). Endoscopic examination and staging systems can help track fluctuations between visits.[18] ▶ Table 32.2 and ▶ Table 32.3 show the Philpott-Javer staging systems devised as a more specific method of tracking all sinus cavities and the olfactory cleft in AFRS. Patients with AFRS appear to show good correlation between subjective and objective measures of disease, especially with reference to olfaction.[44]

32.4.3 Complications: Management

Case Example

A 24-year-old man presented with severe AFRS. Initial assessment revealed grade 4 polyposis bilaterally with evidence of allergic mucin (▶ Fig. 32.3). IgE levels were consistently over 5,000 throughout the course of medical and surgical management. He underwent primary complete bilateral computer-assisted sinus surgery (BiCASS) in 2012 where he was identified to have left-sided orbital and intracranial extension. Despite aggressive topical and oral therapies and appropriate medical management, he continued to have severe allergic mucin and redevelopment of polyposis 3 months after surgical intervention. He underwent revision surgery 1 year later, where he was identified to have redeveloped significant fungus with extensive disease in the left supraorbital ethmoid cells, lateral left frontal recess, and extending into the

Table 32.2 Philpott–Javer endoscopic staging system for allergic fungal rhinosinusitis

Grading	State of mucosa
0	No edema
1–3	Mucosal edema (mild/moderate/severe)
4–6	Polypoid edema (mild/moderate/severe)
7–9	Frank polyps (mild/moderate/severe)

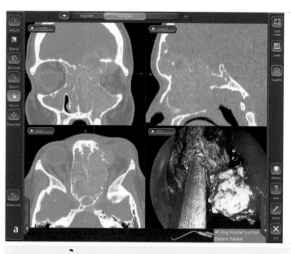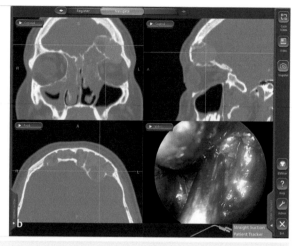

Fig. 32.3 (a, b) Image guidance views at the back of the left frontal recess and in the left frontal sinus.

Table 32.3 Philpott–Javer endoscopic staging system for allergic fungal rhinosinusitis

Sinus cavity	Right	Mucin	Left	Mucin
Olfactory cleft	0–9	1	0–9	1
Frontal	0–9	1	0–9	1
Ethmoid	0–9	1	0–9	1
Maxillary	0–9	1	0–9	1
Sphenoid	0–9	1	0–9	1
Total (maximum score)	50		50	
Bilateral total	100			

crista galli. There was evidence of dehiscence of the anterior and posterior tables of the left frontal sinus. A frontal trephine and wide frontal sinusotomy involving removal of the anterior buttress (nasofrontal beak) were required to access the deep and lateral cavities. Postoperative maintenance therapy included a low-dose oral Prednisone (5 mg) daily, topical Pulmicort via MAD (Mucosal Atomization Device) syringe, and oral itraconazole. Unfortunately the patient was lost to follow-up for 1 year and upon presentation, he was identified to have severe recurrence of AFRS. He was commenced on oral and topical therapy but was again lost to follow-up. He presented in 2015 with left frontal facial swelling and significant left frontal headache. He was subsequently taken to the operating room for revision BiCASS and left frontal resection of a mucocele and fungal mucin. The frontal sinus recess was resected and marsupialized bilaterally and the lateral recess was debrided bilaterally and cleared of inflammatory disease. Despite the use of angled 70- and 90-degree scopes and accompanying angled instrumentation specifically designed for use in the frontal sinus, it was challenging to visualize and completely remove all fungal debris due to its extension laterally within the frontal sinus, as well as the presence of deep cavities harboring the fungal debris. In such cases, it is prudent to utilize angled instrumentation and scopes to visualize and reach such extensive frontal sinus disease in order to ensure complete removal of fungal debris. Postoperatively, the patient did well and at his last visit 6 months postoperatively, he was identified to have completely clear sinus cavities bilaterally, with no evidence of mucin or polyposis.

32.5 Conclusion

Fungal sinus disease involves a spectrum of severity from invasive and potentially fatal infection to benign affectation with poor quality of life and high rates of potential relapse. Ultimately, most scenarios involve the need for some form of surgical debridement; in the frontal sinus, this results in specific challenges for access, and the surgeon tasked with these cases must have the skills and equipment to be able to tackle the varying scenarios to ensure success. In the case of AFRS, long-term follow-up of patients will be needed to maintain control of the disease with an emphasis on compliance for the patients. With increasing understanding of disease endotypes, perhaps the future will see a more focused and patient-centered treatment regimen from the outset.

References

[1] Turner JH, Soudry E, Nayak JV, Hwang PH. Survival outcomes in acute invasive fungal sinusitis: a systematic review and quantitative synthesis of published evidence. Laryngoscope. 2013; 123(5):1112–1118

[2] Valera FC, do Lago T, Tamashiro E, Yassuda CC, Silveira F, Anselmo-Lima WT. Prognosis of acute invasive fungal rhinosinusitis related to underlying disease. Int J Infect Dis. 2011; 15(12):e841–e844

[3] deShazo RD. Fungal sinusitis. Am J Med Sci. 1998; 316(1):39–45

[4] Gillespie MB, O'Malley BW. An algorithmic approach to the diagnosis and management of invasive fungal rhinosinusitis in the immunocompromised patient. Otolaryngol Clin North Am. 2000; 33(2):323–334

[5] Chen CY, Sheng WH, Cheng A, et al. Invasive fungal sinusitis in patients with hematological malignancy: 15 years experience in a single university hospital in Taiwan. BMC Infect Dis. 2011; 11:250

[6] Drakos PE, Nagler A, Or R, et al. Invasive fungal sinusitis in patients undergoing bone marrow transplantation. Bone Marrow Transplant. 1993; 12(3):203–208

[7] Cho HJ, Jang MS, Hong SD, Chung SK, Kim HY, Dhong HJ. Prognostic factors for survival in patients with acute invasive fungal rhinosinusitis. Am J Rhinol Allergy. 2015; 29(1):48–53

[8] deShazo RD, O'Brien M, Chapin K, Soto-Aguilar M, Gardner L, Swain R. A new classification and diagnostic criteria for invasive fungal sinusitis. Arch Otolaryngol Head Neck Surg. 1997; 123(11):1181–1188

[9] McCarthy DS. Bronchiectasis in allergic bronchopulmonary aspergillosis. Proc R Soc Med. 1968; 61(5):503–506

[10] Safirstein BH. Allergic bronchopulmonary aspergillosis with obstruction of the upper respiratory tract. Chest. 1976; 70(6):788–790

[11] Bent JP, III, Kuhn FA. Diagnosis of allergic fungal sinusitis. Otolaryngol Head Neck Surg. 1994; 111(5):580–588

[12] deShazo RD, Swain RE. Diagnostic criteria for allergic fungal sinusitis. J Allergy Clin Immunol. 1995; 96(1):24–35

[13] Philpott CM, Erskine S, Hopkins C, et al. CRES group. Prevalence of asthma, aspirin sensitivity and allergy in chronic rhinosinusitis: data from the UK National Chronic Rhinosinusitis Epidemiology Study. Respir Res. 2018; 19(1):129

[14] Chakrabarti A, Denning DW, Ferguson BJ, et al. Fungal rhinosinusitis: a categorization and definitional schema addressing current controversies. Laryngoscope. 2009; 119(9):1809–1818

[15] DelGaudio JM, Swain RE, Jr, Kingdom TT, Muller S, Hudgins PA. Computed tomographic findings in patients with invasive fungal sinusitis. Arch Otolaryngol Head Neck Surg. 2003; 129(2):236–240

[16] Halderman A, Shrestha R, Sindwani R. Chronic granulomatous invasive fungal sinusitis: an evolving approach to management. Int Forum Allergy Rhinol. 2014; 4(4):280–283

[17] Challa S, Pamidi U, Uppin SG, Uppin MS, Vemu L. Diagnostic accuracy of morphologic identification of filamentous fungi in paraffin embedded tissue sections: correlation of histological and culture diagnosis. Indian J Pathol Microbiol. 2014; 57(4):583–587

[18] Philpott CM, Javer AR, Clark A. Allergic fungal rhinosinusitis: a new staging system. Rhinology. 2011; 49(3):318–323

[19] Meltzer EO, Hamilos DL, Hadley JA, et al. American Academy of Allergy, Asthma and Immunology (AAAAI), American Academy of Otolaryngic Allergy (AAOA), American Academy of Otolaryngology-Head and Neck Surgery (AAO-HNS), American College of Allergy, Asthma and Immunology (ACAAI), American Rhinologic Society (ARS). Rhinosinusitis: establishing definitions for clinical research and patient care. J Allergy Clin Immunol. 2004; 114(6) Suppl:155–212

[20] Ponikau JU, Sherris DA, Kern EB, et al. The diagnosis and incidence of allergic fungal sinusitis. Mayo Clin Proc. 1999; 74(9):877–884

[21] Ferguson BJ. Eosinophilic mucin rhinosinusitis: a distinct clinicopathological entity. Laryngoscope. 2000; 110(5, Pt 1):799–813

[22] Saravanan K, Panda NK, Chakrabarti A, Das A, Bapuraj RJ. Allergic fungal rhinosinusitis: an attempt to resolve the diagnostic dilemma. Arch Otolaryngol Head Neck Surg. 2006; 132(2):173–178

[23] Orlandi RR, Thibeault SL, Ferguson BJ. Microarray analysis of allergic fungal sinusitis and eosinophilic mucin rhinosinusitis. Otolaryngol Head Neck Surg. 2007; 136(5):707–713

[24] Foshee J, Luminais C, Casey J, et al. An evaluation of invasive fungal sinusitis outcomes with subsite analysis and use of frozen section analysis. Int Forum Allergy Rhinol. 2016; 6(8):807–811

[25] Pagella F, De Bernardi F, Dalla Gasperina D, et al. Invasive fungal rhinosinusitis in adult patients: our experience in diagnosis and management. J Craniomaxillofac Surg. 2016; 44(4):512–520

[26] Monroe MM, McLean M, Sautter N, et al. Invasive fungal rhinosinusitis: a 15-year experience with 29 patients. Laryngoscope. 2013; 123(7):1583–1587

[27] Gupta R, Gupta AK. Isolated primary frontal sinus aspergillosis: role of endonasal endoscopic approach. J Laryngol Otol. 2013; 127(3):274–278

[28] Bernardini E, Karligkiotis A, Fortunato S, Castelnuovo P, Dallan I. Surgical and pathogenetic considerations of frontal sinus fungus ball. Eur Arch Otorhinolaryngol. 2017; 274(6):2493–2497

[29] Chen IH, Chen TM. Isolated frontal sinus aspergillosis. Otolaryngol Head Neck Surg. 2000; 122(3):460–461

[30] Kodama S, Moriyama M, Okamoto T, Hirano T, Suzuki M. Isolated frontal sinus aspergillosis treated by endoscopic modified Lothrop procedure. Auris Nasus Larynx. 2009; 36(1):88–91

[31] Mukherji SK, Figueroa RE, Ginsberg LE, et al. Allergic fungal sinusitis: CT findings. Radiology. 1998; 207(2):417–422

[32] Marple BF. Allergic fungal rhinosinusitis: current theories and management strategies. Laryngoscope. 2001; 111(6):1006–1019

[33] Snidvongs K, Pratt E, Chin D, Sacks R, Earls P, Harvey RJ. Corticosteroid nasal irrigations after endoscopic sinus surgery in the management of chronic rhinosinusitis. Int Forum Allergy Rhinol. 2012; 2(5):415–421

[34] Ferguson BJ. Mucormycosis of the nose and paranasal sinuses. Otolaryngol Clin North Am. 2000; 33(2):349–365

[35] Kennedy CA, Adams GL, Neglia JP, Giebink GS. Impact of surgical treatment on paranasal fungal infections in bone marrow transplant patients. Otolaryngol Head Neck Surg. 1997; 116(6, Pt 1):610–616

[36] Saedi B, Sadeghi M, Seilani P. Endoscopic management of rhinocerebral mucormycosis with topical and intravenous amphotericin B. J Laryngol Otol. 2011; 125(8):807–810

[37] Busaba NY, Colden DG, Faquin WC, Salman SD. Chronic invasive fungal sinusitis: a report of two atypical cases. Ear Nose Throat J. 2002; 81(7):462–466

[38] Li Y, Li Y, Li P, Zhang G. Diagnosis and endoscopic surgery of chronic invasive fungal rhinosinusitis. Am J Rhinol Allergy. 2009; 23(6):622–625

[39] Stringer SP, Ryan MW. Chronic invasive fungal rhinosinusitis. Otolaryngol Clin North Am. 2000; 33(2):375–387

[40] D'Anza B, Stokken J, Greene JS, Kennedy T, Woodard TD, Sindwani R. Chronic invasive fungal sinusitis: characterization and shift in management of a rare disease. Int Forum Allergy Rhinol. 2016; 6(12):1294–1300

[41] Klossek JM, Serrano E, Péloquin L, Percodani J, Fontanel JP, Pessey JJ. Functional endoscopic sinus surgery and 109 mycetomas of paranasal sinuses. Laryngoscope. 1997; 107(1):112–117

[42] Marple BF. Allergic fungal rhinosinusitis: a review of clinical manifestations and current treatment strategies. Med Mycol. 2006; 44 Supplement_1:S277–S284

[43] Kuhn FA, Swain R, Jr. Allergic fungal sinusitis: diagnosis and treatment. Curr Opin Otolaryngol Head Neck Surg. 2003; 11(1):1–5

[44] Philpott CM, Thamboo A, Lai L, et al. Olfactory dysfunction in allergic fungal rhinosinusitis. Arch Otolaryngol Head Neck Surg. 2011; 137(7):694–697

33 Frontal Sinus Trauma and Its Management

Ulrik A. Felding and Christian von Buchwald

Abstract

The management of frontal sinus trauma remains controversial. Several aspects regarding the management of frontal sinus fractures defy consensus at present due to the lack of large prospective and/or controlled studies evaluating patient outcomes. The anterior bony wall of the frontal sinuses requires greater force to fracture than any other facial bone, so patients with frontal sinus fractures often have concomitant facial fractures and/or intracranial injuries due to the high energy needed to cause a fracture. Traumatic injury to the nasofrontal outflow tract and the bony boundaries of the frontal sinuses may cause various complications such as cosmetic deformities, cerebrospinal fluid leak, mucocele, or infection that may spread intracranially or into the orbital cavity. The classical standard for managing frontal sinus fractures is the open approach. However, minimally invasive endoscopic procedures are gaining popularity as the primary choice of treatment of frontal sinus fractures. Extensive procedures such as obliteration and cranialization of the frontal sinuses have been favored in the past. Current treatment modalities strive toward preserving the normal function of the sinuses.

Keywords: frontal sinus fracture, frontal recess, cranialization, obliteration, endoscopy, combined procedures, complications

33.1 Epidemiology and Etiology

33.1.1 Anatomy

The frontal sinuses are pneumatized compartments in the frontal bone, which are absent at birth but begin to develop as ethmoidal air cells invaginate the frontal bone around the age of 2 years. Pneumatization of the frontal bone is typically identifiable radiographically at the age of 6 years and is completed by around 15 years of age.[1] The frontal sinuses are the last of the paranasal sinuses to develop and may be partially or completely absent in 5 to 15% of the Caucasian population.[2,3,4] Some populations, for example, Inuits, have a higher prevalence of frontal sinus agenesis (25–45%).[5,6]

The frontal sinuses usually consist of a left and right compartment separated by a septum, which can often deviate from the midline sagittal plane. The frontal sinuses are bordered inferiorly by the sinus floor, and by anterior and posterior walls referred to as "tables." The frontal sinus communicates with the infundibulum via the frontal recess. The narrowest part of this hourglass-shaped connection is the true frontal ostium, which is the beginning of the nasofrontal outflow tract (NFOT), which crucially is a pathway for mucociliary clearance into the middle meatus of the nasal cavity.[1] The NFOT is not a true duct but is a drainage pathway with bony boundaries from the maxillary and ethmoidal bone. Optimum functionality of mucociliary clearance is mandatory for normal sinus function and presupposes an open pathway for clearance of mucus and ventilation of the sinuses. Trauma can cause chronic obstruction of the NFOT leading to mucocele or mucopyocele development, which in severe cases may erode the posterior table and lead to meningitis or encephalitis. Though uncommon, frontal sinus trauma management can be challenging due to the risk of associated displacement of the anterior or posterior tables, cerebrospinal fluid (CSF) leak, impaired mucociliary clearance, and because of a desire to manage using a minimally invasive surgical technique that respects the aesthetic of the forehead region.

33.1.2 Trauma Mechanism

Frontal sinus fractures (FSFs) may be classified into fractures of the anterior table, posterior table, or of both.[7] Isolated anterior table fractures and combined fractures (the anterior table, posterior table, and/or the nasofrontal recess) account for one-third and two-thirds of frontal sinus injuries, respectively.[8] Isolated traumatic fractures of the posterior wall are rare.

The frontal sinuses are involved in only 2 to 15% of all traumatic craniomaxillofacial (CMF) fractures.[9] However, when FSFs do occur, concomitant facial fractures and/or intracranial injuries are commonly present due to the high energy needed to cause a fracture.[2] The anterior bony wall of the adult frontal sinus is relatively thick at 2 to 12 mm, while the posterior wall is thinner at 0.1 to 4.8 mm.[10] The anterior bony table thus requires greater force to fracture than any other facial bone (3.6–7.1 kN corresponding to 367–723 kg of pressure).[11] This is almost twice as much energy as it would take to fracture the mandibular symphysis and almost three times more than is required to fracture the malar eminence of the zygoma.[12] This resilience to injury of the anterior wall may be due to both its thickness and its curved convexity. Both circumferential and radial fractures occur with a tendency for propagation of the fracture toward the orbit.

FSFs most often occur in younger individuals in a predominantly male population as is the case in all CMF fractures. FSFs may be caused by blast, sharp, or blunt trauma to the forehead. The most common trauma mechanism is blunt trauma resulting from motor vehicle accidents (MVA), which comprises 60 to 70% of all FSFs.[10,13] In

MVA, facial injuries are caused by sudden deceleration or acceleration of the steady-state body resulting in high-energy direct facial impact usually to the dashboard and/or steering wheel. The incidence of FSFs has fallen significantly since the introduction of mandatory seat belt and air bag protection in cars in the United States.[10,14] Assault is another cause of FSFs and typically requires the use of a blunt object to fracture the frontal sinus; closed-fist punches alone rarely generate sufficient force.[13] FSFs are also seen in actions of war and may be caused by both blast injury and gunshot wounds.[15] In primary blast injuries, fractures are caused by the shock wave passing through the air-filled paranasal sinuses causing an implosion/explosion effect as the air is first compressed and then re-expanded.[16] However, FSFs resulting from blast injury may also be caused by a secondary blast injury, which is a penetrating injury caused by fragments or by a tertiary blast injury, which is the resulting impact of the head upon the ground, a wall, or other solid objects.

33.2 Clinical Presentation and Investigations

33.2.1 Initial Examination of the Patient

Frontal sinus trauma patients present with a relevant history based on blast, sharp, or blunt trauma to the forehead. In severe cases, the patient may be unresponsive, with further investigations undertaken by the receiving trauma team in respect of other injuries or signs, in the absence of a complete patient history. The symptoms most often associated with FSFs are pain, skin abrasions or lacerations, cosmetic deformity, and CSF leak resulting in CSF rhinorrhea. A thorough clinical examination of a patient suspected of an FSF consists of otoscopy, anterior rhinoscopy, transnasal endoscopy of the nasal cavity, and an examination of the eyes, face, forehead, mouth, and pharynx. The forehead should be cleansed and examined for lacerations and the forehead should be palpated for contour irregularities of the underlying bone. A thorough neurological evaluation of the patient should also be part of the initial examination comprising an evaluation of the forehead sensation and facial nerve motor function. An overall neurological status including Glasgow Coma Scale will be performed initially by the trauma team when indicated.

33.2.2 Imaging and Paraclinical Investigations

A high-resolution computed tomographic (CT) scan is recommended and should be performed when an FSF is suspected. The CT scan should depict the NFOT in all three planes (axial, coronal, and sagittal) and have a slice thickness of ≤ 2 mm[17] (preferably thin-cut slices of 1.0 mm[8]). Involvement of the NFOT is best evaluated in the sagittal plane but may be difficult to discern. The fractures may be classified according to whether the fracture is isolated to the frontal sinuses, displaced or nondisplaced, if it is simple or comminute, if the NFOT is involved, and if there is a CSF leak or not. The patient must not be left unattended during the CT scan.

When the posterior table is involved, nasal endoscopy is indicated in order to exclude CSF leak. Rhinorrhea should be tested for the presence of CSF. A CSF leak is best diagnosed with a beta-2 transferrin (β2T) test.[18] Filter paper patterning (Halo test) and glucose testing are not recommended due to a high percentage of false-positive and false-negative results.[19] Another CSF protein test is beta-trace protein (βTP) testing, which has shown promising results with studies reporting sensitivities and specificities as high as β2 T testing.[20,21,22] However, although βTP testing merits consideration,[18] the technique is still designated for research purposes only and may be unreliable in the setting of renal disease and meningitis.[23,24] MRI is, in general, not indicated in the cases of isolated FSF.

33.3 Management

FSFs are usually classified as either anterior or posterior table fractures, or a combination of both. The choice of treatment modality for FSFs is based on these fracture classifications as well as an evaluation of the displacement of the fracture, the patency of the NFOT, and presence of a CSF leak.[25] The primary end goals of treating FSFs are normal aesthetics of the forehead, absence of CSF leak, and a normal frontal sinus mucociliary function. The three treatment modalities in treating FSFs consist of conservative approach, surgery with preservation of the normal sinus function, and surgery with "removal" of normal sinus function by either obliteration or cranialization. Historically, surgery with obliteration and cranialization of the frontal sinus has been the more popular method. Parallel with technical developments, including the use of CT image guidance in the last couple of decades, another promising development has occurred toward preserving the normal anatomy and function of the frontal sinuses with either conservative treatment or endoscopic approaches—or combining the latter with a minimal external approach.[26]

33.3.1 Surgical Techniques

There are a variety of ways to obtain access to the frontal sinuses and treat FSFs. The classical choice of treatment is an open approach to the frontal sinus. The open approaches include the coronal incision, frontal trephination via a subbrow incision, endoscopy-assisted surgery via brow lift incisions and direct forehead crease incision (possibly using preexisting lacerations).

The traditional approach to repairing a FSF is the coronal incision of the scalp. This procedure provides a wide exposure of the forehead, which facilitates an easier manipulation of bony fragments for optimal reduction and fixation. An incision traversing the vertex from helical root to helical root is performed and is usually followed by an anterior subgaleal dissection to the fracture site where the dissection is then transitioned to a subperiosteal, which exposes the fracture site.[27] Complications, to this quite extensive approach, include scars, alopecia, and loss of sensibility of the forehead due to injury to the supraorbital and supratrochlear nerves.

Frontal sinus trephination is a direct and simple method to access the frontal sinuses, which may be performed by itself or as a supplement to transnasal endoscopy. An incision is performed midway between the glabella and the medial canthus.[26] Once the frontal bone is reached via dissection, a frontal sinusotomy is performed with a small bur. By this approach, the frontal sinus can be evaluated with either a 0- or 30-degree endoscope. Frontal sinus trephination allows surgery of FSFs without the risk of iatrogenic damage to the NFOT. Also, trephination allows the surgeon to access the most lateral parts of the frontal sinuses, which are difficult to reach via an endonasal approach. Bilateral trephination can be performed to facilitate greater visualization of the frontal sinuses. During dissection, care must be taken not to injure the supraorbital neurovascular pedicle and the supratrochlear nerve.

Conventionally, surgeons chose between traditional open approaches (osteoplastic flap, frontal trephination) and purely endoscopic approaches (endoscopic frontal sinusotomy, endoscopic modified Lothrop).[6,7]

However, the combination of trephination with endoscopic techniques is increasingly being utilized.

Endoscopic anterior wall fracture repair may be performed transnasally or transcutaneously via brow lift incisions, which provide access to the fracture site.[8] The endoscopic-assisted open procedure in case of anterior table fracture leading to a cosmetic deformity may be performed months after the trauma. In case of a transcutaneous approach, an access incision for the endoscope and a second working incision are made sagittally, behind the hairline, and the periosteum is lifted over the defect. An implant is inserted in the larger working incision and positioned over the defect for camouflage of the deformity. The implant is stabilized via screws inserted through a stab incision over the fracture site. Transnasal endoscopy provides access to the frontal sinuses without the morbidity of transcutaneous incisions. This minimally invasive approach enables the surgeon to evaluate and maintain patency of the NFOT and allows for endoscopic surveillance postoperatively to monitor for complications, such as recurrent CSF leak or closure of the frontal sinus.[28]

More severe cases of fracture may require obliteration or cranialization of the frontal sinuses. The obliteration procedure destroys normal frontal sinus function by the removal of all mucosa and by plugging the NFOT and the whole frontal sinus with autologous tissue (fat, bone, muscle, and/or pericranium). A coronal incision is performed and a pericranial flap is prepared as described earlier. The entire frontal wall is outlined, drilled out, and removed for later repositioning. This osteoplastic flap procedure exposes the whole frontal sinus. Defining the borders of the frontal wall may be difficult. If the margins are too wide, drilling will result in cranial entry. If it is too narrow, a full exposure of the frontal sinus is not achieved. Techniques for delineating the frontal sinus include sinus probing with a bayonet forceps or transillumination with a light source. A newer technique is 3D modeling of the frontal sinus and surrounding bone using a CT scan.[29] This model is used to make an onlay template, which can be sterilized and used perioperatively to exactly determine the extent of frontal sinus pneumatization. When the frontal bone flap is removed, all the sinus mucosa must meticulously be removed to prevent later development of a mucocele. The frontal ostium and the rest of the frontal sinus are filled with autologous material (usually abdominal fat) and the frontal bone flap is reattached. Another form of obliteration is osteoneogenesis, where the frontal sinus is stripped of its mucosa and left empty to be slowly filled with scar tissue and new bone formation. This "auto-obliteration" carries with it a high risk of infection.[30]

Cranialization is usually reserved for the most severe posterior wall fractures. The posterior table and all mucosa are removed, which allows the brain to herniate into and occupy the frontal sinuses. It has several advantages, for example, wide exposure of the injured area for repair of dural injury and elimination of the sinus with its propensity for infection and mucocele formation.[31] It is crucial to maintain the integrity of the pericranial flap for dural repair and control of CSF leaks.[8]

33.3.2 Surgical Decision-Making

The decision of which treatment the patient should receive is based on variables that include fracture type, fracture displacement/comminution, and CSF leak. The fracture types are anterior wall fracture, posterior wall fracture, and NFOT fracture. These fractures are often combined. As mentioned earlier, the possible treatment options are observation, open reduction and internal fixation, endoscopic-assisted open procedure, transnasal endoscopic repair, and sinus obliteration or cranialization (see ▶ Fig. 33.1 for treatment guidelines).

Nondisplaced anterior and posterior wall fractures with no CSF leaks and no obstruction of the NFOT may be treated conservatively. Transnasal endoscopy is a minimally invasive method that can be used both for reduction of displaced bone segments and for opening an obstructed NFOT. Anterior fractures with more than 2-mm displacement in the sagittal plane should be

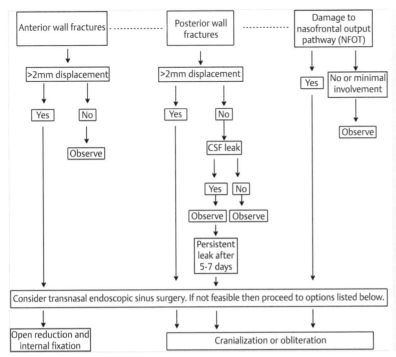

Fig. 33.1 A guideline for primary treatment choice in frontal sinus fractures. Depicted are individual treatment paths for fractures of the anterior wall, posterior wall, and the nasofrontal output pathway, respectively. However, since frontal sinus trauma commonly results in a combination of these fracture types, the primary choice of treatment must be decided based on the specific combination of fractures. Displacement of greater than 2 mm of the anterior and posterior tables is chosen as a cutoff value. Other reports have used displacement greater than the table width as an indication for surgery.

considered for primary transnasal endoscopy. This approach may be used in connection with trephination or coronal flap surgery in difficult cases. Minimally displaced fractures with mild NFOT injuries may be followed clinically with CT scans. If clinically relevant obstruction of the NFOT is present, the patency may be restored via transnasal endoscopic surgery or the frontal sinuses may be obliterated. Open reduction of an anterior fracture with internal fixation can be performed when transnasal endoscopy is unfeasible.

Nondisplaced posterior wall fractures with a CSF leak may be observed for 7 days. If the CSF leak is persistent, the leak may be managed by transnasal endoscopy with overlay of a biodesign graft or by cranialization.[9] Displacement of more than one width of the posterior wall may be treated with either obliteration or cranialization, but even comminuted segments can be treated endoscopically (see Chapter 35).

33.4 Case Example

A 32-year-old man was attacked by a man with an iron rod. He sustained a comminuted frontal table fracture involving the supraorbital rim (▶ Fig. 33.2). The fracture was reduced using an open procedure with a coronal incision (▶ Fig. 33.3). There were no complications.

33.5 Complications: Management

Complications may arise from FSFs, which can range in severity from a slight cosmetic deformity to an intracranial infection. Complications may arise years after the trauma, so a long follow-up period seems reasonable. The follow-up period should be 1 to 2 years. Early complications (< 6 months) may be sinusitis, wound infection, CSF leaks, and meningitis, while late complications (> 6 months) may be CSF leaks, mucopyoceles, intracranial infections, hypesthesia, persistent cosmetic deformity, and chronic pain.[2] A retrospective review of 857 FSF patients revealed complication rates of 10% for 504 operated patients and 3% for 353 conservatively treated patients.[31]

A CSF leak may be present immediately after the trauma or may arise several months after treatment. If present, it increases the long-term risk of meningitis, which is dependent on several variables including status of pneumococcal immunization and patient adherence. Evidence points toward early surgical intervention in all anterior skull base CSF leaks due to long-term risk of meningitis.[32,33,34] However, studies have shown that CSF leaks disappear with conservative treatment in 85% of patients after 7 days.[35] Although surgery would minimize the risk of meningitis, many patients would be operated on unnecessarily (see Chapter 35).

Frontal mucoceles usually arise due to obstruction of the NFOT, which hinders normal mucociliary clearance.[31] Reconstruction and stenting of the NFOT has proven very difficult with the NFOT being prone to restenosis. The primary choice of treatment for a mucocele is transnasal endoscopy utilizing either a Draf IIa, IIb, or III approach. A mucocele may become a mucopyocele if it becomes infected. Prolonged frontal sinus infection may spread

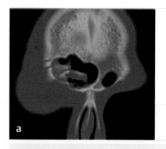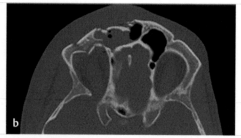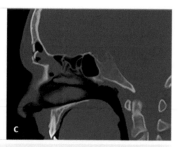

Fig. 33.2 The right frontal sinus anterior wall fracture on a **(a)** coronal, **(b)** axial, and **(c)** sagittal CT scan with a slice thickness of 0.5 mm.

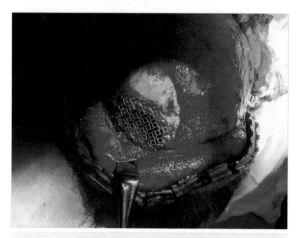

Fig. 33.3 Intraoperative view of open procedure where a coronal incision has been performed. A titanium net has been fixed over the frontal table fracture. Normal internal fixation with plates and screws was not possible in this case due to the fracture being too comminuted. The titanium net is bent around the supraorbital rim of the right orbit.

intracranially via a direct route, by eroding the posterior table, or by intravenous spread of bacteria from the frontal sinus. The veins that drain the frontal sinus have an intimate relation with the dural veins of Breschet, which may lead to an inherent risk of intracranial extension of frontal sinusitis.[36] Infection may also spread to the orbital region and cause pre- and/or postseptal cellulitis.

Bellamy et al showed that there is a fourfold increased risk for serious infection with operative delay beyond 48 hours.[37] However, the patients who were delayed operatively tended to have more severe injuries. The timeliness of an FSF surgery must be based on an estimation of the subacute risk of infection compared with the immediate risk of evolving intracranial or bodily injury.[37]

Chronic pain is also a possible complication of an FSF. Pain may be from the initial trauma or subsequent mucocele and infection. First, it is important to rule out serious intracranial causes such as an intracranial hematoma. Sensory innervation of the frontal sinuses is via the ophthalmic division of the trigeminal nerve, which also gives some dural innervation. This shared innervation may account for the global and referred pain to the scalp associated with frontal sinusitis.[36]

References

[1] Golden B, Jaskolka M, Vescan A, MacDonald K. Evaluation and Management of frontal sinus injuries. In: Fonseca R, Barber H, Powers M, Frost D, eds. Oral and Maxillofacial Trauma. 4th ed. St. Louis, MO: Elsevier; 2013:470–490

[2] Guy WM, Brissett AE. Contemporary management of traumatic fractures of the frontal sinus. Otolaryngol Clin North Am. 2013; 46 (5):733–748

[3] Patel RS, Yousem DM, Maldjian JA, Zager EL. Incidence and clinical significance of frontal sinus or orbital entry during pterional (fronto-temporal) craniotomy. AJNR Am J Neuroradiol. 2000; 21(7):1327–1330

[4] Szilvassy J. Zur variation, Entwicklung and Vererbung der Stirnhohlen. Ann Naturhist Mus Vienna.. 1982; 84:97–125

[5] Hanson CL, Owsley DW. Frontal sinus size in Eskimo populations. Am J Phys Anthropol. 1980; 53(2):251–255

[6] Koertvelyessy T. Relationships between the frontal sinus and climatic conditions: a skeletal approach to cold adaptation. Am J Phys Anthropol. 1972; 37(2):161–172

[7] Holmes S, Perry M. Craniofacial fractures and the frontal sinus. In: Perry M, Holmes S, eds. Atlas of Operative Maxillofacial Trauma Surgery. London, UK: Springer; 2014:673–738

[8] Strong EB. Frontal sinus fractures: current concepts. Craniomaxillofac Trauma Reconstr. 2009; 2(3):161–175

[9] Chaaban MR, Conger B, Riley KO, Woodworth BA. Transnasal endoscopic repair of posterior table fractures. Otolaryngol Head Neck Surg. 2012; 147(6):1142–1147

[10] Strong EB, Pahlavan N, Saito D. Frontal sinus fractures: a 28-year retrospective review. Otolaryngol Head Neck Surg. 2006; 135(5):774–779

[11] Nahum AM. The biomechanics of maxillofacial trauma. Clin Plast Surg. 1975; 2(1):59–64

[12] Rhee JS, Posey L, Yoganandan N, Pintar F. Experimental trauma to the malar eminence: fracture biomechanics and injury patterns. Otolaryngol Head Neck Surg. 2001; 125(4):351–355

[13] Pletcher SD, Goldberg AN. Frontal sinus fractures. In: Lalwani AK, ed. Current Diagnosis & Treatment Otolaryngology: Head and Neck Surgery. 3rd ed. New York, NY: The McGraw-Hill Companies; 2012:302–309

[14] Murphy RX, Jr, Birmingham KL, Okunski WJ, Wasser T. The influence of airbag and restraining devices on the patterns of facial trauma in motor vehicle collisions. Plast Reconstr Surg. 2000; 105(2):516–520

[15] Wordsworth M, Thomas R, Breeze J, Evriviades D, Baden J, Hettiaratchy S. The surgical management of facial trauma in British soldiers during combat operations in Afghanistan. Injury. 2017; 48(1):70–74

[16] Dussault MC, Smith M, Osselton D. Blast injury and the human skeleton: an important emerging aspect of conflict-related trauma. J Forensic Sci. 2014; 59(3):606–612

[17] Schütz P, Ibrahim HHH, Rajab B. Contemporary management of frontal sinus injuries and frontal bone fractures. In: Hosein M, Motamedi K, eds. Contemporary Management of Frontal Sinus Injuries and Frontal Bone Fractures: A Textbook of Advanced Oral and Maxillofacial Surgery. Vol. 2: InTech; 2015. Available at: http://dx.doi.org/10.5772/59096

[18] Oakley GM, Alt JA, Schlosser RJ, Harvey RJ, Orlandi RR. Diagnosis of cerebrospinal fluid rhinorrhea: an evidence-based review with recommendations. Int Forum Allergy Rhinol. 2016; 6(1):8–16

[19] Phang SY, Whitehouse K, Lee L, Khalil H, McArdle P, Whitfield PC. Management of CSF leak in base of skull fractures in adults. Br J Neurosurg. 2016; 30(6):596–604

[20] Arrer E, Meco C, Oberascher G, Piotrowski W, Albegger K, Patsch W. β-Trace protein as a marker for cerebrospinal fluid rhinorrhea. Clin Chem. 2002; 48(6, Pt 1):939–941

[21] McCudden CR, Senior BA, Hainsworth S, et al. Evaluation of high resolution gel. (2)-transferrin for detection of cerebrospinal fluid leak. Clin Chem Lab Med. 2013; 51(2):311–315

[22] Schnabel C, Di Martino E, Gilsbach JM, Riediger D, Gressner AM, Kunz D. Comparison of beta2-transferrin and beta-trace protein for detection of cerebrospinal fluid in nasal and ear fluids. Clin Chem. 2004; 50(3):661–663

[23] Le C, Strong EB, Luu Q. Management of anterior skull base cerebrospinal fluid leaks. J Neurol Surg B Skull Base. 2016; 77(5):404–411

[24] Meco C, Oberascher G, Arrer E, Moser G, Albegger K. Beta-trace protein test: new guidelines for the reliable diagnosis of cerebrospinal fluid fistula. Otolaryngol Head Neck Surg. 2003; 129(5):508–517

[25] Oppenheimer AJ, Sugg KB, Buchman SR. Frontal sinus fractures. In: Taub PJ, Patel PK, Buchman SR, Cohen MN, eds. Ferraro's Fundamentals of Maxillofacial Surgery. New York, NY: Springer New York; 2015:235–246

[26] Patel AB, Cain RB, Lal D. Contemporary applications of frontal sinus trephination: A systematic review of the literature. Laryngoscope. 2015; 125(9):2046–2053

[27] Delaney SW. Treatment strategies for frontal sinus anterior table fractures and contour deformities. J Plast Reconstr Aesthet Surg. 2016; 69 (8):1037–1045

[28] Grayson JW, Jeyarajan H, Illing EA, Cho DY, Riley KO, Woodworth BA. Changing the surgical dogma in frontal sinus trauma: transnasal endoscopic repair. Int Forum Allergy Rhinol. 2017 May;7(5):441–449

[29] Daniel M, Watson J, Hoskison E, Sama A. Frontal sinus models and onlay templates in osteoplastic flap surgery. J Laryngol Otol. 2011; 125(1):82–85

[30] MacBeth R. The osteoplastic operation for chronic infection of the frontal sinus. J Laryngol Otol. 1954; 68(7):465–477

[31] Rodriguez ED, Stanwix MG, Nam AJ, et al. Twenty-six-year experience treating frontal sinus fractures: a novel algorithm based on anatomical fracture pattern and failure of conventional techniques. Plast Reconstr Surg. 2008; 122(6):1850–1866

[32] Bernal-Sprekelsen M, Alobid I, Mullol J, Trobat F, Tomás-Barberán M. Closure of cerebrospinal fluid leaks prevents ascending bacterial meningitis. Rhinology. 2005; 43(4):277–281

[33] Bernal-Sprekelsen M, Bleda-Vázquez C, Carrau RL. Ascending meningitis secondary to traumatic cerebrospinal fluid leaks. Am J Rhinol. 2000; 14(4):257–259

[34] Brodie HA. Prophylactic antibiotics for posttraumatic cerebrospinal fluid fistulae. A meta-analysis. Arch Otolaryngol Head Neck Surg. 1997; 123(7):749–752

[35] Bell RB, Dierks EJ, Homer L, Potter BE. Management of cerebrospinal fluid leak associated with craniomaxillofacial trauma. J Oral Maxillofac Surg. 2004; 62(6):676–684

[36] Metzinger SE, Guerra AB, Garcia RE. Frontal sinus fractures: management guidelines. Facial Plast Surg. 2005; 21(3):199–206

[37] Bellamy JL, Molendijk J, Reddy SK, et al. Severe infectious complications following frontal sinus fracture: the impact of operative delay and perioperative antibiotic use. Plast Reconstr Surg. 2013; 132 (1):154–162

34 Cerebrospinal Fluid Leak in the Frontal Sinus: Endoscopic Management

Hari Jeyarajan, Benjamin K. Walters, and Bradford A. Woodworth

Abstract

Cerebrospinal fluid leaks originating from the frontal sinus pose both diagnostic and therapeutic challenges. Defects result from four primary etiologies: trauma, neoplasia, congenital, and spontaneous. Thorough clinical assessment is critical in correctly identifying the presence and source of a leak. Traditionally, skull base pathology involving the frontal sinus has been managed via open approaches; however, advances in the field have generated increased interest in endoscopic treatment.

Keywords: cerebrospinal fluid leak, encephalocele, frontal sinus, endoscopic sinus surgery, Draf III, anterior table fracture, posterior table fracture, frontal sinus fracture

34.1 Epidemiology and Etiology

Cerebrospinal fluid (CSF) rhinorrhea can develop from defects anywhere along the skull base. Pertaining to the frontal sinus, trauma is by far the most common etiology. Historically, such skull base defects have been approached via an open repair. While endoscopic repair of CSF leaks has evolved to become the standard of care for most defects of the anterior cranial base over the last several decades, there is widespread trepidation in translating this to management of frontal sinus CSF leaks. However, advances in surgical techniques, teaching, and instrumentation have significantly improved access to the frontal sinus. Recent evidence indicates endoscopic repair has at least equivalent outcomes to open approaches and has improved patient morbidity.[1,2,3,4,5,6,7,8,9,10,11,12] The following discussion will review etiologies, preoperative evaluation and diagnosis, surgical approach, postoperative care and complications, and published outcomes for frontal sinus CSF leak management.

34.1.1 Etiologies

Trauma (either accidental or iatrogenic) is by far the most common cause of CSF leaks in the frontal sinus; however, it is essential to understand other less common causes since etiology can greatly influence medical and surgical management, prognosis, and outcomes.

Trauma

Frontal sinus fractures are present in 2 to 15% of all traumatic craniofacial fractures.[13] In cases of frontal sinus trauma, posterior table injuries present with (67%) and without (7–11%) anterior table fractures.[14,15,16,17,18] Presence of posterior table fracture is often associated with dural injuries including pneumocephalus (25–33%), CSF leak (13–25%), and extradural hematoma (10%; ▶ Fig. 34.1, ▶ Fig. 34.2, ▶ Fig. 34.3).[13,18,19,20] While rhinorrhea usually occurs within 48 hours, CSF leaks can present months to years after the injury.[21]

Functional endoscopic sinus surgery (FESS) and frontal craniotomies are the most common causes of iatrogenic frontal injury. While some retrospective series document FESS to be responsible for as much as 46% of traumatic CSF leaks, almost half of these occurred in revision cases and, overall, less than 1% of FESS now results in CSF leak.[11] In fact, prospective series have shown FESS to be a relatively uncommon cause of CSF leak overall.[22] Frontal craniotomy may result in CSF leak if the superior and lateral sinus recesses are entered during removal of the bony plate.[23]

Neoplasia

Both sinonasal and anterior skull base tumors may cause CSF leaks in the region of the frontal sinus through direct erosion of the posterior table or frontal recess (▶ Fig. 34.4, ▶ Fig. 34.5, ▶ Fig. 34.6). Equally, tumor regression from nonsurgical treatment may also result in a delayed leak. Surgical ablation often creates large dural defects necessitating meticulous, multilayered repairs that may fail in up to 11.5% of cases.[24] Leak recurrence can be attributed to technical errors (such as incomplete coverage or tears sustained during elevation), retraction secondary to failure in postoperative packing and support, or devitalization consequent to chemo-/radiotherapy. Wolfe's pericranial flap,[25] once a staple workhorse of open anterior skull base reconstruction, has been plagued by radiation-induced vasculitis, which results in flap loss in as many as 20% of cases.[26,27] This has led many to consider a combination of techniques in difficult cases.[28,29]

Congenital

Technically, congenital skull base defects of the frontal sinus do not exist as the frontal sinus is not present at birth. However, with growth and development of the frontal sinus, defects in the anterior skull base can encroach upon the outflow tract. Congenital defects in the skull base allow for herniation of intracranial contents and the formation of a nasal encephalocele in 1 out of every 4,000 live births.[30,31,32] Persistence of the fonticulus nasofrontalis, prenasal space, or foramen cecum can result in herniation of intracranial contents forming a frontal encephalocele.[31,33] These are classically divided into sincipital/frontoethmoidal types (typically involving the foramen cecum and possessing external nasal components) and basal (typically not involving the foramen cecum and remaining completely intranasal).[30,31,32,34,35] In practice, however, congenital dehiscences can be found at any point in the skull base, with anterior defects requiring comfort with 70-degree endoscopes and angled instrumentation.[5]

Spontaneous

Spontaneous leaks classically occur in middle-aged, obese females as part of a syndrome of idiopathic intracranial hypertension. Chronically increased pressure erodes the skull base causing multiple areas of pitting and erosion. This etiology has the highest rate of encephalocele formation and recurrences following surgical repair compared to other etiologies.[36,37,38,39] Due to high recurrence rate, adjuvant measures to lower chronically elevated intracranial pressure (ICP) is strongly recommended.[40]

34.2 Clinical Presentation and Investigations

While a history of sudden-onset clear rhinorrhea in the setting of antecedent trauma is almost pathognomonic for a CSF leak, establishing such a diagnosis in someone with intermittent nasal drainage and no recollection of head injury is much more challenging. A thorough history and examination including nasal endoscopy is critical in the clinical evaluation. Patients may describe a salty or metallic taste to their drainage as well as headaches (from both high and low ICPs). The presence of an encephalocele may also cause symptoms of nasal obstruction. A history of recurrent meningitis should also raise suspicions, as 30 to 50% are associated with skull base defects.[41,42,43]

A number of diagnostic tools can help in temporally and spatially establishing a diagnosis (▸ Table 34.1). It is important to consider the invasiveness of the test as well as remember that reported sensitivities and specificities are significantly dependent on the patient population studied, defect size, leak flow rate, and individual interpretation of results. As such, we feel that clinical acumen should guide the judicious use of these tests rather than adopting an algorithmic approach.

Although over 70% of traumatic CSF leaks will resolve with conservative management, mounting evidence indicates surgical intervention and formal duraplasty may be indicated for all anterior skull base CSF leaks. Proponents of early endoscopic repair argue that there is no true dural regeneration. The risk of bacterial meningitis increases with time to a lifetime risk of 10 to 37% and mortality of at least 10% with reported cases occurring 48 years after injury.[44,45,46,47,48,49,50] Surgical repair eliminates this risk with overall success rates of at least

Table 34.1 Diagnostic tools for cerebrospinal fluid leak

Technique	Advantages	Disadvantages
Beta-2 transferrin	Noninvasive, accurate, patient can collect during intermittent episodes	Nonlocalizing
Computed tomography (CT)	Noninvasive, excellent bony detail, accessible	Cannot differentiate CSF from soft tissue, bony dehiscence/attenuation may be present without leak
Intrathecal fluorescein	Precise localization, blue light filter may increase sensitivity	Invasive, skull base exposure necessary for precise localization of leak, risks with high concentration or rapid injection
CT cisternogram	Contrast may pool in frontal sinus, excellent bony detail	Invasive, not as diagnostic for intermittent leaks
Magnetic resonance imaging/cisternography	Excellent soft-tissue detail to determine difference between CSF/brain/mucous, noninvasive	Poor bony detail
Radioactive cisternogram	Localizes side of leak, utility for low and intermittent leaks	Imprecise localization, NOT recommended due to high false-positive rate

98%.[11,45,50,51,52] Unfortunately, there are no identifying factors that accurately predict patients most at risk for meningitis after conservative management. Thus, the majority of these individuals would undergo unnecessary surgery.

Timing of definitive repair in adults is dependent on various features. While postponing elective repair of a nonactive leak in the setting of concurrent sinus infection is recommended, it is generally considered that the increased risk of ascending infection mandates not delaying such repair in active leaks. While appropriate perioperative and continued culture-directed postoperative antibiotics with adequate CSF penetration are recommended around the time of surgery, the use of prophylactic antibiotics for leaks is discouraged due to unproven efficacy and risk of selection for resistant organisms.[50] Bleeding diathesis and pharmacological coagulopathy need to be addressed before definitive repair with consideration and patient counseling of associated cardiovascular and cerebrovascular risks. Concerning pediatric patients, uncertainty remains regarding operative timing for nonactive leaks, with the risk of ascending infection counterbalanced against allowing for adequate facial growth in the hope of facilitating instrumentation and visualization. While the rarity of congenital nasal encephaloceles precludes adequate sampling for risk assessment, it appears from case series that the risk of meningitis is low.[5,53,54,55] However, it has been demonstrated to be both feasible and safe to achieve successful repair even in infants.[5,53,55]

Additional preoperative counseling and written consent is required if the use of intrathecal fluorescein is to be considered intraoperatively. Normally introduced via a lumbar drain preoperatively, it dyes the CSF a fluorescent green. Since Kirchner and Proud's first description in 1960,[56] it has been widely utilized for intraoperative localization of dural defects with a sensitivity and specificity of 92.9 and 100%, respectively.[57] However, it is not Food and Drug Administration approved for intrathecal use and has rare but significant risk of seizures and neurotoxicity, as well as other less severe, transient neuropathies. The risk is felt to be largely dose dependent and associated with rapid administration.[58,59,60,61,62]

34.3 Management

Preoperative communication with anesthesia is recommended to optimize operative conditions. Positive pressure ventilation during intubation should be avoided to prevent tension pneumocephalus. We prefer to operate on the patient's right side with the endotracheal tube secured to the patient's left lower lip to avoid interference with surgical access. Prophylactic antibiotics, typically 2-g intravenous ceftriaxone, are recommended. For lumbar drain placement, the patient is placed in the left lateral decubitus position, while 0.1-mL preservative-free 10% fluorescein is placed in 10 mL of the patient's CSF or normal saline, and then subsequently delivered over 10 minutes via the drain. The patient is positioned supine or in Trendelenburg to encourage intracranial circulation of the fluorescein, which should be allowed to circulate for at least 20 minutes prior to endoscopy.[11] Drains are also useful for measuring ICP and withdrawing CSF during encephalocele ablation to assist with retraction and graft placement. Conversely, in cases of large dural defects, it also allows for the transthecal administration of saline during final stages of graft placement to decrease postoperative pneumocephalus.[10,12] Image guidance may be calibrated at this point, and cotton pledgets with decongestant placed in both nostrils. The patient is then prepped and draped in the standard fashion.

34.3.1 Surgical Management

Endoscopic

Endoscopic examination is performed to reevaluate intranasal anatomy as well as potentially visualize the presence and location of fluorescein. This may not be appreciated until better exposure is achieved. The patient is then placed in reverse Trendelenburg to aid with hemostasis for the remainder of the case. Surgical exposure proceeds with standard endoscopic sinus surgery, using through-cutting and powered instruments to avoid mucosal stripping. Exposure of the anterior skull base is achieved by identifying the skull base posteriorly at the sphenoid and diligently dividing the ethmoidal partitions anteriorly to the frontal recess. Here we recommend switching to a reverse 70-degree endoscope with frontal sinus instruments and curved suction to open the frontal recess. A Draf IIb frontal sinusotomy is performed for unilateral defects. For bilateral defects or large skull base lesions, a Draf III procedure may be required. An outside-in approach to the Draf III has been described and can expedite the drilling process when used alone or in combination with the traditional technique.[63] In an effort to decrease postoperative stenosis, mucosal grafts are placed at the anterior aspect of the frontal recess at the close of the Draf III procedure.[64]

Vigilant bipolar hemostasis is essential during reduction of an encephalocele, as dural vessels may retract causing intracranial hemorrhage. We prefer the Procise EZ-View Coblator wand (ArthroCare ENT, Sunnyvale, CA) with dual bipolar and ablate functions for encephalocele reduction and removal of mucosa around the defect. The latter is essential to prevent entrapment of secreting mucosa beneath the repair, which could displace the graft or flap as well as cause a subsequent mucocele.[65] The nasal cavity can be irrigated with clindamycin in order to minimize bacterial contamination and prevent seeding of the grafts.[48]

While various grafting materials have been described, we almost exclusively use porcine small intestine submucosal (SIS) grafts (Biodesign Dural Graft, Cook Medical, Bloomington, IN) for both underlay and/or overlay grafting. It carries no donor site morbidity, does not swell with hydration, and is easy to handle without adhering to itself if crumpled or folded.[66] In the cases where skull base defects are greater than 5 mm, elevated ICP is present, and there is sufficient epidural space, an underlay free bone graft (usually septal or turbinate bone) is used to further strengthen the repair. This is not recommended when reconstructing oncological resections, however, due to the large defect size and risk of osteoradionecrosis with possible adjuvant radiotherapy.

To complete the multilayer duroplasty, an overlay component of SIS, free mucosal graft, or pedicled flap is then positioned over the defect. We prefer utilizing the Hadad–Bassagasteguy nasoseptal flap (NSF)[67] when available, especially for larger defects and high-flow leaks,[50] and have found it capable of reaching up to 3 cm up the posterior table.[9,68] The overlay graft or NSF is then tacked into position with fibrin sealant (Evicel, Johnson & Johnson, Somerville, NJ) and supported with ciprofloxacin-soaked Gelfoam. A 0.5-mm Silastic stent is then placed in the frontal sinus outflow tract to maintain patency as well as prevent inadvertent premature removal of packing. This is followed by a nonlatex gloved cotton sponge (Merocel, Medtronic, Jacksonville, FL) spacer inserted into the anterior aspect of the sphenoid sinus, extending just anterior to the frontal recess such that it fills the entire ethmoid cavity.[9,48] It is subsequently instilled with saline and secured to the septum via a 2–0 Prolene suture.

Prior to extubation, antiemetics are provided, the lumbar drain is opened, and laryngotracheal topical anesthesia is administered to decrease the risk of increased ICP from valsalva and/or coughing. Positive pressure ventilation should be avoided, although the use of multiple packing layers reduces the risk of pneumocephalus.

Extracranial

Open approaches are used when experience and/or materials are limited, and in combination with endoscopic repair for defects that a surgeon may feel are inaccessible in the lateral or superior portions of the posterior table.[48] Frontal trephine may be used to approach the superior limits of the defect, but an osteoplastic flap is recommended if unable to meticulously remove the mucosa.[69,70,71] The nonobliterative approach is recommended in the setting of frontal recess fractures with a substantially intact posterior wall,[72] followed by obliteration if patency is unachievable. The classic indication for obliteration is the presence of bilateral posterior table fractures with small frontal sinuses. Frontal recess mucosa is stripped and abdominal fat is placed within the sinus.

Intracranial

A craniotomy with cranialization of the frontal sinus and frontal lobe retraction may be necessary for patients with large anterior skull base neoplasms, tumors with intracranial extension, multiple comminuted defects, large bilateral defects in a patient with anosmia, badly deformed skull bases, or in the cases where a craniotomy is required for intracranial complication from trauma. Retraction of the frontal lobe may lead to long-term memory issues, edema, epilepsy, anosmia, or intracranial hemorrhage, and increased rates of recurrence.[9]

34.3.2 Endoscopic versus Open Repair

An endoscopic approach with functional sinus preservation allows for optimal assessment of and repair of bony and mucosal injury along with true preservation of functional sinus drainage. Open procedures are associated with more infectious and obstructive complications, often paradoxically caused by the surgeries that were performed to prevent them. Chronic headache occurs after half of open repairs when trauma is the etiology.[73] Cranialization is associated with significant cosmetic issues,[74] resorption of autologous fat,[75,76] and increased risk of

mucocele formation,[77,78] leading to a 25% failure rate.[79] Pericranial flap has a 10 to 17% failure rate in management of traumatic CSF leak.[80] Endoscopy lacks external incisions and provides better frontal sinus drainage pathway clearance, often obviating the need for postsurgical radiological surveillance. Utilization of the current Draf IIB and III techniques also results in a much lower risk of mucocele formation than with open procedures.[81,82]

34.3.3 Postprocedural Care

Patients should be monitored overnight in an ICU with neurological checks. In the case of tumor resection, large encephalocele removal, or altered mental status, a noncontrast head CT should be obtained the next morning to evaluate for cerebral edema or hematoma. Intravenous antibiotics are continued for at least 24 hours. They may be transitioned to oral staphylococcal antibiotics prior to discharge and continued until nasal packing removal, although some studies have not detected any difference in infection rates when comparing perioperative and longer-term postoperative antibiotic use.[83] Patients tend to experience less discomfort and bleeding when the follow-up visit to remove nasal packing is scheduled 9 to 13 days after surgery. Patients may continue to use stool softeners, antitussives, and antiemetics. Activity may be restricted as Valsalva can increase ICP by greater than 25 cm H_2O.[50] Further follow-up visits can be scheduled at 1- to 4-week intervals. Patients should be educated to recognize symptoms of new CSF leak, as many iatrogenic leaks have a delayed presentation. Weight loss counseling is appropriate in order to reduce the risk of recurrence in spontaneous CSF leak patients. Continuous positive airway pressure (CPAP) should be discontinued in the immediate perioperative period, although hypoxia can increase ICP and pressure on the repair site. In the presence of insufficient evidence, we recommend abstaining until removal of packing to confirm success of closure.[50]

34.3.4 Postprocedural Adjuvants

Continued postoperative lumbar drainage in adults has the potential to increase patient morbidity and inpatient stay with complications that are not always predictable. Our conviction is that the success of the repair relies on the successful closure of the defect, and little benefit is achieved in routine drainage. Our practice is to reserve this only for the cases with spontaneous CSF leaks or established hydrocephalus with plan for removal after 2 to 3 postoperative days with adequate control of pressures. Failure to achieve normalcy may require formal diversion with placement of a shunt. In pediatric patients, specific concerns relate more to inability to comply with standard postoperative care instructions[54]; however, numerous case series have noted satisfactory results without drainage.[5,53,55]

34.3.5 Outcomes

While patients with spontaneous CSF leak have the highest risk of surgical failure, the success rate of frontal sinus CSF leak repair is typically 90% or better. As stated earlier, oral acetazolamide and ventriculoperitoneal (VP) shunt to control ICP can decrease the risk of surgical failure in those with spontaneous etiology.[40]

34.4 Case Examples

Case 1: A 20-year-old man presents with self-inflicted gunshot wound and massive posterior trauma, including a right anteriorly telescoped posterior table and severely comminuted left posterior table (▶ Fig. 34.1, ▶ Fig. 34.2, ▶ Fig. 34.3; Video 34.1).

Case 2: A 51-year-old woman with transdural atypical meningioma and involvement of bilateral posterior tables (▶ Fig. 34.4, ▶ Fig. 34.5, ▶ Fig. 34.6; Video 34.2).

34.5 Complications: Management

Even with careful planning and safe technique, complications can occur intraoperatively, postoperatively, or in a delayed fashion. Intraoperatively, significant bleeding can be encountered as well as inadvertent trauma to the globe or the brain. The locations of the anterior ethmoid

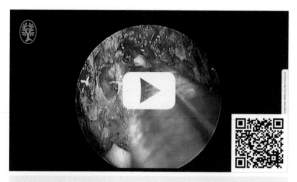

Video 34.1 Post traumatic cerebrospinal fluid (CSF) leak

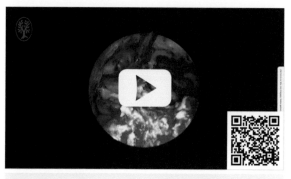

Video 34.2 CSF/Dural repair post resection of meningioma

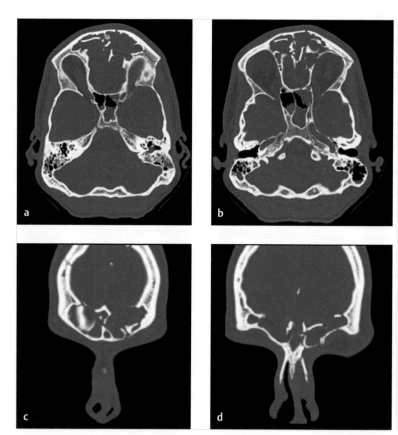

Fig. 34.1 (a,b) Axial and **(c,d)** coronal CT scans of a patient with self-inflicted gunshot wound and severely comminuted posterior table fractures.

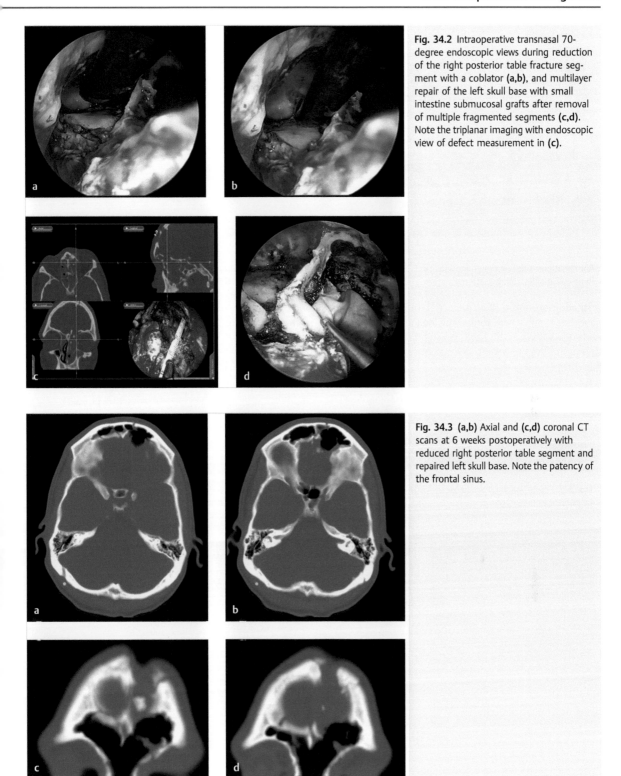

Fig. 34.2 Intraoperative transnasal 70-degree endoscopic views during reduction of the right posterior table fracture segment with a coblator (**a,b**), and multilayer repair of the left skull base with small intestine submucosal grafts after removal of multiple fragmented segments (**c,d**). Note the triplanar imaging with endoscopic view of defect measurement in (**c**).

Fig. 34.3 (**a,b**) Axial and (**c,d**) coronal CT scans at 6 weeks postoperatively with reduced right posterior table segment and repaired left skull base. Note the patency of the frontal sinus.

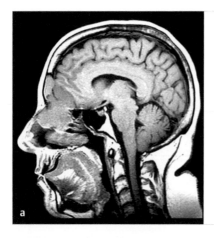
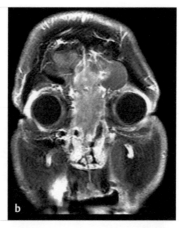

Fig. 34.4 (a) Sagittal and (b) coronal MRI scans of a patient with a transdural atypical meningioma extending through the posterior tables and cribriform plate.

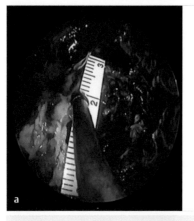
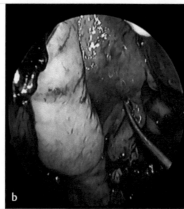
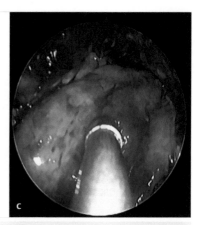

Fig. 34.5 Transnasal endoscopic views following resection of the tumor with defect in anterior skull base including the posterior tables (a) as well as placement of a large nasoseptal flap covering the entire defect (b,c).

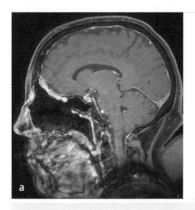
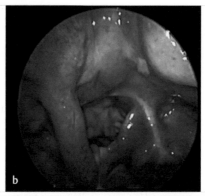
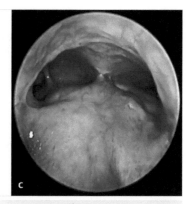

Fig. 34.6 (a) Sagittal MRI scan 2 years post-op showing the length of the flap covering the defect of the posterior table with no tumor recurrence. Postoperative endoscopy shows the (b) posterior and (c) anterior aspects of the nasoseptal flap repair. Note the edge of the flap covers a very large portion of the posterior tables.

artery and sphenopalatine arteries should be appreciated and managed judiciously. If the anterior ethmoid artery retracts and an orbital hematoma forms, ophthalmology should be consulted and a lateral canthotomy and cantholysis performed immediately. Traction on orbital fat may also cause intraorbital hemorrhage due to vessel avulsion. Breach of the orbit may result in orbital muscle or optic nerve damage.[84] Neurosurgical consult is recommended if there is a concern for intracranial bleeding. Careful hemostasis and minimization of mucosal trauma improves visualization and reduces the risk of postoperative epistaxis. The risk of hyposmia is reduced by avoiding excessive removal of the superior turbinates and by dissecting carefully when near the olfactory fila.

Postoperative complications include pneumocephalus, intracranial hypertension (IH), meningitis, and altered mental status. Avoidance of postoperative positive pressure ventilation is important due to risk of tension pneumocephalus. Patients should have careful perioperative neurological observation with urgent cross-sectional imaging obtained for alterations in mental state. Patients are counseled on avoiding use of home CPAP until postoperative removal of packing confirms successful duroplasty. ICP can be managed with elevation of the head of the bed, avoidance of Valsalva, stool softeners, and antiemetics. Lumbar drains placed preoperatively can be used to measure ICP postoperatively in spontaneous CSF leaks in order to determine the need for pressure-lowering therapy.[50] Oral acetazolamide or a VP shunt is used if persistently high pressures are encountered to prevent recurrent or new CSF leaks.[40] VP shunt is typically reserved for recurrent leaks, very high ICP, traumatic brain injuries where ventriculostomies are converted secondary to persistently elevated ICP, and patients who do not respond to acetazolamide.[11] Suspicion of postoperative CSF leak requires prompt surgical re-exploration. Antibiotics and watertight closure will decrease the risk of meningitis. Imaging should be taken for any alteration in mental status or significant change in neurological examination findings.

Delayed frontal sinus stenosis can be avoided by using mucosal-sparing technique, short-term postoperative stenting, mucosal grafting, in-office endoscopic debridements, and maintenance of topical medications. If postoperative inflammation is present, steroid application with nasal irrigations or in Mygind's position may be beneficial. Leak recurrence is more common in spontaneous etiologies, but endoscopic surgery with postoperative control of chronically elevated ICP minimizes this risk.[2] Intraoperative prophylactic opening of sinuses adjacent to the leak site reduces the risk of mucoceles.[48]

34.6 Conclusion

Frontal sinus CSF leaks can be safely and effectively addressed endoscopically. Extracranial or intracranial approaches may be used if necessary. Adequate preoperative evaluation of patient anatomy and disease etiology, as well as appropriate pre- and postoperative patient management can increase the surgical success rate and reduce the risk of intraoperative, postoperative, and delayed complications.

Recommended Readings

Oakley GM, Alt JA, Schlosser RJ, Harvey RJ, Orlandi RR. Diagnosis of cerebrospinal fluid rhinorrhea: an evidence-based review with recommendations. Int Forum Allergy Rhinol. 2016; 6(1):8–16

Ramakrishnan VR, Suh JD, Chiu AG, Palmer JN. Reliability of preoperative assessment of cerebrospinal fluid pressure in the management of spontaneous cerebrospinal fluid leaks and encephaloceles. Int Forum Allergy Rhinol. 2011; 1(3):201–205

Oakley GM, Orlandi RR, Woodworth BA, Batra PS, Alt JA. Management of cerebrospinal fluid rhinorrhea: an evidence-based review with recommendations. Int Forum Allergy Rhinol. 2016; 6(1):17–24

Grayson JW, Jeyarajan H, Illing EA, Cho DY, Riley KO, Woodworth BA. Changing the surgical dogma: transnasal endoscopic repair. Int Forum Allergy Rhinol. 2016; In press

References

[1] Woodworth BA, Palmer JN. Spontaneous cerebrospinal fluid leaks. Curr Opin Otolaryngol Head Neck Surg. 2009; 17(1):59–65

[2] Woodworth BA, Prince A, Chiu AG, et al. Spontaneous CSF leaks: a paradigm for definitive repair and management of intracranial hypertension. Otolaryngol Head Neck Surg. 2008; 138(6):715–720

[3] Woodworth B, Schlosser RJ. Repair of anterior skull base defects and CSF leaks. Op Tech Otolaryngol. 2006; 18:111–116

[4] Woodworth B, Neal JG, Schlosser RJ. Sphenoid sinus cerebrospinal fluid leaks. Op Tech Otolaryngol. 2006; 17:37–42

[5] Woodworth BA, Schlosser RJ, Faust RA, Bolger WE. Evolutions in the management of congenital intranasal skull base defects. Arch Otolaryngol Head Neck Surg. 2004; 130(11):1283–1288

[6] Schuster D, Riley KO, Cure JK, Woodworth BA. Endoscopic resection of intracranial dermoid cysts. J Laryngol Otol. 2011; 125(4):423–427

[7] Roehm CE, Brown SM. Unilateral endoscopic approach for repair of frontal sinus cerebrospinal fluid leak. Skull Base. 2011; 21(3):139–146

[8] Purkey MT, Woodworth BA, Hahn S, Palmer JN, Chiu AG. Endoscopic repair of supraorbital ethmoid cerebrospinal fluid leaks. ORL J Otorhinolaryngol Relat Spec. 2009; 71(2):93–98

[9] Jones V, Virgin F, Riley K, Woodworth BA. Changing paradigms in frontal sinus cerebrospinal fluid leak repair. Int Forum Allergy Rhinol. 2012; 2(3):227–232

[10] Blount A, Riley K, Cure J, Woodworth BA. Cerebrospinal fluid volume replacement following large endoscopic anterior cranial base resection. Int Forum Allergy Rhinol. 2012; 2(3):217–221

[11] Banks CA, Palmer JN, Chiu AG, O'Malley BW, Jr, Woodworth BA, Kennedy DW. Endoscopic closure of CSF rhinorrhea: 193 cases over 21 years. Otolaryngol Head Neck Surg. 2009; 140(6):826–833

[12] Alexander NS, Chaaban MR, Riley KO, Woodworth BA. Treatment strategies for lateral sphenoid sinus recess cerebrospinal fluid leaks. Arch Otolaryngol Head Neck Surg. 2012; 138(5):471–478

[13] Chaaban MR, Conger B, Riley KO, Woodworth BA. Transnasal endoscopic repair of posterior table fractures. Otolaryngol Head Neck Surg. 2012; 147(6):1142–1147

[14] Delaney SW. Treatment strategies for frontal sinus anterior table fractures and contour deformities. J Plast Reconstr Aesthet Surg. 2016; 69(8):1037–1045

[15] Pawar SS, Rhee JS. Frontal sinus and naso-orbital-ethmoid fractures. JAMA Facial Plast Surg. 2014; 16(4):284–289

[16] Rice DH. Management of frontal sinus fractures. Curr Opin Otolaryngol Head Neck Surg. 2004; 12(1):46–48

[17] Stanwix MG, Nam AJ, Manson PN, Mirvis S, Rodriguez ED. Critical computed tomographic diagnostic criteria for frontal sinus fractures. J Oral Maxillofac Surg. 2010; 68(11):2714–2722

[18] Strong EB, Pahlavan N, Saito D. Frontal sinus fractures: a 28-year retrospective review. Otolaryngol Head Neck Surg. 2006; 135(5):774–779

[19] Gossman DG, Archer SM, Arosarena O. Management of frontal sinus fractures: a review of 96 cases. Laryngoscope. 2006; 116(8):1357–1362

[20] Sataloff RT, Sariego J, Myers DL, Richter HJ. Surgical management of the frontal sinus. Neurosurgery. 1984; 15(4):593–596

[21] Zlab MK, Moore GF, Daly DT, Yonkers AJ. Cerebrospinal fluid rhinorrhea: a review of the literature. Ear Nose Throat J. 1992; 71(7):314–317

[22] Jones V, Virgin F, Riley K, Woodworth BA. Changing paradigms in frontal sinus cerebrospinal fluid leak repair. Int Forum Allergy Rhinol. 2012; 2(3):227–232

[23] Meetze K, Palmer JN, Schlosser RJ. Frontal sinus complications after frontal craniotomy. Laryngoscope. 2004; 114(5):945–948

[24] Harvey RJ, Parmar P, Sacks R, Zanation AM. Endoscopic skull base reconstruction of large dural defects: a systematic review of published evidence. Laryngoscope. 2012; 122(2):452–459

[25] Wolfe SA. The utility of pericranial flaps. Ann Plast Surg. 1978; 1 (2):147–153

[26] Price JC, Loury M, Carson B, Johns ME. The pericranial flap for reconstruction of anterior skull base defects. Laryngoscope. 1988; 98 (11):1159–1164

[27] Neligan PC, Mulholland S, Irish J, et al. Flap selection in cranial base reconstruction. Plast Reconstr Surg. 1996; 98(7):1159–1166, discussion 1167–1168

[28] Chaaban MR, Chaudhry A, Riley KO, Woodworth BA. Simultaneous pericranial and nasoseptal flap reconstruction of anterior skull base defects following endoscopic-assisted craniofacial resection. Laryngoscope. 2013; 123(10):2383–2386

[29] Eloy JA, Choudhry OJ, Christiano LD, Ajibade DV, Liu JK. Double flap technique for reconstruction of anterior skull base defects after craniofacial tumor resection: technical note. Int Forum Allergy Rhinol. 2013; 3(5):425–430

[30] Rahbar R, Resto VA, Robson CD, et al. Nasal glioma and encephalocele: diagnosis and management. Laryngoscope. 2003; 113(12):2069–2077

[31] Tirumandas M, Sharma A, Gbenimacho I, et al. Nasal encephaloceles: a review of etiology, pathophysiology, clinical presentations, diagnosis, treatment, and complications. Childs Nerv Syst. 2013; 29(5):739–744

[32] Hoving EW. Nasal encephaloceles. Childs Nerv Syst. 2000; 16(10–11):702–706

[33] Di Ieva A, Bruner E, Haider T, et al. Skull base embryology: a multidisciplinary review. Childs Nerv Syst. 2014; 30(6):991–1000

[34] Suwanwela C, Suwanwela N. A morphological classification of sincipital encephalomeningoceles. J Neurosurg. 1972; 36(2):201–211

[35] Suwanwela C, Hongsaprabhas C. Fronto-ethmoidal encephalomeningocele. J Neurosurg. 1966; 25(2):172–182

[36] Schlosser RJ, Woodworth BA, Wilensky EM, Grady MS, Bolger WE. Spontaneous cerebrospinal fluid leaks: a variant of benign intracranial hypertension. Ann Otol Rhinol Laryngol. 2006; 115(7):495–500

[37] Schick B, Ibing R, Brors D, Draf W. Long-term study of endonasal duraplasty and review of the literature. Ann Otol Rhinol Laryngol. 2001; 110(2):142–147

[38] Hubbard JL, McDonald TJ, Pearson BW, Laws ER, Jr. Spontaneous cerebrospinal fluid rhinorrhea: evolving concepts in diagnosis and surgical management based on the Mayo Clinic experience from 1970 through 1981. Neurosurgery. 1985; 16(3):314–321

[39] Gassner HG, Ponikau JU, Sherris DA, Kern EB. CSF rhinorrhea: 95 consecutive surgical cases with long term follow-up at the Mayo Clinic. Am J Rhinol. 1999; 13(6):439–447

[40] Chaaban MR, Illing E, Riley KO, Woodworth BA. Spontaneous cerebrospinal fluid leak repair: a five-year prospective evaluation. Laryngoscope. 2014; 124(1):70–75

[41] Adriani KS, van de Beek D, Brouwer MC, Spanjaard L, de Gans J. Community-acquired recurrent bacterial meningitis in adults. Clin Infect Dis. 2007; 45(5):e46–e51

[42] Tebruegge M, Curtis N. Epidemiology, etiology, pathogenesis, and diagnosis of recurrent bacterial meningitis. Clin Microbiol Rev. 2008; 21(3):519–537

[43] Verma N, Savy LE, Lund VJ, Cropley I, Chee R, Seneviratne SL. An important diagnosis to consider in recurrent meningitis. JRSM Short Rep. 2013; 4(9):2042533313486640

[44] Meco C, Oberascher G. Comprehensive algorithm for skull base dural lesion and cerebrospinal fluid fistula diagnosis. Laryngoscope. 2004; 114(6):991–999

[45] Schick B, Weber R, Kahle G, Draf W, Lackmann GM. Late manifestations of traumatic lesions of the anterior skull base. Skull Base Surg. 1997; 7(2):77–83

[46] Friedman JA, Ebersold MJ, Quast LM. Persistent posttraumatic cerebrospinal fluid leakage. Neurosurg Focus. 2000; 9(1):e1

[47] Ziu M, Savage JG, Jimenez DF. Diagnosis and treatment of cerebrospinal fluid rhinorrhea following accidental traumatic anterior skull base fractures. Neurosurg Focus. 2012; 32(6):E3

[48] Schlosser RJ, Bolger WE. Nasal cerebrospinal fluid leaks: critical review and surgical considerations. Laryngoscope. 2004; 114(2):255–265

[49] Bernal-Sprekelsen M, Bleda-Vázquez C, Carrau RL. Ascending meningitis secondary to traumatic cerebrospinal fluid leaks. Am J Rhinol. 2000; 14(4):257–259

[50] Oakley GM, Orlandi RR, Woodworth BA, Batra PS, Alt JA. Management of cerebrospinal fluid rhinorrhea: an evidence-based review with recommendations. Int Forum Allergy Rhinol. 2016; 6(1):17–24

[51] Psaltis AJ, Schlosser RJ, Banks CA, Yawn J, Soler ZM. A systematic review of the endoscopic repair of cerebrospinal fluid leaks. Otolaryngol Head Neck Surg. 2012; 147(2):196–203

[52] Bernal-Sprekelsen M, Alobid I, Mullol J, Trobat F, Tomás-Barberán M. Closure of cerebrospinal fluid leaks prevents ascending bacterial meningitis. Rhinology. 2005; 43(4):277–281

[53] Castelnuovo P, Bignami M, Pistochini A, Battaglia P, Locatelli D, Dallan I. Endoscopic endonasal management of encephaloceles in children: an eight-year experience. Int J Pediatr Otorhinolaryngol. 2009; 73 (8):1132–1136

[54] Kanowitz SJ, Bernstein JM. Pediatric meningoencephaloceles and nasal obstruction: a case for endoscopic repair. Int J Pediatr Otorhinolaryngol. 2006; 70(12):2087–2092

[55] Woodworth B, Schlosser RJ. Endoscopic repair of a congenital intranasal encephalocele in a 23 months old infant. Int J Pediatr Otorhinolaryngol. 2005; 69(7):1007–1009

[56] Kirchner FR, Proud GO. Method for the identification and localization of cerebrospinal fluid, rhinorrhea and otorrhea. Laryngoscope. 1960; 70:921–931

[57] Raza SM, Banu MA, Donaldson A, Patel KS, Anand VK, Schwartz TH. Sensitivity and specificity of intrathecal fluorescein and white light excitation for detecting intraoperative cerebrospinal fluid leak in endoscopic skull base surgery: a prospective study. J Neurosurg. 2016; 124(3):621–626

[58] Guimarães RE, Stamm AE, Giannetti AV, Crosara PF, Becker CG, Becker HM. Chemical and cytological analysis of cerebral spinal fluid after intrathecal injection of hypodense fluorescein. Rev Bras Otorrinolaringol (Engl Ed). 2015; 81(5):549–553

[59] Placantonakis DG, Tabaee A, Anand VK, Hiltzik D, Schwartz TH. Safety of low-dose intrathecal fluorescein in endoscopic cranial base surgery. Neurosurgery. 2007; 61(3) Suppl:161–165, discussion 165–166

[60] Tabaee A, Placantonakis DG, Schwartz TH, Anand VK. Intrathecal fluorescein in endoscopic skull base surgery. Otolaryngol Head Neck Surg. 2007; 137(2):316–320

[61] Seth R, Rajasekaran K, Benninger MS, Batra PS. The utility of intrathecal fluorescein in cerebrospinal fluid leak repair. Otolaryngol Head Neck Surg. 2010; 143(5):626–632

[62] Banu MA, Kim JH, Shin BJ, Woodworth GF, Anand VK, Schwartz TH. Low-dose intrathecal fluorescein and etiology-based graft choice in endoscopic endonasal closure of CSF leaks. Clin Neurol Neurosurg. 2014; 116:28–34

[63] Chin D, Snidvongs K, Kalish L, Sacks R, Harvey RJ. The outside-in approach to the modified endoscopic Lothrop procedure. Laryngoscope. 2012; 122(8):1661–1669

[64] Conger BT, Jr, Riley K, Woodworth BA. The Draf III mucosal grafting technique: a prospective study. Otolaryngol Head Neck Surg. 2012; 146(4):664–668

[65] Smith N, Riley KO, Woodworth BA. Endoscopic Coblator™-assisted management of encephaloceles. Laryngoscope. 2010; 120(12):2535–2539

[66] Illing E, Chaaban MR, Riley KO, Woodworth BA. Porcine small intestine submucosal graft for endoscopic skull base reconstruction. Int Forum Allergy Rhinol. 2013; 3(11):928–932

[67] Hadad G, Bassagasteguy L, Carrau RL, et al. A novel reconstructive technique after endoscopic expanded endonasal approaches: vascular pedicle nasoseptal flap. Laryngoscope. 2006; 116(10):1882–1886

[68] Virgin F, Barañano CF, Riley K, Woodworth BA. Frontal sinus skull base defect repair using the pedicled nasoseptal flap. Otolaryngol Head Neck Surg. 2011; 145(2):338–340

[69] Guggenheim P. Indications and methods for performance of osteoplastic-obliterative frontal sinusotomy with a description of a new method and some remarks upon the present state of the are of external frontal sinus surgery. Laryngoscope. 1981; 91(6):927–938

[70] Goodale RL, Montgomery WW. Technical advances in osteoplastic frontal sinusectomy. Arch Otolaryngol. 1964; 79:522–529

[71] Goodale RL, Montgomery WW. Anterior osteoplastic frontal sinus operation. Five years' experience. Ann Otol Rhinol Laryngol. 1961; 70:860–880

[72] Gerbino G, Roccia F, Benech A, Caldarelli C. Analysis of 158 frontal sinus fractures: current surgical management and complications. J Craniomaxillofac Surg. 2000; 28(3):133–139

[73] Adelson R, Wei C, Palmer JN. Atlas of Endoscopic and Sinonasal Skull Base Surgery. Philadelphia, PA: Elsevier; 2013:337–356

[74] Emara TA, Elnashar IS, Omara TA, Basha WM, Anany AM. Frontal sinus fractures with suspected outflow tract obstruction: a new approach for sinus preservation. J Craniomaxillofac Surg. 2015; 43(1):1–6

[75] Gonty AA, Marciani RD, Adornato DC. Management of frontal sinus fractures: a review of 33 cases. J Oral Maxillofac Surg. 1999; 57(4):372–379, discussion 380–381

[76] Dolan R. Facial plastic, reconstructive, and trauma surgery. New York, NY: Marcel Dekker; 2004

[77] Rodriguez ED, Stanwix MG, Nam AJ, et al. Twenty-six-year experience treating frontal sinus fractures: a novel algorithm based on anatomical fracture pattern and failure of conventional techniques. Plast Reconstr Surg. 2008; 122(6):1850–1866

[78] Poetker D, Smith TL. Endoscopic treatment of the frontal sinus outflow tract in frontal sinus trauma. Oper Tech Otolaryngol Head Neck Surg. 2006; 17(1):66–72

[79] Steiger JD, Chiu AG, Francis DO, Palmer JN. Endoscopic-assisted reduction of anterior table frontal sinus fractures. Laryngoscope. 2006; 116(10):1936–1939

[80] Archer JB, Sun H, Bonney PA, et al. Extensive traumatic anterior skull base fractures with cerebrospinal fluid leak: classification and repair techniques using combined vascularized tissue flaps. J Neurosurg. 2016; 124(3):647–656

[81] Illing EA, Cho Do Y, RIley KO, Woodworth BA. Draf III mucosal graft technique: long-term results. Int Forum Allergy Rhinol. 2016; 6(5):514–517

[82] Conger BT, Jr, Illing E, Bush B, Woodworth BA. Management of lateral frontal sinus pathology in the endoscopic era. Otolaryngol Head Neck Surg. 2014; 151(1):159–163

[83] Lauder A, Jalisi S, Spiegel J, Stram J, Devaiah A. Antibiotic prophylaxis in the management of complex midface and frontal sinus trauma. Laryngoscope. 2010; 120(10):1940–1945

[84] Rene C, Rose GE, Lenthall R, Moseley I. Major orbital complications of endoscopic sinus surgery. Br J Ophthalmol. 2001; 85(5):598–603

Section V

Controversial Topics in Current Practice

35 The Use of Flaps in Frontal Sinus
   Surgery   *268*

36 Osteitis and the Frontal Sinus   *275*

37 Extreme Lateral Lesions: What Is the
   Limit of Endoscopic Surgery?   *282*

38 Use of Image Guidance Technology:
   Mandatory or Not   *299*

39 Balloon Technology in the Frontal
   Sinus: Useful or Gimmick   *304*

40 Minimum versus Maximal Surgical
   Sinusotomy   *314*

41 Patient-Reported Outcome Measures
   and Outcomes in Frontal Sinus
   Surgery: Do They Make a Difference?   *320*

42 Symptoms of Frontal Sinus Disease:
   Where Is the Evidence?   *325*

43 Anatomy and Classification of
   Frontoethmoidal Cells   *333*

44 To Drill or Not to Drill   *340*

45 Indications for Operating the Frontal
   Sinus: Primary Surgery or Always
   Second Line?   *344*

46 Economic and Quality-of-Life
   Evaluation of Surgery and Medical
   Treatment for Chronic Rhinosinusitis   *351*

47 Training Models and Techniques in
   Frontal Sinus Surgery   *358*

48 Augmented Reality in Frontal Sinus
   Surgery   *363*

49 Robotic Surgery: Beyond DaVinci   *366*

50 Pathophysiology of the Failed
   Frontal Sinus and Its Implications for
   Medical Management   *371*

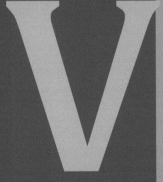

35 The Use of Flaps in Frontal Sinus Surgery

Nadim Khoueir and Philippe Herman

Abstract

The golden principle of endoscopic sinus surgery is mucosal preservation. Exposed bone is known to induce osteitis with secondary neo-osteogenesis, scarring, and stenosis. The main concern in frontal Draf IIb and III procedures is a significant rate of restenosis. Leaving extensive exposed bone after drilling is one of the major factors that contribute to postoperative failure. Since mucosa cannot be preserved during these procedures, local mucoperiosteal flaps are presented as an attractive alternative. Vascularized flaps are associated with fast re-epithelialization and integration with the underlying surface that might reduce the inflammatory stenotic process. The posterior-based nasoseptal and turbinoseptal flaps are harvested to cover the posterior wall of the cavity, while the lateral-based nasoseptal flap is used to cover the anterior wall. Two cadaver studies and two clinical reports show the feasibility of such flaps in a single or double fashion. The limited results of the clinical studies are promising with a reported low rate of postoperative failure. However, comparative studies in homogenous groups are needed in the future in order to have definite conclusion on the efficacy of local mucoperiosteal flaps in Draf IIb and III procedures.

Keywords: frontal sinus, frontal drilling, Draf IIb, Draf III, nasoseptal flap, septoturbinal flap

35.1 Published Evidence

35.1.1 Background

Frontal sinus surgery is still challenging despite advances in endoscopic approaches, instrumentations, and image guidance systems. This is because of the complex anatomy, the large anatomical variation of the frontal recess, and the location of the frontal recess behind the frontal beak.[1] Endoscopic surgery approach to the frontal sinus is based on the comprehensive classification that was proposed by Draf in 1992.[2] Variable outcome is reported in the literature based on surgery extent, surgeon experience, indications, and follow-up. This chapter aims to focus on mucosal flaps in endoscopic frontal surgery by exposing controversies regarding its potential added value and available techniques.

There are few papers selectively focused on end results of Draf IIb, possibly because most surgeons favor Draf III since it provides a wider view and a larger passage for instruments. In a personal series that was presented in 2007,[3] the rate of closure of the drainage pathway was significantly higher for Draf IIb as compared with Draf III,

38 versus 4% at 1-year follow-up, respectively. In 2012, Eloy et al[4] reported on a series of four cases with a modification of the Draf IIb designed to overcome the risk of drainage pathway stenosis by removing the interfrontal septum. This technique was also reported by Al Kadah and Schick[5]: all the patients maintained an air-filled frontal sinus, but with the closure of the nasal outflow in one case out of nine.

Long-term results of Draf III procedures, performed without the use of flaps, vary a lot in the literature. A short review of the evidence available during the last decade shows a rate of failure of 23% for Shirazi et al[6] in a series of 97 consecutive cases, of 10% in a series of 77 consecutive patients by Tran et al,[7] and of 14% in a systematic review reporting on 18 studies including 612 patients.[8] Risk factors for Draf III failure reported in the literature include ostium size at surgery,[7] AFS (allergic fungal rhinosinusitis),[9] recalcitrant *staphylococcus aureus* infection,[9] and EMCRS (eosinophilic mucin chronic rhinosinusitis).[10]

35.1.2 Rationale for Flaps

In Draf IIb and III procedures, extensive drilling results in exposed bone around the newly created ostium. In 2004, an animal study showed that drilling is associated with neo-osteogenesis and recess stenosis.[11] Exposed bone and subsequent neo-osteogenesis is believed to be a critical factor that contributes to closure of largely opened sinus.[12] When mucosa is not preserved, osteitic bone results from inflammation associated with healing. It also stimulates progressive osteoblastic activity with subsequent neo-osteogenesis and ostium narrowing.[13]

A number of strategies have been used to overcome this issue. Frontal sinus stenting with soft or firm material for different period of time showed variable success rate.[14] Application of topical treatment such as mitomycin C or steroids drops has been used with no significant effect.[15] Covering exposed bone with mucosal grafts was proposed in Draf III with promising results. Conger et al demonstrated a 100% success rate in 27 patients as defined by a reduction of ostium size not more than 50%.[16] Hildenbrand et al reported a 94% success rate in 24 patients using the same technique.[17] Another option recently reported is the use of local mucoperiosteal flaps to speed up mucosal healing and prevent scarring. Vascularized flaps are associated with fast re-epithelialization and integration with the underlying surface that might reduce osteitis, scarring, and neo-osteogenesis.[18] When mucosa cannot be preserved, these flaps could be used in order to overcome one of the major factors that contribute to ostium restenosis.

35.1.3 Literature Review and Surgical Techniques

Mucoperiosteal flaps in endoscopic frontal surgery were first described by Wormald in 2002 in a series of 64 patients with a success rate of 82%.[19] Local axillary flap was used in Draf IIa procedures in order to prevent the lateralization of the head of the middle turbinate. Technically, a superior incision is made approximately 8 mm above the axilla of the middle turbinate starting approximately 6 mm posterior to the axilla. This incision is continued vertically to the level of the axilla. The inferior incision runs around the axilla onto the middle turbinate and is continued for 2 mm posteriorly along the medial aspect of the middle turbinate. After flap elevation to its medial base, it is tucked between the middle turbinate and septum.[19]

The first description of mucosal flaps for Draf III procedures was reported at the 2012 meeting of the American Academy by DeConde et al in a cadaver study.[20] They described two flaps taken either from the medial aspect of the upper middle turbinate or from the area of the septal window in order to cover the posterior raw surface of the Draf III cavity. Later on, the first use of flaps in the living was reported by Seyedhadi et al,[21] who again aimed to cover the posterior wall of a Draf III procedure with a septal flap: results were satisfactory but included only four patients with a 3-month follow-up. The same concept has been developed for Draf IIb procedures, and a recent paper sampling patients from two separate institutions revealed an unexpected rate of success in 93% of the procedures with the help of a septoturbinal flap on a series of 46 patients.[22] Those early works were interesting but left the bone of the anterior wall of the Draf IIb and III drainage pathway uncovered, which might allow scarring and progressive stenosis. In order to cover the whole exposed bone, AlQahtani et al[18] designed and performed on cadavers a double flap to cover both the posterior and the anterior walls of the Draf III drainage pathway. They advised elevating a posteriorly based nasoseptal flap on one side and a laterally based nasoseptal flap on the other side and demonstrated the possibility to cover all the exposed bone. For the posteriorly based flap, the posterior incision starts at the septum 1 cm posterior to the anterior edge of the middle turbinate down to the level of its inferior limit. The incision is directed forward to a level parallel to the maxillary line and then backward and upward to a level parallel to the middle turbinate axilla. At this point, an inverted U-shaped incision is directed to the axilla laterally (▶ Fig. 35.1). Careful subperiosteal dissection is carried out posteriorly until reaching the first olfactory fiber to facilitate mobilization of the flap. The laterally based flap will be described later. Those flaps are obviously vascularized flaps, although pedicles might be difficult to define, since the septal branch of the anterior ethmoidal artery is usually cut during the dissection of

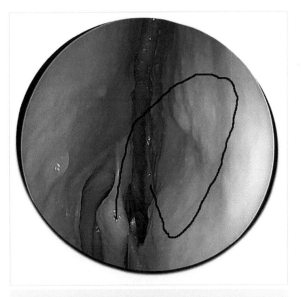

Fig. 35.1 The dark line shows the incision limits of the posterior-based nasoseptal flap.

the floor of the frontal sinus just ahead of the first olfactory filet, while the lateral based flap might be supplied by branches of the facial artery.

We performed a dissection in order to experiment the design of the septoturbinal and lateral-based nasoseptal flaps, shown in ▶ Fig. 35.2 and ▶ Fig. 35.3. In ▶ Fig. 35.2, which is a left side, the dotted line shows the design of a posteriorly based septoturbinal flap. An inverted U-shaped incision is made from the leading edge of the middle turbinate, across the axilla of the middle turbinate, following the lacrimal bone onto the roof of the nasal cavity and down to the septum where the incision should be bent backward to allow the rotation of the flap. Then the septoturbinal flap is harvested from the incision posteriorly until the first olfactory fiber is reached, that is, after transection of the most anterior branch of the anterior ethmoidal artery, and stored in the olfactory cleft. It will be unfolded in the end of the procedure to cover the posterior wall. ▶ Fig. 35.3 presents the drawing of the incision for a lateral-based nasoseptal flap. Notice that the landmarks are more difficult to understand in a complex 3D anatomy. The easiest way is to identify the most anterior part of the olfactory cleft under the nasion anteriorly, and the upper projection in the olfactory cleft of the axilla of the middle turbinate posteriorly: this defines the width of the pedicle of the flap. Medially, two vertical lines are drawn on 2 cm to delineate the septal portion of the flap, while laterally the flap needs to be freed until the dorsum of the inferior turbinate following posteriorly the so-called maxillary line, just posterior to the uncinated process, and anteriorly a parallel line at a distance defined by the width of the pedicle. In the end of the procedure, this flap will be slightly twisted to cover

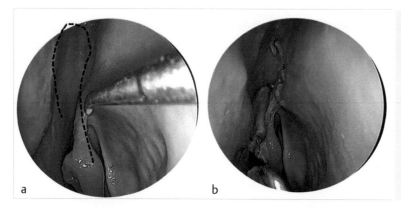

Fig. 35.2 Septoturbinal flap elevation. **(a)** The dotted line shows the incision limits. **(b)** The flap is elevated until reaching the first olfactory fiber and stored in the olfactory cleft.

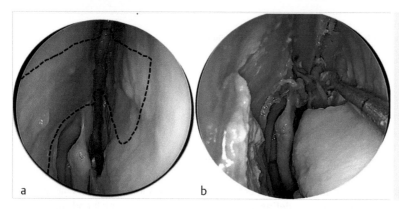

Fig. 35.3 Lateral-based septoturbinal flap elevation. **(a)** The dotted line shows the incision limits. Note that the septal portion does not overlap with the septoturbinal flap. **(b)** The flap is elevated and based on the lateral nasal wall just superior to the head of the inferior turbinate.

the anterior wall of the Draf cavity. Looking at ▶ Fig. 35.2 and ▶ Fig. 35.3, it can be clearly seen that the two flaps do not overlap, which allows raising both flaps on the same side. This differs from the flaps described by AlQahtani et al[18] that do overlap and cannot be used hypothetically as double flaps in a unilateral Draf IIb procedure. Technical aspects regarding these flaps are elicited in ▶ Table 35.1.

35.2 Controversies and Opinions

35.2.1 Promising Outcome for Flaps

The available literature is limited to two cadaveric studies[18,20] and two clinical series[21,22] that mainly show on one hand the feasibility of local mucoperiosteal flaps in Draf IIb and III procedures where these pedicled flaps can be harvested to cover the exposed bone without compromising their vascularization. On the other hand, the results of the clinical studies[21,22] are promising although they cover a limited number of patients. Achieving good results with flaps could be expected since it is designed to suppress one of the major factors implicated in ostium restenosis: exposed bone with subsequent osteitis, scarring, and neo-osteogenesis. This concept is not new to endoscopic sinus surgery that has evolved into a mucosa preservation approach in order to avoid exposed bone and optimize healing. Preserving the mucosa by using

through-cutting instruments and powered microdebriders is considered the gold standard resulting in improved surgical outcomes.[23,24] Since mucosa cannot be preserved in Draf IIb and III procedures, it will be replaced by using these local mucoperiosteal flaps.

35.2.2 Recommendation for Future Studies

However, these studies are insufficient to show the superiority of using the flaps in Draf IIb and III procedures. Further randomized controlled studies are needed in order to reach definite conclusions. Clinical case series often mix patients with frontal disease of various etiologies: benign tumors like osteoma or inverted papilloma, inflammatory diseases that may have very different prognosis and are most of the time ranked as chronic rhinosinusitis with or without polyposis, without any reference to Samter or cystic fibrosis disease. This mixture of different pathologies may seriously flaw comparative studies that should include homogeneous subgroups.

Review of the literature reveals different outcome selection when defining failure and success of Draf III procedures. Failure is considered by some authors a completely blocked ostium based on follow-up endoscopies.[12,25,26] Others defined it as more than 50[1,27] or 60%[9] reduction in the section surface area of the recess compared to that at the end of the surgery. Schlosser et al classified the ostium

Table 35.1 Special considerations for local mucoperiosteal flaps in frontal sinus surgery

	Difficulty points	Technical hints
Septoturbinal flap	Difficulty to raise the flap from the middle turbinate	Keep the turbinate steady (no luxation) for dissection
	Injury of the flap with the drill	Store in the olfactory cleft
	Would not conform to the posterior wall	Bend the inferior incision of the septum backward
	Reduced exposure of the frontal sinus floor	Do not hesitate to cut the septal branch of the anterior ethmoidal artery
Posterior-based nasoseptal flap	Injury of the flap with the drill	Store in the olfactory cleft
	Reduced exposure of the frontal sinus floor	Do not hesitate to cut the septal branch of the anterior ethmoidal artery
	Overlaps with lateral-based flap	Contralateral elevation
Lateral-based nasoseptal flap	Narrow pedicle	Roof of nasal fossa should be incised at the nasion anteriorly and upon the axilla posteriorly
	Obscures vision upward	Flap should be elevated up to the roof of the inferior turbinate
	Impairs entry in the nasal fossa	Endoscopic septoplasty should be performed on demand to enlarge access and vision

into patent, stenotic, or closed based on the ability to incorporate a 3-mm suction tip into the cavity.[28] Anderson and Sindwani in a systematic review of Draf III procedure classified failure as the need for any revision surgery on the frontal sinus.[8] This heterogeneity in outcome definition makes it difficult to compare the results of different series and obviates the need to conduct comparative studies using the same outcome for both groups.

35.2.3 Flaps Feasibility

In our institution, we have been using septoturbinal flaps to cover the posterior border of Draf IIb and III cavities for the last 4 years. We participated with another institution to publish a series of 46 consecutive patients undergoing Draf IIb and septoturbinal flap with a success rate of 93%.[22] For the last 2 years, we have adopted a double-flap approach by adding a lateral-based septoturbinal flap to also cover the anterior border of Draf IIb and III cavities. Our clinical experience looks promising based on the improved healing process during the postoperative period. However, we noted some rare critical situations where flap usage is compromised:

- Distorted anatomy in previously operated patients especially in the case of wide septal window, extensive fibrosis, and middle turbinectomy. In the Draf IIb series, 2 out of 48 patients were excluded because of difficult distorted anatomy and inability to raise the flap.[22]
- Unhealthy mucosa in patients having a severe diffuse polyposis.

- Small anteroposterior diameter limiting the usage of double flaps that may obstruct the lumen of the cavity.
- Narrow roof limiting the space to perform inverted U incision in lateral-based nasoseptal flap.

35.2.4 Illustrative Cases

Case 1: Single Flap in Draf IIB

A 77-year-old man presented with frontal headache, mild anterior rhinorrhea, and purulent discharge from a fistula at the level of the nasion. A sinus CT showed a left pansinusitis of dental origin with a left frontal pyocele that eroded the anterior wall of the left frontal sinus and the interfrontal septum (▶ Fig. 35.4). A complete left endoscopic sinus surgery was performed under general anesthesia with extraction of teeth numbers 15 and 16. A left Draf IIb procedure allowed drainage of the left frontal pyocele. A septoturbinal flap was elevated to cover the posterior edge of the cavity. The flap was secured with a silicone roll that was removed at 3 weeks. The fistula healed spontaneously and the patient remained asymptomatic at 2-year follow-up. ▶ Fig. 35.5 shows a patent left Draf IIb cavity at 2 years with evidence of a well-integrated posterior flap.

Case 2: Double Flaps in Draf IIC

A 48-year-old woman was referred to our department for a right frontal sinusitis caused by obstructive frontoethmoidal osteoma. A right anterior ethmoidectomy and

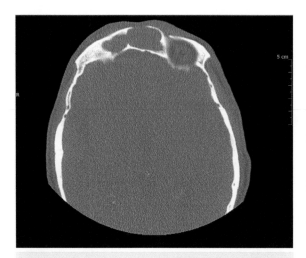

Fig. 35.4 Case 1: Axial sinus CT scan showing a right frontal pyocele with erosion of the anterior table.

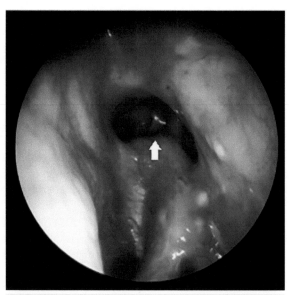

Fig. 35.5 Case 1: Nasal endoscopy at 2-year follow-up revealing a patent right Draf IIb cavity. We can see the septoturbinal flap that is well integrated on the posterior edge (*white arrow*).

Draf IIc were performed under general anesthesia in order to expose and remove the osteoma with subsequent drainage of the frontal sinus. A septoturbinal flap and a lateral-based nasoseptal flap were harvested from the right side to cover the posterior and anterior edges of the Draf IIc cavity, respectively. The flaps were secured with a silicone roll that was removed at 3 weeks. At 6-month follow-up, nasal endoscopy showed a patent cavity with well-integrated anterior and posterior flaps (▶ Fig. 35.6).

Case 3: Double Flaps in Draf III

A 38-year-old man with a history of AERD (aspirin exacerbated respiratory disease) underwent several years ago a bilateral endoscopic sinus surgery with extensive mucosal stripping. He was referred for recurrent rhinosinusitis with extensive scarring and multiple mucoceles in the right sphenoid sinus, right Onodi cell, and left frontal sinus. A revision endoscopic sinus surgery was performed under general anesthesia with Draf III procedure allowing drainage of the mucocele. A left septoturbinal flap and right lateral-based nasoseptal flap were elevated to cover the posterior and anterior edge of the Draf III cavity, respectively. The flaps were secured with a silicone roll that was removed at 3 weeks. At 1-year follow-up, the patient was asymptomatic treated with budesonide sinus rinse. Nasal endoscopy showed a patent Draf III cavity with well-integrated flaps while the thickening of the diseased mucosa is obvious (▶ Fig. 35.7).

Case 4: Difficult Flap Elevation

A 65-year-old woman presented with a right orbital cellulitis and frontal headache. A sinus CT revealed a right

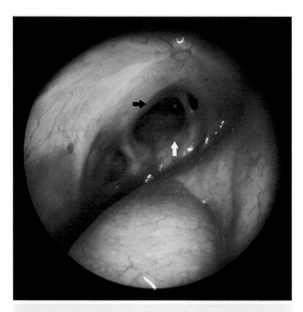

Fig. 35.6 Case 2: nasal endoscopy at 6-month follow-up revealing a patent right Draf IIc cavity. Unilateral double flaps were elevated: a septoturbinal flap (*white arrow*) covering the posterior edge and a lateral-based nasoseptal flap covering the anterior edge (*black arrow*).

frontal pyocele with erosion of the posterior wall of the frontal sinus and the right orbital roof. The frontal recess was obstructed by a type 4 frontal cell (▶ Fig. 35.8). A Draf

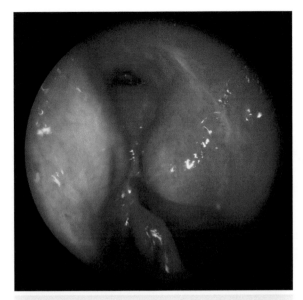

Fig. 35.7 Case 3: Nasal endoscopy at 1-year follow-up revealing a patent right Draf III cavity. A septoturbinal flap and a lateral-based nasoseptal flap were used to cover the Draf III cavity edges. We can see that the flaps are thick probably related to a diseased mucosa in AERD (aspirin-exacerbated respiratory disease).

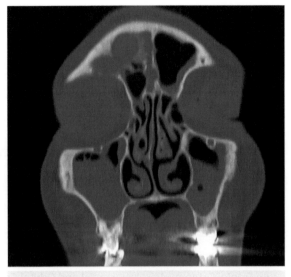

Fig. 35.8 Case 4: Coronal sinus CT shows a right frontal pyocele and a type 4 frontal cell with erosion of the orbital roof.

- Are bilateral flaps better than ipsilateral flaps?
- Are flaps efficient in all indications of Draf IIb and III?
- Are flaps superior to mucosal grafts?

IIc procedure was performed under general anesthesia, allowing the opening of the type 4 frontal cell with drainage of the frontal pyocele. Elevation of the right lateral-based nasoseptal flap was compromised because of a narrow roof making the inverted **U** incision impossible. The flap was sacrificed and a single septoturbinal flap was elevated to cover the posterior wall of the cavity.

35.3 Surgical Tips

- Raise the flap at the beginning of the surgery.
- Store the lateral flap at the level of the inferior turbinate and posterior flap in the olfactory cleft to avoid damage during drilling.
- Available studies show the cadaveric and clinical feasibility of local mucoperiosteal flaps in Draf IIb and III procedures.
- Rare clinical situations where flap usage is compromised.
- Promising results in limited clinical studies with low level of evidence.
- Need for randomized controlled studies in homogenous group to compare the outcome of Draf IIB and III with and without flaps.

35.4 Unanswered Questions

- Do local mucoperiosteal flaps improve the outcome of Draf IIb and III procedures?
- Are double flaps superior to single flaps?

References

[1] Wormald PJ. Salvage frontal sinus surgery: the endoscopic modified Lothrop procedure. Laryngoscope. 2003; 113(2):276–283

[2] Draf W. Endonasal micro-endoscopic frontal sinus surgery: the Fulda concept. Oper Tech Otolaryngol Head Neck Surg. 1991; 2:234–240

[3] Sauvaget E, El Bakkouri W, Bayonne E, Kania R, Tran Ba Huy P, Herman P. Long-term outcome of the frontal sinus surgery using Draf procedure. 6th European Congress of Oto-Rhino-Laryngology Head and Neck Surgery (EUFOS). July 2007

[4] Eloy JA, Friedel ME, Kuperan AB, Govindaraj S, Folbe AJ, Liu JK. Modified mini-Lothrop/extended Draf IIB procedure for contralateral frontal sinus disease: a case series. Int Forum Allergy Rhinol. 2012; 2 (4):321–324

[5] Al Kadah B, Schick B. Endonasal modification of the frontal sinus drainage type IIb according to Draf. Eur Arch Otorhinolaryngol. 2015; 272(8):1961–1965

[6] Shirazi MA, Silver AL, Stankiewicz JA. Surgical outcomes following the endoscopic modified Lothrop procedure. Laryngoscope. 2007; 117(5):765–769

[7] Tran KN, Beule AG, Singal D, Wormald P-J. Frontal ostium restenosis after the endoscopic modified Lothrop procedure. Laryngoscope. 2007; 117(8):1457–1462

[8] Anderson P, Sindwani R. Safety and efficacy of the endoscopic modified Lothrop procedure: a systematic review and meta-analysis. Laryngoscope. 2009; 119(9):1828–1833

[9] Naidoo Y, Bassiouni A, Keen M, Wormald PJ. Long-term outcomes for the endoscopic modified Lothrop/Draf III procedure: a 10-year review. Laryngoscope. 2014; 124(1):43–49

[10] Khong JJ, Malhotra R, Selva D, Wormald PJ. Efficacy of endoscopic sinus surgery for paranasal sinus mucocele including modified endoscopic Lothrop procedure for frontal sinus mucocele. J Laryngol Otol. 2004; 118(5):352–356

[11] Rajapaksa SP, Ananda A, Cain TM, Oates L, Wormald PJ. Frontal ostium neo-osteogenesis and restenosis after modified endoscopic Lothrop procedure in an animal model. Clin Otolaryngol Allied Sci. 2004; 29 (4):386–388

[12] Gross CW, Schlosser RJ. The modified Lothrop procedure: lessons learned. Laryngoscope. 2001; 111(7):1302–1305

[13] Lee JT, Kennedy DW, Palmer JN, Feldman M, Chiu AG. The incidence of concurrent osteitis in patients with chronic rhinosinusitis: a clinicopathological study. Am J Rhinol. 2006; 20(3):278–282

[14] Rains BM, III. Frontal sinus stenting. Otolaryngol Clin North Am. 2001; 34(1):101–110

[15] Chan KO, Gervais M, Tsaparas Y, Genoway KA, Manarey C, Javer AR. Effectiveness of intraoperative mitomycin C in maintaining the patency of a frontal sinusotomy: a preliminary report of a double-blind randomized placebo-controlled trial. Am J Rhinol. 2006; 20 (3):295–299

[16] Conger BT, Jr, Riley K, Woodworth BA. The Draf III mucosal grafting technique: a prospective study. Otolaryngol Head Neck Surg. 2012; 146(4):664–668

[17] Hildenbrand T, Wormald PJ, Weber RK. Endoscopic frontal sinus drainage Draf type III with mucosal transplants. Am J Rhinol Allergy. 2012; 26(2):148–151

[18] AlQahtani A, Bignami M, Terranova P, et al. Newly designed double-vascularized nasoseptal flap to prevent restenosis after endoscopic modified Lothrop procedure (Draf III): laboratory investigation. Eur Arch Otorhinolaryngol. 2014; 271(11):2951–2955

[19] Wormald PJ. The axillary flap approach to the frontal recess. Laryngoscope. 2002; 112(3):494–499

[20] DeConde AS, Vorasubin N, Thompson CF, Suh JD. Rotation flaps after Draf procedure: a cadaver study. Otolaryngol Head Neck Surg. 2012; 147(2) s uppl:255–259

[21] Seyedhadi S, Mojtaba MA, Shahin B, Hoseinali K. The Draf III septal flap technique: a preliminary report. Am J Otolaryngol. 2013; 34 (5):399–402

[22] Fiorini FR, Nogueira C, Verillaud B, Sama A, Herman P. Value of septo-turbinal flap in the frontal sinus drill-out type IIb according to draf. Laryngoscope. 2016; 126(11):2428–2432

[23] Levine HL. Endoscopic sinus surgery: reasons for failure. Oper Tech Otolaryngol–Head Neck Surg. 1995; 6:176–179

[24] Kennedy DW, Senior BA. Endoscopic sinus surgery: a review. Prim Care. 1998; 25(3):703–720

[25] Weber R, Draf W, Kratzsch B, Hosemann W, Schaefer SD. Modern concepts of frontal sinus surgery. Laryngoscope. 2001; 111(1):137–146

[26] Metson R, Gliklich RE. Clinical outcome of endoscopic surgery for frontal sinusitis. Arch Otolaryngol Head Neck Surg. 1998; 124 (10):1090–1096

[27] Dubin MG, Kuhn FA. Endoscopic modified Lothrop (Draf III) with frontal sinus punches. Laryngoscope. 2005; 115(9):1702–1703

[28] Schlosser RJ, Zachmann G, Harrison S, Gross CW. The endoscopic modified Lothrop: long-term follow-up on 44 patients. Am J Rhinol. 2002; 16(2):103–108

36 Osteitis and the Frontal Sinus

Christos Georgalas

Abstract

There is increased recognition of the high prevalence of osteitic changes affecting the bony framework of the frontal sinuses in patients with frontal chronic rhinosinusitis (CRS) with or without nasal polyps. However, their assessment, clinical significance, and optimal management remain controversial. A number of studies have confirmed that there is a clear correlation between radiological and endoscopic CRS burden, as measured with Lund–Mckay computed tomography and endoscopic grading system and osteitis. However, there is little or no correlation between symptom severity and osteitis, with no evidence of worse quality of life (QOL) or more nasal symptoms or headache in such patients. The number of previous surgeries appears to be closely correlated with the extent of sinusitis, although it is not clear if that is a direct or a secondary association. Global Osteitis Scoring Scale (GOSS) is a novel validated composite grading system—measuring the extent and severity of osteitis. There is no or limited role for antibiotics or steroids, and, just as for biofilms, radical surgical removal of osteitic bone may be the only solution available for end-stage disease.

36.1 Introduction

There is a subgroup of patients with frontal sinusitis whose symptoms persist despite maximal medical and surgical management. These patients with "difficult-to-treat rhinosinusitis," as defined in the new European Position Paper on Chronic Rhinosinusitis and Nasal Polyps,[1] often have areas of bony thickening and remodeling within their frontal sinuses. Such areas have been alternatively described as osteitis, ostitis, or (neo)osteogenesis. The presence of such areas in the frontal sinus presents diagnostic and treatment challenges for the surgeon, and its optimal management remains unknown.

36.2 Epidemiology and Etiology

36.2.1 Definitions

Terms that describe inflammation of the sinonasal bony framework associated with radiologically visible abnormities include "osteitis," "osteomyelitis," "hyperostosis," "bone hyperplasia," "bone remodeling," and "neo-osteogenesis." As there is no marrow space ("myelos") in the flat bones around the sinus, we feel that the term osteomyelitis is not appropriate. Equally, while hyperostosis and neo-osteogenesis are often present, they are not always the main or even the predominant feature. In this review, we will be using the term **osteitis** in order to describe the bony changes associated with chronic inflammation in patients with chronic rhinosinusitis (CRS) with nasal polyposis (CRSwNP) and CRS without nasal polyposis (CRSsNP).

36.2.2 Histology: Pathophysiology

A number of animal studies[2,3,4,5,6] have demonstrated a link between experimentally induced rhinosinusitis and chronic inflammation of the bony middle turbinate as well as the ethmoid and maxillary sinus bony walls.

Four early human studies focused on the pathological findings of bony inflammation in patients with CRS. Kennedy et al[7] used radiolabelled tetracycline to assess bone remodeling of the ethmoid sinus and demonstrated higher bone activity with increased bone resorption and marked neo-osteogenesis in sinusitis patients compared with normal controls. Pathologically, this corresponded to new bone formation, fibrosis, and the presence of inflammatory cells. Similar results were found by Giacchi et al,[8] who also assessed the bone of ethmoid sinus of CRS patients and compared it with control patients undergoing a cerebrospinal fluid leak repair. He found periosteal thickening and increased osteoblastic–osteoclastic activity, disruption of organized lamellar bone, and formation of immature woven bone. Interestingly, the extent of bony remodeling was found to correlate with radiologically defined disease severity, with more advanced bony changes associated with higher Lund–Mackay (L-M) scores on CT. Histological samples of patients with rhinosinusitis were also analyzed by Lee et al,[9] who found pathological evidence of osteitis in 53% of their samples, ranging from 6.7% in those undergoing primary surgery to 58% in patients having revision endoscopic sinus surgery (ESS). He also showed new bone formation in patients with CRS, with increased osteoid production and osteoblastic activity. Finally, Cho et al[10] showed thickening of the periosteum and osteoblastic–osteoclastic activity in patients with CRS.

It is fair to say that what these studies demonstrated is that patients with chronic sinusitis tend to have new bone formation, fibrosis, inflammatory cell infiltration, periosteal thickening, and a varying degree of increased osteoblastic–osteoclastic activity, as shown by the disruption of organized lamellar bone and formation of immature woven bone. Patients with a history of an acute frontal sinusitis, complicated, for example, by Pott's puffy tumor or frontocutaneous fistula, may show relatively early osteitic changes, suggesting that the presence of purulence may be a triggering factor (▶ Fig. 36.1, ▶ Fig. 36.2).

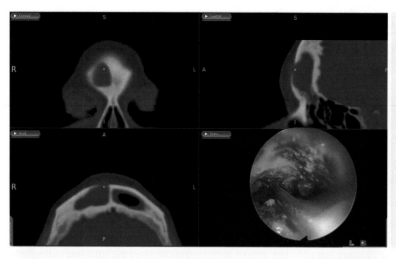

Fig. 36.1 Intraoperative navigation image of a female patient with a 2-year history of frontal sinusitis with headache who has had a middle meatal antrostomy a year ago and presented with a 1-month history of frontal swelling (Pott's puffy tumor). Note the anterior frontal plate defect and the prominent osteitis especially on the right frontal recess.

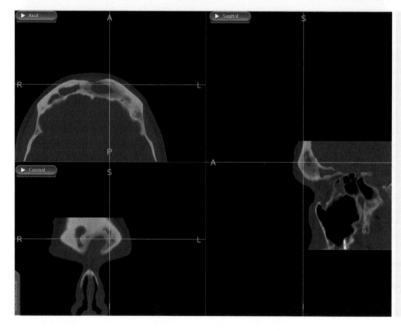

Fig. 36.2 Intraoperative navigation image of a male patient with history of chronic frontal sinusitis, operated twice and who presents with a frontocutaneous fistula. Note the extensive presence of osteitis

However, as surgeons we often come across patients with minimal or no history of inflammation of the sinus who have extensive osteitis in the frontal sinus. In such patients, the presence of osteitis is difficult to reconcile with the above pathophysiology—suggesting that other mechanisms may be at play. In patients where permanent drains have been placed through the frontal sinus (often from a previous era when that was commonplace), the presence of severe osteitic changes surrounding the semi-ossified and blocked drain is a constant finding.

36.2.3 Allergy

A number of studies have shown an association between osteitis and tissue and serum eosinophilia.[11,12,13] However, in patients with frontal sinusitis undergoing Draf III, this has not been shown to be the case. A study specifically measuring osteitis after Draf III[14] demonstrated that the presence of osteitis preoperatively was the single stronger predictive factor of neo-osteogenesis after surgery, with no correlation with allergy or eosinophilia.

36.2.4 Bacteriology

This chronic low-grade inflammation does not seem to be associated with direct bacterial invasion, as no group until now has been able to demonstrate bacteria in the bone. Rather, it seems to both be stimulated by and act as a "depot" of inflammatory cytokines,[15,16] which ensure the persistence of disease, even when the mucosa is either treated medically or removed. It is not unusual to see extensive areas of osteitis in the frontal sinus, especially around the frontal recess, following the resolution of an acute frontal sinusitis—often frustrating any attempts at surgery and delaying resolution or even resulting in chronicity. Acute frontal sinusitis especially with Pott's puffy tumor is a typical example (▶ Fig. 36.1). Such cases demonstrate that an acute bacterial infection may trigger a long-term process associated with bony resorption and remodelling in the frontal sinus.

36.2.5 Biofilms

Like osteitis, the presence of biofilms represents an end stage of chronic inflammation. Biofilm serves as a reservoir for bacteria and is associated with eosinophilic inflammation, which has been shown to be correlated with osteitis.[12] A number of studies, with more prominent that of Dong et al,[17] have demonstrated that and ever more relevantly showed that the volume of biofilms correlated with the severity of osteitis as measured with the Global Osteitis Scoring Scale (GOSS).

36.2.6 Incidence

Studies using CT, using various criteria to define osteitis, showed that the incidence of radiological changes in patients with CRS ranged between 4%,[18] 36%,[9] and 40%.[19] Both the study by Lee et al and the study by Richtsmeier et al found an increased incidence of osteitis in patients with higher L-M score, while another study found a greater incidence in patients undergoing revision surgery. Using the GOSS, we found that the incidence of osteitis was 33% in a nonoperated CRS group compared to 75% in the operated CRS group ($p < 0.001$).[19] Interestingly, there was an almost linear relation between the mean Global Osteitis Score and the number of previous surgeries, rising from 1.6 in patients with no previous surgeries to 3.6

in patients who had undergone one sinus procedure to 15.5 in patients with two previous operations to 31.5 in patients with more than six previous sinus surgeries ($p < 0.001$; ▶ Fig. 36.3) However, and although such a strong and linear association strongly suggests causation, there is always the possibility that it is a secondary association, with surgery acting as a proxy marker of more severe, resistant disease.

36.3 Clinical Presentation and Investigations

36.3.1 Radiological Features

Radiology is, for the vast majority of patients, the diagnostic modality of choice.

Radiological Features in CT

In most studies, and certainly in current clinical practice, CT scan is the modality of choice in order to evaluate the presence and extent of osteitis in patients with CRS. Hence, osteitis is, almost always, a radiological diagnosis, confirmed occasionally with pathological specimens taken during surgery. Radiological as well as clinical features can help, in most cases, to differentiate CRS osteitis from other bone diseases such as Paget's disease or metabolic bone disease, as well as fibrous dysplasia (▶ Fig. 36.4). In the case of patients with CRSwNP or CRSsNP, it is important to record the presence and the extent of osteitic changes. To such effect, a composite grading system has been devised (GOSS) that assesses bone thickness, the extent of involvement for each sinus, and the number of sinuses involved.[19] Osteitis is defined as loss of bone definition/hyperostosis/new bone

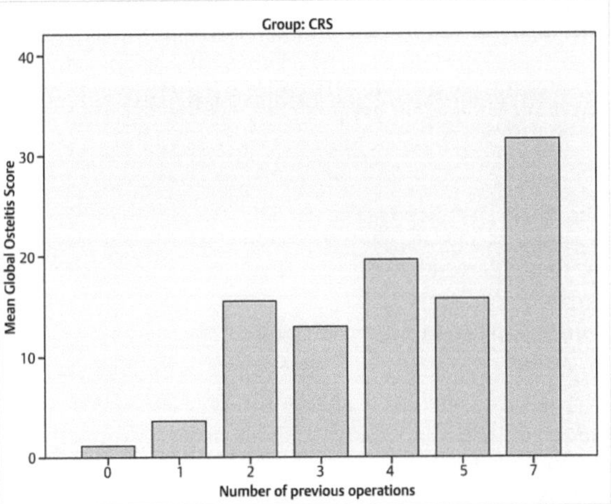

Fig. 36.3 Correlation between number of previous sinus procedures and GOSS (Global Osteitis Scoring Scale) osteitis score. (Adapted from Georgalas et al.[19])

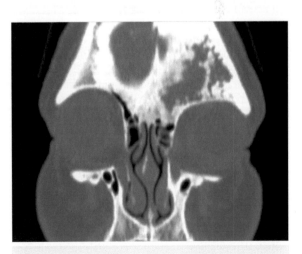

Fig. 36.4 Fibrous dysplasia in the left frontal sinus of a young male patient.

formation or signal heterogeneity. The area of maximal thickness of each osteitic focus is measured.

The scoring per sinus is as follows:

- *Grade 1*: Less than 50% of the sinus walls involved AND osteitis less than 3-mm wide.
- *Grade 2*: Less than 50% of the sinus walls involved AND 3 to 5 mm wide.
- *Grade 3*: Less than 50% of the sinus walls involved AND wider than 5 mm OR more than 50% of the sinus wall involved AND less than 3-mm-wide osteitic changes.
- *Grade 4*: More than 50% of the sinus wall involved AND 3 to 5 mm wide.
- *Grade 5*: More than 50% of the sinus wall AND thicker than 5 mm.

In this way, each sinus is given a grading ranging from 0 to 5. The scores of all 10 sinuses (right and left frontal, anterior ethmoid, posterior ethmoid, maxillary, and sphenoid) are added, producing a composite score (range: 0–50). We have shown that grading using this scale is easy to perform (usually 2–3 minutes per patient) and gives reproducible results. We found that inter-rater variability was low, and the agreement between different assessors, using intraclass correlation coefficient, was excellent (0.947). The best agreement was found for the maxillary sinuses and the lowest for the ethmoids. Using this grading scale, an almost linear correlation between L-M score and GOS was demonstrated.[19]

Radiological Features on SPECT

Bone scintigraphy is considered the method of reference for the diagnosis of bone inflammation, although it is used rarely in everyday clinical practice. Two studies have assessed CRS patients with single-photon emission computed tomography (SPECT) scans: In the first study, 36 patients awaiting surgery for CRS underwent SPECT with technetium-99 m methylene diphosphonate. Thirty-two of 36 patients were positive (increased uptake in the ethmoid sinus), and this result was confirmed with pathological findings in 31 (bone changes from lamellar to woven in the face of the bulla).[20]

Another study showed that 19 out of 24 patients with CRS had positive bone scintigraphy, with more positive results in patients with radiologically more extensive sinusitis.[21] However, SPECT is much more costly and exposes the patient to much higher doses of radiation than CT; hence, it is almost never used in the clinical practice for the diagnosis and grading of osteitis.

36.3.2 Clinical Implications

Although one would expect osteitis to be associated with more severe symptoms, this has not been shown. In our study,[19] there was no correlation between nasal RSOM (rhinosinusitis outcome measure) scores and the presence of osteitis. Specifically, using VAS (Visual Analog Scale) to assess headache, there was no correlation between osteitis severity and headache.[19]

Similar results were found in a subsequent study from the United States, which used the RSDI (Rhinosinusitis Disability Index) and CSS (Chronic Sinusitis Survey) patient-reported outcome measures to assess patients with CRS and osteitis and failed to show any worse baseline QOL scores in patients with osteitis.[22]

Disease burden (radiologically and endoscopically defined disease severity): Unlike subjective symptoms, radiologically defined abnormalities are more extensive in sinusitis patients with osteitis. Both L-M scores and endoscopic scores have been shown to be correlated with osteitis, in a number of studies.[19] Many studies[9,19,23] have confirmed the link between revision surgery and duration of symptoms with osteitis, although it remains unclear if this is a primary or secondary association (underlying disease severity being the common factor). However, it is clear that the burden of disease is highly correlated with the presence and extent of osteitis.

36.3.3 Prognostic Factor

It appears that osteitis is an independent negative prognostic factor after ESS for CRS, in terms of both endoscopic grading of the outcome and QOL improvement after ESS.[22] A number of studies have shown that patients with osteitis are at a higher risk of revision surgery, both generally[23] and specifically, revision surgery in the frontal sinus, in the form of revision Draf III.[14] Specifically, the study by Ye et al showed that the single most important factor associated with neo-ostium stenosis after Draf III was the presence preoperatively of neo-osteogenesis (osteitis) as measured by the GOSS. That study, which assessed 25 patients undergoing Draf III at least 12 months postoperatively, showed that while asthma, eosinophil count, L-M score, or previous surgery were not correlated with neo-ostium stenosis, the preoperative Global Osteitis Score was negatively associated with the cross-sectional area of neo-ostium a year after surgery, as measured by CT.

36.4 Management

The management of osteitic bone in patients with CRS remains controversial.

Antibiotics (oral and intravenous): The use of long-term antibiotics, especially macrolides, has been advocated in CRS, not only (or even primarily) for their antibacterial properties but also in view of their direct anti-inflammatory action.[24,25] However, a recent large randomized multicenter trial has put doubts on it,[26] which is also reflected in the 2012 European Position Paper on Rhinosinusitis Guidelines[1] and even more forcefully in the recent ICARS guidelines.[27] Unfortunately, the evidence of long-term antibiotics in osteitis is even more scarce. Its advocates use the example of long bone osteomyelitis to suggest that intravenous administration of antibiotics can produce high enough levels in the bone to clear an infection.[28,29] However, both studies suffer from methodological problems, number of participants, and lack of control group, while even more importantly, it is difficult to support such an intervention conceptually, when (exactly as for biofilms) no group has yet demonstrated the presence of active, alive bacteria within areas of sinus osteitis.

Surgery: The idea of removing all involved bone, through drilling and the performance of radical procedures either endoscopic (Draf III[30]) or open (frontal sinus obliteration), is an attractive one. In the relevant chapters, the role of radical surgery of the frontal sinus in the form of Draf III in patients with recalcitrant frontal CRS is discussed; however, its role in patients with osteitis is less well defined. Indeed, a recent study showed worse surgical outcomes in patients with osteitis,[22] while we should not forget that there is a direct correlation between the number of surgeries and osteitis.[19] Correlation does not equal causation, however, and it could be that this is a secondary association, with both osteitis and number of surgeries serving as surrogate markers of severe disease. Just like biofilms represent an end point of irreversible disease, the presence of osteitis seems to be also associated with end-stage disease. Like biofilm, osteitis is part of disease load and it could be important to maximally remove osteitic bone when present. It is not always possible to remove all osteitic bone from the lateral walls of the sphenoid or maxillary sinuses, but in the frontal sinuses, the results from both literature[31] and our experience have been that aggressive removal of osteitis bone may be useful, through either radical endoscopic approaches such as Draf III or an external, osteoplastic approach.

36.5 Case Example

A young male patient with a long history of recalcitrant chronic frontal sinusitis associated with immunosuppression and multiple previous endoscopic procedures presented with chronic frontal headache and purulent discharge. Endoscopic examination confirmed the presence of pus, and on CT imaging, there was evidence of frontal sinus opacification with osteitis and a small lateral mucocele with posterior frontal plate erosion (Video 36.1; ▶ Fig. 36.5).

A decision was taken to drain the frontal sinuses via a Draf IIb procedure with drilling of the osteitis occupying the anterior ethmoids and also the right frontal recess. The operation was successful, with opening of the mucocele and removal of the bone blocking the frontal recess (▶ Fig. 36.6).

However, the symptoms recurred and there was both endoscopic and CT evidence of obstruction of the right frontal recess (▶ Fig. 36.7). The patient underwent a Draf III

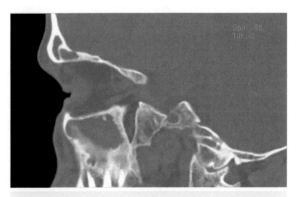

Fig. 36.5 Lateral frontal sinus mucocele with posterior wall erosion in a patient with chronic frontal sinusitis who has been operated multiple times.

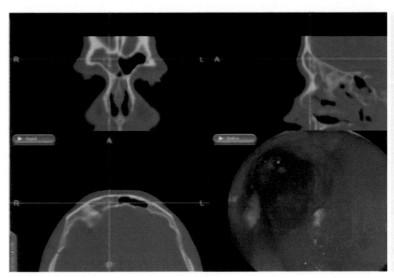

Fig. 36.6 Endoscopic and navigation intraoperative view during a Draf IIb procedure in the previous patient (Live Surgery).

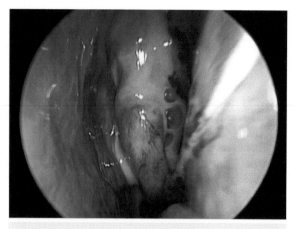

Fig. 36.7 Endoscopic view of the right nasal cavity with mucopurulent secretions and recurrence of the right frontal sinusitis in the previous patient.

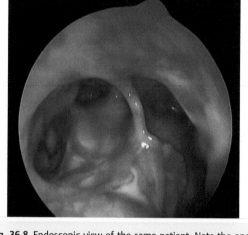

Fig. 36.8 Endoscopic view of the same patient. Note the open neo-ostium and the reappearance of healthy mucosa.

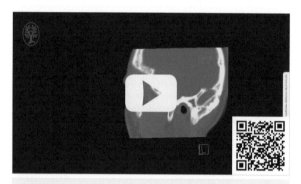

Video 36.1 Case example Osteitis – Draf IIb performed as part of live surgery on a patient with frontal sinusitis

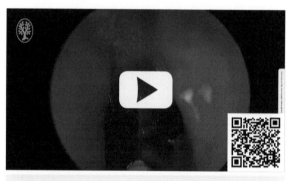

Video 36.2 Case example – Draf III performed in the same patient following osteitis recurrence

procedure, with extensive removal of osteitis bone (Video 36.2). A year later, the patient was free of symptoms while endoscopy confirmed a healthy, healed mucosa with patent wide neo-ostium (▶ Fig. 36.8).

36.6 Summary

Osteitis is increasingly recognized as a common factor in the cases of recalcitrant or difficult-to-treat rhinosinusitis. We do know that the number and extent of previous surgeries is associated with osteitis and that it is predictive of worse postoperative outcomes; however, the role, if any, of antibiotics or radical surgery in its management remains undefined.

36.7 Key Points

The method of choice for the diagnosis of osteitis is the CT, where osteitic bone appears as heterogeneous, irregular bone with areas of growth and destruction.

A variety of grading scales has been described—the GOSS is a validated composite scale incorporating bony thickness, extent, and number of sinus involved.

There is ample evidence that osteitis is associated with more extensive disease on both CT and endoscopically.

There is no evidence that osteitis is linked with more debilitating symptoms or worse QOL.

There is some evidence that the presence of osteitis can be associated with worse outcome following surgery.

References

[1] Fokkens WJ, Lund VJ, Mullol J, et al. European Position Paper on Rhinosinusitis and Nasal Polyps 2012. Rhinol Suppl. 2012; 23:1–298

[2] Westrin KM, Norlander T, Stierna P, Carlsöö B, Nord CE. Experimental maxillary sinusitis induced by Bacteroides fragilis. A bacteriological and histological study in rabbits. Acta Otolaryngol. 1992; 112 (1):107–114

[3] Norlander T, Forsgren K, Kumlien J, Stierna P, Carlsöö B. Cellular regeneration and recovery of the maxillary sinus mucosa. An experimental study in rabbits. Acta Otolaryngol Suppl. 1992; 492:33–37

[4] Bolger WE, Leonard D, Dick EJ, Jr, Stierna P. Gram negative sinusitis: a bacteriologic and histologic study in rabbits. Am J Rhinol. 1997; 11 (1):15–25

[5] Khalid AN, Hunt J, Perloff JR, Kennedy DW. The role of bone in chronic rhinosinusitis. Laryngoscope. 2002; 112(11):1951–1957

[6] Antunes MB, Feldman MD, Cohen NA, Chiu AG. Dose-dependent effects of topical tobramycin in an animal model of Pseudomonas sinusitis. Am J Rhinol. 2007; 21(4):423–427

[7] Kennedy DW, Senior BA, Gannon FH, Montone KT, Hwang P, Lanza DC. Histology and histomorphometry of ethmoid bone in chronic rhinosinusitis. Laryngoscope. 1998; 108(4, Pt 1):502–507

[8] Giacchi RJ, Lebowitz RA, Yee HT, Light JP, Jacobs JB. Histopathologic evaluation of the ethmoid bone in chronic sinusitis. Am J Rhinol. 2001; 15(3):193–197

[9] Lee JT, Kennedy DW, Palmer JN, Feldman M, Chiu AG. The incidence of concurrent osteitis in patients with chronic rhinosinusitis: a clinicopathological study. Am J Rhinol. 2006; 20(3):278–282

[10] Cho SH, Min HJ, Han HX, Paik SS, Kim KR. CT analysis and histopathology of bone remodeling in patients with chronic rhinosinusitis. Otolaryngol Head Neck Surg. 2006; 135(3):404–408

[11] Tran KN, Beule AG, Singal D, Wormald P-J. Frontal ostium restenosis after the endoscopic modified Lothrop procedure. Laryngoscope. 2007; 117(8):1457–1462

[12] Snidvongs K, McLachlan R, Chin D, et al. Osteitic bone: a surrogate marker of eosinophilia in chronic rhinosinusitis. Rhinology. 2012; 50 (3):299–305

[13] Mehta V, Campeau NG, Kita H, Hagan JB. Blood and sputum eosinophil levels in asthma and their relationship to sinus computed tomographic findings. Mayo Clin Proc. 2008; 83(6):671–678

[14] Ye T, Hwang PH, Huang Z, et al. Frontal ostium neo-osteogenesis and patency after Draf III procedure: a computer-assisted study. Int Forum Allergy Rhinol. 2014; 4(9):739–744

[15] Clement S, Vaudaux P, Francois P, et al. Evidence of an intracellular reservoir in the nasal mucosa of patients with recurrent Staphylococcus aureus rhinosinusitis. J Infect Dis. 2005; 192(6):1023–1028

[16] Plouin-Gaudon I, Clement S, Huggler E, et al. Intracellular residency is frequently associated with recurrent Staphylococcus aureus rhinosinusitis. Rhinology. 2006; 44(4):249–254

[17] Dong D, Yulin Z, Xiao W, et al. Correlation between bacterial biofilms and osteitis in patients with chronic rhinosinusitis. Laryngoscope. 2014; 124(5):1071–1077

[18] Richtsmeier WJ. Top 10 reasons for endoscopic maxillary sinus surgery failure. Laryngoscope. 2001; 111(11, Pt 1):1952–1956

[19] Georgalas C, Videler W, Freling N, Fokkens W. Global Osteitis Scoring Scale and chronic rhinosinusitis: a marker of revision surgery. Clin Otolaryngol. 2010; 35(6):455–461

[20] Catalano PJ, Dolan R, Romanow J, Payne SC, Silverman M. Correlation of bone SPECT scintigraphy with histopathology of the ethmoid bulla: preliminary investigation. Ann Otol Rhinol Laryngol. 2007; 116 (9):647–652

[21] Saylam G, Görgülü O, Korkmaz H, Dursun E, Ortapamuk H, Eryilmaz A. Do single-photon emission computerized tomography findings predict severity of chronic rhinosinusitis: a pilot study. Am J Rhinol Allergy. 2009; 23(2):172–176

[22] Bhandarkar ND, Mace JC, Smith TL. The impact of osteitis on disease severity measures and quality of life outcomes in chronic rhinosinusitis. Int Forum Allergy Rhinol. 2011; 1(5):372–378

[23] Telmesani LM, Al-Shawarby M. Osteitis in chronic rhinosinusitis with nasal polyps: a comparative study between primary and recurrent cases. Eur Arch Otorhinolaryngol. 2010; 267(5):721–724

[24] Ragab SM, Lund VJ, Scadding G. Evaluation of the medical and surgical treatment of chronic rhinosinusitis: a prospective, randomised, controlled trial. Laryngoscope. 2004; 114(5):923–930

[25] Fokkens W, Lund V, Mullol J, European Position Paper on Rhinosinusitis and Nasal Polyps group. European position paper on rhinosinusitis and nasal polyps 2007. Rhinol Suppl. 2007; 20(20):1–136

[26] Videler WJ, Badia L, Harvey RJ, et al. Lack of efficacy of long-term, low-dose azithromycin in chronic rhinosinusitis: a randomized controlled trial. Allergy. 2011; 66(11):1457–1468

[27] Orlandi RR, Kingdom TT, Hwang PH, et al. International Consensus Statement on Allergy and Rhinology: Rhinosinusitis. Int Forum Allergy Rhinol. 2016; 6 Suppl 1:S22–S209

[28] Tovi F, Benharroch D, Gatot A, Hertzanu Y. Osteoblastic osteitis of the maxillary sinus. Laryngoscope. 1992; 102(4):426–430

[29] Schaberg MR, Anand VK, Singh A. Hyperostotic chronic sinusitis as an indication for outpatient intravenous antibiotics. Laryngoscope. 2010; 120 Suppl 4:S245

[30] Georgalas C, Hansen F, Videler WJM, Fokkens WJ. Long terms results of Draf 3 procedure. Rhinology. 2011; 49(2):195–201

[31] Zhao YC, Wormald P-J. Biofilm and osteitis in refractory chronic rhinosinusitis. Otolaryngol Clin North Am. 2017; 50(1):49–60

37 Extreme Lateral Lesions: What Is the Limit of Endoscopic Surgery?

Cem Meco, Suha Beton, and Hazan Basak

Abstract

Continuous progress achieved in endoscopic techniques has dramatically changed the way we can approach extreme lateral lesions of the frontal sinuses. Driven by the eventual objective of causing less morbidity without compromising outcomes, endoscopic surgery nowadays can address most far lateral frontal sinus lesions even in large and well-pneumatized sinuses. An array of sophisticated endoscopic techniques added to Draf procedures can be used to achieve this goal. In order to adequately manipulate in the extreme lateral portion, orbital content needs to be suspended laterally with intact periorbita, after removing superomedial restricting orbital bones with appropriate instrumentation. At this moment, transection of the anterior ethmoidal artery, which is the only medial attachment of periorbita, plays a crucial role. This provides a wide access route to the most lateral portion of the frontal sinus, opening the area extensively for satisfactory visualization and manipulation around the lesions and their bony attachments. Thus, laterally located, especially benign frontal pathologies like mucoceles, fibro-osseous lesions, inverted papillomas, dura lesions, and others could be managed effectively. This evolution of divergence from established external surgical approaches is a result of achieving equal, if not better, outcomes with endoscopic surgery, while avoiding skin incisions and osteoplastic techniques that could cause problems. Nevertheless, one must not forget that external open approaches have withstood the test of time as elegant gold standard approaches and will always have their place for managing extreme lateral frontal lesions, especially for malignant neoplastic diseases or, if adequate instrumentation and expertise are not available to utilise endoscopic approaches.

Keywords: frontal sinus, endoscopic surgery, extreme lateral pathology, Draf procedures, periorbital suspension, orbital transposition

37.1 Published Evidence

Traditionally, extreme lateral lesions of the frontal sinuses have been managed by external approaches that require skin incisions and integrate osteoplastic techniques. Throughout the evolution of modern rhinology, such approaches were required due to the technical inability to visualize and reach this portion of the aerated sinonasal tract, which also constitutes the most lateral aspect of the sinonasal anterior skull base. Especially in well-aerated sinuses, the exposure, as well as the ability to manipulate around lesions of this far lateral area, was impossible through an endonasal endoscopic route until recently. Thus, external osteoplastic techniques were well developed over time and became the classical way of addressing extreme lateral lesions of the frontal sinuses. Today, these open approaches also establish the benchmark of outcome measures to evaluate results of any other possible approach.

37.1.1 Traditional External Approaches for Far Lateral Lesions

For inflammatory diseases and benign tumors of the lateral frontal sinuses when standard endonasal endoscopic techniques fall short, the regular approach is the osteoplastic frontal sinus (OFS) approach.[1,2,3] With this approach, not only the extreme lateral portion, but also the whole frontal sinus can be managed perfectly by addressing the pathology with maximum exposure, then removing and drilling out the entire frontal sinus mucosa, followed by abdominal fat obliteration of the sinus. This approach actually targets the interior borders of the frontal sinus; thus, if not necessarily required according to managed pathology and the case, fat obliteration could be utilized optionally without producing a nonfunctional sinus, provided that the outflow pathway is intact.[4,5,6] Apart from this approach, in some instances, a lateral frontal sinus trephination through a small skin incision may also be helpful to reach a lateral lesion in the most direct way. Nevertheless, the narrow burr hole access to the lateral frontal sinus limits visualized manipulation, hence its limited utility only in selected cases for observing and biopsy taking or otherwise introducing an additional instrument to facilitate a combined (external and endonasal) multiportal approach.

For malignant tumors of the lateral frontal sinuses, which also constitute the most lateral aspect of the sinonasal anterior skull base, craniofacial techniques originally described in the 1960s[7] and their modifications like the subcranial approach according to Raveh et al establish the basis of treatment. This latter approach was developed in the late 1970s, primarily for addressing craniofacial anomalies and frontobasal trauma, and then eventually modified to manage tumor resections.[8,9] In contrast to neurosurgical transcranial approach, this approach exposes the whole anterior skull base, including the sphenoidal and clival planes, as well as both orbital roofs avoiding frontal lobe retraction. The extended exposure also of the extreme lateral portion of the frontal sinuses as well as the whole paranasal sinuses provides

Table 37.1 Complications associated with external open approaches to the frontal sinus

Intraoperative	Exposure of orbital fat
	Unintentional fracture of the anterior wall of the frontal sinus
	Incorrect placement of the anterior wall
	Dural exposure or dural injury due to the anterior flap being too large
	Dural injury in the course of disease removal
	Superior sagittal sinus injury due to a too large anterior flap
Postoperative	Obvious scarring along the incision line
	Depression or embossment of the anterior table causing unattractive cosmetic deformity along the osteotomy line or along the whole surface of the frontal bony flap due to instability, infection, and concomitant resorption
	Persistent numbness of the supraorbital and frontal region
	Supraorbital neuralgia
	Cerebrospinal fluid leak, meningitis, encephalitis
	Development of mucoceles

an effective en bloc tumor removal without facial incisions, ending with frontal sinus cranialization.

The two main above-mentioned external approaches, the OFS and the subcranial approach provide perfect exposure to the entire frontal sinuses and supraorbital cells along the orbital roof, including the most lateral aspect of the frontal sinuses in the presence of extreme lateral lesions. Nevertheless, these procedures could be associated with some degree of morbidity as listed in ▶ Table 37.1.[3,4,10,11]

37.1.2 Endonasal Endoscopic Surgery and Evolution of Lateral Disease Management

On the other hand, due to the minimal invasive nature of endonasal endoscopic surgery (EES) techniques and driven by the eventual objective of causing less morbidity without compromising outcomes, new surgical concepts have emerged in the last decades. Accompanied by continuous technological development, but more importantly parallel to our better understanding of the complex anatomy of the frontal recess as well as the characteristics of the pathologies that affect frontal sinuses and its drainage pathways, endonasal endoscopic approaches to the frontal sinuses have developed to be utilized in a stepwise manner for distinct indications.[12] The foundation of this stepwise approach to the frontal sinuses has been classified by Draf.[4,5] Frontal sinus Draf procedures gradually enable a wider opening to the frontal sinuses. They improve endoscopic ease of access and enhance manipulation capability around the lesions to an extent and at the end they leave an adequate drainage pathway

postoperatively. Particularly, Draf III median drainage, also called endoscopic modified Lothrop procedure (EMLP), achieves the largest opening into the frontal sinuses. This opening has been used to address various frontal sinus pathologies also beyond the scope of chronic rhinosinusitis, including benign solid tumors according to the established guidelines for management of sinonasal tumors.[13] Over time, the fundamental rules that were set to manage each different type of lesion along the whole sinonasal cavity except frontal sinuses (due to limited visualization and manipulation) have gradually become obsolete as the stepwise frontal approaches have been utilized to treat lesions of this difficult-to-reach region.

The advent of image-guided navigated surgery (IGNS) and dedicated frontal endoscopic instrumentation in the form of either curved or double-curved instruments or powered drills played an important role in this development. This led to changes in treatment paradigms of especially benign frontal disorders and pathologies like mucoceles, fibro-osseous lesions, inverted papillomas (IPs), and others that have a lateral extension. ▶ Fig. 37.1 shows the outside projection of the lateral extent of a curved powered drill through a standard Draf III opening in such a patient.

Mucoceles

One of the earliest benign lesions that EES was utilized to manage a laterally extending disease was mucocele. Regarding mucoceles of the lateral frontal sinus and supraorbital recess, instead of the practice in the 1980s and 1990s,[14] preliminary data in 2004 suggested that ESS provided adequate drainage and helped avoid external approaches.[15] Similarly in 2005, Anand et al revised their

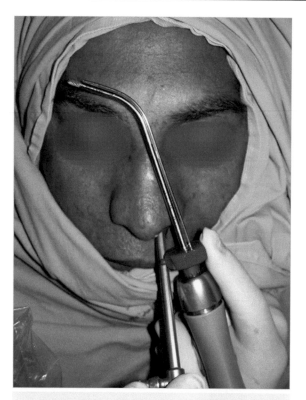

Fig. 37.1 Outside projection view of the lateral extent of a curved powered drill introduced from the contralateral side through a Draf III opening.

first 710 IGNS cases and reported that in all patients with frontal mucocele, surgery should be attempted endoscopically using IGNS because of the low morbidity of the procedure, and only if it is unsuccessful, should the patients with risk factors for failure be considered for osteoplastic flap (OPF) surgery.[16] Furthermore, the changing paradigm in recent modern treatment algorithms clearly shows the advantages of ESS approaches even in frontal sinus wall dehiscence and extrasinus mucocele extensions.[17]

Fibro-osseous Lesions

Frontal sinus fibro-osseous lesions and in particular osteomas that require a surgical resection according to the guidelines[13] yielded another area of management paradigm in the direction of ESS procedures over the years. In an early case series from 1990s, EES was proffered if sufficient frontal sinus access could be achieved endonasally, the osteoma was placed medially to a virtual sagittal plane through the lamina papyracea, and the tumor base was at the inferior part of the posterior frontal sinus wall.[18] Later on in 2005, Chiu et al described a grading scale for osteomas, in which they felt grade III and IV tumors, which included osteomas with anterior or superior attachments within the frontal

sinus (grade III), tumors that extended lateral to a sagittal plane through the lamina papyracea (grade III), and tumors that filled the entire frontal sinus (grade IV) would be best managed with the aid of an OPF rather than endonasally.[12,19] In addition, Bignami et al found that ESS could not be applied in osteomas with intracranial extension, large orbital involvement, erosion of the anterior or posterior wall, or when the anteroposterior diameter of the frontal sinus is less than 10 mm.[20] Nevertheless, in 2009, Seiberling et al[21] reported that they were able to remove a good portion of grade III and IV tumors by utilizing a Draf III procedure; Ledderose et al[22] also reported similar findings. A setback in applying ESS in some huge osteomas in these studies was simply the increased surgical time it would take to remove the tumor endonasally with relatively weak curved drills that are needed for cavitation. Additionally, as mentioned by Rokade and Sama, previous meningitis or cerebrospinal fluid (CSF) leak, extensive intracranial extension, and significant supraorbital component with lateral orbital mucoceles could make the cases more challenging for ESS.[23] Georgalas et al, in light of their experience, reviewed the contraindications of endonasal approaches of frontal osteomas[24] and set out as absolute contraindications just the extended erosion of the anterior frontal plate. Due to the improved access provided by the Draf III procedure, if not all, the vast majority of frontal sinus osteomas can nowadays be endoscopically managed regardless of their size, lateral extent, and intraorbital involvement, all these being no more considered absolute contraindications.[25]

Inverted Papillomas

IP involving the frontal sinuses would be exclusively addressed with an external approach in the past. The treatment algorithm has undergone a complex evolution that still continues. Proper preoperative evaluations, precise determination of the sites of tumor origin and attachment during the operation, meticulous use of subperiosteal dissection in the involved areas, wide removal of tumor origin along the subperiosteal plane, drilling the underlying bone, and complete removal of all diseased mucosa with creation of wide cavities for long-term regular follow-ups constitute the key elements of successful endoscopic management today.[12,13,26,27,28,29] Frontal sinuses pose an extra challenge due to narrow access achieved to this anatomically restricted area by causing difficult visualization and manipulation of the lesions. Nevertheless, advanced endoscopic techniques like Draf III facilitate in most instances adequate entry to set the goals of IP surgery. This is especially true in the cases where the tumors expand or prolapse into the frontal rather than involve the frontal sinus mucosa itself. However, massive involvement of the frontal and supraorbital recess, as well as far lateral and posterior wall involvement, constitutes the points of debate nowadays that may necessitate external approaches.

Cerebrospinal Fluid Leaks

An important practice change regarding management of dural defects along the posterior wall of frontal sinuses and frontal sinus outflow tract has also occurred over the decades. Formally, external approaches were accepted to be the primary choice of approach for any frontal sinus-related CSF leak or dural dehiscence of any cause from traumatic fractures to congenital defects as well as those arising from tumor erosion or iatrogenic origin.[1,2,3,8,9] These techniques principally intend to obliterate or ablate the frontal sinus while achieving a watertight closure of dural defects. Nevertheless, despite these attempts to eliminate aerated frontal sinuses at the end, due to regrowth of mucosa, mucocele formation up to 10% necessitates continuing imaging follow-up.[3] On the other hand, experiences gained with endoscopic Draf procedures that gradually enable a wider opening to the frontal sinuses led surgeons to apply already established endonasal duraplasty techniques to frontal sinus posterior wall and outflow tract as well and also to supraorbital recess dural lesions in selected cases with more than 90% success rates.[30,31,32,33,34,35,36] Better visualization and effective manipulation offered by these advanced endoscopic frontal sinus procedures make their use feasible in most of the patients while maintaining the structure and function of the sinus and minimizing early and late complications. The major limiting factor in most of the reported series was extreme extension superiorly or laterally within the posterior table beyond the reach of current instrumentation. In those cases with lesions especially located in the far lateral portion of the frontal sinuses, EES was combined mostly with a frontal trephine when needed. In a case series of 24 lateral frontal CSF leaks originating laterally to the plane of the lamina papyracea, Conger et al[37] reported only 1 (4%) trephine-assisted repair to support lateral placement of the graft, showing the capabilities of endoscopic technique through standard Draf procedures and a 70-degree endoscope, as well as other dedicated instruments.

37.1.3 Evolution of Far Lateral Frontal Sinus Surgery: Exploring Limits of ESS

Regardless of the pathology addressed within the frontal sinuses whether a mucocele, fibro-osseous lesion, IP, dura lesion, or others, the irresistible rise of EES through the application of Draf procedures over time aroused the curiosity to investigate the lateral limits of pure endoscopic approaches. In a cadaver study, Becker et al[38] demonstrated that lateral instrumentation and visualized reach (VR) to manipulate the lesions increase significantly as the frontal sinus opening increases from Draf IIa to

Draf III. There was no statistical difference between visualization and instrumentation in the lateral direction within each Draf procedure group. Nevertheless, for more important lateral VR with two pieces of equipment (endoscope and an instrument), the obstructive anatomy was found to be the lamina papyracea of the orbit and this anatomic obstacle could be overcome when the frontal sinus opening was enlarged. In the largest Draf III opening, the most lateral border of the frontal sinus was always visualized, but only in 64% could the instruments reach this border and a VR was possible in 54% of cases.

In case of frontal neoplasia surgery, accessing the lateral bony attachment with a drill would be a requirement to drill out tumor bed for disease eradication. Thus, Timperley et al[39] attempted to define the lateral limits of the Draf III approach using a 70-degree diamond bur under a 70-degree endoscope view in a cadaver study, where 50% of the cadaver's frontal sinuses had lateral pneumatization beyond the virtual midorbital line. In 95% of the sinuses, they were able to access the most lateral extent of the posterior and anterior walls. However, the inferior wall, forming the orbital roof was accessible in 35% of the sinuses overall, representing the most challenging area of the frontal sinus to reach via an endoscopic approach and the key finding from this study. Orbital roof access was only in 10% beyond the midline pneumatized sinuses and thus was dependent on pneumatization. Another finding was the significant correlation between the anteroposterior distance (APD) between the outer periosteum and the olfactory fossa and the distance reached on the orbital roof beyond the midline. Along the orbital roof, apart from the lateral reach also to the posterior, the orbitocranial cleft of the supraorbital recess poses difficulty to control for adequate manipulation and resection, as the space between the bony walls gets narrower than the drill or other instruments, if one approaches anteriorly. It has been reported that even with bone removal the management of the cleft between the dura and the periorbita in this region may be tricky and may require open approaches oncoming from superior.[40] Additionally, for addressing orbital roof lesions and lateral frontal sinus disease, transorbital endoscopic approaches solely or in combination with endonasal endoscopic hybrid techniques were also described with good results.[41,42]

Previous cadaver studies[38,39] clearly demonstrated that the lateral reach can be achieved by using standard Draf procedures and the lamina papyracea was found to be the anatomical obstacle limiting the extent of these approaches. In a case presentation, our group reported in 2014[43] a frontal cholesteatoma located extremely laterally that was even extending to the middle cranial fossa and inner periosteum of the temporalis muscle, as can be seen in ▶ Fig. 37.2. As the cholesteatoma had already eroded the bony orbital roof, we managed the case through an exclusively endonasal

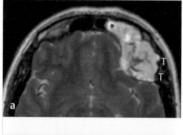
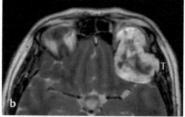
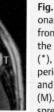
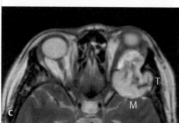
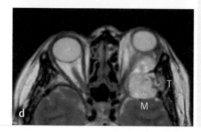

Fig. 37.2 Axial T2-weighted magnetic resonance imaging (MRI) scans of the left frontal cholesteatoma, showing disease at the midlateral portion of the frontal sinus (*), extending far laterally to the inner periosteum of the temporalis muscle (T) and posteriorly to the middle cranial fossa (M). (a–d) Serial scans illustrate the outspread of the lesion from cranially to caudally.

endoscopic approach by removing the lamina papyracea and transecting the anterior ethmoidal artery (AEA), which allowed us to suspend the periorbita laterally to have adequate exposure with VR, a technique that we have been using occasionally since 2010 for various pathologies.

Furthermore, in an effort to overcome the limitation created by the medial orbital wall and improve endoscopic lateral access, Poczos et al[44] conducted another cadaver study by adding the medial and superior orbital decompression (MSOD) to standard Draf III procedures. They removed the bony medial superior wall of the orbit while preserving the periorbita, nevertheless posteriorly up to the level of the AEA, leaving it intact. Even without the transection of AEA, they demonstrated that with this modification they had better access and visualization beyond the midorbital line compared to Draf III alone. In total, the lateral extent of the entire frontal sinus was accessed under visualization in 85% of their cadaver sinuses by the addition of MSOD. Although this finding was slightly lower than reported by Timperley et al,[39] it was much higher than the 54% reported by Becker et al,[38] both using only Draf III approach, showing the impact of MSOD.

Role of Anterior Ethmoidal Artery Transection

On the other hand, in addition to removal of the medial and superior walls of the orbit, the AEA plays a crucial role in achieving the greatest amount of lateral suspension of periorbita that would create the widest lateral exposure and VR as demonstrated by our case presentation.[43] As AEA is the only anatomical structure holding the periorbita medially, its coagulation and transection enable the maximum possible suspension of periorbita laterally with malleable retractors, opening a wide corridor to the most lateral portion of the frontal sinus and supraorbital recess. Actually, transection of the AEA to

suspend the periorbita laterally is a very well-developed procedure that has been safely used during external approaches as for external ethmoidectomies. Traditionally, through skin incisions like Lynch incision,[45] the periorbita is elevated, exposing the medial orbital wall and the supraorbital roof in a subperiosteal plane back to the AEA at the frontoethmoidal suture. Ligation and transection of the AEA and if needed posterior ethmoidal artery allow the orbital contents to fall away laterally, aiding with further exposure according to the aim of surgery planned, like anterior skull base or optic nerve exposure. From these external medial transorbital approaches, it is a known fact that lateral retraction of the periorbita is a safe procedure. Moving further from these experiences, a similar concept could also be safely utilized through the route of endonasal endoscopic approaches to overcome the anatomic limitations, which would enable control of the far lateral frontal sinus and supraorbital recess regions.

Throughout the evolution of endoscopic techniques, one of the early limited applications of this concept was reported by Nicolai et al[46] for the eradication of IP from the supraorbital cells with limited lateral extension back in 2006. During the conversion phase of IP surgeries from predominantly external approaches to endonasal approaches, they were cautious to bind themselves to limited lateral extent, but they clearly described coagulation and sectioning of the AEA, drilling the upper part of the lamina papyracea and lateral displacement of the orbital content for better endonasal exposure of the IP involvement site.

However, the first big case series managed with this concept was reported by Karligkiotis et al.[47] They utilized a technique that they called endoscopic endonasal orbital transposition to manage 24 patients who had various frontal lesions lateral to the plane of the lamina papyracea. They were able to achieve complete control of the lesion's boundaries in each case, even if the lesion was located in the far lateral portion of the frontal sinus or into the supraorbital recess. According to the needs of each case, they differently associated Draf IIb, Draf III, and endoscopic lateralization of the orbit along with the use of double-angled instruments and, if needed, binostril approach by using the contralateral nasal fossa as described by Liu et al.[48] With this tailored approach that transposes the orbita laterally, they were able to gain more space and reach the far lateral aspect of the frontal sinus by passing over the orbit with dedicated instruments. The median follow-up time was 40.6 months and they reported 20.8% frontal stenosis that required a revision surgery.

As mentioned earlier with the frontal cholesteatoma case[43] and as reported in different studies,[49,50] we have also been using the endoscopic lateralization of the orbit to expose lesions at the far lateral portion of the frontal sinus as well as the supraorbital recess. Up to now, we have operated on 29 cases with a minimum follow-up of 7 months and mean follow-up of 37.7 months. Apart from addressing mucoceles, fibro-osseous lesions, and IPs that were reported by Karligkiotis et al,[47] in our series as shown in ▶ Table 37.2, we had additionally managed six CSF leaks, and single cases of frontal cholesteatoma, foreign body removal (cranioplasty material), mesenchymal tumor, and histiocytosis X tumor resections with success. According to the requirements of each case to adequately expose and manage lesions optimally, either the Draf IIb or III procedure was utilized to facilitate endonasal endoscopic periorbital suspension.

Being the first reported malignant disease managed with this purely endoscopic technique in this difficult-to-reach area, the mesenchymal tumor and histiocytosis X patients are being followed up 42 and 19 months, respectively, with no evidence of disease. These were both female patients who rejected skin incision for an external biopsy. Thus, although the initial goal of the surgery in both patients was to get a definitive histopathology to facilitate further multidisciplinary treatment protocols, which were also done, due to the wide exposure achieved during surgery, we were able to achieve complete tumor removal and drill out the tumor bed in both cases. Nevertheless, regarding the whole group, the patency of the very large opening achieved during initial surgeries did not remain stable in 24.1% of the 29 patients, who developed a stenosis that required a revision surgery in a median follow-up time of 37.7 months.

37.2 Controversies and Opinions

The optimal management of the far lateral frontal sinus lesions has increasingly been a key topic of discussion among the scientific community. This is mainly due to controversies between foreseeable results of the established classical external procedures and the promising intrusion of the minimally invasive endonasal approaches

that avoid skin incisions and osteoplastic techniques in the endoscopic era. The continuous evolution of the EES techniques with better understanding of the anatomy and disease pathophysiology and the never-ending exponential developments in instrumentation like more powerful drills and sophisticated navigation systems constantly improve our abilities to push our limits forward and revise our management guidelines. The published evidence summarized here demonstrates that most of the earlier limitations for EES to address many far lateral frontal sinus and supraorbital recess pathologies have either become obsolete or are not valid anymore.

Furthermore, the pathophysiology of each disease process should also be encountered. For inflammatory and benign diseases of the far lateral frontal sinus that are refractory to or inaccessible to endoscopic approaches, the OPF approach will always have its place. However, for example, for a far laterally extended mucocele, instead of an external OPF technique, nowadays it is much wiser to create a wide marsupialization and a large cavity with complete removal of interfrontal septations to see all borders through a Draf III median drainage from which we can always control the inside in the follow-ups. In such a case, doing an OPF without obliteration would expose the patient to the same questionable postoperative long-term drainage and aeration problems as in the EES approach, but instead, doing an OPF with fat obliteration would surely not rule out a self-created iatrogenic mucocele in the long term.[3,6,10,11]

The same is also true for laterally extending osteomas, as today most of the earlier contraindications except wide anterior frontal wall erosion are no more absolute contraindications regardless of size, extent, and intraorbital involvement of the osteoma.[12] However, as mentioned earlier, some conditions like intracranial involvement and others could make EES more challenging.[23,24,25] Nevertheless, endoscopic inaccessibility is probably no more a valid reason, as sophisticated techniques combining the Draf procedures with maneuvers suspending or transposing the orbita laterally give direct access even in most extreme lateral cases.[43,47,49,50] Additionally, as the industry is now producing much faster and powerful curved drills that are required for cavitation before dissecting osteoma from neighboring structures, the setback to apply EES for not slowing down the surgery has also become outdated, further avoiding an OPF approach and possible fat obliteration as well as omitting skin incisions.

Among all other benign lesions, the hottest ongoing debate is perhaps on the management of patients with far lateral frontal IPs, because of the chance of malignant transformation in case of a residual or recurrent disease. The standard external approaches naturally give a direct access for disease eradication, but they still pose all the problems mentioned earlier. Besides, in well-pneumatized sinuses, drilling at the narrow edges between the anterior skull base and the orbital roof could be very

Table 37.2 Data of patients operated for far lateral frontal sinus lesions using endonasal endoscopic periorbital suspension technique in addition to Draf procedures at the Department of Otolaryngology Head and Neck Surgery, Ankara University, since 2010

Patient	Gender	Age (y)	Indication	Draf	Year	Follow-up (mo)
1	M	10	Traumatic cerebrospinal fluid (CSF) leak	III	2013	63
2	M	7	Traumatic CSF leak	IIB	2014	53
3	M	12	Traumatic CSF leak	IIB	2015	42
4	F	11	Traumatic CSF leak	III	2015	41
5	M	20	Traumatic CSF leak	III	2018	7
6	F	53	Spontaneous CSF leak	III	2016	31
7	M	31	Mucocele	IIB	2010	102
8	M	38	Mucocele	III	2013	67
9	F	33	Mucocele	III	2016	30
10	F	37	Mucocele	III	2016	31
11	M	52	Mucocele	III	2017	15
12	F	44	Mucocele	III	2017	17
13	M	25	Osteoma	III	2015	40
14	M	34	Osteoma	III	2016	29
15	M	18	Osteoma	III	2017	12
16	M	47	Osteoma	IIB	2017	12
17	M	36	Osteoma	III	2017	17
18	M	20	Fibrous dysplasia	III	2011	89
19	M	19	Fibrous dysplasia	III	2015	41
20	F	40	Fibrous dysplasia	III	2016	31
21	M	28	Fibrous dysplasia	IIB	2018	7
22	F	61	Inverted papilloma	IIB	2013	63
23	M	28	Inverted papilloma	III	2014	52
24	M	72	Inverted papilloma	III	2015	40
25	F	77	Inverted papilloma	IIB	2017	15
26	F	51	Frontal cholesteatoma	III	2014	54
27	F	43	Mesenchymal tumor	III	2014	53
28	F	39	Histiocytosis X	III	2016	28
29	M	28	Foreign body/cranioplasty	III	2017	12
						Mean: 37.7

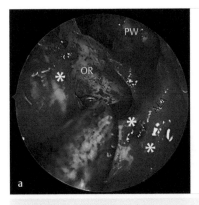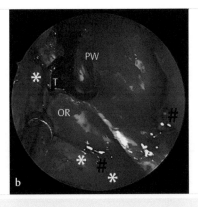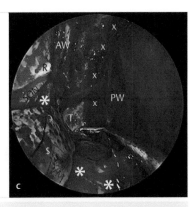

Fig. 37.3 Technique of periorbital suspension on the right side pictured under the lateral vision of a 45-degree endoscope. **(a)** View of the frontal sinus posterior wall (PW) and the frontal recess area after Draf III procedure and resection of the lamina papyracea, demonstrating how the anterior ethmoidal artery (AEA) is holding the periorbita (*) intact medially, although the curved suction is trying to push laterally. The bony orbital roof (OR) hinders the view and access to the lateral frontal sinus. **(b)** Lateral view from the frontal recess after transection of the AEA showing medial and lateral transected AEA buds (#) and much more effective lateral displacement of the intact periorbita (*) with suction. Start of the bony OR removal and lateral frontal sinus exposure (T). **(c)** Lateral view of the fully exposed most lateral portion of the frontal sinus (T) during dissection with an instrument seen from the midline frontal sinus after complete removal of the bony OR up to the level of the orbital rim (R) while protecting the superior orbital nerve (SON) and the periorbita (*) suspended inferolaterally with a brain spatula ($). Posterior (PW) and anterior (AW) frontal walls including their narrow lateral junction (x) is under complete visualized reach.

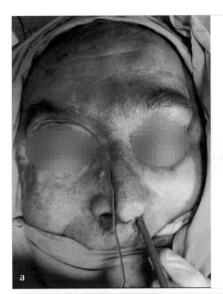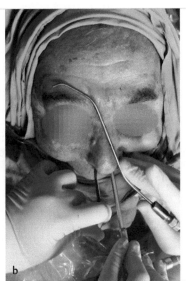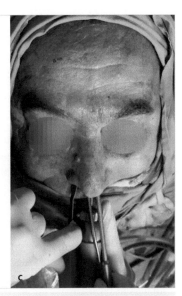

Fig. 37.4 Intraoperative situs of the same inverted papilloma patient in ▶ Fig. 37.3 showing endonasal endoscopic transillumination of the right frontal sinus as well as dedicated instrumentation and their binostril four-hand handling. **(a)** Outside projection view of the malleable brain spatula used for retracting periorbita inferolaterally. **(b)** Outside projection view of a double-curved suction after Prof. Kucuk. **(c)** Application of a binostril four-hand endoscopic surgery while using a malleable retractor, double-curved suction, and the curved powered drill for drilling out far lateral frontal sinus.

challenging, still carrying a risk for residual and recurrent disease, which also explains the failure rates in this cohort.[3,10,11] However, as demonstrated in ▶ Fig. 37.3 and ▶ Fig. 37.4 in a recurrent IP case, after performing a Draf III opening, the AEA can be identified and transected, the lamina papyracea and superior orbital roof removed, and

the periorbita could be laterally suspended with a brain spatula to access, manipulate, and remove all frontal and supraorbital disease and drill out all adjacent bony borders no matter how lateral they are through both nostrils. ▶ Fig. 37.5 shows the preoperative imaging showing the far lateral IP involvement and the postoperative 40th-

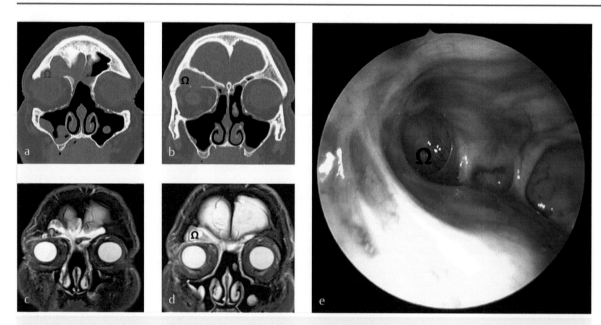

Fig. 37.5 Preoperative imaging and postoperative control endoscopy of an already three times operated recurrent inverted papilloma patient. (a,b) Coronal computed tomography (CT) and (c,d) coronal T2-weighted magnetic resonance imaging (MRI) showing right far lateral frontal sinus (Ω) disease involvement and (e) illustration of a postoperative 40th-month endoscopic view of that very lateral portion of the right frontal sinus with no evidence of disease.

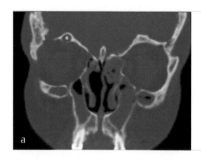
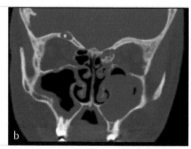

Fig. 37.6 Coronal computed tomography (CT) scans of the right-sided isolated lateral supraorbital cell mucocele. (a,b) Isolated lateral supraorbital mucocele (*) that no patent pathway for an aerated functional cavity can be created on the right side.

month endoscopic view of that very lateral portion of the frontal sinus with no evidence of disease. Thus, in all IP patients in whom we have applied this technique of periorbital suspension on top of Draf III, it clearly enabled us to eradicate all disease even from the most far lateral frontal sinus region, while at the end leaving a functional aerated cavity for endoscopic follow-ups.[49,50] Using the same procedure they call orbital transposition, Karligkiotis et al[47] reported similar results. Although experiences are limited to a few centers, the reported outcomes are very promising for the integrity of this evolving concept in comparison to benchmark outcomes of external approaches.

The same approach can also be used to reach out isolated lateral supraorbital cell mucoceles, where there is no hope of creating a pathway for an aerated functional cavity like the case shown in ▶ Fig. 37.6. In such a case, surgery aims to reach and open the mucocele from below as demonstrated in ▶ Fig. 37.7, aspirate the content, and

drill out the bony walls to remove all mucosae to prohibit recurrence. Naturally, this could also have been achieved through an external approach, but that would surely risk more operative morbidity like a dural tear, as the angle of attack would be more tangent to the anterior skull base, in addition to all earlier mentioned possible postoperative frontal sinus problems.

A completely different point of discussion is the management of malignant disease involving the far lateral frontal sinus. In this region, due to the narrow cleft with the posterior table, the tumor involves the anterior skull base in most instances. It is mandatory to know that, if surgery will be a part of the curative treatment, the first attempt should be the definitive one and aim at an R_0 resection in order to provide the best survival outcomes. There is no argument that external approaches and in particular craniofacial resection would facilitate this goal the best in nearly all cases. Nevertheless, in case of suspicion of malignancy and lack of histopathological

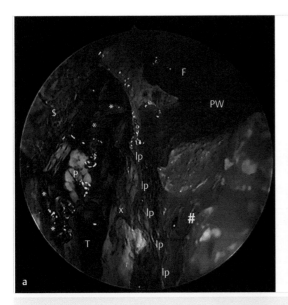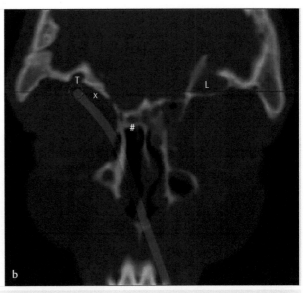

Fig. 37.7 Technique of periorbital suspension for isolated lateral supraorbital mucocele on the right side. **(a)** Endoscopic view of the frontal sinus posterior wall (PW) and frontal sinus (F) after Draf III procedure and attachment of resected lamina papyracea (lp) to the anterior skull base between ethmoidal roof (#) and medial orbital roof (x), as well as the periorbita (*) being suspended laterally with a malleable retractor ($) exposing the targeted supraorbital cell (T), whose inferior orbital wall was drilled to remove mucoid pus (P). As the next step then, the mucosal lining of the cell will be removed and drilled to avoid further mucocele development. **(b)** The navigated coronal trajectory to the isolated supraorbital cell (T) through the plane of lamina papyracea, avoiding anterior skull base at ethmoidal roof (#) and medial orbital roof (x). The red circle indicates the tip of navigation probe shown with a green line. Additionally, one can see another isolated lateral supraorbital mucocele on the left side (L).

diagnosis, first a biopsy would be required to reach a definitive diagnosis. Of course, a lateral frontal sinus trephination or an OPF could accomplish this task; nevertheless, these may disturb the dissection planes and cause a tumor to spread to the skin by disrupting barriers through direct skin incisions. Thus, in suitable cases and when required instrumentation and expertise are available, one can attempt to use the natural aerated tract of sinonasal cavity to reach this far lateral region to take a biopsy and even do more through EES.

In our case load, we had some limited experience with extremely confined selected malignancies, where the preoperative diagnosis was unknown and a biopsy was initially required. The imaging of one can be seen in ▶ Fig. 37.8. It illustrates a left-sided far lateral frontal sinus lesion with irregular bony erosions and a solid consistency requiring diagnostic biopsy due to persistent local symptoms. However, the 39-year-old woman rejected having an external approach through skin incisions in the first hand, only for getting a biopsy and eventually resection to avoid any possible visible scar and frontal sensation loss without knowing the definitive histopathology. Instead, she authorized us to take the biopsy using EES with informed consent of the possibility to convert to an open approach. By utilizing a Draf III combined with periorbital suspension, it was possible to expose and take a biopsy from the lesion adequately as could be seen in ▶ Fig. 37.9, whose frozen section and later the

definitive histopathology revealed histiocytosis X. At that point, as we were already there, we decided to completely remove the lesion and drill its tumor bed, which was also possible without a hurdle endonasally. The case was then presented at the tumor board meeting and after being further investigated, the patient had two cycles of systemic chemotherapy. ▶ Fig. 37.10 shows the postoperative MRI scans and 18th-month endoscopy of the tumor bed, both revealing no evidence of tumor. As demonstrated in this example, EES may also play a role in the diagnostic and treatment algorithm of limited and highly selected malignant lesions of the far lateral frontal sinuses.

Another controversial area is the management of extreme lateral lesions that may even go beyond the borders of the frontal sinuses. Nearly all published literature report on external approaches for good reasons, when extreme lateral pathologies are considered. There are only anecdotal reports on the sole use of EES for extreme lateral lesions. As demonstrated earlier, the far lateral borders of the frontal sinuses can be perfectly exposed when required, by removal of the medial and superior bony orbital walls, which are the major limiting factor of the lateral endoscopic approach, and transection of the AEA that enables maximal lateral displacement of intact periorbita, after performing a Draf III opening. This facilitates the pathway to the most lateral portion of the frontal sinus in almost all cases. Then principally the nature

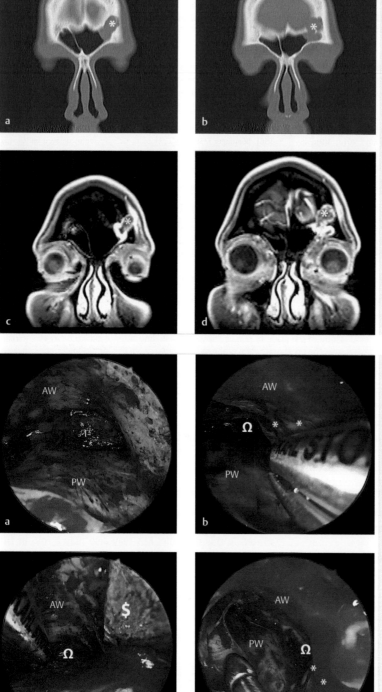

Fig. 37.8 Imaging of a suspicious left-sided far lateral frontal sinus lesion (*) with persistent local symptoms. **(a,b)** Coronal computed tomography (CT) scans show irregular bony erosions and **(c,d)** coronal magnetic resonance imaging (MRI) scans illustrate the solid consistency of the lateral portion of the lesion indicating the need for a diagnostic biopsy.

Fig. 37.9 Endoscopic view of the left frontal sinus far lateral lesion and visualized reach through periorbital suspension. **(a)** Exposition of the tumor (T) between the anterior and posterior frontal walls at the lateral corner through Draf III and taking a biopsy. **(b)** Drilling out the lamina papyracea and the orbital roof (*) for better exposition of the tumor bed (Ω). **(c)** After periorbital suspension with a malleable retractor ($), optimal conditions for best manipulation of the drill and other instruments to resect and drill out the tumor bed (Ω) completely. **(d)** Endoscopic view of the frontal sinus and tumor bed (Ω) after complete resection of the lesion. (AW, anterior wall; PW, posterior wall.)

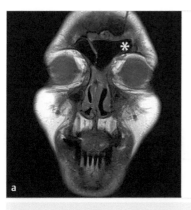 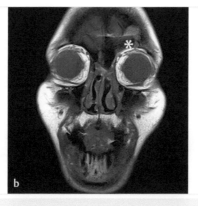 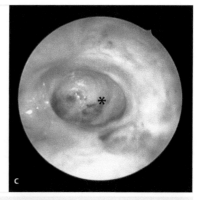

Fig. 37.10 **(a,b)** Postoperative coronal T1-weighted magnetic resonance imaging (MRI) scans and **(c)** the endoscopic view of the 18th-month follow-up reveal no evidence of tumor at the left frontal sinus lateral attachment site (*).

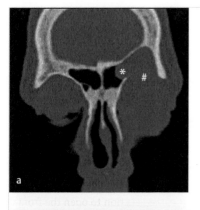 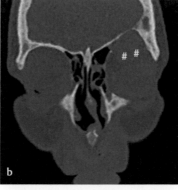

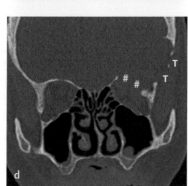

Fig. 37.11 Coronal computed tomography (CT) scans showing left frontal cholesteatoma that extends far lateral to the inner periosteum of the temporalis muscle (T) and posterior to the level of orbital apex. **(a)** The most medial portion of the lesion (*) and the eroded orbital roof (#). **(b,c)** A more posterior display of the complete absence of bony orbital roof (#), as well as the anterior ethmoidal artery region (Ω) holding the periorbita in its place medially. **(d)** The most lateral portion of the lesion that has eroded the lateral skull bones in the pterional region and reached to the inner periosteum of the temporalis muscle (T).

of the pathology and aims of surgical management dictate how extreme lateral we can visualize, manipulate, and be able to achieve our goals by using a purely endoscopic approach. ▸ Fig. 37.11 and ▸ Fig. 37.12 demonstrate, respectively, the coronal CT and MRI of such an extreme laterally situated frontal cholesteatoma that extends posterolaterally to the middle cranial fossa and the inner periosteum of the temporalis muscle in the pterional region, as also can be appreciated in axial MRI scans in ▸ Fig. 37.2. Like in a radical cavity surgery of the temporal bone, in this case, the aim of surgery was to create a large frontal opening to aerate the cavity while removing as much matrix as possible. ▸ Fig. 37.13

illustrates the major steps of the purely endoscopic dissection. As the slowly expanding disease had already eroded all the bone along its contact areas including the orbital roof, lateral frontal sinus, anterior and middle cranial fossa dura, it was possible to push away the periorbita laterally and the frontal lobe dura posteriorly to reach most of the disease right from the beginning. However, the real access up to the level of the middle cranial fossa and temporalis muscle was achieved after the transection of AEA and suspending the periorbita inferolaterally, which created an incredibly wide exposure, helping us to achieve our goals. The postoperative first-year MRI in ▸ Fig. 37.14 reveals the patency of the extremely lateral

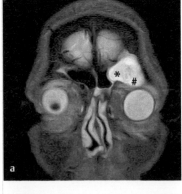
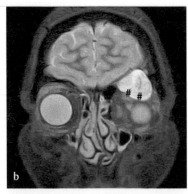
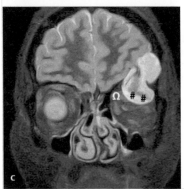
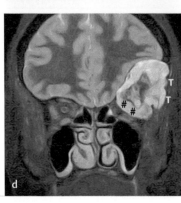

Fig. 37.12 Coronal T2-weighted magnetic resonance imaging (MRI) scans display left frontal cholesteatoma extending far lateral to the inner periosteum of the temporalis muscle (T) and posteriorly to the level of the orbital apex. **(a)** The most medial portion of the lesion (*) and the disease pushing orbita superiorly (#). **(b,c)** A more posterior display of the intrusion of the lesion into the orbit (#) along the whole orbital roof, pushing the globe anteriorly, as well as the anterior ethmoidal artery region (Ω) that holds the periorbita in its place medially. **(d)** The most lateral portion of the lesion (T) reaching to the inner periosteum of the temporalis muscle in the pterional region and the lesion pushing the orbital apex (#).

aerated cavity through the midline drainage, while ▶ Fig. 37.15 shows an endoscopic examination at the second year and diffusion-weighted MRI control at almost the fourth year, both with no evidence of disease.

The lateral frontal sinus and the supraorbital recess pose a highly challenging area for picking the optimal approach. Although controversies exist, we believe that advanced EES techniques provide a safe and effective treatment option in properly selected cases, as demonstrated.

37.3 Unanswered Questions

The lateral limits of endoscopic approaches continue to expand with improved techniques, equipment, and experience, which will surely continue to evolve. The current data suggest that inaccessibility of the far lateral frontal sinus is nowadays no more the major problem for EES to adequately address the lesions in this region. Nevertheless, due to the limited number of reported cases, it is very hard to clearly establish the updated objective restrictions for its application. Thus, considering also the rarity of these lesions in the daily practice, multicenter prospective assessments are needed to gather data of large series, in an attempt to establish the actual place and limitations of its use to address the far lateral and even the extreme lateral lesions of the frontal sinuses. Until then, taking into account patient's specific anatomy and the caregiver's experience and resources, a patient-

and disease-oriented balanced approach should be decided for the optimal best personalized management.

A more relevant unanswered question regarding ESS being used for addressing the far lateral lesions of the frontal sinus by using advanced techniques seems to be the stenosis of the frontal sinusotomy. Keeping the frontal sinus drainage pathway patent in the long term has always been a challenge even for the simple EES. As a rule, the key to success lies in preservation of mucosa along the frontal recess. Nevertheless, the extensive surgeries aiming the far lateral sinus are in their nature associated with significant mucosal damage. In our series, and also in other reported series where the periorbita was retracted laterally to have access to far lateral frontal sinus, this problem occurred in about 21 to 24% of the cases, requiring a second procedure for revision.[47,49] Although these rates fall into the range of expected failures when nothing more than a Draf III is performed,[12] better results are surely needed. To achieve this, in general, perhaps use of mucosal flaps to cover the bare bone of the recess area could be a solution, which should be studied and answered.

Another unanswered emerging topic to be studied is the use of transorbital endoscopic approaches.[41,42] If the recess area is not affected by the disease and works properly, in order to reach an extreme lateral lesion of the frontal sinus and beyond, an endoscopic transorbital approach with nearly invisible small blepharoplasty incisions and avoiding bony destruction of the osteoplastic

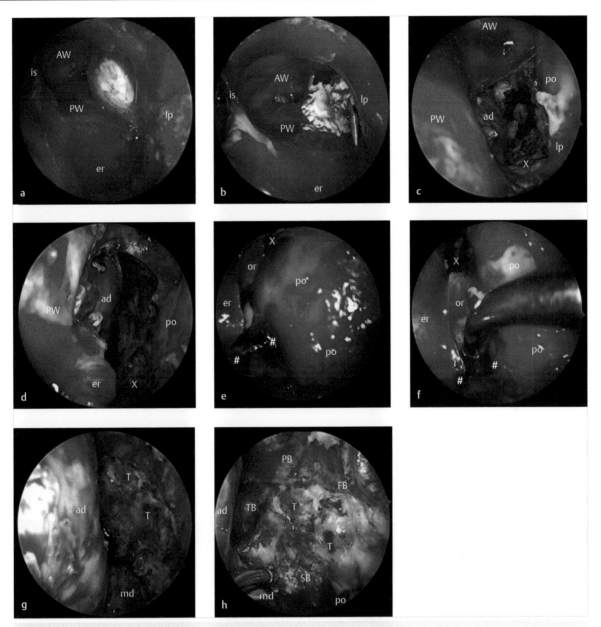

Fig. 37.13 Endoscopic views looking with a 45-degree endoscope to the left side and illustrating the major steps of the purely endoscopic dissection. **(a)** Left frontal sinus posterior bony wall (PW), anterior bony wall (AW), superior attachment of the interfrontal septum (is), lamina papyracea (lp), and ethmoidal roof (er), as well as the medially bulging lesion (*) after performing a Draf III procedure before lesion removal. **(b)** Demonstration of the beginning of lesion resection and **(c)** a close-up view to the lateral as the lesion is being removed (X) and a deeper lateral space is created while exposing the anterior fossa dura (ad) and the superior portion of the periorbita (po) without bony covering. **(d)** The maximum opening and removal that could be achieved through the Draf III approach, also showing the inferior limit (X) of visualized reach in a narrow cleft between the ethmoid roof (er) and the medial remnant of the superior orbital roof bone, inhibiting further access inferiorly along the superior periorbita (po). **(e,f)** Demonstration of the periorbital suspension technique, where the lamina papyracea is completely removed, and the periorbita (po) and the anterior ethmoidal artery, which is bipolar cauterized and transected between its medial and lateral ends (#), are completely exposed. This enables inferolateral retraction of the periorbita and further removal of the medial bony remnant of the superior orbital roof (or) carefully up to the limit of the ethmoidal roof (er). **(g)** The wide opening achieved by this technique throughout which one can straightforwardly go deeper to the most lateral, inferior, and posterior portion of the lesion, exposing the anterior fossa dura (ad), middle fossa dura (md), and the inner periosteum of the temporalis muscle (T) enabling fine dissection on all surfaces and clefts. **(h)** Further close-up look to the extreme lateral border of resection, the inner surface of the pterional region of the skull, consisting of squamous portion of the temporal bone (TB), parietal bone (PB), frontal bone (FB), and greater wing of sphenoid bone (SB). One can also see the inner periosteum of the temporalis muscle (T) at areas where bone is completely eroded, as well as anterior (ad) and middle cranial fossa (md) dura and orbital roof periorbita (po) on the edges.

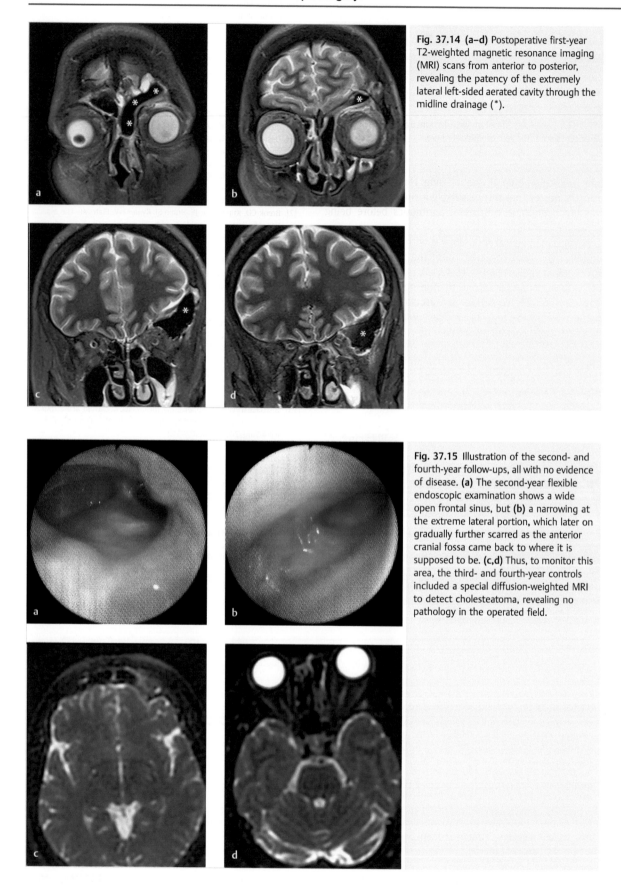

Fig. 37.14 (a–d) Postoperative first-year T2-weighted magnetic resonance imaging (MRI) scans from anterior to posterior, revealing the patency of the extremely lateral left-sided aerated cavity through the midline drainage (*).

Fig. 37.15 Illustration of the second- and fourth-year follow-ups, all with no evidence of disease. **(a)** The second-year flexible endoscopic examination shows a wide open frontal sinus, but **(b)** a narrowing at the extreme lateral portion, which later on gradually further scarred as the anterior cranial fossa came back to where it is supposed to be. **(c,d)** Thus, to monitor this area, the third- and fourth-year controls included a special diffusion-weighted MRI to detect cholesteatoma, revealing no pathology in the operated field.

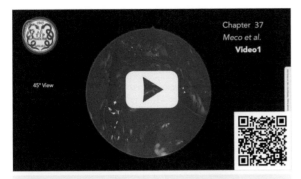

Video 37.1 Far lateral right frontal recurrent inverted papilloma.

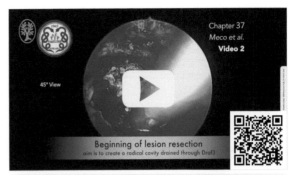

Video 37.2 Frontal cholesteatoma. Extending far lateral to middle cranial fossa and temporalis muscle.

techniques could offer more than lateral trephination of the frontal sinus and be a viable option in the spectrum of our armamentarium. On the other hand, with advanced EES applications, we are already capable of maintaining the patency of the frontal sinus outflow tract in the majority of patients, which in return allows postoperative endoscopic surveillance to monitor recurrent disease. Especially in benign tumor patients with essentially healthy mucosa, one may not want to lose this important advantage.

In the conquest of exploring the lateral limits of EES, although there are ongoing debates on management controversies and there exists no widespread consensus, we believe that the examples given in this chapter provide a good basis for understanding the considerable capability of endoscopic techniques to manage pathologies located at the far lateral frontal sinuses. In centers where adequate experience is accumulated in the existence of dedicated instrumentation and infrastructure, these advanced and sophisticated EES techniques offer us just an additional armamentarium in managing this difficult-to-reach area by overcoming accessibility issues.

It is also important to remember that external approaches today still establish the mainstream standard of care in most of the instances for addressing extreme far lateral lesions of the frontal sinuses. Nevertheless, in optimal conditions, advanced applications of EES could also offer comparable results to these while offering less morbidity. Without being dogmatic, it is our task to evaluate the advantages and disadvantages of all possible treatment options and target the optimal management for each specific patient and condition. At the end, each patient is unique regarding their sinus pneumatization pattern, frontal drainage pathway, and involvement and attachment site of their pathologies, in combination with the nature and biology of the specific disease process being treated, which as a whole clearly show the need for a personalized treatment protocol.

References

[1] Tato JM, Bergaglio OE. Surgery of frontal sinus. Fat grafts: new technique. Otolaryngologica. 1949; 3:1

[2] Hardy JM, Montgomery WW. Osteoplastic frontal sinusotomy: an analysis of 250 operations. Ann Otol Rhinol Laryngol. 1976; 85(4, Pt 1):523–532

[3] Weber R, Draf W, Keerl R, et al. Osteoplastic frontal sinus surgery with fat obliteration: technique and long-term results using magnetic resonance imaging in 82 operations. Laryngoscope. 2000; 110 (6):1037–1044

[4] Draf W. Endonasal micro-endoscopic frontal sinus surgery: the Fulda concept. Oper Tech Otolaryngol Head Neck Surg. 1991; 2:243–40

[5] Draf W. Endonasal sinus drainage type I–III. In: Kountakis S, Senior B, Draf W, eds. The Frontal Sinus. Berlin: Springer-Verlag; 2005:219–232

[6] Javer AR, Sillers MJ, Kuhn FA. The frontal sinus unobliteration procedure. Otolaryngol Clin North Am. 2001; 34(1):193–210

[7] Ketcham AS, Wilkins RH, Vanburen JM, Smith RR. A combined intracranial facial approach to the paranasal sinuses. Am J Surg. 1963; 106:698–703

[8] Raveh J, Laedrach K, Speiser M, et al. The subcranial approach for fronto-orbital and anteroposterior skull-base tumors. Arch Otolaryngol Head Neck Surg. 1993; 119(4):385–393

[9] Fliss DM, Zucker G, Cohen A, et al. Early outcome and complications of the extended subcranial approach to the anterior skull base. Laryngoscope. 1999; 109(1):153–160

[10] Ulualp SO, Carlson TK, Toohill RJ. Osteoplastic flap versus modified endoscopic Lothrop procedure in patients with frontal sinus disease. Am J Rhinol. 2000; 14(1):21–26

[11] Isa AY, Mennie J, McGarry GW. The frontal osteoplastic flap: does it still have a place in rhinological surgery? J Laryngol Otol. 2011; 125 (2):162–168

[12] Georgalas C, Fokkens W. Approaches to the frontal sinus. In: Georgalas C, Fokkens W, eds. Rhinology and Skull Base Surgery: From the lab to the operating room—an evidence based approach. New York, NY: Thieme Medical Publishers; 2013:376–409

[13] Lund VJ, Stammberger H, Nicolai P, et al. European Rhinologic Society Advisory Board on Endoscopic Techniques in the Management of Nose, Paranasal Sinus and Skull Base Tumours. European position paper on endoscopic management of tumours of the nose, paranasal sinuses and skull base. Rhinol Suppl. 2010; 22:1–143

[14] Bockmühl U, Kratzsch B, Benda K, Draf W. Paranasal sinus mucoceles: surgical management and long term results. Laryngorhinootologie. 2005; 84(12):892–898

[15] Chiu AG, Vaughan WC. Management of the lateral frontal sinus lesion and the supraorbital cell mucocele. Am J Rhinol. 2004; 18(2):83–86

[16] Anand VK, Hiltzik DH, Kacker A, Honrado C. Osteoplastic flap for frontal sinus obliteration in the era of image-guided endoscopic sinus surgery. Am J Rhinol. 2005; 19(4):406–410

[17] Sama A, McClelland L, Constable J. Frontal sinus mucocoeles: new algorithm for surgical management. Rhinology. 2014; 52(3):267–275

[18] Schick B, Steigerwald C, el Rahman el Tahan A, Draf W. The role of endonasal surgery in the management of frontoethmoidal osteomas. Rhinology. 2001; 39(2):66–70

[19] Chiu AG, Schipor I, Cohen NA, Kennedy DW, Palmer JN. Surgical decisions in the management of frontal sinus osteomas. Am J Rhinol. 2005; 19(2):191–197

[20] Bignami M, Dallan I, Terranova P, Battaglia P, Miceli S, Castelnuovo P. Frontal sinus osteomas: the window of endonasal endoscopic approach. Rhinology. 2007; 45(4):315–320

[21] Seiberling K, Floreani S, Robinson S, Wormald PJ. Endoscopic management of frontal sinus osteomas revisited. Am J Rhinol Allergy. 2009; 23(3):331–336

[22] Ledderose GJ, Betz CS, Stelter K, Leunig A. Surgical management of osteomas of the frontal recess and sinus: extending the limits of the endoscopic approach. Eur Arch Otorhinolaryngol. 2011; 268(4):525–532

[23] Rokade A, Sama A. Update on management of frontal sinus osteomas. Curr Opin Otolaryngol Head Neck Surg. 2012; 20(1):40–44

[24] Georgalas C, Goudakos J, Fokkens WJ. Osteoma of the skull base and sinuses. Otolaryngol Clin North Am. 2011; 44(4):875–890, vii

[25] Turri-Zanoni M, Dallan I, Terranova P, et al. Frontoethmoidal and intraorbital osteomas: exploring the limits of the endoscopic approach. Arch Otolaryngol Head Neck Surg. 2012; 138(5):498–504

[26] Minovi A, Kollert M, Draf W, Bockmühl U. Inverted papilloma: feasibility of endonasal surgery and long-term results of 87 cases. Rhinology. 2006; 44(3):205–210

[27] Carta F, Verillaud B, Herman P. Role of endoscopic approach in the management of inverted papilloma. Curr Opin Otolaryngol Head Neck Surg. 2011; 19(1):21–24

[28] Lombardi D, Tomenzoli D, Buttà L, et al. Limitations and complications of endoscopic surgery for treatment for sinonasal inverted papilloma: a reassessment after 212 cases. Head Neck. 2011; 33(8):1154–1161

[29] Selleck AM, Desai D, Thorp BD, Ebert CS, Zanation AM. Management of frontal sinus tumors. Otolaryngol Clin North Am. 2016; 49(4):1051–1065

[30] Woodworth BA, Schlosser RJ, Palmer JN. Endoscopic repair of frontal sinus cerebrospinal fluid leaks. J Laryngol Otol. 2005; 119(9):709–713

[31] Anverali JK, Hassaan AA, Saleh HA. Endoscopic modified Lothrop procedure for repair of lateral frontal sinus cerebrospinal fluid leak. J Laryngol Otol. 2009; 123(1):145–147

[32] Becker SS, Duncavage JA, Russell PT. Endoscopic endonasal repair of difficult-to-access cerebrospinal fluid leaks of the frontal sinus. Am J Rhinol Allergy. 2009; 23(2):181–184

[33] Purkey MT, Woodworth BA, Hahn S, Palmer JN, Chiu AG. Endoscopic repair of supraorbital ethmoid cerebrospinal fluid leaks. ORL J Otorhinolaryngol Relat Spec. 2009; 71(2):93–98

[34] Jones V, Virgin F, Riley K, Woodworth BA. Changing paradigms in frontal sinus cerebrospinal fluid leak repair. Int Forum Allergy Rhinol. 2012; 2(3):227–232

[35] Illing EA, Woodworth BA. Management of frontal sinus cerebrospinal fluid leaks and encephaloceles. Otolaryngol Clin North Am. 2016; 49(4):1035–1050

[36] Grayson JW, Jeyarajan H, Illing EA, Cho D-Y, Riley KO, Woodworth BA. Changing the surgical dogma in frontal sinus trauma: transnasal endoscopic repair. Int Forum Allergy Rhinol. 2017; 7(5):441–449

[37] Conger BT, Jr, Illing E, Bush B, Woodworth BA. Management of lateral frontal sinus pathology in the endoscopic era. Otolaryngol Head Neck Surg. 2014; 151(1):159–163

[38] Becker SS, Bomeli SR, Gross CW, Han JK. Limits of endoscopic visualization and instrumentation in the frontal sinus. Otolaryngol Head Neck Surg. 2006; 135(6):917–921

[39] Timperley DG, Banks C, Robinson D, Roth J, Sacks R, Harvey RJ. Lateral frontal sinus access in endoscopic skull-base surgery. Int Forum Allergy Rhinol. 2011; 1(4):290–295

[40] Harvey RJ, Sheahan PO, Schlosser RJ. Surgical management of benign sinonasal masses. Otolaryngol Clin North Am. 2009; 42(2):353–375

[41] Lim JH, Sardesai MG, Ferreira M, Jr, Moe KS. Transorbital neuroendoscopic management of sinogenic complications involving the frontal sinus, orbit, and anterior cranial fossa. J Neurol Surg B Skull Base. 2012; 73(6):394–400

[42] Kopelovich JC, Baker MS, Potash A, Desai L, Allen RC, Chang EH. The hybrid lid crease approach to address lateral frontal sinus disease with orbital extension. Ann Otol Rhinol Laryngol. 2014; 123(12):826–830

[43] Mulazimoglu S, Basak H, Tezcaner ZC, Meco BC, Beton S, Meco C. Endonasal endoscopic management of giant frontal sinus and supraorbital cholesteatoma extending far back to the middle fossa and temporal muscle. In: Stammberger H, Mokry M, eds. Jahrestagung der Gesellschaft für Schädelbasischirurgie Programm and Abstract Book. Vienna: GSB; 2014:59

[44] Poczos P, Kurbanov A, Keller JT, Zimmer LA. Medial and superior orbital decompression: improving access for endonasal endoscopic frontal sinus surgery. Ann Otol Rhinol Laryngol. 2015; 124(12):987–995

[45] Lynch RC. The technique of a radical frontal sinus operation which has given me the best results. Laryngoscope. 1921; 31(1):1–5

[46] Nicolai P, Tomenzoli D, Lombardi D, Maroldi R. Different endoscopic options in the treatment of inverted papilloma. Op Tech Otolaryngol.. 2006; 17(2):80–86

[47] Karligkiotis A, Pistochini A, Turri-Zanoni M, et al. Endoscopic endonasal orbital transposition to expand the frontal sinus approaches. Am J Rhinol Allergy. 2015; 29(6):449–456

[48] Liu JK, Mendelson ZS, Dubal PM, Mirani N, Eloy JA. The modified hemi-Lothrop procedure: a variation of the endoscopic endonasal approach for resection of a supraorbital psammomatoid ossifying fibroma. J Clin Neurosci. 2014; 21(12):2233–2238

[49] Meco C, Beton S, Basak H, et al. Periorbital suspension for management of far lateral frontal sinus lesions. Rhinology. 2016; 54 Suppl 25:397

[50] Meco C, Beton S, Basak H, et al. Periorbital suspension for endonasal endoscopic access to the lateral portion of the frontal anterior skull base. J Neurol Surg B Skull Base. 2017; 78 Suppl S1:S68–S69

38 Use of Image Guidance Technology: Mandatory or Not

Judd H. Fastenberg, Marvin P. Fried, and Waleed M. Abuzeid

Abstract

Image-guided surgery (IGS) is an important adjunct tool that may help surgeons perform safer and more comprehensive frontal sinus surgery. IGS is not a substitute for sound knowledge of anatomy, critical decision-making, or technical expertise. However, for well-trained otolaryngologists, it may help increase surgeon confidence and reduce fear of misadventure into hazardous areas such as the orbit and brain. Although the technology has become commonplace throughout the United States and Europe, the use of IGS is not mandatory or the standard of care and should be used on a case-by-case basis at the discretion of the operating surgeon. Continued research is necessary to define the impact of IGS on patient outcomes and cost, as well as to guide meaningful use of the technology moving forward.

Keywords: frontal sinus, image guidance, navigation, rhinosinusitis

38.1 Introduction

Image-guided surgery (IGS) represents one of the most significant advances in sinus surgery since the inception of the endoscopic approach in the mid-1980s. The technology was initially developed for neurosurgery in the late 1980s[1,2] with its first use in endoscopic sinus surgery (ESS) occurring in 1994 as described by Anon and colleagues.[3] Since that time, the use of IGS has expanded dramatically across multiple surgical specialties, though ESS represents a leading indication for the use of the technology. Whereas IGS was initially employed only by tertiary referral centers for revision or complex sinus cases in which the distortion of anatomy was anticipated, systems can now be found in hospitals and ambulatory surgery centers throughout the United States and Europe.[4] There has been a concurrent development in surgeon experience and comfort with the use of IGS leading to the implementation of this technology in a greater percentage of cases.[5,6]

Image guidance systems for ESS may be either electromagnetic or optically based. Systems typically consist of a computer workstation, a tracking system, and specially designed navigation instruments for use during surgery. Computed tomography (CT) scans, which are more commonly used in ESS, are typically noncontrast and formatted in the axial plane with 1 mm or thinner cuts. Magnetic resonance (MR) images can also be acquired as high-resolution axial cuts and these images are merged with the CT scan axial images to maximize bone and soft-tissue detail. The patient's imaging is loaded preoperatively and then calibrated to the patient just before beginning surgery. Once registered correctly, the intraoperative location of navigation instruments is displayed in real time on the patients imaging in the axial, coronal, and sagittal planes. Several systems are commercially available for purchase.

38.1.1 Indications

To date, there are no explicit guidelines for the use of IGS in ESS. Since 2002, the American Academy of Otolaryngology - Head and Neck Surgery's position statement has endorsed IGS for complex procedures involving the paranasal sinuses or skull base at the discretion of the operating surgeon.[7] Importantly, the use of IGS is *not* considered the standard of care and is recommended as an option that should be based on clinical judgment and applied on a case-by-case basis. The academy lists seven relative indications for use of IGS. This includes pathology involving the frontal sinus, as well as distorted anatomy, revision cases, and disease abutting the skull base (▶ Table 38.1).

The frontal sinus is widely considered the most technically demanding sinus to address during ESS. This is due to the complex anatomy of the sinus, the acute nasofrontal angle, as well as the proximity to critical structures such as the orbit, skull base, olfactory fossa, and orbit. Distorted anatomy that is the result of chronic inflammation or previous surgery may also contribute to technical difficulty and increased risk of complications during frontal sinus surgery.[8] In a survey administered by the American Rhinologic Society in 2010, 71% of otolaryngologists responded that they regarded primary frontal sinus exploration as a relative or absolute indication for IGS. This percentage increased to 96 and 98% for revision frontal sinus exploration and modified Lothrop procedures, respectively.[5]

Table 38.1 Position statement: Intraoperative use of computer-aided surgery (approved 2002, revised 2014)[7]

Indications for use of image-guided surgery
1. Revision sinus surgery
2. Distorted sinus anatomy of development, postoperative, or traumatic origin
3. Extensive sinonasal polyposis
4. Pathology involving the *frontal*, posterior ethmoid, and sphenoid sinuses
5. Disease abutting the skull base, orbit, optic nerve, or carotid artery
6. CSF rhinorrhea or conditions where there is a skull base defect
7. Benign and malignant sinonasal neoplasms

Abbreviation: CSF, cerebrospinal fluid.

38.1.2 Applications

IGS has applications for both endoscopic and external approaches to the frontal sinus. Importantly, the technology should not be relied upon in submillimeter decision-making near critical structures since current IGS platforms are only accurate to within 2 mm.[9]

In regard to the endoscopic approach, IGS facilitates maximizing the dimensions of the frontal sinusotomy by promoting a more complete frontal dissection during ESS. Using navigation instruments, intraoperative localization can help avoid the misidentification of structures such as frontal cells, supraorbital ethmoid cells, and agger nasi cells for the frontal recess or sinus—errors that may contribute to primary surgical failure.[10] Indeed, IGS may often facilitate the complete dissection of the aforementioned structures. IGS may also be used to define final frontal recess dimensions during extended procedures such as Draf IIa, IIb, and III frontal sinusotomy, during which localization of critical anatomic structures such as the orbit, skull base, and vascular structures including the anterior ethmoid artery is particularly important.[8] The Draf III sinusotomy, specifically, is performed in a select patient population whose sinonasal anatomy is commonly distorted due to multiple prior surgeries and ongoing sinonasal inflammation. As a result, during this procedure, IGS may be especially helpful to the surgeon in identifying important anatomy and defining the full extent of the nasofrontal beak, therefore assisting in the safe and efficient opening of a wide Lothrop cavity.[11]

While advances in endoscopy have led to a general decrease in the use of external approaches to the frontal sinus, procedures such as frontal sinus trephination and osteoplastic flaps may still play a role in the treatment of certain disease processes. The most common scenario in this regard is a lesion involving the superior or lateral frontal sinus that is inaccessible by endoscopic approach. As opposed to using surface anatomy alone, IGS may be used to design a precise frontal sinus trephination through which a surgeon may introduce endoscopes and instruments into the frontal sinus to accurately target lesions such as fibro-osseous lesions, lateral mucoceles, or type III or IV frontal cells. This may be done as part of either an external-only or a combined open and endoscopic "above-and-below" approach. The increased accuracy afforded by IGS has likely expanded the utility of trephination, helping many patients to avoid the morbidity of traditional osteoplastic flaps, and has allowed for the approach to be used in other procedures such as frontal sinus obliteration, treatment of posterior table fractures, lateral frontal sinus biopsies, as well as intersinus septectomies, which some have described as a method to address unilateral frontal sinus disease by diverting drainage to the contralateral outflow tract.[12]

When an osteoplastic flap is necessary, IGS may similarly be used to map out the bony edges of the sinus prior to cutting into bone.[13] This increased precision helps minimize the high risk of complications with frontal bony cuts, including dural exposure, dural injury with CSF leak, and orbital fat exposure, as well as ensuring that the osteoplastic flap is as large as safely possible to ensure a greater chance of surgical success.[8,14,15] Mapping with IGS has been found to be more accurate and quicker than other techniques, such as 6-foot Caldwell radiography and transillumination.[16]

38.2 Published Evidence

Several studies directed at IGS use in ESS have been performed to analyze associated complication rates, revision rates, patient quality-of-life outcomes, cost, and medicolegal aspects of care.[17,18,19,20,21,22,23] The majority of these studies do not focus on frontal sinus surgery, specifically. Despite this breadth of research efforts, there is still a general paucity of high-level evidence. The 2016 International Consensus Statement on Rhinosinusitis determined the aggregate grade of evidence to be "D."[24] Two important factors that have limited IGS-related research are the need for large sample sizes and ethical issues affecting study accrual. Power analyses have indicated that, to show a statistical difference in complication rates with IGS, for example, thousands of subjects would need to be prospectively enrolled.[25] Furthermore, if a surgeon feels that IGS is indicated for a particular patient based on his or her expert opinion, it would present a significant ethical issue to randomize that patient away from IGS in a prospective trial.[26]

38.2.1 Complications

While the potential for safer surgery with IGS is clear, the findings of several studies investigating complication rates with IGS during ESS have been inconsistent. A 2013 evidence-based review by Ramakrishnan and colleagues demonstrated that the use of IGS has not clearly been shown to decrease surgical complications or improve surgical outcomes.[21] Based on this review, there was determined to be a preponderance of benefit versus harm based on C-level quality of evidence, making the use of IGS for reduction of complications an "option." Importantly, the authors noted that study design limitations may have contributed to a lack of significant findings. A different meta-analyses of 13 relevant studies reported that IGS may contribute to a decreased rate of major complications and total complications when the data were pooled.[23]

38.2.2 Revision Rate

The impact of IGS on revision rates is similarly unclear. In 2002, Fried and colleagues reviewed 160 subjects and demonstrated a significantly higher need for revision surgery among those in the non-IGS group as compared to the IGS group.[17] These findings run in contrast to a similar study published a year earlier, as well as two more recent meta-analyses, all of which found no significant difference in revision rates with and without IGS.[19,23,27]

38.2.3 Clinical and Quality-of-Life Outcomes

Several studies have compared subject quality-of-life outcomes after ESS with and without the use of IGS.[8] A retrospective chart review by Tabaee and colleagues found no difference in the 20-item sinonasal outcome test (SNOT-20) scores at least 6 months after sinus surgery.[22] A second prospective, nonrandomized study demonstrated improved 31-item Rhinosinusitis Outcome Measure (RSOM-31) scores 6 months after ESS with IGS.[18] However, a similar study demonstrated no difference in visual analog scale (VAS) scores 12 months after surgery.[25] Importantly, a tendency to use IGS for more complex cases may offer an explanation for these inconsistent findings.

38.2.4 Medicolegal Concerns

As with many new technologies, questions exist regarding the medicolegal ramifications of IGS. For example, although IGS is not explicitly described as the standard of care for sinus surgery, it is unclear whether recovery is more likely against a surgeon with a complication who did not use the technology. Although a 2013 study by Eloy and colleagues showed that the use of IGS did not contribute to ESS litigation or outcomes from 2004 to 2013, there is a general paucity of literature regarding this topic.[20]

38.2.5 Cost

Last but not least, IGS has been shown to increase the overall cost of ESS. A 2001 study by Gibbons and colleagues demonstrated that IGS was, on average, 6.7% more expensive than similar non-IGS surgeries.[19] This is due to the cost of the navigation system, the need for additional equipment, and added operative time, although this may be secondary to the time needed to set up the guidance system in the beginning of the case.[28] Despite this increased cost, taking into consideration the potential reduction in need for revision surgery, IGS may, in fact, reduce the overall cost of care.[29]

38.3 Controversies and Opinions

IGS is an important adjunct tool that may help surgeons perform safer and more comprehensive frontal sinus surgery. IGS is not a substitute for sound knowledge of anatomy, critical decision-making, or technical expertise. However, for well-trained otolaryngologists, it may help increase surgeon confidence and reduce fear of misadventure into hazardous areas such as the orbit and brain.

38.3.1 Indications

Although the technology has become commonplace throughout the United States and Europe, the use of IGS is not mandatory or the standard of care and should be used on a case-by-case basis at the discretion of the operating surgeon. It is the authors' opinion that the technology is best utilized for cases involving complex pathology or distorted frontal sinus anatomy, such as revision cases or Lothrop cavities. Triplanar navigation views for **Patient 1** and **Patient 2** (see ▶ Fig. 38.1 and ▶ Fig. 38.2), who had a left anterior ethmoid osteoma obstructing the left frontal sinus outflow tract and a biethmoidal and bifrontal inverting papilloma requiring a Draf III sinusotomy, respectively, are two such examples. It is imperative that surgeons not rely on IGS alone for critical decision-making and maintain proficiency with alternative skills.

38.3.2 Surgical Training

The potential harm of IGS is relatively limited. However, it is important to consider the potential impact of the technology on surgical training. Care must be taken to ensure that new surgical trainees do not become over-reliant on IGS and, consequently, less proficient in alternative techniques that may be necessary if the technology malfunctions or is unavailable during surgery.

The technique of ESS lies in the hands of the surgeon performing the procedure. As the region of the frontal recess and sinuses is complex, the surgeon supervising the trainee can have a better appreciation of the anatomy and procedure as it progresses. Navigation thus becomes critical to the training process.

38.3.3 Future Use

With several technological improvements with navigation on the horizon, it is the authors' opinion that use of IGS will continue to expand in frontal sinus surgery. For example, future image guidance systems may have the ability to update in real time, removing tissue from the displayed scan as the surgeon resects the corresponding anatomy. Recent developments also permit the surgeon to trace the proposed route of dissection to the frontal recess on triplanar images, and to have this route superimposed on the endoscopic view to "guide" the dissection. Specialized navigation instruments, including guidewires that precisely confirm balloon positioning and flexible suctions, are already available. This may contribute to increased applications for IGS in office-based rhinology procedures.

38.4 Unanswered Questions

Despite considerable effort, the true impact of IGS is still largely unknown. As suggested by the inconsistent and often conflicting study findings described in the

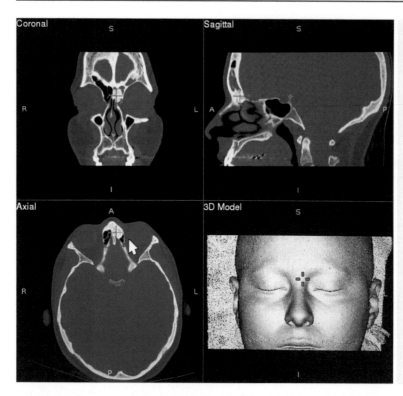

Fig. 38.1 Patient 1: Triplanar navigation view of a left anterior ethmoid osteoma obstructing the left frontal sinus outflow tract.

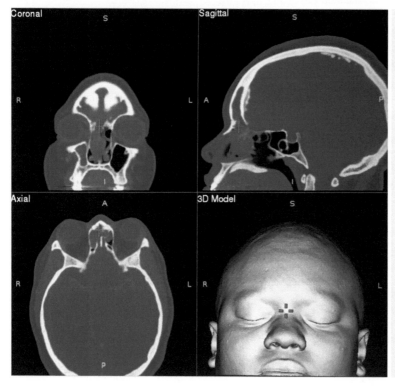

Fig. 38.2 Patient 2: Triplanar navigation view of a large bifrontal, biethmoidal inverted papilloma treated with a Draf III sinusotomy.

"Published Evidence" section of this chapter, continued research is necessary to define the significance of IGS to surgical outcomes, quality-of-life outcomes, complications, revision rates, cost, medicolegal issues, surgeon confidence, and surgical training, as well as to guide use of the technology in the future.

References

[1] Roberts DW, Strohbehn JW, Hatch JF, Murray W, Kettenberger H. A frameless stereotaxic integration of computerized tomographic imaging and the operating microscope. J Neurosurg. 1986; 65(4):545–549

[2] Friets EM, Strohbehn JW, Hatch JF, Roberts DW. A frameless stereotaxic operating microscope for neurosurgery. IEEE Trans Biomed Eng. 1989; 36(6):608–617

[3] Anon JB, Lipman SP, Oppenheim D, Halt RA. Computer-assisted endoscopic sinus surgery. Laryngoscope. 1994; 104(7):901–905

[4] Fried MP, Parikh SR, Sadoughi B. Image-guidance for endoscopic sinus surgery. Laryngoscope. 2008; 118(7):1287–1292

[5] Justice JM, Orlandi RR. An update on attitudes and use of image-guided surgery. Int Forum Allergy Rhinol. 2012; 2(2):155–159

[6] Orlandi RR, Petersen E. Image guidance: a survey of attitudes and use. Am J Rhinol. 2006; 20(4):406–411

[7] AAO-HNS. Position Statement: Intra-Operative Use of Computer Aided Surgery. 2014. Available at: http://www.entnet.org/content/intra-operative-use-computer-aided-surgery. Accessed October 1, 2016

[8] Oakley GM, Barham HP, Harvey RJ. Utility of image-guidance in frontal sinus surgery. Otolaryngol Clin North Am. 2016; 49(4):975–988

[9] Metson R, Gliklich RE, Cosenza M. A comparison of image guidance systems for sinus surgery. Laryngoscope. 1998; 108(8, Pt 1):1164–1170

[10] Chiu AG, Vaughan WC. Revision endoscopic frontal sinus surgery with surgical navigation. Otolaryngol Head Neck Surg. 2004; 130 (3):312–318

[11] Anderson P, Sindwani R. Safety and efficacy of the endoscopic modified Lothrop procedure: a systematic review and meta-analysis. Laryngoscope. 2009; 119(9):1828–1833

[12] Sowerby LJ, MacNeil SD, Wright ED. Endoscopic frontal sinus septectomy in the treatment of unilateral frontal sinusitis: revisiting an open technique. J Otolaryngol Head Neck Surg. 2009; 38(6):652–654

[13] Carrau RL, Snyderman CH, Curtin HB, Weissman JL. Computer-assisted frontal sinusotomy. Otolaryngol Head Neck Surg. 1994; 111 (6):727–732

[14] Hardy JM, Montgomery WW. Osteoplastic frontal sinusotomy: an analysis of 250 operations. Ann Otol Rhinol Laryngol. 1976; 85(4, Pt 1):523–532

[15] Sindwani R, Metson R. Impact of image guidance on complications during osteoplastic frontal sinus surgery. Otolaryngol Head Neck Surg. 2004; 131(3):150–155

[16] Melroy CT, Dubin MG, Hardy SM, Senior BA. Analysis of methods to assess frontal sinus extent in osteoplastic flap surgery: transillumination versus 6-ft Caldwell versus image guidance. Am J Rhinol. 2006; 20(1):77–83

[17] Fried MP, Moharir VM, Shin J, Taylor-Becker M, Morrison P. Comparison of endoscopic sinus surgery with and without image guidance. Am J Rhinol. 2002; 16(4):193–197

[18] Javer AR, Genoway KA. Patient quality of life improvements with and without computer assistance in sinus surgery: outcomes study. J Otolaryngol. 2006; 35(6):373–379

[19] Gibbons MD, Gunn CG, Niwas S, Sillers MJ. Cost analysis of computer-aided endoscopic sinus surgery. Am J Rhinol. 2001; 15(2):71–75

[20] Eloy JA, Svider PF, D'Aguillo CM, Baredes S, Setzen M, Folbe AJ. Image-guidance in endoscopic sinus surgery: is it associated with decreased medicolegal liability? Int Forum Allergy Rhinol. 2013; 3(12):980–985

[21] Ramakrishnan VR, Orlandi RR, Citardi MJ, Smith TL, Fried MP, Kingdom TT. The use of image-guided surgery in endoscopic sinus surgery: an evidence-based review with recommendations. Int Forum Allergy Rhinol. 2013; 3(3):236–241

[22] Tabaee A, Hsu AK, Shrime MG, Rickert S, Close LG. Quality of life and complications following image-guided endoscopic sinus surgery. Otolaryngol Head Neck Surg. 2006; 135(1):76–80

[23] Dalgorf DM, Sacks R, Wormald PJ, et al. Image-guided surgery influences perioperative morbidity from endoscopic sinus surgery: a systematic review and meta-analysis. Otolaryngol Head Neck Surg. 2013; 149(1):17–29

[24] Orlandi RR, Kingdom TT, Hwang PH. International consensus statement on allergy and rhinology: rhinosinusitis executive summary. Int Forum Allergy Rhinol. 2016; 6 Suppl 1:S3–S21

[25] Tschopp KP, Thomaser EG. Outcome of functional endonasal sinus surgery with and without CT-navigation. Rhinology. 2008; 46 (2):116–120

[26] Smith TL, Stewart MG, Orlandi RR, Setzen M, Lanza DC. Indications for image-guided sinus surgery: the current evidence. Am J Rhinol. 2007; 21(1):80–83

[27] Sunkaraneni VS, Yeh D, Qian H, Javer AR. Computer or not? Use of image guidance during endoscopic sinus surgery for chronic rhinosinusitis at St Paul's Hospital, Vancouver, and meta-analysis. J Laryngol Otol. 2013; 127(4):368–377

[28] Reardon EJ. Navigational risks associated with sinus surgery and the clinical effects of implementing a navigational system for sinus surgery. Laryngoscope. 2002; 112(7, Pt 2) Suppl 99:1–19

[29] Masterson L, Agalato E, Pearson C. Image-guided sinus surgery: practical and financial experiences from a UK centre 2001–2009. J Laryngol Otol. 2012; 126(12):1224–1230

39 Balloon Technology in the Frontal Sinus: Useful or Gimmick

Claire Hopkins and Roland Hettige

Abstract

Since the inception of sinus ostial balloon dilatation in 2005, there has been a fivefold increase in the number of frontal sinus procedures in the United States, although the overall rates of sinus surgery remain relatively stable. Most outcome studies using balloon techniques have selected patients with limited sinus disease without nasal polyps; in these groups, outcomes appear to be comparable to endoscopic sinus surgery (ESS) and the technique may facilitate surgery in an office setting without general anesthesia. The role of balloon dilatation in the presence of nasal polyps or more extensive sinus disease remains unclear. There is no role for the use of the technology in the setting of a patient with a normal sinus computed tomography (CT) scan.

Keywords: balloon dilatation, minimally invasive sinus techniques, office-based procedures

39.1 Published Evidence

As case series of balloon sinus procedures started to emerge in the published literature, certain bodies tasked with commissioning these rhinological procedures argued that level 4 evidence alone could not be used to form conclusions regarding the comparative efficacy of balloon sinuplasty (BSP) to functional endoscopic sinus surgery (FESS). Conflict occurred when the procedure was marketed directly to consumers at a time when many believed the technology was yet unproven.[1] The small, nonblinded, nonrandomized clinical studies (e.g., the CLinical Evaluation to confirm sAfety and efficacy of sinuplasty in the paRanasal sinuses or CLEAR study)[2] were criticized for their apparent methodological flaws,[3,4,5,6,7,8,9,10,11,12,13] which left insufficient comparative follow-up data on ostial patency and health outcomes.[14]

Therefore, in this section, the authors analyze the evidence from systematic reviews, randomized controlled trials (RCTs), and nonrandomized comparative trials in greater detail.

39.1.1 Level 1 Evidence

One systematic review conducted in 2012 entitled "Balloon sinus ostial dilation for treatment of chronic rhinosinusitis"[14] reviewed evidence from one RCT, three nonrandomized comparative studies, and nine case series. It concluded that the evidence was insufficient to determine the effect of balloon technology on outcomes, citing that the randomized clinical trial comparing BSP to FESS was inadequately powered and did not evaluate differences in outcomes between the two treatments.

A Cochrane review on balloon sinus dilatation published in 2011,[15] containing only one small RCT,[9] noted at the time that there was insufficient evidence to recommend balloon dilation over conventional ESS. However, the same conclusion was also relevant to the 2014 Cochrane review comparing medical with surgical intervention for chronic rhinosinusitis (CRS)[16]; at that time, there was insufficient level 1 evidence to demonstrate benefit of any sinus surgery over medical treatment.

Batra et al, in 2011, performed a comprehensive literature review regarding balloon catheter technology in rhinology[17] and noted that the significant study design flaws from the available studies prevented the pooling of effectiveness data. Even though the largest published observational cohort studies demonstrated the ability to achieve ostia patency for up to 2 years, because the selection criteria for these studies were not clearly defined, it was not possible to extrapolate these data reliably to the general population with CRS.

With regard to stand-alone RCTs, the Randomized Evaluation of Maxillary Antrostomy versus Ostial Dilation Efficacy through Long-Term Follow-Up (REMODEL) trial was an industry-sponsored, multicentered effort, comparing stand-alone in-office balloon dilation with traditional ESS under general anesthesia (GA) with follow-up between 1 and 2 years for patients with CRS recalcitrant to medical therapy.[18] A total of 105 patients with recurrent acute sinusitis or chronic sinusitis in whom maximal medical therapy had failed were randomized to balloon ostial dilation or FESS. Balloon ostial dilation was performed with the Entellus device. FESS consisted of maxillary antrostomy and uncinectomy with or without anterior ethmoidectomy. The primary outcomes were the change in the 20-Item Sinonasal Outcome Test (SNOT-20) score at 6-month follow-up, and the mean number of debridements performed postoperatively. Secondary outcomes included recovery time, complication rates, and rates of revision surgery.

REMODEL was a statistically powered trial (sufficient to detect group differences) that demonstrated noninferiority of balloon dilation to ESS for improvement of symptoms of CRS using the SNOT-20, and superiority of balloon dilation over ESS for a reduction in postoperative debridements (0.1 vs. 1.2 per patient, $p < 0.0001$). A total of 135 patients were treated in the study, of which 130 (96%) were followed to 1 year postprocedure.

Secondary endpoints demonstrated that balloon dilation and ESS resulted in similar rates of ostial patency, revision surgery, complications, and reduction in the number of rhinosinusitis episodes. Work productivity was also improved similarly after balloon dilation and ESS. Moreover, patients who underwent balloon dilation

Table 39.1 Main Outcomes of Randomized Evaluation of Maxillary Antrostomy versus Ostial Dilation Efficacy through Long-Term Follow-Up (REMODEL) randomized controlled trial (RCT)

Overall outcomes	Balloon dilation (mean or %)	FESS (mean or %)	p value	Balloon dilation vs. FESS
Primary endpoints				
1-y change in SNOT-20	−1.59	−1.60	< 0.001	Balloon dilation non-inferior to FESS
Number of debridements per patient	0.2	1	< 0.00-01	Balloon dilation superior to FESS
Secondary outcomes (recovery and short term)				
Technical success	99.3%	99.4%	NS	No significant difference between study arms
Patients discharged with nasal bleeding	32%	56%	0.009	Balloon dilation significantly better than FESS
Recovery time (d)	1.7	5	< 0.00-01	Balloon dilation significantly better than FESS
Duration of prescription of pain medications (d)	1.0	2.8	< 0.00-01	Balloon dilation significantly better than FESS
Secondary outcomes (1 y)				
Change in number of rhinosinusitis episodes per patient	−4.2	−3.7	NS	No significant difference between study arms
Ostial patency	91.9%	97.4%	NS	No significant difference between study arms
Mean reduction of activity impairment due to CRS	68%	76%	NS	No significant difference between study arms
Mean reduction in overall work impairment due to CRS	72%	80%	NS	No significant difference between study arms
Complications	0%	0%	NS	No significant difference between study arms
Revision surgery rate	1.4%	1.6%	NS	No significant difference between study arms

Abbreviations: CRS, chronic rhinosinusitis; FESS, functional endoscopic sinus surgery; SNOT-20, 20-Item Sinonasal Outcome Test.

had faster recovery times (1.6 vs. 4.8 days, *p* = 0.001), less postoperative nasal bleeding, and shorter duration of prescription pain medication use compared with the patients who underwent ESS (*p* = 0.001; see ▶ Table 39.1 for the main outcomes of the REMODEL trial).

This RCT addressed many of the previously noted limitations in the body of evidence for balloon sinus dilation. Critics stated, however, that the trial was unblinded and did not have blinded outcome assessment for the symptom-based outcomes or the secondary clinical outcomes.[14] There was also some evidence of differential dropout, with larger numbers of patients withdrawing from the FESS group following randomization (21 vs. 4%).

The authors of the REMODEL trial also reported a meta-analysis conducted on patient-level data from 358 patients (846 sinuses) who had undergone stand-alone balloon dilation for medical recalcitrant CRS, again with follow-up periods of up to 2 years[18] (see ▶ Table 39.2). The results of this meta-analysis of six stand-alone balloon dilation studies demonstrated that balloon dilation resulted in

statistically significant and clinically meaningful improvements in sinus symptoms that were durable up to 2 years after treatment. The meta-analysis also confirmed the REMODEL results with regard to the benefits of quick recovery time, low rates of postoperative debridement, and a shorter duration for use of prescription pain medications in patients undergoing balloon dilation.

Additional outcomes showing statistically significant improvements after balloon dilation were reductions in workdays/school days missed, homebound days, physician/nurse visits for sinus problems, acute infections, and antibiotic courses. Procedural pain scores were low, demonstrating high tolerance for the procedure, when performed under local anesthesia (LA). The revision surgery rate was not statistically different from that observed in either arm of the REMODEL trial. Clearly, there now existed statistically powered level 1 evidence supporting the safety and efficacy of balloon dilation compared with the standard of care (ESS) for patients with medically recalcitrant CRS.

Table 39.2 Main outcomes from meta-analyses of standalone balloon sinus dilation studies

Trials and patient numbers	Patient population and study design	Key findings

358 adult patients (846 sinuses) from 6 clinical studies:
• *REMODEL RCT*
• *XprESS MultiSinus*
• *XprESS Maxillary Pilot*
• *RELIEF*
• *FinESS Registry*
• *BREATHE*
	Multicenter (38 distinct sites):
	• Patients with chronic or recurrent acute uncomplicated rhinosinusitis who met criteria for medically necessary FESS and underwent standalone balloon dilation with Entellus devices
	• Follow-up (FU) from 6 mo to 2 y based on study protocols
	• Outcomes:
	  - Technical success
	  - Change in sinus symptoms (20-Item Sinonasal Outcome Test [SNOT-20])
	  - Postoperative debridements per patient
	  - Revision rates
	  - Recovery outcomes
	  - Procedural pain
	  - Health care utilization
	  - Work limitations
	• No differences in patient baseline characteristics between studies
	• Some outcomes compared with REMODEL FESS arm ($n = 61$)
		1-y FU compliance: 93.2% (314/337); 18-mo compliance: 100% (37/37); 2-y compliance: 96.1% (74/77)
		Results:
		• Technical success: 97.5% (825/846 sinuses)
		• Changes in symptom scores (mean SNOT-20) from baseline were statistically significant and clinically meaningful (≥ 8) at all FU time periods and not statistically different from FESS
		• Symptom improvement was maintained from 1-wk through 2-y FU
		• Mean number of debridements/patient = 0.16
		• No statistically significant difference in 12-mo revision rates (REMODEL 1.4%, meta-analysis 5 pooled studies 3.2%) compared with FESS (1.7%)
		• Recovery time (return to normal daily activities) = 1.4 d
		• Patients discharged with nasal bleeding = 13.8%
		• Patients with postoperative nausea = 12.7%
		• Duration of prescription pain medication use = 0.8 d
		• Duration of OTC pain medication use = 1.5 d
		• Procedure pain = 2.6 on scale of 0 (no pain) to 10
		• RSI: statistically significant improvements ($p < 0.0001$) in missed work/school days, homebound days, MD/nurse visits, acute infections, and antibiotic courses at 1 y after compared with 1 y preceding balloon dilation
		• Work limitations questionnaire: statistically significant improvements from baseline in 4 of 5 domains (time management, mental/interpersonal, output, and productivity loss) through 2-y FU
		Subgroup analyses:
		• Statistically significant ($p < 0.0001$) and clinically meaningful (≥ 8) change in SNOT-20 scores from baseline to 12-mo FU for patients with:
		  - CRS ($n = 191$) and RARS ($n = 52$)
		  - With ($n = 97$) and without ($n = 211$) ethmoid disease
		• No differences between subgroups
		1-y FU compliance: 96.3% (130/135; 18-mo compliance: 100% (66/66); 24-mo compliance: 100% (25/25)

Abbreviations: CRS, chronic rhinosinusitis; FESS, functional endoscopic sinus surgery; OTC, over-the-counter; RARS, recurrent acute rhinosinusitis; RSI, relative strength index.

In addition to the REMODEL trial, the other RCTs that have been published comparing balloon sinus dilation with FESS[9,10,11,12,13,19] have substantiated the positive findings of the REMODEL trial, and the evidence is scrutinized below.

The RCT by Marzetti et al[12] compared balloon ostial dilation (unspecified device) with FESS in the treatment of sinus headaches ($n = 83$). Forty-four patients were randomized to conventional ESS and 35 to balloon ostial dilation. In the balloon dilation group, 23 patients were "only frontal sinus balloon" patients, in which balloon catheters were the only tools used for frontal sinusotomy, and 12 were "hybrid," in which balloon catheters and traditional ESS were used concurrently. Unfortunately, it was not specified how patients were selected for these groups. FESS treatment was administered on participants in both groups, but specific data were not reported by the study authors. At 6 months of follow-up, scores on the SNOT-22 improved from 28.6 at baseline to 7.8 in the ESS group and 27.3 at baseline to 5.3 in the balloon ostial dilation group, with a statistically significant reduction in both groups ($p < 0.001$). At 6 months of follow-up, headache scores based on the visual analog score (VAS) improved from 6.5 to 5.4 in the ESS group and from 7.1 at baseline to 1.2 in the balloon ostial dilation group ($p < 0.001$). The authors did not report other patient-relevant outcomes, such as the number of headache days or use of pain medications following treatment. Limitations of this study included the small number of patients who received balloon ostial dilation, which limits the generalizability of study results, and the lack of blinding of both patients and clinical assessors. In addition, there were various concurrent surgical procedures conducted in both treatment and control groups, which made it difficult to properly assess the treatment effects of balloon ostial dilation.

In contrast, a recent single-blinded study[20] comparing sinus balloon dilatation with a sham procedure (placebo treatment) found no statistically significant difference in outcomes at 6 months, in terms of reduction in SNOT-22 scores or headache severity scores, in patients with a diagnosis of "sinus headaches" but without evidence of sinonasal disease on computed tomography (CT). This study suggests that there may be a significant placebo effect for any interventional procedure for "sinus headache," and caution should be exercised in such patients. Balloon dilatation should not be used in patients with normal CT imaging.[21]

Bizaki et al[19] compared 92 patients (balloon dilation in office, $n = 50$; FESS, $n = 42$) and studied their 1-year patient-reported quality-of-life (QOL) outcomes. The authors concluded that stand-alone balloon dilation was as effective as FESS in the treatment of CRS in patients with maxillary sinus disease, with or without anterior ethmoid disease, who failed medical therapy and met the criteria for medically necessary FESS. However, some criticisms were leveled at the use of patient-reported outcome measures (PROMS) and their tendency for recall bias,[14] despite their widespread validation for use in rhinology.[22] In contrast to this, a small RCT in 2011 ($n = 20$) reported physiological outcomes only,[23] comparing randomly assigned patients to removal of the uncinate process via FESS or balloon sinus ostial dilation as a stand-alone procedure. The main outcome measures were CO_2 concentration in the sinuses and maximum sinus pressure, both intended to be surrogate measures for sinus ventilation. The CO_2 concentration decreased in both study arms to a similar degree. The mean maxillary sinus pressure on inspiration decreased in the FESS group but did not change in the balloon sinus ostial dilation group.

In 2012, an RCT randomized 24 patients to sinuplasty as a hybrid procedure or FESS,[10] and again there were no differences noted at 6 months in terms of SNOT-20 scores or saccharine clearance times. However, this study was heavily criticized for being underpowered and adverse events were not reported. Bozdemir et al's small study ($n = 10$ patients with nasal polyposis), in which one side was treated with FESS and the other with balloon sinus ostial dilation,[24] had all the procedures performed by the same surgeon. A polypectomy was performed prior to FESS or balloon sinus ostial dilation in all patients. Outcome measures included sinus patency, as measured by CT scan (Lund–MacKay [LM] classification) or repeat endoscopy (McKay grading). At 10 days following the procedure, there were improvements in both groups on measures of patency, but no differences between the groups, suggesting noninferiority of BSP compared to FESS.

39.1.2 Nonrandomized Studies

Seven prospective, multicenter, controlled, and single-arm studies also demonstrated statistically significant sinus symptom improvement over baseline for patients treated with balloon dilation that was consistent and durable at follow-up periods from 1 month to 2 years.[2,4,5,6,21,25,26] Within this body of evidence, reported follow-up of more than 1 year for 122 patients was undertaken within the Optimization and Refinement of technique in In-Office Sinus dilation (ORIOS II) study for outcomes of sinus symptom improvement and revision rates.[26] The combined ORIOS and RELIEF trials contained 314 patients in 26 centers, with feasibility rates of 92%, demonstrating a clinically and statistically significant reduction in SNOT-20 at 6 months of follow-up, a clinically and statistically significant reduction in LM score, and return to normal activity at 2.2 days.

Koskinen et al, in a retrospective controlled trial, compared success of BSP to standard FESS procedures and reported slightly better outcomes for FESS in acute exacerbations and in patients with occupational or CRS-related risk factors,[27] but no effect of allergic rhinitis and previously diagnosed nasal polyps on patient outcomes.

However, these nonrandomized studies have been criticized due to certain methodological limitations, such as a limited number of patients, a heterogenous study population, no primary health outcomes reported, limited follow-up, and a retrospective study design. There is no randomization or blinding in a retrospective study design; therefore, it is difficult to control for bias and confounders. Also, retrospective studies are limited by the accuracy of the medical records reviewed or the recall ability of patients when filling out a study questionnaire.

Much of the evidence included studies that enrolled patients with very limited sinus disease, or undertook BSP in only primary cases. Therefore, the clinical applicability and generalization to a wider population with a background of CRS should be done so with caution.

39.2 Controversies and Opinions

Surgeons increasingly recognize the importance of preserving the mucosa and restoring normal sinus physiology. The more anatomical and physiological methods of reopening and enlarging natural drainage pathways of the sinuses are the basis of modern FESS. A cadaveric study, first conducted in 2005 by Bolger and Vaughan, demonstrated that balloon dilatation of the frontal sinus ostia was a feasible technique.[20] A number of other studies since then have demonstrated the application of this technique in clinical practice, with successful frontal sinus ostia cannulation rates ranging from around 92 to 96% in a mixture of operating room (OR) and office-based procedures.[2,3,21,28] Balloon sinus ostial dilation has been proposed as an alternative or adjunct to standard endoscopic surgery for use in the frontal, maxillary, and sphenoid sinuses. The technology uses a balloon with fixed maximum external diameter, inflated to very high pressures, to dilate the bony ostia of the sinuses. It works by

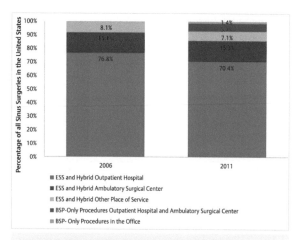

Fig. 39.1 A chart to show the increase in popularity of balloon sinus procedures (BSP) as a percentage of total sinus surgeries in the United States, from 2006 to 2011.[7,30]

inducing microfractures in the surrounding bony lamellae, rather than by cutting or removing the mucosa.

Balloon techniques may therefore be considered a relatively less invasive treatment than traditional cutting instruments. However, balloon dilatation was perhaps wrongly promoted as an alternative to endoscopic techniques; it should be viewed as a new tool rather than as an entirely novel procedure, with the indications for intervention remaining largely unchanged. With the evolution of technology and practice, balloon sinus ostial dilation can be performed under LA in an office setting, leading to potentially significant cost savings to the health care economy, enhanced patient recovery, and, perhaps, a lower threshold for intervention. As a consequence, there has been concern that generous remuneration in an office environment could lead to inappropriate selection of patients and significant controversy regarding its place in our surgical repertoire.

Despite these fears, the overall number of sinus surgery procedures per head of population with CRS[29] has remained stable. However, balloon procedures have gained in popularity with an increasing market share in recent years (see ▸ Fig. 39.1), with a fivefold increase in the number of frontal sinus procedures being performed from 2006 to 2011 in the United States.[30]

As with any instrument used in sinus surgery, balloon sinus dilation is only as good as the surgeon performing it. It is crucial to state that the choice of surgical instrumentation should not change the indications for sinus surgery, with the aim of achieving durable access to a previously obstructed or inflamed sinus with mucosal preservation. This can be achieved with the balloon technique in selected cases. Patient selection is paramount to the success of any sinus procedure and is the responsibility of the operating surgeon; poor selection cannot be blamed on an instrument. Any patient with persistent symptoms, endoscopic evidence of disease, and/or

radiological findings of CRS on CT scanning who fails to respond to maximum medical therapy, as recommended by accepted guidelines such as the European Position Paper on Rhinosinusitis (EPOS) 2020 guidelines,[31] may subsequently benefit from surgical intervention; the choice of balloon technology or conventional instrumentation is then based on discussion between the patient and the surgeon.

39.2.1 Diffuse versus Localized CRS

A recent study utilized an international, multidisciplinary panel of experts in CRS to rank 624 different scenarios and their appropriateness for ESS.[32] For adult patients with uncomplicated CRS without nasal polyps, ESS can be appropriately offered when the CT LM score is ≥ 1 and there has been a minimum trial of a topical intranasal corticosteroid plus either a short course of a broad-spectrum/culture-directed systemic antibiotic or the use of a prolonged course of systemic low-dose anti-inflammatory antibiotic with a posttreatment total SNOT-22 score ≥ 20.

Overall, patients with anterior mucosal disease involving the maxillary and frontal, with only limited disease in the anterior ethmoid sinuses, would be considered the "ideal" candidates for balloon dilation alone. The importance of surgically addressing ethmoid disease remains controversial; certain investigators have anecdotally noted ethmoid disease resolution in some patients when peripheral sinuses were dilated without ethmoidectomy.

There is limited support for this concept in the literature. Chan et al[33] studied five patients with chronic frontal sinusitis who had failed medical management and also presented with ipsilateral anterior ethmoid sinusitis. After balloon dilation of the frontal stenosed ostia without ethmoidectomy, all patients showed complete radiographic clearing of both the dilated frontal sinus and the anterior ethmoid sinus. Stankiewicz et al demonstrated that patients with both maxillary and anterior ethmoid disease had statistically and clinically significant improvement in QOL with just maxillary dilation.[34] Karanfilov et al reviewed 203 patients who underwent BSP, 102 of which had ethmoidal disease, and reported complete radiographic resolution by dilating peripheral sinuses without ethmoidectomy.[21] Of course, these trials were nonrandomized without a control arm, and it is conceivable that there would be resolution of disease in all sinuses without any surgical intervention; controlled trials and a better understanding of the natural history of early-stage CRS are therefore essential before advocating widespread use of balloon dilatation as a first line of management in such cases. It is the current practice of the authors to perform a conventional frontoethmoidectomy when there is evidence of extensive ethmoidal disease on CT, with balloon dilatation being reserved for more limited but persistent sinus disease.

39.2.2 Polyp Disease

For many surgeons, the presence of polyposis is a relative contraindication to balloon dilatation. Most studies supporting the use of balloon sinus ostial dilation used predominantly nonpolyp patients with limited sinus disease, and, therefore, we do not have evidence to support whether the efficacy seen in those studies is generalizable to patients with more extensive disease or CRS with nasal polyp (CRSwNP). Office-based polypectomy techniques may be combined with balloon techniques; however, as a key aim of surgery in CRSwNP involves optimizing access to topical therapies, these patients may not achieve comparable longer-term outcomes. Certainly, cannulation may be more challenging in the presence of nasal polyps.

39.2.3 Miscellaneous Uses

Although acute rhinosinusitis does not frequently require surgical management, in the presence of complications or failure of medical therapy, it is sometimes necessary to intervene. In the acutely infected setting in particular, dilatation of the acutely obstructed ostia without tissue removal would seem to be an ideal adjunct to treatment, with a lower potential risk of iatrogenic stenosis than other endoscopic techniques. There are small case series or single case reports published in the literature that describe the successful application of balloon technology in the frontal sinuses in acute frontal sinusitis,[35] Pott's puffy tumor, and frontal sinusitis, treated with retrograde balloon dilatation via mini-trephination.[36] The procedure may be performed at the bedside in a high-dependency unit, in patients with suspected sinogenic intracranial complications to facilitate collection of microbiology samples.

The management of recurrent acute rhinosinusitis (RARS), defined by at least four acute episodes per year separated by symptom-free intervals, remains contentious, but ESS for RARS can significantly reduce utilization of antibiotics and health care expenditure, as well as reduce risk of both antibiotic-related morbidity and the development of bacterial resistance.[37]

Another setting where BSP may be ideal is for recurrent sinus barotrauma, with frontal recess narrowing. Occupations that are particularly prone to these symptoms can include frequent flyers (i.e., pilots, cabin crew, or travelling business passengers) and divers. In the literature, balloon sinus ostial dilation has found limited roles in other specific circumstances such as in patients with frontal sinus mucocoeles[15,16,38] or in sinogenic headaches.[12]

39.2.4 Contraindications

BSP may not be appropriate for all chronic and recurrent sinusitis patients.[39,40] Patients with extensive CRS, allergic fungal disease, or suspected neoplasm are unlikely to be considered for balloon sinus dilatation as the principal modality. In addition to this, clinical studies have typically excluded patients with eosinophilic disease, severe septal deviation, cystic fibrosis, Samter's triad, and facial trauma.[41] When dealing with any solid tissue pathology within the frontal sinus, it is unlikely that the access gained via ballooning of the natural ostia will be sufficient to allow histopathological sampling or extirpate the disease fully.

If bony thickening or osteitis is present in the context of severe disease, this may limit access or the impact of balloon dilatation at pressures that are safe to use within the frontal recess. The converse is also true, with any dehiscence of the orbital wall or skull base placing balloon dilatation at a higher risk of causing complications.

Caution with ballooning should be exercised in the pediatric cohort, as the frontal sinus does not develop until the age of 5 to 6 years. Increased technical failure rates reflect this in studies with a pediatric population.[42,43] Contraindications may also be evident in 5 to 10% of patients who have hypoplastic or underdeveloped frontal sinuses, and hence careful note of the CT scan should be made preoperatively.

As with FESS, balloon sinus dilatation should not be offered in the absence of comprehensive medical treatment, in accordance to the EPOS guidance.[31]

39.2.5 Preoperative Preparation

Informed consent should be sought in the same manner as that obtained for conventional ESS, particularly as at times it may become necessary to change to conventional instrumentation during a procedure.

Careful preoperative review of sinus CT scans in three different planes and access to the images intraoperatively are essential for successful placement of the balloon. Sinus navigation can be a helpful adjunct in complex or revision cases, but it is not usually a requirement, especially in primary cases.

Assessment should be made of the uncinate attachment, which determines the drainage pathway of the frontal sinus. If the uncinate process inserts onto the lamina papyracea (type A, which is most common), forming a recessus terminalis, then the drainage of the frontal recess is into the middle meatus, medial to the uncinate insertion. The balloon or guidewire may hit a "hard stop" in the terminal recess and should be directed more medially. If the uncinate inserts onto the roof of the ethmoid (type B) or the middle turbinate (type C), then the frontal recess drains into the infundibulum, lateral to the uncinate insertion; in such cases, the balloon can be directed slightly more laterally.

Furthermore, the presence of any frontoethmoidal cells may cause difficulty in locating the frontal recess. These are anterior ethmoid cells that pneumatize the frontal recess and may cause obstruction or persistent disease,[44]

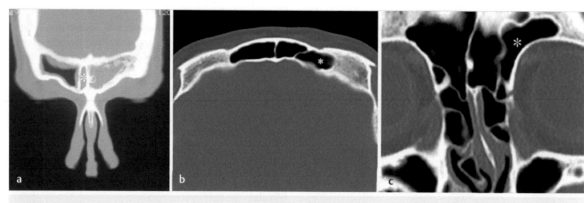

Fig. 39.2 **(a)** Coronal computed tomography (CT) slice demonstrating intersinus septal cell (*yellow asterisk*) that can be mistaken for frontal sinus. **(b)** Axial and **(c)** coronal CT slice demonstrating supraorbital ethmoid cell (*white asterisk*) that can easily be mistaken for frontal sinus, as it will transilluminate due to contact with the anterior table. It is found lateral to the vertical partition on the coronal sequences.

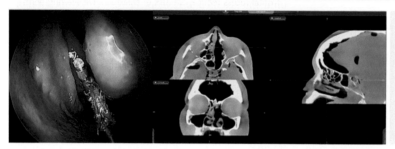

Fig. 39.3 An example of the integrated operative view and computed tomography (CT) scan display from a navigable balloon system, to help guide the clinician on balloon catheter deployment in real time.

and are among reasons cited in the literature for cannulation failure in addition to significant osteoneogenesis.[45] Often when such cells are present, the balloon or guidewire may preferentially cannulate the frontoethmoidal cell (see ▶ Fig. 39.2). Any cell that pneumatizes to the anterior table of the frontal bone will transilluminate, and this may cause confusion if a supraorbital or anterior frontoethmoidal cell is cannulated. Dilatation of these cells rather than the frontal recess may then further compromise the true frontal sinus drainage pathway. It is the authors' practice to undertake conventional dissection of the frontal recess in the presence of complex anatomy, although careful interpretation of the imaging and the use of image guidance may facilitate the use of the balloon (see ▶ Fig. 39.3).

39.2.6 Training Requirements

The attraction of this technique is that it entails a relatively short learning curve, compared to other frontal sinus procedures, with a fairly low risk of complications. This may encourage some surgeons to manage frontal sinus pathology where they would not have done if merely armed with conventional techniques. However, there are no studies comparing the training time required to learn frontal BSP versus performing a Draf II procedure.

The major medical device companies provide training on models, in cadaveric labs, and on site, in vivo (see ▶ Fig. 39.4, ▶ Fig. 39.5, and ▶ Fig. 39.6). The authors would recommend a minimum of 10 cases performed successfully under GA before attempting to perform balloon sinus dilation in a patient under LA. Also, with slight differences between each company's devices, some experience of the setup and techniques would be preferable prior to use under LA.

There is increasing interest in balloon techniques being performed under LA in the outpatient or "office" setting, using topical, local infiltration with or without sedation. The suggested benefits include reduced cost, operating time, and morbidity to the patient in whom a GA is avoided.[4,21,25] The authors perceive that the future area of growth for balloon sinus ostial dilation is likely to be in those cases with limited anteriorly based mucosal disease where a short "balloon-only" procedure under LA can be performed safely, effectively, and cost-efficiently, or in the drainage of acute frontal sinusitis resulting in a lower risk of iatrogenic disease.

39.2.7 Complications

A number of large series of patients who underwent balloon sinus dilation with long-term follow-up have been recently published. Balloon sinus dilation appears to be a very safe procedure with a 0 to 0.1% major complication rate.[4,5,6,11,18,19,21,25,46,47,48,49] This compares well with the historic FESS complication rate of approximately 1% with

1 in 1,500 FESS cases resulting in an overt cerebrospinal fluid (CSF) leak.[50] Meta-analysis[18] suggests 32% of patients report nasal bleeding after BSP compared with 56% after conventional ESS.

Single case reports in the literature mention rare complications including dural lesions resulting in CSF leak,[7,17,46] orbital lesions of the lamina papyracea,[17,46,51,52] and intraoperative cardiac arrest.[53] In the sinuplasty registry,[3] two CSF leaks have been recorded in hybrid procedures, both of which were in the fovea ethmoidalis region. There were no apparent major adverse events in this study attributed to the balloon itself. Only one case of CSF leak after frontal BSP was reported in the Manufacturer and User Facility Device Experience (MAUDE)

adverse event report database by the Food and Drug Administration (FDA) in 2006, again caused by a traditional instrument in a hybrid procedure.[54] Similarly, Tomazic et al[55] reported a case of CSF leak in a 36-year-old patient who underwent an isolated BSP procedure of the frontal sinus. The thin lateral lamella of the cribriform plate was penetrated with the tip of the sinus catheter while attempting to dilate the frontal recess. Postoperative examination confirmed a circumscribed brain herniation indicative of trauma to the surface of the brain.

With the drive to reduce production costs and increase simplicity of use, there has been a trend of reduced emphasis on correct placement (image-guided surgery being an exception), from fluoroscopy, to transillumination to tactile feedback alone, which may increase the risk of complications. Some of the more recently introduced products have replaced a flexible guidewire with a more rigid probe or guide catheter that is placed directly through the frontal recess; this may increase the risk of skull base penetration if incorrectly positioned.

39.3 Unanswered Questions

39.3.1 Cost-Effectiveness

Currently in the authors' institution, the benefits of BSP as a "hybrid procedure" are not significant enough to justify the extra costs in the OR during standard ESS. Although tariffs and rates may vary by region, the estimated cost of disposables consumed for each balloon sinus ostial dilation case in the United Kingdom works out to be around £1,000. However, a U.K. cost-effectiveness analysis[56] suggested around £150 saving for an in-office or outpatient procedure under LA compared with FESS under GA. Further societal indirect costs could be reduced with an earlier return to work for the patient, and less outpatient visits for debridement, although the necessity of debridement in routine FESS is not clearly established.[57]

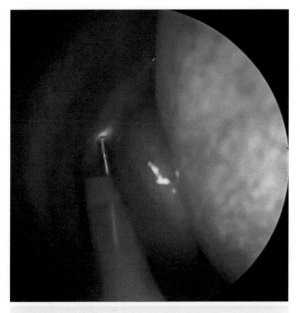

Fig. 39.4 Insertion of catheter and illuminated guidewire to locate the right frontal ostium.

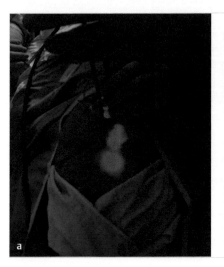
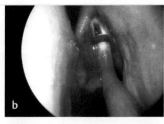
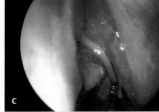

Fig. 39.5 External visualization of frontal sinus illumination confirming placement of light-tipped guidewire (**a**) with simultaneous endoscopic view (**b, c**).

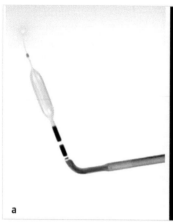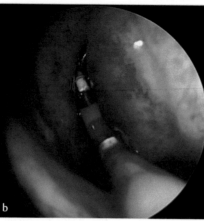

a b

Fig. 39.6 (a) Simulation of the balloon catheter dilation. **(b)** Balloon catheter dilation in vivo.

In times of economic restraint, it is important to justify the extra disposable costs; use in an office setting is likely to be cost-effective, but use in an OR environment may not be. So far, there is no evidence to support a shift in the threshold for intervention in CRS (i.e., failed maximal medical therapy with evidence of residual sinus disease remains the indication for ESS as for BSP). This technique may be seen as a useful adjunct or tool but is unlikely to replace current surgical practice in the OR.

39.3.2 Extrapolation to Wider Patient Cohort

With nearly 10 years of clinical studies, including recent meta-analysis and the long-term results from the statistically powered, randomized controlled REMODEL trial comparing balloon dilation with FESS, the body of evidence is sufficient and consistent to support that balloon dilation within the frontal sinus is a reliable, safe, and efficacious technique with results comparable to ESS for selected CRS patients who have failed medical management.

Careful patient selection is essential, as with any sinus procedure. However, whether patients with disease limited to the maxillary and frontal sinuses, with only mild ethmoidal involvement, need any surgical management remains to be fully evaluated, and a trial with a control arm of nonsurgical management is urgently required.

The authors note the limitations of this technique in CRSwNP cases, in complex frontal sinus anatomy where there is greater risk of damage to the skull base or failure to cannulate, in extensive ethmoidal disease (i.e., complete opacification of anterior ethmoids/or posterior ethmoid disease), in revision cases, or in the presence of osteoneogenesis. Revision cases are also more challenging with balloon technology.

References

[1] Catalano PJ. Use of a novel osmotic self-expanding dilation device for the treatment of sinusitis. Otorinolaringol. 2016; 66(2):26–30

[2] Weiss RL, Church CA, Kuhn FA, Levine HL, Sillers MJ, Vaughan WC. Long-term outcome analysis of balloon catheter sinusotomy: two-year follow-up. Otolaryngol Head Neck Surg. 2008; 139(3) Suppl 3: S38–S46

[3] Levine HL, Sertich AP, II, Hoisington DR, Weiss RL, Pritikin J, PatiENT Registry Study Group. Multicenter registry of balloon catheter sinusotomy outcomes for 1,036 patients. Ann Otol Rhinol Laryngol. 2008; 117(4):263–270

[4] Gould J, Alexander I, Tomkin E, Brodner D. In-office, multisinus balloon dilation: 1-Year outcomes from a prospective, multicenter, open label trial. Am J Rhinol Allergy. 2014; 28(2):156–163

[5] Albritton FD, IV, Casiano RR, Sillers MJ. Feasibility of in-office endoscopic sinus surgery with balloon sinus dilation. Am J Rhinol Allergy. 2012; 26(3):243–248

[6] Brodner D, Nachlas N, Mock P, et al. Safety and outcomes following hybrid balloon and balloon-only procedures using a multifunction, multisinus balloon dilation tool. Int Forum Allergy Rhinol. 2013; 3 (8):652–658

[7] Tomazic PV, Stammberger H, Koele W, Gerstenberger C. Ethmoid roof CSF-leak following frontal sinus balloon sinuplasty. Rhinology. 2010; 48(2):247–250

[8] Kuhn FA, Church CA, Goldberg AN, et al. Balloon catheter sinusotomy: one-year follow-up: outcomes and role in functional endoscopic sinus surgery. Otolaryngol Head Neck Surg. 2008; 139(3) Suppl 3: S27–S37

[9] Plaza G, Eisenberg G, Montojo J, Onrubia T, Urbasos M, O'Connor C. Balloon dilation of the frontal recess: a randomized clinical trial. Ann Otol Rhinol Laryngol. 2011; 120(8):511–518

[10] Achar P, Duvvi S, Kumar BN. Endoscopic dilatation sinus surgery (FEDS) versus functional endoscopic sinus surgery (FESS) for treatment of chronic rhinosinusitis: a pilot study. Acta Otorhinolaryngol Ital. 2012; 32(5):314–319

[11] Cutler J, Bikhazi N, Light J, Truitt T, Schwartz M, REMODEL Study Investigators. Standalone balloon dilation versus sinus surgery for chronic rhinosinusitis: a prospective, multicenter, randomized, controlled trial. Am J Rhinol Allergy. 2013; 27(5):416–422

[12] Marzetti A, Tedaldi M, Passali FM. The role of balloon sinuplasty in the treatment of sinus headache. Otolaryngol Pol. 2014; 68(1):15–19

[13] Hathorn IF, Pace-Asciak P, Habib AR, Sunkaraneni V, Javer AR. Randomized controlled trial: hybrid technique using balloon dilation of the frontal sinus drainage pathway. Int Forum Allergy Rhinol. 2015; 5(2):167–173

[14] BlueCross BlueShield Association. Balloon sinus ostial dilation for treatment of chronic rhinosinusitis. Technol Eval Cent Assess Program Exec Summ. 2013; 27(9):1–3

[15] Ahmed J, Pal S, Hopkins C, Jayaraj S. Functional endoscopic balloon dilation of sinus ostia for chronic rhinosinusitis. Cochrane Database Syst Rev. 2011; 7(7):CD008515

[16] Rimmer J, Fokkens W, Chong LY, Hopkins C. Surgical versus medical interventions for chronic rhinosinusitis with nasal polyps. Cochrane Database Syst Rev. 2014; 12(12):CD006991

[17] Batra PS, Ryan MW, Sindwani R, Marple BF. Balloon catheter technology in rhinology: Reviewing the evidence. Laryngoscope. 2011; 121 (1):226–232

[18] Chandra RK, Kern RC, Cutler JL, Welch KC, Russell PT. REMODEL larger cohort with long-term outcomes and meta-analysis of standalone balloon dilation studies. Laryngoscope. 2016; 126(1):44–50

[19] Bizaki AJ, Taulu R, Numminen J, Rautiainen M. Quality of life after endoscopic sinus surgery or balloon sinuplasty: a randomized clinical study. Rhinology. 2014; 52(4):300–305

[20] Bolger WE, Vaughan WC. Catheter-based dilation of the sinus ostia: initial safety and feasibility analysis in a cadaver model. Am J Rhinol. 2006; 20(3):290–294

[21] Karanfilov B, Silvers S, Pasha R, Sikand A, Shikani A, Sillers M, ORIOS2 Study Investigators. Office-based balloon sinus dilation: a prospective, multicenter study of 203 patients. Int Forum Allergy Rhinol. 2013; 3(5):404–411

[22] Hopkins C, Philpott C, Crowe S, et al. Identifying the most important outcomes for systematic reviews of interventions for rhinosinusitis in adults: working with Patients, Public and Practitioners. Rhinology. 2016; 54(1):20–26

[23] Kutluhan A, Şalvız M, Bozdemir K, et al. The effects of uncinectomy and natural ostial dilatation on maxillary sinus ventilation: a clinical experimental study. Eur Arch Otorhinolaryngol. 2011; 268(4):569–573

[24] Bozdemir K, Kutluhan A, Çetin H, Yalçıner G, Bilgen AS. Comparison of outcomes of simple polypectomy plus balloon catheter dilatation versus functional endoscopic sinus surgery in nasal polyposis: a preliminary study. Am J Rhinol Allergy. 2011; 25(3):198–200

[25] Levine SB, Truitt T, Schwartz M, Atkins J. In-office stand-alone balloon dilation of maxillary sinus ostia and ethmoid infundibula in adults with chronic or recurrent acute rhinosinusitis: a prospective, multi-institutional study with-1-year follow-up. Ann Otol Rhinol Laryngol. 2013; 122(11):665–671

[26] Sikand A, Silvers SL, Pasha R, et al. ORIOS 2 Study Investigators. Office-based balloon sinus dilation: 1-year follow-up of a prospective, multicenter study. Ann Otol Rhinol Laryngol. 2015; 124(8):630–637

[27] Koskinen A, Penttilä M, Myller J, et al. Endoscopic sinus surgery might reduce exacerbations and symptoms more than balloon sinuplasty. Am J Rhinol Allergy. 2012; 26(6):e150–e156

[28] Bikhazi N, Light J, Truitt T, Schwartz M, Cutler J, REMODEL Study Investigators. Standalone balloon dilation versus sinus surgery for chronic rhinosinusitis: a prospective, multicenter, randomized, controlled trial with 1-year follow-up. Am J Rhinol Allergy. 2014; 28 (4):323–329

[29] Truven Health Analytics. MarketScan studies: abbreviated bibliography. Available at: http://sites.truvenhealth.com/bibliography/2014TruvenHealthMarketScanBibliography.pdf. Accessed January 22, 2014

[30] Svider PF, Sekhsaria V, Cohen DS, Eloy JA, Setzen M, Folbe AJ. Geographic and temporal trends in frontal sinus surgery. Int Forum Allergy Rhinol. 2015; 5(1):46–54

[31] Fokkens WJ, Lund VJ, Hopkins C, et al. European position paper on rhinosinusitis and nasal polyps 2020. Rhinology. 2020; 58 Suppl S29:1–464

[32] Rudmik L, Soler ZM, Hopkins C, et al. Defining appropriateness criteria for endoscopic sinus surgery during management of uncomplicated adult chronic rhinosinusitis: a RAND/UCLA appropriateness study. Rhinology. 2016; 54(2):117–128

[33] Chan Y, Melroy CT, Kuhn FA. Is Anterior Ethmoid Disease Really Responsible for Chronic Frontal Sinusitis? Annual Meeting of the American Rhinologic Society Annual Meeting, Chicago, IL, September 2008

[34] Stankiewicz J, Tami T, Truitt T, Atkins J, Liepert D, Winegar B. Trans-antral, endoscopically guided balloon dilatation of the ostiomeatal complex for chronic rhinosinusitis under local anesthesia. Am J Rhinol Allergy. 2009; 23(3):321–327

[35] Hopkins C, Noon E, Roberts D. Balloon sinuplasty in acute frontal sinusitis. Rhinology. 2009; 47(4):375–378

[36] Wexler DB. Frontal balloon sinuplasty via minitrephination. Otolaryngol Head Neck Surg. 2008; 139(1):156–158

[37] Bhandarkar ND, Mace JC, Smith TL. Endoscopic sinus surgery reduces antibiotic utilization in rhinosinusitis. Int Forum Allergy Rhinol. 2011; 1(1):18–22

[38] Eloy JA, Friedel ME, Eloy JD, Govindaraj S, Folbe AJ. In-office balloon dilation of the failed frontal sinusotomy. Otolaryngol Head Neck Surg. 2012; 146(2):320–322

[39] Mistry S, Kumar B. Balloon sinuplasty for an acute frontal sinus mucocele. J Surg Case Rep. 2011; 2011(11):6

[40] Cohen AN. Suitability for balloon sinuplasty procedure. Los Angeles Sinus Surgeon. February 24, 2014. Available at https://web.archive.org/web/20150414111418/http://losangelessinussurgeon.com/blog/Suitability-for-Balloon-Sinuplasty-Procedure.html. Accessed April 13, 2015

[41] ClinicalTrials.gov. Safety and Efficacy of Balloon Sinuplasty in Pediatric Sinusitis (INTACT). July 10, 2012. Accessed April 13, 2015

[42] Ramadan HH, McLaughlin K, Josephson G, Rimell F, Bent J, Parikh SR. Balloon catheter sinuplasty in young children. Am J Rhinol Allergy. 2010; 24(1):e54–e56

[43] Ramadan HH. Safety and feasibility of balloon sinuplasty for treatment of chronic rhinosinusitis in children. Ann Otol Rhinol Laryngol. 2009; 118(3):161–165

[44] Bent JP, Cuilty-Siller C, Kuhn FA. The frontal cell as a cause of frontal sinus obstruction. Am J Rhinol. 1994; 8(4):185–191

[45] Heimgartner S, Eckardt J, Simmen D, Briner HR, Leunig A, Caversaccio MD. Limitations of balloon sinuplasty in frontal sinus surgery. Eur Arch Otorhinolaryngol. 2011; 268(10):1463–1467

[46] Melroy CT. The balloon dilating catheter as an instrument in sinus surgery. Otolaryngol Head Neck Surg. 2008; 139(3) Suppl 3:S23–S26

[47] Hathorn I, Habib AR, Santos RD, Javer A. The safety and performance of a maxillary sinus ostium self-dilation device: a pilot study. Int Forum Allergy Rhinol. 2014; 4(8):625–631

[48] Stankiewicz J, Truitt T, Atkins J, et al. Two-year results: transantral balloon dilation of the ethmoid infundibulum. Int Forum Allergy Rhinol. 2012; 2(3):199–206

[49] Koskinen A, Myller J, Mattila P, et al. Long-term follow-up after ESS and balloon sinuplasty: comparison of symptom reduction and patient satisfaction. Acta Otolaryngol. 2016; 136(5):532–536

[50] Hopkins C, Browne JP, Slack R, et al. Complications of surgery for nasal polyposis and chronic rhinosinusitis: the results of a national audit in England and Wales. Laryngoscope. 2006; 116(8):1494–1499

[51] Batra PS. Evidence-based practice: balloon catheter dilation in rhinology. Otolaryngol Clin North Am. 2012; 45(5):993–1004

[52] Özkiriş M, Akin İ, Özkiriş A, Aydin R, Saydam L. Orbital complication of balloon sinuplasty. J Craniofac Surg. 2014; 25(2):499–501

[53] Hughes N, Bewick J, Van Der Most R, O'Connell M. A previously unreported serious adverse event during balloon sinuplasty. BMJ Case Rep. 2013; 2013

[54] U.S. Food and Drug Administration. Manufacturer and User Facility Device Experience (MAUDE) Database. Silver Spring, MD: FDA; 2006

[55] Tomazic PV, Stammberger H, Braun H, et al. Feasibility of balloon sinuplasty in patients with chronic rhinosinusitis: the Graz experience. Rhinology. 2013; 51(2):120–127

[56] Taghi AS, Khalil SS, Mace AD, Saleh HA. Balloon Sinuplasty: balloon-catheter dilation of paranasal sinus ostia for chronic rhinosinusitis. Expert Rev Med Devices. 2009; 6(4):377–382

[57] Green R, Banigo A, Hathorn I. Postoperative nasal debridement following functional endoscopic sinus surgery, a systematic review of the literature. Clin Otolaryngol. 2015; 40(1):2–8

40 Minimum versus Maximal Surgical Sinusotomy

Anne E. Getz and Todd T. Kingdom

Abstract

One of the first surgical challenges encountered after making a recommendation for endoscopic sinus surgery (ESS) is determining the extent of surgery. This is perhaps most true of the frontal sinus where underoperating can result in insufficient control of disease and persistent symptoms, while overoperating can result in unnecessary surgery, increase the risk of iatrogenic scarring, and place undue risk upon surrounding structures in an anatomically unforgiving location. This chapter reviews the evidence available for performing frontal sinus balloon sinuplasty, Draf I, IIa, IIb, and III frontal sinusotomies. It also presents controversies, opinions, and unanswered questions on the topic of extent of frontal sinus surgery.

Keywords: frontal sinusotomy, minimal frontal sinusotomy, maximal frontal sinusotomy, balloon sinuplasty, Draf I, Draf IIa, Draf IIb, Draf III

40.1 Published Evidence

One of the first surgical challenges encountered after making a recommendation for endoscopic sinus surgery (ESS) is determining the extent of surgery. This is perhaps most true of the frontal sinus where underoperating can result in insufficient control of disease and persistent symptoms, while overoperating can result in unnecessary surgery, increase the risk of iatrogenic scarring, and place undue risk upon surrounding structures in an anatomically unforgiving location. Historically, Messerklinger assigned great importance to the concept of anatomic configuration in the pathogenesis of chronic rhinosinusitis (CRS).[1]

Key to the determination of appropriate surgical extent is consideration of the underlying disease process. The simplest distinction is inflammatory versus noninflammatory etiology. In the former, postoperative delivery of anti-inflammatory topical therapy has become an important goal of surgical intervention. In noninflammatory cases such as barosinusitis or obstructing mucocele, a more directed approach may be adequate. The optimal extent of surgery likely differs between these two clinical scenarios.

DeConde et al[2] studied the outcomes of complete versus targeted sinus surgery in a prospective observational cohort of 311 patients. They found that patients with a diagnosis of aspirin sensitivity, asthma, nasal polyposis, or history of prior sinus surgery were offered more complete surgery. Mean improvement in postoperative outcomes measured with the 22-item Sinonasal Outcome Test (SNOT-22) and Brief Smell Identification Test (B-SIT) were found to be significantly greater in patients undergoing complete sinus surgery. Thus, these data suggest extent of surgery, or degree of "completeness," might be important. One might tend to extrapolate these data to the frontal sinus and conclude complete surgery translates to "maximal" opening of the ostium. Caution is required as the DeConde et al review did not provide data unique to frontal sinusotomy. Isolating the outcomes of frontal sinus surgery is complicated as ESS most often addresses more than one sinus, and thus the available evidence for frontal-specific outcomes is limited. We will briefly review the best available evidence for the various surgical techniques commonly used to surgically manage the frontal sinus.

40.1.1 Balloon Dilation

Generally speaking, balloon dilation of the frontal sinus offers the opportunity to achieve durable sinus outflow tract dilation while sparing tissue in the process. Fracturing and displacement of obstructing frontal recess cells and/or dilation of soft-tissue stenosis in a minimally invasive fashion are theoretical advantages of this technique. The largest study to date examining balloon dilation of the frontal sinuses in an office setting reported successful dilation in 251 of 268 sinuses (93.7%), with 5 frontal sinuses (2%) requiring revision.[3] Though overall improvement in SNOT-20 and computed tomography (CT) scores was reported, outcomes specific to the frontal sinus were not provided. In addition, information on frontal ostium size postdilation was not given. Hathorn et al[4] evaluated frontal sinus ostial patency following balloon dilation compared to a Draf IIa frontal sinusotomy. They reported 100% patency in both groups ($n = 30$ patients, 60 frontal sinuses) at 3-month follow-up. Twenty-two patients were evaluated at 1 year following surgery and 100% of the frontal sinus ostia evaluated were patent. The authors reported no difference in ostial size between the two techniques at all time points assessed. Patient-reported outcomes and CT scores following surgery were not provided.

The available evidence suggests balloon dilation of the frontal sinus may create an ostial size equivalent to that created with the Draf IIa technique, but comparison to the more extensive approaches (Draf IIb, Draf III) is not possible. The data for balloon dilation of the frontal sinus, particularly for sinus-specific outcomes and measures, are simply too limited to draw conclusions.

40.1.2 Draf I

A recent prospective observational study of 226 patients sought to determine the efficacy of anterior or total ethmoidectomy without frontal sinusotomy ($n = 196$) versus frontal sinusotomy ($n = 30$) in improving quality-of-life (QOL) measures and adjunct medical therapy usage in patients with chronic frontal sinusitis.[5] The results of this study demonstrated that QOL outcomes as measured by the SNOT-22 were comparable for patients treated with ethmoidectomy alone and those treated with frontal sinusotomy. Both cohorts demonstrated significant improvements in their postoperative Lund–MacKay endoscopy scores, although the frontal sinusotomy group demonstrated a higher magnitude of improvement ($p = 0.023$). Both groups had significant and comparable improvements in oral steroid and oral antibiotic use postoperatively. Key differences did exist, however, between the two groups. The frontal sinusotomy group had a significantly higher prevalence of nasal polyposis, prior surgery, asthma, and aspirin intolerance. The authors conclude that in patients with frontal CRS without nasal polyposis, prior surgery, asthma, or aspirin intolerance, ethmoidectomy alone without instrumentation of the frontal sinus outflow tract can achieve similar QOL improvements and comparable decreases in the use of oral steroid and antibiotic use as frontal sinusotomy. This study suggests a "minimal" approach to frontal sinus disease; in other words, ethmoidectomy alone is adequate in select patient populations.

An earlier retrospective study[6] examined the efficacy of anterior ethmoidectomy alone in the treatment of chronic frontal sinusitis. Seventy-seven patients (121 frontal sinuses) with chronic frontal sinusitis underwent a Draf I procedure and 88.5% demonstrated resolution of disease of the frontal sinuses. Of the 11.5% who demonstrated persistence of disease, 8.5% required revision surgery for symptom control. Failure of disease control was associated with aspirin intolerance, presence of both nasal polyposis and asthma, and identification of interfrontal sinus septal cells.

These are the only known studies addressing the efficacy of ethmoidectomy alone versus frontal sinusotomy for treatment of chronic frontal sinusitis.

40.1.3 Draf IIa

The existing outcome data for Draf IIa consist of case series and are thus level IV. These studies employ a range of objective and subjective outcome collection, many of which do not use validated disease-specific measures.[7] Despite these limitations, most patients reported symptomatic improvement (68.5–92%). Endoscopic patency rates in the last 10 years improved to an average of mid-80% (67.6–92%).

Of note, the available data on Draf IIa frontal sinusotomy outcomes span 25 years. It is important to note that many advances have occurred during this time frame including the emphasis on mucosal-sparing technique, introduction of the microdebrider, high-definition cameras, image-guidance systems, topical steroid irrigations, and drug-eluting stents.[7] These most probably account in some way to the overall trend in improvement in symptoms and patency over time.

Sinusotomy size does appear to be a determinant of success as defined by patency rate and symptom improvement. Several Draf IIa studies have investigated size as a predictor of such outcomes.[8,9,10] These studies found that a sinusotomy less than 4.5 mm was significantly more likely to stenose. Critical review of the patient-specific anatomic limits on preoperative imaging is thus critical in guiding the extent of the sinusotomy.

Mucosal preservation is a tenant of ESS that is especially critical in the narrow confines of the frontal recess. An early case series of Draf IIa frontal sinusotomies in which the drill was employed in 50% of cases found a high rate (40%) of stenosis—a rate much higher than recently reported outcomes.[11]

Regarding the effect of inflammatory status on patency rates, there is somewhat surprisingly no evidence that correlates the severity of inflammatory disease with stenosis.[9,12]

40.1.4 Draf IIb

Very few studies have directly assessed the efficacy of the Draf IIb technique. The main limitation with the currently available data is the lack of clear differentiation between use of the Draf IIa and Draf IIb techniques within the patient cohorts. This is problematic and makes drawing significant conclusions nearly impossible. Kikawada et al[13] published outcomes for a small group undergoing extended endoscopic frontal sinus surgery (Draf III: 22 patients; Draf IIb: 12 patients) with at least 12-month follow-up. They reported a 42% patency rate for the Draf IIb group and 88% for the Draf III group. They did not provide information on intraoperative ostium size, extent of surgery, postoperative ostium size, or comorbidities such as presence of nasal polyps, asthma, or aspirin sensitivity.

Turner et al[14] recently published their experience with a total of 22 Draf IIb procedures in 18 patients. They reported patency in 20 of 22 sides at a mean follow-up of 16.2 months. Patency was defined as the ability to pass a 3-mm standardized curved suction during postoperative endoscopy. The most common indication for selecting this approach in their hands was chronic frontal sinusitis due to a lateralized middle turbinate remnant, mucocele, or postoperative synechiae. Interestingly, the authors point out that the decision to not proceed with the more extensive Draf III was primarily due to anatomic limitations or a desire to avoid mucosal injury associated with drilling.

The Draf IIb technique is likely an underused approach; however, the lack of outcome data makes it difficult to know where it should fall within the options we have for frontal sinusotomy. Patient selection appears important, but direct comparison to the Draf III technique (maximal frontal sinusotomy) outcomes is not possible at this time.

40.1.5 Draf III

Similar to the Draf IIa literature, data supporting Draf III are level IV consisting predominantly of case series.[7]

The Draf III approach was designed in the early 1990s[15] as an alternative to frontal sinus obliteration and is largely employed now as a salvage procedure for patients failing more conservative surgical options. The true limits of the Draf III are from the first olfactory fiber posteriorly to the periosteum laterally and anteriorly. Reports of successful long-term outcomes have described dimensions of approximately 20 × 20 mm.

Decrease in size of the opening is observed for up to 2 years after surgery and thus long-term follow-up is important for accurate assessment of success. Several studies reporting long-term outcomes following Draf III exist. One study of 229 patients reports patency rates of up to 97% after an average of 45 months and a low revision rate for persistence of symptoms of 5.2%.[16] Other reports have been somewhat less impressive with a mean stenosis of 33% of the cross-sectional area at 1 year and a 29.9% revision rate,[17] and in another study, 43% of cases stenosing by greater than 50% of the initial area at 6 months.[18]

Patient-reported outcomes reflect objective findings of patency. Naidoo et al[16] found 47% of patients to be asymptomatic following surgery and 27% to have mild symptoms only. The authors speculate this may be due to the large area of the neo-ostia and facilitation of topical medical therapy and irrigation delivery, and dimensions more forgiving to circumferential scarring.

An earlier retrospective study by the same group[19] evaluated a total of 339 patients undergoing primary, revision and Draf III frontal sinusotomy to assess risk factors that may help determine which patient would benefit from which procedure. Patients with underlying asthma and polyposis, as well as narrow frontal ostia (<4 mm) and extensive radiological disease (Lund–Mackay [LM] score > 16) were found to have a high failure rate following standard ESS. Although none of these risk factors alone were significant, the risk of requiring a Draf III procedure increased with each additional factor. Specifically, there was a 10% ($p = 0.16$) risk of requiring a Draf III for CRS with nasal polyposis (CRSwNP) alone, 22% ($p = 0.014$) for CRSwNP and asthma, 67% ($p = 0.0002$) for CRSwNP, asthma, and LM > 16, and 75% ($p = 0.0012$) for CRSwNP, asthma, LM > 16, and frontal ostia < 4 mm. The authors concluded that a primary Draf III procedure should thus be given consideration in certain patient groups.

40.2 Controversies and Opinions

- The optimal frontal sinusotomy size cannot be known and will vary based on a number of clinical and patient factors including anatomy, inflammatory status, surgical technique utilized, and disease pathology.
- Though the size of the surgically created ostium appears important, it is the "state" of the mucosa that likely determines the outcome.
- Outcomes are based on subjective QOL questionnaires, not on objective data such as sinus patency of endoscopy.
- It is difficult to parse out the effect on outcomes of frontal sinusotomy alone when it is often done in conjunction with other procedures. This is a major limitation in interpreting the currently available best evidence.
- The available evidence shows that for the vast majority of patients, more conservative and limited surgical techniques (balloon dilation, Draf I, Draf IIa) will be sufficient to address uncomplicated frontal recess and frontal sinus disease.
- A Draf IIb approach is a reasonable option for accessing mucoceles, addressing a lateralized middle turbinate remnant, or unilateral frontal disease.
- The use of a drill during any frontal sinusotomy other than a Draf III should be avoided since stenosis rates may be higher due to mucosal injury.
- A Draf III approach should be preferred in the setting of severe osteitis, extensive nasal polyposis with frontal sinus involvement, and in revision cases after failed conservative frontal sinusotomy.
- Recent experience and opinion has suggested a Draf III procedure might be the preferred approach as primary surgery for a select group of patients with more severe disease and anatomic constraints. However, this requires additional analysis of clinical outcomes and remains an area of controversy.
- When local topical drug delivery is a main objective of postsurgical treatment, a larger sinusotomy may be advantageous; however, there is not yet robust evidence to fully support this position.

40.3 Case Studies

40.3.1 Case 1

A 43-year-old woman presents with left forehead and periorbital pain. She had undergone sinus surgery several years prior. CT showed opacification of the left frontal sinus with a lateralized middle turbinate remnant (▶ Fig. 40.1a–c). A Draf IIb was performed on the left side to decompress a frontal sinus mucocele. Follow-up at 4 years after surgery demonstrated a widely patent frontal sinus (▶ Fig. 40.2). This case highlights the value of a Draf IIb approach for unilateral and isolated disease in the

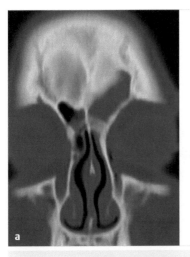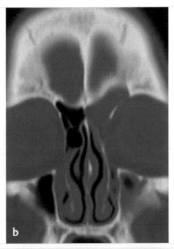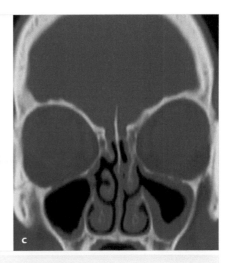

Fig. 40.1 (a–c) Coronal sinus computed tomography (CT) showing opacification of the left frontal sinus suggestive of mucocele formation and a lateralized middle turbinate remnant as the cause of obstruction.

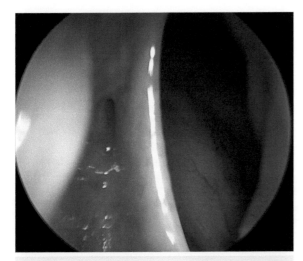

Fig. 40.2 Endoscopic (30-degree endoscope) view 4 years after surgery showing a widely patent left frontal sinus.

setting of a known anatomic issue, that is, lateralized middle turbinate remnant. The procedure was performed without the use of a drill. A more aggressive Draf III would have been unnecessary.

40.3.2 Case 2

A 61-year-old woman presents with headache and frontal sinusitis based on CT imaging after 3 prior surgeries. CT revealed opacification of the left frontal sinus with severe osteitis/osteoneogenesis (▶ Fig. 40.3). Though largely unilateral disease, a Draf III was performed to more thoroughly address the postoperative changes and diffuse osteoneogenesis. Endoscopy at 1 year (▶ Fig. 40.4) and CT at 3 years (▶ Fig. 40.5) after surgery revealed a widely patent surgical cavity. With the presence of significant

osteoneogenesis, the size of the surgical ostium was likely a critical determinant of success in this case, thus the reason for the Draf III approach. In this case, a Draf IIb approach would have been unsuccessful in our opinion.

40.3.3 Case 3

A 32-year-old woman with CRSwNP and aspirin-exacerbated respiratory disease (AERD) presents with progressive nasal polyposis and symptoms after two prior surgeries. CT showed poorly controlled disease in the frontal recess and sinus bilaterally (▶ Fig. 40.6). Though amenable to more conservative approaches, such as a Draf IIa or IIb, a Draf III was performed. She has been maintained on high-volume topical steroid irrigations and aspirin desensitization, and endoscopy at 1 year after surgery demonstrated excellent control of disease with a widely patent surgical cavity (▶ Fig. 40.7). This case highlights the evolving important role for the Draf III technique in cases of CRSwNP in the setting of multiple comorbidities and risk factors (i.e., AERD, asthma, and eosinophilia).

40.4 Unanswered Questions

- Lack of rigorous evidence and outcome data (level IV) complicates analysis and the ability to draw concrete conclusions about the optimal extent of surgery for frontal sinusotomy.
- Published data suggest the optimal ostial size for long-term patency is 4 to 5 mm; however, this is based on results using the Draf IIa technique. Extrapolation to more extended techniques is problematic.
- It is very difficult to accurately attribute patient symptoms to the presence or absence of frontal sinus disease based on CT and/or endoscopy. This presents a major

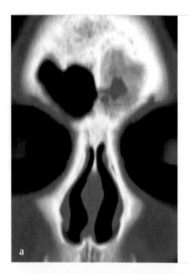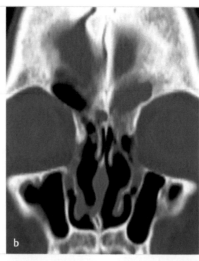

Fig. 40.3 (a,b) Coronal computed tomography (CT) showing left frontal sinusitis with severe osteoneogenesis.

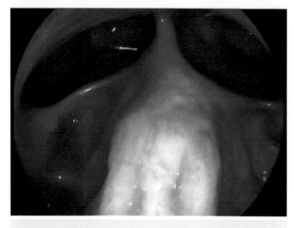

Fig. 40.4 Endoscopy (45-degree endoscope) showing a well-healed and patent frontal sinus.

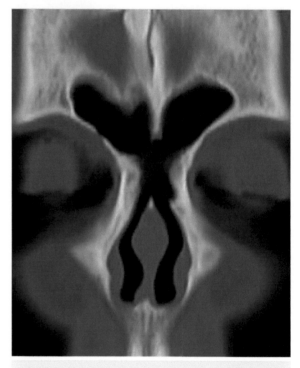

Fig. 40.5 Computed tomography (CT) at 3 years after surgery showing well-aerated frontal sinus.

challenge to interpreting causation and clinical outcomes.

- The possible link or association between ostium size, frontal patency and symptom improvement, and disease control remains a critical unanswered question.
- Attempts to maximize the size of the frontal sinusotomy should not be pursued at the expense of preserving functional mucosa. Understanding the delicate balance between aggressive techniques for optimal tissue removal and ostium size with preservation of mucosa remains a significant challenge.
- Although the size of the frontal sinusotomy likely plays a role in postoperative patency, it is also likely that the underlying disease process greatly influences outcomes. We currently do not have enough data to answer this important question.
- No data exist on the impact of tissue eosinophilia or osteoneogenesis on frontal sinus stenosis after frontal sinusotomy.

- A Draf III may give the largest frontal sinusotomy, but it remains unclear whether this impacts or drives clinical outcomes across all situations or patient profiles.
- Consistent with trends in the field of rhinology, we have seen our practice gradually shift toward employing the Draf III more often and earlier in the treatment algorithm for frontal sinusitis. The ideal application of this technique requires continued study.

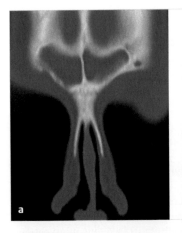
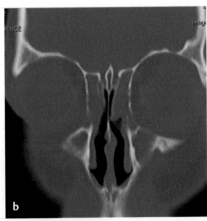

Fig. 40.6 (a,b) Preoperative sinus computed tomography (CT) showing severe frontal recess and frontal sinus disease after prior surgeries.

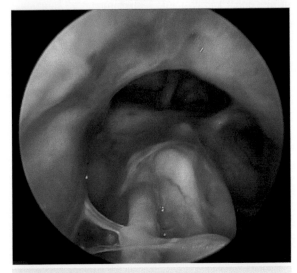

Fig. 40.7 Nasal endoscopy at 1 year after surgery demonstrating excellent control of disease with a widely patent surgical cavity.

References

[1] Stammberger H, Posawetz W. Functional endoscopic sinus surgery. Concept, indications and results of the Messerklinger technique. Eur Arch Otorhinolaryngol. 1990; 247(2):63–76

[2] DeConde AS, Suh JD, Mace JC, Alt JA, Smith TL. Outcomes of complete vs targeted approaches to endoscopic sinus surgery. Int Forum Allergy Rhinol. 2015; 5(8):691–700

[3] Karanfilov B, Silvers S, Pasha R, Sikand A, Shikani A, Sillers M, ORIOS2 Study Investigators. Office-based balloon sinus dilation: a prospective, multicenter study of 203 patients. Int Forum Allergy Rhinol. 2013; 3(5):404–411

[4] Hathorn IF, Pace-Asciak P, Habib AR, Sunkaraneni V, Javer AR. Randomized controlled trial: hybrid technique using balloon dilation of the frontal sinus drainage pathway. Int Forum Allergy Rhinol. 2015; 5(2):167–173

[5] Abuzeid WM, Mace JC, Costa ML, et al. Outcomes of chronic frontal sinusitis treated with ethmoidectomy: a prospective study. Int Forum Allergy Rhinol. 2016; 6(6):597–604

[6] Becker SS, Han JK, Nguyen TA, Gross CW. Initial surgical treatment for chronic frontal sinusitis: a pilot study. Ann Otol Rhinol Laryngol. 2007; 116(4):286–289

[7] DeConde AS, Smith TL. Outcomes after frontal sinus surgery: an evidence-based review. Otolaryngol Clin North Am. 2016; 49(4):1019–1033

[8] Chandra RK, Palmer JN, Tangsujarittham T, Kennedy DW. Factors associated with failure of frontal sinusotomy in the early follow-up period. Otolaryngol Head Neck Surg. 2004; 131(4):514–518

[9] Naidoo Y, Wen D, Bassiouni A, Keen M, Wormald PJ. Long-term results after primary frontal sinus surgery. Int Forum Allergy Rhinol. 2012; 2(3):185–190

[10] Hosemann W, Kühnel T, Held P, Wagner W, Felderhoff A. Endonasal frontal sinusotomy in surgical management of chronic sinusitis: a critical evaluation. Am J Rhinol. 1997; 11(1):1–9

[11] Wigand ME, Hosemann WG. Endoscopic surgery for frontal sinusitis and its complications. Am J Rhinol. 1991; 5(3):85–89

[12] Askar MH, Gamea A, Tomoum MO, Elsherif HS, Ebert C, Senior BA. Endoscopic management of chronic frontal sinusitis: prospective quality of life analysis. Ann Otol Rhinol Laryngol. 2015; 124(8):638–648

[13] Kikawada T, Fujigaki M, Kikura M, Matsumoto M, Kikawada K. Extended endoscopic frontal sinus surgery to interrupted nasofrontal communication caused by scarring of the anterior ethmoid: long-term results. Arch Otolaryngol Head Neck Surg. 1999; 125(1):92–96

[14] Turner JH, Vaezeafshar R, Hwang PH. Indications and outcomes for Draf IIB frontal sinus surgery. Am J Rhinol Allergy. 2016; 30(1):70–73

[15] Draf W. Endonasal micro-endoscopic frontal sinus surgery: the Fulda concept. Oper Tech Otolaryngol Head Neck Surg. 1991; 2:234–240

[16] Naidoo Y, Bassiouni A, Keen M, Wormald PJ. Long-term outcomes for the endoscopic modified Lothrop/Draf III procedure: a 10-year review. Laryngoscope. 2014; 124(1):43–49

[17] Ting JY, Wu A, Metson R. Frontal sinus drillout (modified Lothrop procedure): long-term results in 204 patients. Laryngoscope. 2014; 124(5):1066–1070

[18] Casiano RR, Livingston JA. Endoscopic Lothrop procedure: the University of Miami experience. Am J Rhinol. 1998; 12(5):335–339

[19] Naidoo Y, Bassiouni A, Keen M, Wormald PJ. Risk factors and outcomes for primary, revision, and modified Lothrop (Draf III) frontal sinus surgery. Int Forum Allergy Rhinol. 2013; 3(5):412–417

41 Patient-Reported Outcome Measures and Outcomes in Frontal Sinus Surgery: Do They Make a Difference?

Yujay Ramakrishnan, M. Reda El Badawey, and Sean Carrie

Abstract

Patients are increasingly taking a prominent role in the care they receive. Therefore, patient-centric assessment of outcomes in the form of patient-reported outcome measures (PROMs) is steadily accompanying the traditional clinical ways of measuring the effects of treatment on the patient. PROMs, which measure health-related quality of life, are self-rated and refer to a single time point or clearly defined preceding period. The impact of a clinical intervention can be determined by comparing PROMs pre- and posttreatment. These have a particular relevance in the field of rhinology as the primary aim of treatment is to improve quality of life. Various PROMs have been utilized within sinus surgery over the years, both generic and disease specific. The role of PROMs in frontal sinus surgery is unclear as isolated frontal sinus surgery is performed rarely. Usually frontal sinus surgery is carried out as a part of functional endoscopic sinus surgery where other sinuses are treated concurrently. In addition, the rarity of isolated frontal sinus disease, coupled with heterogeneity in pathophysiology and treatment options, renders any comparison of studies challenging. The scope of this chapter is to summarize the studies on this issue, including any opinions and controversies. It also raises the question of whether the current disease-specific PROMs in rhinology are "fit for purpose" in frontal sinus surgery.

Keywords: sinusitis, frontal sinus surgery, quality of life, patient-reported outcomes

41.1 Published Evidence

Historically there is little in the literature relating to specific frontal sinus surgery outcome measures. Those in existence are broadly based on general rhinological and generic symptoms.

41.1.1 Patient-Reported Outcome Measures in Rhinology

Patient-reported outcome measures (PROMs) in rhinology can be generic or disease specific, with each having their own strengths and weaknesses. They can also facilitate comparative audit (of different treatments or providers), thus improving provision for health care.

Generic PROMs include the 36-item short-form survey (SF-36) and Glasgow Benefit Inventory (GBI). **SF-36** is a multipurpose, 36-item survey measuring eight domains of health: physical functioning, role limitations due to physical health, bodily pain, general health perceptions, vitality, social functioning, role limitations due to emotional problems, and mental health. Chronic rhinosinusitis (CRS) has been shown to adversely affect quality of life (QOL) on SF-36.[1] The GBI is a validated generic QOL instrument that has been used extensively in the field of otolaryngology. It is a postintervention questionnaire that measures change in health status following interventions. In functional and cosmetic septorhinoplasty,[2] functional endoscopic sinus surgery (FESS),[3] and septoplasty,[4] improvements in GBI have all been noted. As this is a postintervention questionnaire, baseline pretreatment data of the patient cohort (e.g., symptom severity) are not collected. Therefore, these may not be controlled for in comparative studies.

Various validated rhinology-specific PROMs have been reported in the modern literature. In 1995, Piccirillo et al reported the use of a 31-item rhinosinusitis outcome measure (RSOM-31), which contains both general and rhinosinusitis-specific questions.[5] This was subsequently condensed into the validated 20-Item Sinonasal Outcome Test (SNOT-20), containing 20 nose, sinus, and general points.[5] Two further points that were felt to be extremely important in QOL reporting by CRS patients, that is, nasal obstruction and loss of sense of taste and smell, were added, resulting in the SNOT-22 questionnaire.[6] Based on their appraisal of the available measures, Morley and Sharp[7] concluded that SNOT-22 was the most suitable tool in terms of reliability, validity, responsiveness, and ease of use. It is however worth noting the lack of correlation between SNOT-22 scores and endoscopic and radiological scores (Lund–Mackay) in certain studies.[8] The largest published outcome study to date in CRS utilized SNOT-22 to prospectively measure outcomes of 3,128 patients in the National Comparative Audit of Surgery for Chronic Rhinosinusitis and Nasal Polyposis.[9] SNOT-22 scores significantly reduced with surgery and this was maintained across a 5-year period.[9]

The importance of PROMs in CRS is underlined in a recent study that explored factors that impact a patient's choice to pursue sinus surgery. Interestingly, baseline SNOT-22 severity was more effective at predicting treatment modality selection than a variety of other measures including personality traits, risk aversion, degree of social support, economic factors, and the patient–physician relationship.[10]

41.1.2 Patient-Reported Outcome Measures in Frontal Sinus Treatment

Although PROMs have been used extensively in a range of surgical procedures for CRS, there is a paucity of literature relating to frontal sinus disease treatment. Of the data that are available, the studies often lack controls with significant heterogeneity in terms of patient population, treatment, and outcome measures.

▶ Table 41.1 summarizes the studies relating to frontal sinus disease treatment. It is worth noting that there were no studies measuring PROMs in external approaches to the frontal sinus.

One of the recurring themes that emerge about measuring PROMs in frontal sinus treatment is the hybrid nature of the surgical procedures, where other sinuses are treated concurrently (be it through balloon dilatation[11,15] or FESS[18]). As a result, it is difficult to differentiate the direct impact of the frontal intervention alone. The majority of studies used the older SNOT-20 instead of the more recent SNOT-22.

Different frontal sinus interventions have been evaluated. In early studies of balloon sinus dilatation (BSD) of the frontal sinus,[11,17] there was no comparator group, so definitive conclusions could not be made about the efficacy of frontal sinus BSD. Subsequent studies incorporated a control group (FESS, BSD, Draf frontal sinus drillout, medical treatment). The only randomized controlled trial of frontal sinus BSD versus Draf I to date for CRS polyps is by Plaza et al.[13] All the patients underwent hybrid procedures, which included a minimum of maxillary antrostomy, anterior ethmoidectomy, posterior ethmoidectomy, and sphenoidotomy. The Visual Analog Score (VAS) and Rhinosinusitis Disability Index (RSDI) statistically improved in both groups following treatment. As the first prospective comparative analysis of BD and FESS, it has many strengths that include using validated outcome tools, low attrition rate, and long follow-up. However, the study had no power analysis and although statistical significance was reported, confidence intervals and p-values were often omitted. Given the hybrid nature of the surgical procedures, it was also challenging to differentiate the direct impact of the frontal intervention from concurrent ethmoidectomy.

Abuzeid et al[19] compared the impact of FESS ± frontal sinusotomy in CRS. They found a comparable SNOT-22 improvement between the two groups. However, the cohort undergoing frontal sinusotomy had a higher proportion of revision FESS, asthma, nasal polyps, and aspirin sensitivity.

The impact of conservative versus surgical treatment (Draf IIb) was evaluated in those who had undergone surgery before.[14] All patients with recurrent chronic frontal sinusitis had undergone at least one FESS ± Draf I/IIa procedure prior to being enrolled in the study. The surgical group underwent a Draf IIb, while the conservative group was treated with topical steroid spray and oral macrolides. The total SNOT-20 score was significantly lower in the surgical group compared to the conservative group at 6 and 12 months. On the face of it, it would appear that surgery is superior to conservative treatment in those who had undergone prior surgery. However, both groups were not matched; there was no randomization and patients decided on their surgical intervention. This study underscores the need to carefully evaluate the data before making any definitive conclusions.

The impact of frontal sinus intervention in different patient cohorts has also been evaluated. Aspirin-exacerbated respiratory disease (AERD), eponymously referred to as Samter's triad, is characterized by nasal polyps, asthma, and sensitivity to cyclooxygenase-1 (COX-1) inhibiting drugs. Patients with AERD typically have more severe sinonasal disease compared to aspirin-tolerant patients. Although various studies have suggested that more extensive sinus surgery in AERD patients reduces the need for revision surgery,[20,21] the outcome specifically related to the frontal sinus has not been addressed until the recent paper by Morrissey et al.[22] This paper reported that complete sphenoethmoidectomy, maxillary antrostomy, and endoscopic modified Lothrop procedure (EMLP) are successful in a significant majority of patients with AERD and CRS with nasal polyps (CRSwNP). Although SNOT-22 was measured, details on these outcomes were not described in this paper or in a subsequent paper by the same authors evaluating outcomes of revision modified Lothrop.[23]

41.2 Controversies and Opinions

Although PROMs are useful in frontal sinus surgery, their usefulness has to be interpreted with caution. First, it is rare to have isolated frontal sinus disease. Any intervention usually has to address other diseased sinuses concurrently. Managing the disease in all the affected sinuses is central to the improvement in QOL for those patients.

Second is the difficulty in assessing outcomes of intervention due to significant disease heterogeneity. The existing model of categorizing CRS based on phenotype (CRS without nasal polyps [CRSsNP], CRSwNP, fungal sinusitis, and AERD) is over-simplistic. As more is discerned about CRS endotypes, this new categorization will influence the accuracy of PROMs to inform future decision-making. Finally, there are certain frontal sinus pathologies, for example, uncomplicated mucoceles, where PROMs (SNOT-22) are minimally affected, yet still require surgery to correct the underlying disease process.[24]

A further factor is the difficulty in defining the "minimal clinically important difference" (MCID) in PROMs for a particular disease. The MCID is the minimal change in symptom or QOL after a given intervention that is perceptible and relevant to the individual patient. In SNOT-22, for example, the MCID is 9 points. This is a

Table 41.1 Summary of studies

Study	Cohort	Type frontal sinus surgery			Additional surgery	PROM	Comments
		Balloon	Hybrid	Draf			
Bolger et al[11] Clinical Evaluation to Confirm Safety and Efficacy of Sinuplasty in the Paranasal Sinuses (CLEAR) United States	• 109 CRSsNP • Single arm (no control) BSD (frontal/sphenoid/maxillary) + concomitant ethmoidectomy (52%) • Follow-up: 24 wk	Yes	Yes (52%)		BSD maxillary, sphenoid sinus + concomitant ethmoidectomy (52%)	SNOT-20	SNOT-20 scores improved in balloon-only and hybrid groups
Kuhn et al[12] 1-y follow-up of Clinical Evaluation to Confirm Safety and Efficacy of Sinuplasty in the Paranasal Sinuses (CLEAR) United States	• 66 CRSsNP • Single arm (no control) BSD (frontal/sphenoid/maxillary) + concomitant ethmoidectomy • Follow-up: 1 y	Yes	Yes		BSD maxillary, sphenoid + concomitant ethmoidectomy	SNOT-20	SNOT-20 improved in balloon-only and hybrid groups Patients undergoing concomitant ethmoidectomy have higher baseline SNOT-20 but derive greater benefit from surgery at 1 y
Plaza et al[13] Spain	• 32 CRS polyps (Samter's triad excluded) • RCT frontal BSD vs. Draf I (all either MMA, ethmoidectomy, or sphenoidotomy) • Follow-up: 12 mo	Yes	Yes	Draf I	All either MMA, ethmoidectomy, or sphenoidotomy	VAS, RSDI	VAS and RSDI improved in both groups Limitations: • Unpowered • Reporting bias: no between-group analysis for VAS and RSDI • No confidence interval and *p*-values • Hybrid procedure: unable to differentiate direct impact of frontal intervention from concurrent ethmoidectomy
Ma et al[14] China	• Recurrent chronic frontal sinusitis • Prospective case control (revision surgery) • 51 Draf IIb vs. 34 medical • Follow-up: 12 mo			Draf IIb		SNOT-20	SNOT-20 markedly improved in Draf IIb compared to medical treatment Limitation: patient-selected treatment
Abreu et al[15]	• CRS, *n* = 13 • BSD (10 frontal, 10 maxillary sinus, 4 sphenoid sinus) • Follow-up: 6 months					SNOT-20	No SNOT-specific results for frontal BSD

ElBadawey et al[16] United Kingdom	• 2 arms (*n* = 33)
	   – Retrospective (*n* = 19)
	   – Prospective (*n* = 7)
	 • Pathology: CRSsNP and CRSwNP (both groups), mucocele (retrospective group)
		Yes	Yes	Draf III	FESS	GBI, SNOT-22	Frontal sinus surgery, as an isolated procedure or part of FESS, has shown benefit in all GBI domains and physical domain of SNOT-22

Table 41.1 (continued) Summary of studies

Study	Cohort	Type frontal sinus surgery			Additional surgery	PRO-M	Comments
		Balloon	Hybrid	Draf			

	• Treatment: frontal BSD, frontal BSD + FESS, frontal recess clearance (FRC), Draf III
	• Mean follow-up:
	  - Retrospective: 3 mo
	  - Prospective: 12 mo						

Sikand et al[17] United States	• CRS (10% polyp) • N = 122 • Multicenter, prospective • Single arm: BSD under local anaesthesia (LA)—frontal, maxillary, and sphenoid sinuses • Follow-up: 52 + wk	LA			BSD maxillary and sphenoid sinuses	SN0-T-20	SNOT-20 improved at 1 y Limitations: medical therapy not standardized across sites
Deconde et al[18] United States and Canada	• Prospective • Multicenter • Primary or revision surgery • Complete FESS (bilateral frontosphenoethmoidectomy, MMA) n = 147 vs. targeted FESS (n = 164) • Follow-up: 6 + mo		Yes	Draf II/III	FESS	SNO-T-22	Significantly greater SNOT-22 improvement with complete surgery (5.9 unit) vs. targeted FESS Limitations: • Observational bias • Only minor SNOT-22 improvement • Not generalizable (4 rhinological centers)
Abuzeid et al[19] United States and Canada	Prospective multicenter CRS FESS (including FS) n = 196 vs. FESS (excluding FS) n = 30 Follow-up: FESS (FS +) 12.6 FESS FS(−) 13.8		Yes	Draf II/III	FESS ± FS	SNO-T-22	SNOT-22 improvement comparable between groups, but the cohorts differ (revision FESS, asthma, nasal polyps, aspirin sensitivity more common in FS group) Revision surgery 2.6% in FS + group, 0% in FS− group

Abbreviations: BSD, balloon sinus dilatation; CRS, chronic rhinosinusitis; CRSsNP, CRS without nasal polyps; CRSwNP, CRS with nasal polyps; FESS, functional endoscopic sinus surgery; FS, frontal sinusotomy; GBI, Glasgow Benefit Inventory; MMA, middle meatal antrostomy; RSDI, Rhinosinusitis Disability Index; RCT, randomized controlled trial; SNOT-22, 22-Item Sinonasal Outcome Test; VAS, Visual Analog Score.

population-derived mean rather than an individual one. Therefore, what may represent a clinically important change will vary among individuals and any improvement in PROMs postintervention may not reflect the patient's expectation of success. Despite noticeable improvement in PROMs and/or disease clearance endoscopically and radiologically, certain domains in PROMs that are important to the patient may not have altered (despite a reduction in overall scores). Therefore, further research needs to be carried out to define clinically significant improvement in PROMs, on an individual level.

The existing studies, frequently retrospective, contain small numbers, are unpowered, and employ different PROMs. To date, the largest prospective outcome study in CRS utilized SNOT-22 to measure outcomes in over 3,000 patients (National Comparative Audit of Surgery for Chronic Rhinosinusitis and Nasal Polyposis).[9] Larger corroborative prospective databases using standardized PROMs will strengthen the statistical and clinical accuracy of PROMs in frontal sinus surgery. We do recognize that this may be undermined by disease, patient, and treatment heterogeneity among the different centers, and every effort should be made to harmonize these.

The authors believe that the greatest utility of PROMs is to stratify patients based on disease severity and to provide an indicative chance of success. This will in turn improve the patient–physician shared decision-making process. Indeed, this has been the case in a recent study where patients with a preoperative SNOT-22 score of greater than 30 had a greater than 70% chance of achieving the MCID, while those with preoperative score of less than 20 failed to achieve a mean improvement greater than the MCID.[25] Reaching an MCID does not equate to a cure, as patients are likely to be left with a measurable disease burden, remain symptomatic postoperatively, and potentially a higher risk of revision surgery.

Given the limitations of various PROMs including SNOT-22, it may be worthwhile developing a specific PROM for frontal sinus surgery. However, the authors accept this is challenging given that symptoms attributable to the frontal sinus can be relatively nonspecific.

41.3 Unanswered Questions

1. Rinologists should be encouraged in the uptake of PROMs as a routine part of clinical practice.
2. The development of a specific outcome measure for frontal sinus disease should be a priority.

Despite the limitations from existing studies of the utility of PROMs in frontal sinus surgery, it is clear that worsening disease-specific QOL (rather than objective measures such as CT or endoscopy scores) is an important metric to patients, which influences the treatment choices they pursue. Therefore, strong consideration should be given to incorporating PROMs into routine clinical practice. Considerable uncertainty exists in patient selection for frontal sinus procedures underpinned by a lack of clear understanding of etiopathophysiology of inflammatory sinus disease. Furthermore, the choice of surgical approach for frontal sinus disease is variable and unclear. In order for such questions to be addressed, further multicenter studies are necessary. The development of a PROM with particular relevance for frontal sinus surgery may be helpful.

References

[1] Gliklich RE, Metson R. The health impact of chronic sinusitis in patients seeking otolaryngologic care. Otolaryngol Head Neck Surg. 1995; 113(1):104–109

[2] McKiernan DC, Banfield G, Kumar R, Hinton AE. Patient benefit from functional and cosmetic rhinoplasty. Clin Otolaryngol Allied Sci. 2001; 26(1):50–52

[3] Mehanna H, Mills J, Kelly B, McGarry GW. Benefit from endoscopic sinus surgery. Clin Otolaryngol Allied Sci. 2002; 27(6):464–471

[4] Calder NJ, Swan IRC. Outcomes of septal surgery. J Laryngol Otol. 2007; 121(11):1060–1063

[5] Piccirillo JF, Merritt MG, Jr, Richards ML. Psychometric and clinimetric validity of the 20-Item Sino-Nasal Outcome Test (SNOT-20). Otolaryngol Head Neck Surg. 2002; 126(1):41–47

[6] Hopkins C, Gillett S, Slack R, Lund VJ, Browne JP. Psychometric validity of the 22-item Sinonasal Outcome Test. Clin Otolaryngol. 2009; 34 (5):447–454

[7] Morley AD, Sharp HR. A review of sinonasal outcome scoring systems: which is best? Clin Otolaryngol. 2006; 31(2):103–109

[8] Hopkins C, Browne JP, Slack R, Lund V, Brown P. The Lund-Mackay staging system for chronic rhinosinusitis: how is it used and what does it predict? Otolaryngol Head Neck Surg. 2007; 137(4):555–561

[9] Hopkins C, Browne JP, Slack R, et al. The national comparative audit of surgery for nasal polyposis and chronic rhinosinusitis. Clin Otolaryngol. 2006; 31(5):390–398

[10] Steele TO, Rudmik L, Mace JC, DeConde AS, Alt JA, Smith TL. Patient-centered decision making: the role of the baseline SNOT-22 in predicting outcomes for medical management of chronic rhinosinusitis. Int Forum Allergy Rhinol. 2016; 6(6):590–596

[11] Bolger WE, Brown CL, Church CA, et al. Safety and outcomes of balloon catheter sinusotomy: a multicenter 24-week analysis in 115 patients. Otolaryngol Head Neck Surg. 2007; 137(1):10–20

[12] Kuhn FA, Church CA, Goldberg AN, et al. Balloon catheter sinusotomy: one-year follow-up: outcomes and role in functional endoscopic sinus surgery. Otolaryngol Head Neck Surg. 2008; 139(3) Suppl 3: S27–S37

[13] Plaza G, Eisenberg G, Montojo J, Onrubia T, Urbasos M, O'Connor C. Balloon dilation of the frontal recess: a randomized clinical trial. Ann Otol Rhinol Laryngol. 2011; 120(8):511–518

[14] Ma Y, Wang T, Zhang X, et al. Efficacy of the modified endoscopic frontal sinus surgery for recurrent chronic frontal sinusitis. Indian J Otolaryngol Head Neck Surg. 2014; 66(3):248–253

[15] Abreu CB, Balsalobre L, Pascoto GR, Pozzobon M, Fuchs SC, Stamm AC. Effectiveness of balloon sinuplasty in patients with chronic rhinosinusitis without polyposis. Rev Bras Otorrinolaringol (Engl Ed). 2014; 80(6):470–475

[16] ElBadawey MR, Alwaa A, ElTaher M, Carrie S. Quality of life benefit after endoscopic frontal sinus surgery. Am J Rhinol Allergy. 2014; 28 (5):428–432

[17] Sikand A, Silvers SL, Pasha R, et al. ORIOS 2 Study Investigators. Office-based balloon sinus dilation: 1-year follow-up of a prospective, multicenter study. Ann Otol Rhinol Laryngol. 2015; 124(8):630–637

[18] DeConde AS, Suh JD, Mace JC, Alt JA, Smith TL. Outcomes of complete vs targeted approaches to endoscopic sinus surgery. Int Forum Allergy Rhinol. 2015; 5(8):691–700

[19] Abuzeid WM, Mace JC, Costa ML, et al. Outcomes of chronic frontal sinusitis treated with ethmoidectomy: a prospective study. Int Forum Allergy Rhinol. 2016; 6(6):597–604

[20] McFadden EA, Kany RJ, Fink JN, Toohill RJ. Surgery for sinusitis and aspirin triad. Laryngoscope. 1990; 100(10, Pt 1):1043–1046

[21] Jankowski R, Pigret D, Decroocq F. Comparison of functional results after ethmoidectomy and nasalization for diffuse and severe nasal polyposis. Acta Otolaryngol. 1997; 117(4):601–608

[22] Morrissey DK, Bassiouni A, Psaltis AJ, Naidoo Y, Wormald P-J. Outcomes of modified endoscopic Lothrop in aspirin-exacerbated respiratory disease with nasal polyposis. Int Forum Allergy Rhinol. 2016; 6(8):820–825

[23] Morrissey DK, Bassiouni A, Psaltis AJ, Naidoo Y, Wormald P-J. Outcomes of revision endoscopic modified Lothrop procedure. Int Forum Allergy Rhinol. 2016; 6(5):518–522

[24] Rudmik L, Soler ZM, Mace JC, DeConde AS, Schlosser RJ, Smith TL. Using preoperative SNOT-22 score to inform patient decision for Endoscopic sinus surgery. Laryngoscope. 2015; 125(7):1517–1522

[25] Hopkins C, Rudmik L, Lund VJ. The predictive value of the preoperative Sinonasal Outcome Test-22 score in patients undergoing endoscopic sinus surgery for chronic rhinosinusitis. Laryngoscope. 2015; 125(8):1779–1784

42 Symptoms of Frontal Sinus Disease: Where Is the Evidence?

Zara M. Patel

Abstract

Symptoms of pressure or pain over the frontal sinus region are common, and can be from a vast array of etiologies. Despite the layperson and many primary physicians defaulting to a presumed diagnosis of frontal sinusitis, sinus inflammation or infection is often not the cause. Symptoms in this region can be from sinusitis, primary headache disorders such as migraine, temporomandibular joint disorders, trigeminal neuralgia, and many other sources. The key to effective management of frontal sinus symptoms lies in correct diagnosis and keeping a broad differential until objective evidence such as CT, MRI, and nasal endoscopy can lead the practitioner to the true etiology. Even with correct diagnosis, controversies in management of these symptoms remain.

Keywords: frontal sinus, frontal sinusitis, frontal sinus surgery, endoscopic sinus surgery, frontal sinus pain, headache, migraine, neuralgia

42.1 Published Evidence

Pain or pressure in and around the frontal region is often assumed to be from infection or inflammation of the frontal sinuses. Patients often come in complaining of a "sinus headache" and unfortunately this phrase is propagated by emergency room doctors, primary care physicians, pharmaceutical companies in their advertisements, and even some general otolaryngologists. Certainly sometimes this is the case, and appropriate treatment for rhinosinusitis can commence. The evidence, however, suggests that often symptoms felt in this region are not actually from the sinuses themselves. The job of the physician treating these patients is to know how to appropriately diagnose the true etiology of these symptoms in order to begin the correct therapy.

There is a paucity of literature correlating symptoms to sinus disease in this region. The best study evaluating pain in patients with an established radiological diagnosis of frontal sinus disease was done by DelGaudio et al in 2005.[1] They identified 207 patients with frontal disease, and found that 84% of mucocele patients, 29% of patients who had chronic rhinosinusitis with polyps (CRSwNP), and 59% of patients with chronic sinusitis without polyps (CRSsNP) experienced frontal pain. Interestingly, when the nonmucocele patients were combined and stratified, the subcategory that demonstrated the highest proportion of pain was those with mild to moderate mucosal thickening. This confirms a fact that has been demonstrated multiple times in our literature: severity of radiological disease does not necessarily correlate to patient symptomatology.[2]

This was again confirmed in reviewing the comparison of Lund-Mackay score (LMS) and Sinonasal Outcome Test-22 (SNOT-22) scores,[18] which do not correlate, but also the exact opposite was true in CRSsNP patients; the lower LMS consistently reported higher "pain" scores on their SNOT-22 scores.

Multiple societies have published diagnostic criteria concerning pain associated with rhinosinusitis. The American Academy of Otolaryngology–Head and Neck Surgery (AAOHNS) has published a clinical practice guideline, and both Canadian and European societies have published similar criteria, all stating approximations of the idea that pain can be present in acute rhinosinusitis (ARS) if associated with purulent nasal discharge, and even in the setting of chronic rhinosinusitis (CRS) if associated with purulent nasal discharge or nasal obstruction as well as an objective finding of CRS on nasal endoscopy or imaging.[3,4,5]

The International Classification of Headache Disorders from the International Headache Subcommittee (IHS) also supplies criteria for diagnosing headaches associated with sinusitis, and they have gone so far as to say that CRS is not a valid cause of headache or facial pain unless that disease relapses into an acute state.[6]

It is important for the emergency room doctor, primary care physician, and otolaryngologist to remember that even severe frontal pain and pressure coupled with purulent drainage is not necessarily a bacterial sinusitis. If a patient has these symptoms for less than 7 to 10 days, the likelihood that this is an acute viral rhinosinusitis (AVRS) is much more likely.[3] Although many physicians and patients feel compelled to diagnose a bacterial infection when symptoms are more severe, there is no evidence to validate this idea.[3] If either the symptoms last longer than 10 days without beginning to resolve or there is initial improvement and then a worsening in symptoms ("double-worsening"), then an acute bacterial rhinosinusitis (ABRS) is more likely.[3] Impending complications of ABRS such as orbital or intracranial involvement are important to watch out for, but this is different than simply having more severe frontal pain/pressure without any other symptoms or signs of those possible complications.

Allergic rhinitis is associated with nasal obstruction and drainage, but patients will often also report surrounding facial pain and pressure in spite of not having any true sinus involvement when imaged.[7] Nasal endoscopy and computed tomography (CT) scan are often very helpful in establishing, both for the practitioner and the patient, that these are simply referred symptoms without true frontal sinus disease.

Of the most common other diagnoses that can cause similar symptoms as rhinosinusitis in the frontal region, which include multiple primary headache syndromes, neurogenic disorders, surrounding musculoskeletal derangements, and odontogenic problems, migraine has been the most frequently missed diagnosis. When evaluating patients with headache that patients originally attributed to their sinuses in a tertiary care rhinologic practice, after demonstrating a normal nasal endoscopy and CT scan, 58% of these patients went on to be diagnosed with migraine.[8] Alternately, from a neurologic perspective, the Sinus Allergy and Migraine Headache Study (SAMS) was conducted on a similar patient population—those self-identifying as having "sinus headache"—and found that 63% of those patients had migraine based on the IHS criteria.[9]

The other significant group of primary headache disorders that are often confused with CRS or ABRS are the trigeminal cephalalgias, which include cluster headache, hemicrania continua, paroxysmal hemicrania, and many more. The main diagnostic confusion arises from the trigeminal symptoms these patients exhibit, including nasal congestion, rhinorrhea, epiphora, and conjunctival erythema and edema. These are signs the layperson typically associates with sinus problems, and therein lies the challenge.[9]

The main musculoskeletal diagnoses that can cause pressure and pain overlying the frontal region are tension-type headache and temporomandibular joint disorders. The musculature overlying this region is connected to the temporomandibular joint as well as all the other muscles overlying the scalp, quite commonly causing referred pain to this region.[9]

Most neurologic, neurogenic, temporomandibular, or odontogenic associated alternate diagnoses can be distinguished from true frontal rhinosinusitis if a careful history and complete neurological and head and neck physical examination is performed.[10]

Barosinusitis and recurrent acute rhinosinusitis (RARS) are two diagnoses that have little evidence correlating what we consider true "sinus disease" with symptoms, let alone specifically within the frontal sinus region.

One study performed on Danish pilots showed that over the course of 1 year, 30% reported one or more episodes of barosinusitis, and a study by Rudmik et al demonstrated some anatomic findings associated with barosinusitis, but neither of these studies looked specifically at or demonstrated findings regarding the frontal sinus.[11,12] Symptoms generally are limited to events where rapid changes in air pressure occur, such as when descending in an airplane or when deep sea diving. Barosinusitis will be discussed in more depth in a separate chapter in this book.

RARS similarly suffers from a paucity of literature on the subject, specifically regarding the frontal region. However, guideline-based criteria suggest we should diagnose this entity when patients have symptoms and signs of ABRS at least four times within a 12-month period with a relative lack of sinus symptoms at baseline between episodes.[13] The diagnosis can be a difficult one to establish, as often the patient will be between episodes when at the doctor's office and a sinus CT will be clear in these intervening periods of time. Unfortunately, the one anatomic study suggesting the correlation between specific anatomic variants and RARS only looked at data points including Haller's cells, concha bullosa, and septal deviation, but did not look specifically at variations in frontal anatomy.[14]

Finally, somewhere between the diagnostic categories of frontal pressure and pain caused by sinonasal disease and that caused by neurogenic pain syndromes lies the diagnosis of contact point headache. Originally described as Sluder's neuralgia, there are many theories about why and how mucosa touching mucosa may be irritating enough to cause such significant pain and pressure. Although no high-level evidence exists to bolster this theory, multiple small cohort studies have described the phenomenon and reported subsequent resolution of symptoms after removal of contact points.[15] The relationship between mucosal contact points and associated pain and pressure often becomes even more theoretical when the location of those symptoms are in the frontal region, apparently referred upward from whichever contact point is occurring within the nasal cavity (see Box 42.1).

> ## Box 42.1 Possible diagnoses causing symptoms in the frontal sinus region
>
> Bacterial frontal rhinosinusitis
> Viral frontal rhinosinusitis (upper respiratory infection)
> Allergic rhinitis
> Migraine
> Trigeminal autonomic cephalalgias (cluster headache, paroxysmal hemicrania, etc.)
> Tension-type headache
> Temporomandibular joint disorders
> Atypical neuralgia (trigeminal or other nerve)
> Barosinusitis
> Recurrent acute rhinosinusitis
> Contact point headache

42.2 Controversies and Opinions

Within the differential described earlier, true controversy can be found surrounding RARS, contact point headaches, and barosinusitis. Of these three, most rhinologic experts would agree that the diagnoses of RARS and barosinusitis exist—the controversy only begins when discussing appropriate management. However, even the idea of whether or not contact point headache exists has been strongly debated.

- Although small prospective studies exist showing benefit from treating patients with contact point headaches, the studies have no control groups, low numbers, and no high-level evidence exists to justify the diagnosis. We also know that many patients without any pain or pressure have contact points on endoscopy or CT.[16] Thus, we are left to our own clinical acumen to reason if this diagnosis is a real one, and how to treat it. What some experts have suggested and what we do in our center is to use a step-by-step protocol to establish how much a contact point may be affecting a patient. At the initial visit, after the usual anesthetic and decongestant spray has been applied to both nostrils, we evaluate the patient's pain before and after this generalized application. We then use a cotton-tip applicator doused in the same solution to apply this directly to the contact point and leave this within the patient's nose for approximately 5 to 10 minutes. We have found that this methodology will cause a dramatic decrease in symptoms within a subset of patients. If this is the case, then we have the patient return to our office and forego the general spray, but instead only apply the anesthetic solution directly to the contact point. If we again obtain a significant decrease in symptomatology, we use this as our indication that a true contact point headache exists, and we will take that patient to surgery to remove the contact point. We have found good success and consistent results with this method.

42.3 Case Examples

42.3.1 Case 1

A 64-year-old man, with coronary artery disease but otherwise healthy, presents with many years' history of left frontal sinus pain and pressure. He has seen multiple otolaryngologists and neurologists. He has had sinus surgery performed once in the past, with no change in symptoms, and has been told by all subsequent otolaryngologists that his sinuses are clear and this is a primary headache disorder. He has been tried on over 20 different neurologic medications, including triptans, tricyclics, pregabalin, etc., by neurologists to obtain control of this headache, and none have had any effect. He is quite desperate for relief, and comes to see if the author may have any different opinion or anything else to offer in the form of treatment.

Nasal endoscopy (▶ Fig. 42.1): The patient was found to have a contact point with surrounding inflamed mucosa between his left middle turbinate and an ethmoid cell that had not been removed during his first sinus surgery, which was confirmed on CT (▶ Fig. 42.2). We placed anesthetic at the contact point between his middle turbinate and remnant ethmoid septation and at both visits, the patient had a dramatic response and decrease in his headache. (He began crying in the office from a sense of relief from the pain that he had constantly experienced for the past 6 years.)

We moved forward and performed very selective surgery to remove this contact point (▶ Fig. 42.3). He had an increase in headache for the first week after surgery and then, as surgical inflammation resolved, his headache went away completely. He has now been headache free for the last 15 months.

- The controversy surrounding RARS has to do with the appropriate management. There is an increasing body

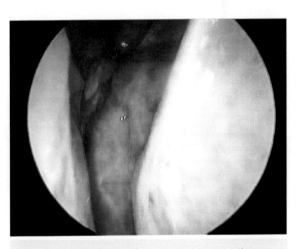

Fig. 42.1 Nasal endoscopy demonstrating contact point between left middle turbinate and ethmoid cell.

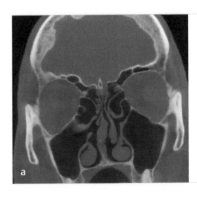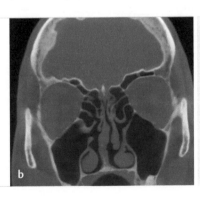

Fig. 42.2 (a,b) Coronal CT cuts demonstrating contact point between left middle turbinate and ethmoid cell.

of literature suggesting that these patients improve with surgical intervention in the same manner that patients do with CRS.[17] However, extent of surgery remains unexplained and can vary widely between practitioners, with some opening all sinuses and others only performing very limited sinus surgery. This pertains to a discussion about frontal rhinosinusitis, because a CT will not necessarily show disease, and symptoms may be all the surgeon has to go by. The tertiary sinus surgeons within our practice have differing methods of treating these patients. The author will open all sinuses each time she operates on a patient with RARS, as she cannot depend on imaging to show him which sinuses are specifically involved in each relapse, and often the area of facial pain and pressure described by the patient is broad and vague. Another senior surgeon in our practice will only address maxillary and ethmoids when treating RARS, and only addresses the frontal sinuses if a patient has a complaint that their pressure is in that specific location. As we currently have no literature to determine which is best, and we both have obtained good results in our patients, both seem to be reasonable options.

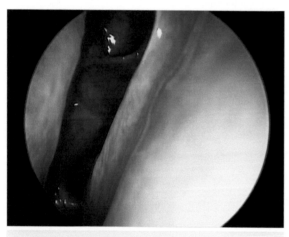

Fig. 42.3 Postoperative nasal endoscopy.

42.3.2 Case 2

The patient is a 34-year-old man who was previously healthy, but over the last 2 years has been having recurrent sinus infections. He notes that he has five to six episodes in a year and always has to take antibiotics to recover from these episodes. After he takes the medication, he feels very well again and returns to baseline, but eventually will relapse. His symptoms when he has these episodes are foul smelling and colored drainage out of his nose and postnasally, severe nasal obstruction and extreme fatigue, but he does not experience too much facial pressure or pain.

Nasal endoscopy (in between episodes): Within normal limits, no pus/polyps (▶ Fig. 42.4, ▶ Fig. 42.5, and ▶ Fig. 42.6).

We took the patient for complete sinus surgery, opening all sinuses. He is now doing well, is 7 months out from surgery, and has not had any relapses, compared to the prior 7 months during which time he suffered from three sinus infections.

Post-OP Nasal Endoscopy (▶ Fig. 42.7a,b)

- Similarly, barosinusitis appears to be well accepted among rhinologists as a true entity, but again controversy arises when discussing management. Similarly to RARS, some will opt to only open the maxillary and ethmoid sinuses and others will open all sinuses. The author follows the same logic when treating barosinusitis as when treating RARS. As the scan is clear and it appears to be anatomic predisposing factors the author is trying to modify, he moves forward with opening all sinuses in these patients, and has had excellent results.

42.3.3 Case 3

The patient is a 55-year-old woman with an extremely sensitive case of what appears to be barosinusitis. She is unable to drive into the mountains to go skiing with her family, she is unable to fly at all, and when the barometric pressure changes in her environment (such as when a storm front approaches), she has an exquisitely tender deep ache within her sinus cavities in the frontal region.

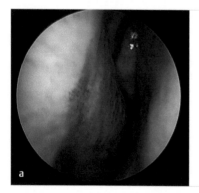
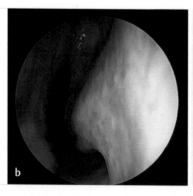

Fig. 42.4 (a,b) Normal nasal endoscopy in a patient with recurrent acute rhinosinusitis when between symptomatic episodes.

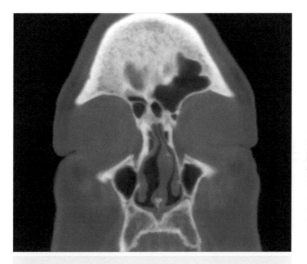

Fig. 42.5 Coronal section of a CT scan in a patient with recurrent acute rhinosinusitis, demonstrating septal deviation and intersinus frontal septal cell as well as supra-agger frontal cells, crowding the outflow of the frontal sinuses.

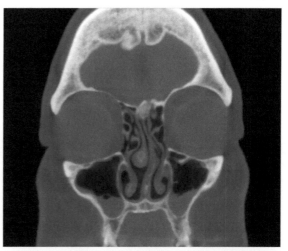

Fig. 42.6 Coronal section of a CT scan in a patient with recurrent acute rhinosinusitis, demonstrating septal deviation and a Haller (infraorbital ethmoid) cell narrowing the natural drainage pathway of the maxillary sinus.

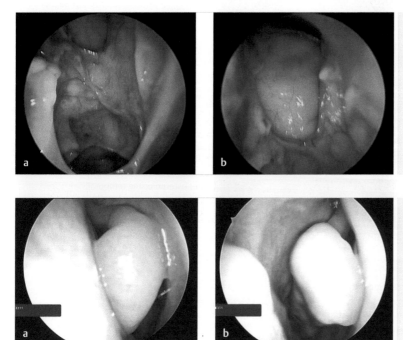

Fig. 42.7 (a,b) Nasal endoscopy after surgery demonstrating widely patent sinuses in a patient with recurrent acute rhinosinusitis.

Fig. 42.8 (a,b) Nasal endoscopy of a patient with barosinusitis, demonstrating mildly edematous leading edge of the middle turbinates but otherwise clear.

Nasal endoscopy: Within normal limits, no pus/polyps although some mild edema of the leading edge of the middle turbinate bilaterally (▶ Fig. 42.8 and ▶ Fig. 42.9).

We took her to surgery and opened all her sinuses (▶ Fig. 42.10). She has recovered well, and now, 3 months later, is asymptomatic and is able to fly and enjoy trips to the mountain with her family and is being taught how to snowboard by her 15-year-old son.

• The final controversy, and one for which we have absolutely no evidence to discuss, is the patient with minimal disease on CT. This is the patient who comes with significant facial pain or pressure in the frontal sinus region and a CT scan is obtained, and there appears to be some very mild mucosal thickening but no frank opacification and no occlusion of the frontal recess. This is a patient for whom many of us believe these minor findings cannot explain their significant symptomatology, but this becomes difficult to explain to a patient when they are sent a radiology report that notes "sinus disease" within the frontal sinus. Not only is it difficult to convince them,

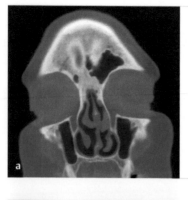

Fig. 42.9 (a,b) Coronal sections of CT scan in a patient with barosinusitis demonstrating clear but crowded sinuses.

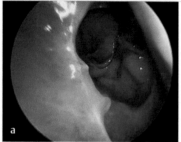
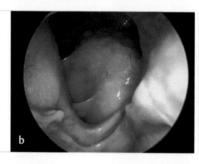

Fig. 42.10 (a,b) Postoperative nasal endoscopy demonstrating widely patent sinuses in a patient with barosinusitis.

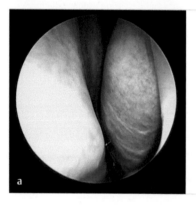
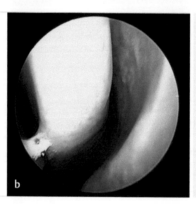

Fig. 42.11 (a,b) Normal nasal endoscopy in a patient with facial pressure and intermittent nasal drainage.

but also we really have no basis in the literature to either support or refute intervention, whether it is medical or surgical, that would be directed toward sinusitis in this patient population. The author's own treatment method varies based on individual findings such as other anatomic factors, whether the patient has had surgery before and whether the author feels the patient has reasonable expectations of which symptoms we think we can improve and which we cannot.

42.3.4 Case 4

A 43-year-old woman comes in with significant complaints of frontal headache, which she is convinced is a "sinus headache," persistent pressure between her eyes, and intermittent nasal drainage.

Nasal endoscopy (▶ Fig. 42.11): Within normal limits, no pus/polyps.

Although the CT scan ▶ Fig. 42.12 shows scant mucosal thickening intermittently throughout the sinuses, in particular within the frontal sinus, we do not believe symptoms of the severity which she describes could be related to these minimal findings. We recommend a trial of rizatriptan to be taken when she feels a headache coming on. She returned to us indicating the rizatriptan was helpful in treating not only her headache but also the pressure between her eyes and nasal drainage. We referred her on to a neurologist so that they can work with her to establish a preventive migraine medication regimen so she does not have to take an abortive migraine medication so many times throughout the month.

42.3.5 Case 5

A 50-year-old man presents with 1-month onset of sudden, sharp, stabbing pain across his temple, forehead, and

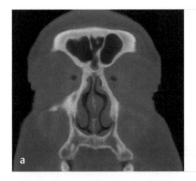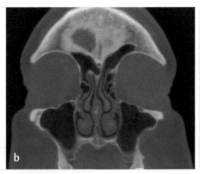

Fig. 42.12 (a,b) Coronal sections of a CT in a patient with scant mucosal thickening in the frontal sinus and trace thickening within ethmoids and maxillary sinuses with significant facial pressure and pain.

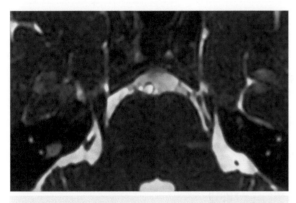

Fig. 42.13 Axial section of an MRI demonstrating vascular compression of the left trigeminal nerve.

mid face region only on the left side. He was told by his primary doctor that this was likely a sinus infection and was given multiple courses of antibiotics before being referred to our clinic.

CT is clear and nasal endoscopy is within normal limits.

MRI shows clear compression of the trigeminal nerve by accompanying artery (▶ Fig. 42.13).

The patient was referred to our neurosurgical colleagues who took the patient for vascular decompression of the trigeminal nerve. The surgery was successful and the patient's facial pain resolved.

42.4 Unanswered Questions

The main questions that remain in the topic of frontal sinus symptomatology are the following:
- How can we get patients to the correct diagnosis and appropriate treatment faster and with less delay in referral to the correct specialist?
- Does contact point headache truly exist, and if so, what is the appropriate diagnostic workup and management?
- What is the appropriate management for patients with RARS?
- What is the appropriate treatment for patients with barosinusitis?

- What is the significance of minimal sinus disease on CT, and how should we manage these patients?

References

[1] DelGaudio JM, Wise SK, Wise JC. Association of radiological evidence of frontal sinus disease with the presence of frontal pain. Am J Rhinol. 2005; 19:167–173

[2] Bhattacharyya N. A comparison of symptom scores and radiographic staging systems in chronic rhinosinusitis. Am J Rhinol. 2005; 19:175–179

[3] Rosenfeld RM, Piccirillo JF, Chandrasekhar SS, et al. Clinical practice guideline (update): adult sinusitis. Otolaryngol Head Neck Surg. 2015; 152:S1–s–39

[4] Fokkens WJ, Lund VJ, Mullol J, et al. European Position Paper on Rhinosinusitis and Nasal Polyps 2012. Rhinology Suppl. 2012;3:1–298

[5] Desrosiers M, Evans GA, Keith PK, et al. Canadian clinical practice guidelines for acute and chronic rhinosinusitis. J Otolaryngol Head Neck Surg. 2011; 40 Suppl 2:S99–S193

[6] Headache Classification Subcommittee of the International Headache Society. The International Classification of Headache Disorders. 2nd edition. Cephalalgia. 2004; 24 Suppl 1:9–160

[7] Brook CD, Kuperstock JE, Rubin SJ, Ryan MW, Platt MP. The association of allergic sensitization with radiographic sinus opacification. Am J Rhinol Allergy. 2017; 31:12–15

[8] Perry BF, Login IS, Kountakis SE. Nonrhinologic headache in a tertiary rhinology practice. Otolaryngol Head Neck Surg. 2004; 130:449–452

[9] Eross E, Dodick D, Eross M. The Sinus, Allergy and Migraine Study (SAMS). Headache. 2007; 47:213–224

[10] Patel ZM, Setzen M, Poetker DM, DelGaudio JM. Evaluation and management of "sinus headache" in the otolaryngology practice. Otolaryngol Clin North Am. 2014; 47:269–287

[11] Boel NM, Klokker M. Upper respiratory infections and barotrauma among commercial pilots. Aerosp Med Hum Perform. 2017; 88:17–22

[12] Rudmik L, Muzychuk A, Oddone Paolucci E, Mechor B. Chinook wind barosinusitis: an anatomic evaluation. Am J Rhinol Allergy. 2009; 23: e14–e16

[13] Bhattacharyya N, Grebner J, Martinson NG. Recurrent acute rhinosinusitis: epidemiology and health care cost burden. Otolaryngol Head Neck Surg. 2012; 146:307–312

[14] Alkire BC, Bhattacharyya N. An assessment of sinonasal anatomic variants potentially associated with recurrent acute rhinosinusitis. Laryngoscope. 2010; 120:631–634

[15] Patel ZM, Kennedy DW, Setzen M, Poetker DM, DelGaudio JM. "Sinus headache": rhinogenic headache or migraine? An evidence-based guide to diagnosis and treatment. Int Forum Allergy Rhinol. 2013; 3:221–230

[16] Herzallah IR, Hamed MA, Salem SM, Suurna MV. Mucosal contact points and paranasal sinus pneumatization: does radiology predict headache causality? Laryngoscope. 2015; 125:2021–2026

[17] Costa ML, Psaltis AJ, Nayak JV, Hwang PH. Medical therapy vs surgery for recurrent acute rhinosinusitis. Int Forum Allergy Rhinol. 2015; 5 (8):667–673

[18] Meltzer EO, Hamilos DL. Rhinosinusitis diagnosis and management for the clinician: a synopsis of recent consensus guidelines. Mayo Clin Proc. 2011;86(5):427–443

43 Anatomy and Classification of Frontoethmoidal Cells

Tomasz Gotlib, Anshul Sama, and Christos Georgalas

Abstract

The complex anatomy of the frontal recess has always evaded classification: A number of attempts have been made to identify and name in a structured way the way in which the various cells, septa, and bony protrusions interact in the area of the anterior ethmoid, frontal beak, and frontal ostium in order to produce the frontal recess. In this chapter, we aim to provide a review of these attempts, from the earliest to the latest, and to suggest a more simple way, descriptive of naming these cells.

Keywords: frontal recess, frontal sinus cells, frontoethmoidal cells, Kuhn cells, frontobullar cell, suprabullar cell, supraorbital cell

43.1 Introduction

The term "frontal recess" was introduced by Killian.[1] Mosher described the connection between frontal sinus and anterior ethmoids as a nontubular structure, contained within the frontal recess, an inverted funnel–shaped space.[2]

The anterior boundary of this funnel begins below the frontal beak and continues along the medial surface of the frontal process of the maxillary bone (agger nasi), down to the level of the middle turbinate attachment. It extends from the lamina papyracea laterally to the upper part of the vertical lamella of the middle turbinate and lateral lamella of the cribriform plate medially. The upper boundary of the frontal recess extends along the skull base to the anterior wall of the ethmoidal bulla (if it reaches the skull base).[3] Posterior border of the frontal recess is delineated by the anterior wall of the ethmoidal bulla[3] or, according to some authors, by the basal lamella of the middle turbinate.[4]

43.2 Published Evidence

Van Alyea gave a detailed description of the frontal recess, and defined "frontal cell" as any cell that encroaches upon the frontal recess or frontal sinus.[5]

He described most of the currently known "frontal cells"; however, definitions and nomenclature of these cells have been evolving. Recently, it was suggested to name these air spaces "frontoethmoidal cells."[3] The most constant cell of the frontal recess is the agger nasi cell, which is found in 78 to 94% of patients.[6,7] Other cells are highly variable, and may pneumatize into the frontal sinus.[5]

The transition between the frontal sinus and recess is not clearly delineated. This is why it is preferred to use the term "opening" instead of ostium, describing a two-dimensional structure.[3] This also implies that in some cases it can be difficult to classify a frontoethmoidal cell as pneumatizing or not pneumatizing into the frontal sinus.

Bent and Kuhn limited the definition of frontal cells to those pneumatizing above the agger nasi (▶ Table 43.1).[8]

In this publication, the origin of pneumatization or the anteroposterior extent of the cells was not discussed. However, in 1996, inspired by the studies of van Alyea, Kuhn[9] extended this classification by adding the following:

- Agger nasi cell.
- Frontal bullar cells (FBC).
- Suprabullar cells (SBC).
- Supraorbital cells (SOEC).
- Interfrontal sinus septal cells.

However, again, no detailed description of the newly described cells was given.

Wormald et al suggested a modification of this classification, based on the embryological fact that no cell isolated within the frontal sinus could exist, by defining the K3 cell (frontal cell type III) as extending less than half of the sinus' vertical height, and K4 cell more than half of it.[10] In 2004, Lee et al used the original extended Kuhn classification to analyze 50 1-mm axial CT scans with coronal and sagittal reconstructions.[11] Detailed definition of each cell type was included this time (▶ Table 43.2). The authors suggested division of the cells into anterior, posterior, and medial. Anterior cells included agger nasi cell and frontal cell types 1 to 4 (▶ Fig. 43.1 and ▶ Fig. 43.2). The posterior wall of these cells is described as "free partition in the frontal recess," not the skull base. In contrast, the posterior cells' anterior wall is also bounded by the free partition in the frontal recess, but posterior/superior wall is the skull base. Posterior cells include FBC, SBC, and SOEC (▶ Fig. 43.2). Interfrontal sinus septal cell is the only "medial" cell in this classification. Its main part, by definition, is located within the frontal sinus (▶ Table 43.2). Recessus terminalis (TR or

Table 43.1 Frontal cell types I to IV according to Bent et al.[8]

Type I	Single frontal recess cell above the agger nasi cell
Type II	Tier of cells in the frontal recess above the agger nasi cells
Type III	Single massive cell pneumatizing the cephalad into the frontal sinus
Type IV	Single isolated cell within the frontal sinus

Table 43.2 Frontal pneumatization pattern definitions and criteria

Frontal recess cell description

Agger nasi cell

- "The most anterior ethmoid cell"
- Swelling along the lateral nasal wall anterior to middle turbinate vertical attachment (endoscopic view)
- Pneumatization of the agger nasi region
- Well seen on sagittal and coronal CT images

Frontal cell, type 1

- Single anterior ethmoid cell above the agger nasi cell
- Posterior wall is not skull base; posterior wall is free partition in the frontal recess
- Well seen on coronal and sagittal CT images

Frontal cell, type 2

- Tier of 2 or more anterior ethmoid cells that pneumatize above the agger nasi cell
- Posterior wall is not skull base; posterior wall is free partition in the frontal recess
- Well seen on coronal and sagittal CT images

Frontal cell, type 3

- Single large anterior ethmoid cell above the agger nasi cell
- Pneumatizes along the inner aspect of the anterior frontal sinus table from the anterior frontal recess
- Extends far into true frontal sinus; superior wall (cap) inserts upon the inner aspect of the anterior frontal sinus table (seen on sagittal CT image)
- Posterior wall is not skull base; posterior wall is free partition in the frontal recess
- Well seen on coronal and sagittal CT images

Frontal cell, type 4

- Apparently isolated cell within the frontal sinus and above the agger nasi cell
- Appears as an "air bubble" on coronal CT scan
- Appears as a "balloon on a string" on sagittal CT scan
- The anterior/inferior margin is the anterior frontal sinus table or the frontal sinus floor
- The posterior boundary is the cell wall, not the posterior frontal sinus table
- Identification requires both sagittal and coronal CT images

Supraorbital ethmoid cell

- Ethmoid cell that extends over the orbit from the frontal recess
- May be single or multiple
- May mimic the appearance of a septate frontal sinus
- Opens into the lateral aspect of the frontal recess (this opening is lateral and posterior to the true frontal sinus ostium)
- Identification requires review of both axial and coronal CT images

Frontal bullar cell

- Ethmoid cell above the ethmoid bulla

Table 43.2 (continued) Frontal pneumatization pattern definitions and criteria

Frontal recess cell description

- Pneumatizes along the skull base into the frontal sinus from the posterior frontal recess

- Posterior wall is anterior cranial fossa skull base (frontal sinus posterior table)

- Anterior border must extend into the frontal sinus

- Located behind the true frontal sinus pneumatization tract

- May represent pneumatization of the anterior wall of the ethmoidal bulla (bulla lamella)

- May cause convexity in the floor of the frontal sinus

- Well seen on sagittal CT

Suprabullar cell

- Ethmoid cell above the ethmoid bulla

- Superior wall is the anterior cranial fossa skull base

- Anterior border does not extend into frontal sinus

- May represent pneumatization of the anterior wall of the ethmoidal bulla (bulla lamella)

- Well seen on sagittal CT

- Bears close resemblance to the suprabullar recess (CT alone is inadequate to distinguish between the suprabullar cell and the suprabullar recess)

Interfrontal sinus septal cell

- Pneumatization of the frontal sinus septum

- Drains into one frontal recess

- Associated with pneumatized crista galli

- Well seen on axial and coronal sinus CT

Recessus terminalis

- The superior uncinate process attaches laterally to the orbit, below the internal frontal ostium

- Frontal sinus drains directly into the middle meatus

- Often associated with the agger nasi cell

- Well seen on the coronal sinus CT

Source: From Lee et al.[12]

terminal recess) was also included into the classification; however, authors stated that it is not a frontal recess cell. Descriptions of the cells also defined their extension into the frontal sinus. Kuhn type 4 cell (▶ Fig. 43.3) was characterized as follows: "appear as isolated cells in the frontal sinus, and they drain through a narrow channel to the region above the ANC." Thus, it was not described as a separate isolated cell without any connection to the frontal recess.

Authors of European Position Paper on the Anatomical Terminology of the Internal Nose and Paranasal Sinuses (2014) suggested classifying "frontoethmoidal cells" as anterior, posterior, medial, or lateral, with respect to the frontal recess/inner walls of the frontal sinus.[3] Using a further definition of high and low, this can be adapted to define frontobullar cells as posterior high and suprabullar cells as posterior low. Similarly, K1 cells become anterior low and K3 cells anterior high.

Wormald et al modified the classification of Lee and Kuhn (▶ Table 43.3). This classification, named "International Frontal Sinus Anatomy Classification" (IFAC), divides the frontoethmoidal cells into three major groups (anterior, posterior, and medial) with regard to the frontal sinus drainage pathway (FSDP).[4]

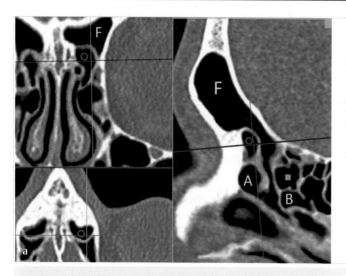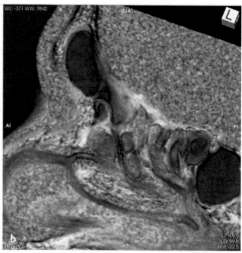

Fig. 43.1 (a) Multiplanar and **(b)** 3D reconstruction of the frontal recess. Frontoethmoidal cells according to Kuhn, IFAC, and modified European Anatomy paper classifications (*red circle*: K1 cell/supra-agger cell/anterior low cell; *green box*: nonapplicable/suprabullar cell/posterior low cell; A, agger nasi cell; B, ethmoidal bulla; F, frontal sinus).

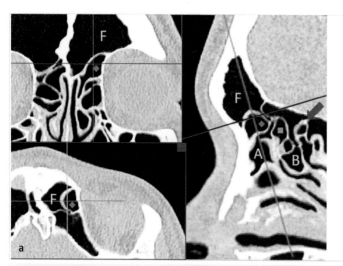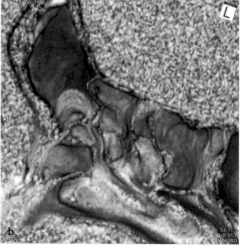

Fig. 43.2 (a) Multiplanar and **(b)** 3D reconstruction of the frontal recess. Frontoethmoidal cells according to Kuhn, IFAC, and modified European Anatomy paper classifications (*orange diamond*: K3 cell/supra-agger frontal cell/anterior high cell; *green box*: nonapplicable/suprabullar cell/posterior low cell; *purple cross*, supraorbital ethmoid cell/supraorbital ethmoid cell/supraorbital cell; F, frontal sinus; B, ethmoidal bulla; A, agger nasi cell; *red arrow*: anterior ethmoidal artery).

Frontal cell classification (as described by Kuhn) was simplified. K1 and K2 are assigned as supra-agger cells and K3 and K4 as supra-agger frontal cells. The definitions of these cells are less precise and their posterior boundary is not clearly specified; however, it is depicted on the figures exemplifying each cell type (free partition of the frontal recess). Classifications of the cells according to their position with regard to FSDP can raise problems as in some patients with massive inflammatory changes it is not possible to find FSDP even using adjusted multiplanar reconstruction (MPR) of thin-slice CT.

43.3 Controversies and Opinions

Although the lateral frontoethmoideal cells were mentioned in the European anatomical paper, they were not described in this document. The lateral cells extend from the inner surface of the frontal process of the maxillary bone, or anterior table of the frontal sinus to the skull base posteriorly, pushing FSDP medially and/or anteriorly (▶ Fig. 43.4).[12] They may pneumatize to the bony canal of the anterior ethmoidal artery. They are unclassifiable using the Kuhn and IFAC classifications, but are defined as lateral cells in our

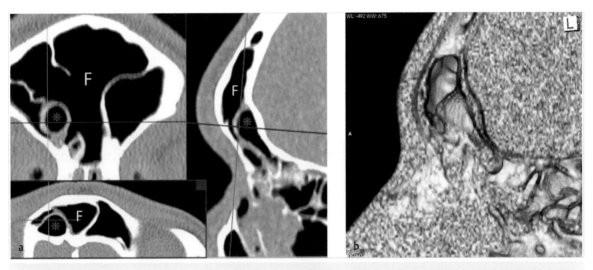

Fig. 43.3 **(a)** Multiplanar and **(b)** 3D reconstruction of the frontal recess. Frontoethmoidal cells according to Kuhn, IFAC, and modified European Anatomy paper classifications (*red asterisk*: frontobullar cell/suprabullar frontal cell/posterior high cell; F, frontal sinus).

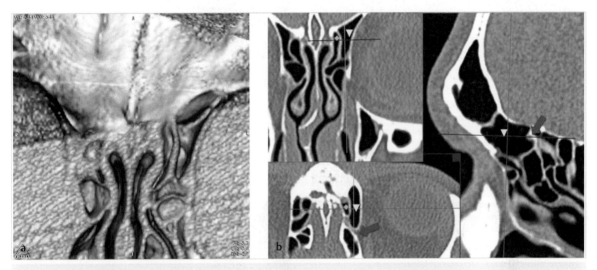

Fig. 43.4 **(a)** 3D reconstruction and **(b)** multiplanar reconstruction of the frontal recess. (*Yellow triangle*: lateral frontoethmoidal cell [unclassifiable according to Kuhn and IFAC classifications]/lateral cell [modified European Anatomy paper classification]; *green diamond*: frontal sinus drainage pathway; *red arrow*: anterior ethmoidal artery).

suggested modified version of the European Anatomy classification. Another cells that have been recently described are paramedian cells, which are medially based cells not attached to the interfrontal sinus septum.[13]

Pianta et al presented agger-bullar classification (ABC), which divides the anterior ethmoids into two compartments with regard to FSDP: anterior agger compartment and posterior bullar compartment.[13] Frontoethmoidal cells were also divided depending on penetration into the frontal sinus, and relation to the insertion of the uncinate process. The number of cells in each compartment is counted. This classification represents a novel approach toward describing frontoethmoidal cells. It gives an overview of all of the air spaces within the frontal recess, and provides different type of information helpful during the surgery, compared to the Kuhn and IFAC classifications. However, its use in everyday practice does not seem easier.

Table 43.3 Kuhn's classification,[11] International Frontal Sinus Anatomy Classification (IFAC),[4] European Anatomical Position Paper Classification (as modified by the authors)[3]

		Kuhn classification	IFAC classification	Modified European Position Paper classification
Cell type	**Definition**		**Cell name**	**Cell name**
Anterior cells (push the drainage pathway of the frontal sinus medial, posterior, or posteromedially)	Cell that sits either anterior to the origin of the middle turbinate or directly above the most anterior insertion of the middle turbinate into the lateral nasal wall	Agger nasi	Agger nasi cell	Agger nasi
	Anterolateral ethmoidal cell, located above the agger nasi cell (not pneumatizing into the frontal sinus)	K1/K2	Supra-agger cell	Anterior low cell
	Anterolateral ethmoidal cell that extends into the frontal sinus. A small supra-agger frontal cell will only extend into the floor of the frontal sinus, whereas a large supra-agger frontal cell may extend significantly into the frontal sinus and may even reach the roof of the frontal sinus	K3, K4	Supra-agger frontal cell	Anterior high cell
Posterior cells (push the drainage pathway anteriorly)	Cell above the bulla ethmoidalis that does not enter the frontal sinus	Suprabullar	Suprabullar cell	Posterior-low cell
	Cell that originates in the suprabullar region and pneumatizes along the skull base into the posterior region of the frontal sinus. The skull base forms the posterior wall of the cell	Frontobullar	Suprabullar frontal cell	Posterior-high cell
	An anterior ethmoid cell that pneumatizes around, anterior to, or posterior to the anterior ethmoidal artery over the roof of the orbit. It often forms part of the posterior wall of an extensively pneumatized frontal sinus and may only be separated from the frontal sinus by a bony septation	Supraorbital	Supraorbital ethmoid cell	Supraorbital cell
Medial cells (push the Drainage pathway laterally)	Medially based cell of the anterior ethmoid or the inferior frontal sinus, attached to or located in the interfrontal sinus septum, associated with the medial aspect of the frontal sinus outflow tract, pushing the drainage pathway laterally and frequently posteriorly	Frontal septal cell	Frontal septal cell	Medial cell
Lateral cells (push the drainage pathway medially)	The lateral cells extend from the inner surface of the frontal process of the maxillary bone to the skull base posteriorly, pushing frontal sinus drainage pathway medially and/or anteriorly	Not defined	Not defined	Lateral cell
	Medially based cell of the anterior ethmoid or the inferior frontal sinus, not attached to the interfrontal sinus septum, pushing the drainage pathway laterally and frequently posteriorly	Not defined	Not defined	Paramedian cell

Ideal classification should be simple, precise, including all frontoethmoidal cell types, and improve communication between the surgeons. However, the frontoethmoidal cells are so highly variable that regardless of which classification is used, finding of unclassifiable air space is very likely. Like in many instances, nature evades our attempts at classification, and one should always keep an open mind and be prepared to be surprised.

References

[1] Killian G. Die Killian'sche radicaloperation chronischer Sternhohleneiterungen: II. Weiteres kasuistisched material und zusammenfassung. Arch Laryngol Rhin.. 1903; 13:59

[2] Mosher HP. The applied anatomy and intranasal surgery of the ethmoid labyrinth. Trans Am Laryngol Assoc. 1912; 34:25–39

[3] Lund VJ, Stammberger H, Fokkens WJ. European position paper on the anatomical terminology of the internal nose and paranasal sinuses. Rhinol Suppl. 2014(24):1–34

[4] Wormald PJ, Hoseman W, Callejas C, et al. The International Frontal Sinus Anatomy Classification (IFAC) and Classification of the Extent of Endoscopic Frontal Sinus Surgery (EFSS). Int Forum Allergy Rhinol. 2016; 6(7):677–696

[5] Van Alyea OE. Frontal cells: an anatomic study of these cells with consideration of their clinical significance. Arch Otolaryngol. 1941; 34:11–23

[6] Landsberg R, Friedman M. A computer-assisted anatomical study of the nasofrontal region. Laryngoscope. 2001; 111(12):2125–2130

[7] Cho JH, Citardi MJ, Lee WT, et al. Comparison of frontal pneumatization patterns between Koreans and Caucasians. Otolaryngol Head Neck Surg. 2006; 135(5):780–786

[8] Bent JP, Cuilty-Siller C, Kuhn FA. The frontal cell as a cause of frontal sinus obstruction. Am J Rhinol. 1994; 8:185–191

[9] Kuhn FA. Chronic frontal sinusitis: The endoscopic frontal recess approach. Oper Tech Otolaryngol Head Neck Surg. 1996; 7:222–229

[10] Wormald PJ, Chan SZ. Surgical techniques for the removal of frontal recess cells obstructing the frontal ostium. Am J Rhinol. 2003; 17 (4):221–226

[11] Lee WT, Kuhn FA, Citardi MJ. 3D computed tomographic analysis of frontal recess anatomy in patients without frontal sinusitis. Otolaryngol Head Neck Surg. 2004; 131(3):164–173

[12] Gotlib, T, Kołodziejczyk, P, Kuźmińska, M, Bobecka–Wesołowska, K, Niemczyk, K. Three-dimensional computed tomography analysis of frontoethmoidal cells: A critical evaluation of the International Frontal Sinus Anatomy Classification (IFAC). Clin Otolaryngol. 2019; 44: 954– 960

[13] Pianta L, Ferrari M, Schreiber A, et al. Agger-bullar classification (ABC) of the frontal sinus drainage pathway: validation in a preclinical setting. Int Forum Allergy Rhinol. 2016; 6(9):981–989

44 To Drill or Not to Drill

Alfonso Santamaría-Gadea, Isam Alobid, and Manuel Bernal-Sprekelsen

Abstract

This chapter addresses the current indications for a Draf type III/endoscopic modified Lothrop procedure, its results, and particularly features related to potential restenosis as well as the cases in which this approach might be discussed as a primary surgery.

Keywords: endoscopic sinus surgery, frontal sinus, drill-out, Draf type III, endoscopic modified Lothrop procedure

44.1 Published Evidence

The endoscopic approach of the frontal sinus is one of the most challenging surgeries in endoscopic sinus surgery. The difficulty of access, the vast anatomical variations, and the close proximity to the orbit and the anterior cranial fossa make the frontal sinus a real challenge.[1,2,3]

The frontal sinus drilling procedures—also known as Draf type III and modified Lothrop, or drillout procedure—are not usually considered the first-line management of the frontal sinus in chronic rhinosinusitis (CRS). A clearance of the frontal recess with an appropriate removal of the ethmoidal cells restores the drainage of the outflow tract and the mucociliary clearance of the frontal sinus in most patients.[4,5] However, in patients with severe stages of CRS, such as nasal polyposis, with NSAIDs Exacerbated Respiratory Disease (N-ERD), or in laterally extended mucoceles, the Draf type III could be indicated as a primary surgery.

In patients with mild or moderate symptoms and frontal sinus involvement, an accurate and careful opening of the frontal recess with clearance of the drainage pathways is usually recommended in the form of a Draf I or IIa. This includes a complete anterior ethmoidectomy, preserving as much as possible the mucosa of frontal opening, particularly avoiding circular damage to the mucosa. Nonetheless, some patients may develop more problems in the frontal sinus than before the surgery.[5,6] Despite achieving an adequate opening of the frontal sinus and ethmoidal cells, restenosis can occur. Scarring, mucosal inflammation, lateralization of the middle turbinate, osteoneogenesis, and fibrosis are mechanisms that may compromise long-term frontal opening patency. Achieving a wide opening of the frontal sinus is one of the main objectives of surgery. In the literature, it has been hypothesized that mucosal preservation at the level of the frontal infundibulum may help reduce the incidence of subsequent blockage of the frontal sinus drainage.[7,8,9] Although it is a non–evidence based hypothesis, this thinking is derived from the high rates of failure with mucosal damage observed with external approaches.[10] In patients with persistent symptoms and frontal sinus disease, a more aggressive approach may be required.[4,5,7]

Thus, the questions that have to be answered are the following:

- What are the indications for the endoscopic drilling of the frontal sinus?
- In which cases would the endoscopic drilling of the frontal sinus be recommended as a primary surgery?
- Does the drillout procedure reduce the need of revision surgeries?
- Is the drillout procedure potentially related to a higher rate of complication?

44.2 Indications for Drilling Approaches of the Frontal Sinus

Since the endoscopic drilling of the frontal sinus was first described by Draf in 1991[11] and its application by Gross et al in 1995,[12] many reports analyzing the results, effects, and complications have been published. The classic indications of the drilling of the frontal sinus, as established by Draf, are shown in ▶ Table 44.1.[6]

According to the literature, the most frequent indication of performing a Draf type III is recalcitrant CRS. In most of these cases, the Draf type III has been considered as salvage surgery after failure of the primary, more conservative surgery of the frontal. In 2009, Anderson and Sindwani published one of the largest meta-analyses about patients who underwent drilling of the frontal sinus. Eighteen studies were analyzed (evidence level II-2 or II-3), containing data of 612 patients, with an average follow-up of 28.5 months. The number of previous surgeries in each patient was not presented in the revision. The authors report that the indications for drilling of the frontal sinus were similar to those of frontal sinus osteoplastic flap obliteration. The most common reasons for a Draf type III were chronic refractory frontal sinusitis and

Table 44.1 The classic indications of the drilling of the frontal sinus

Indications drill frontal sinus	• Difficult revision surgery • Risk factors (asthma, aspirin intolerance, ASA triad) • Benign and malignant tumors • Kartagener's syndrome • Ciliary immotility syndrome • Mucoviscidosis
Indications not to drill frontal sinus	• First surgery • No risk factors • Benign tumors

Source: Draf.[6]

mucocele formation, with a rate of 75.2 and 21.3%, respectively.[13]

However, there are other series[14] in which a Draf type III is performed as a primary surgery in some patients, although there are no accepted and generalized criteria for its application. Some authors try to evaluate whether a particular subset of patients with CRS would benefit from a primary Draf type III of the frontal sinus. A group of 339 patients with CRS were evaluated by Naidoo et al in 2013. All patients underwent a nondrilling approach (Draf I or IIa) as a primary surgery and a drilling approach (Draf III) if symptoms persisted despite the first surgery. The accumulation of nasal polyposis, asthma, Lund–Mackay scores greater than 16, and frontal ostium size less than 4 mm led to an increasing probability of requiring a drilling approach for the frontal sinus. The authors concluded that this group of patients would benefit from a primary Draf type III.[15]

Apart from CRS, the second most common cause for frontal sinus drilling is a frontal mucocele in which a drillout is also usually performed as a rescue surgery. However, there are also other, less frequent causes that may require a Draf type III as a primary surgery. A study on 120 patients with Draf III was reported by Eloy et al in 2011. In this series, the indications for drilling out the frontal sinus for a mucocele or a CRS were also the most frequent, 14 and 74%, respectively. In all cases, the Draf type III was indicated as a salvage surgery. Only in the case of benign (7.5%) or malignant tumors (0.5%) was the frontal sinus drilled as a primary surgery. Apart from being necessary for a complete resection of the malignant tumor, the authors explain that there is another reason to drill out the frontal sinus, namely, to prevent blockage of the frontal sinus due to the postoperative radiotherapy.[16]

In almost all the literature, frontal sinus drilling approaches are performed in the cases where nondrilling approaches have failed. More studies are required to compare patients with similar characteristics (high-risk patients), to identify those in whom frontal sinus drilling might be indicated as the primary surgery.

44.3 Results of Drilling Approaches of the Frontal Sinus

To evaluate the most suitable approach for frontal sinus disease, it is also important to know the results of frontal sinus drilling approaches. Many series of patients who have undergone such a surgery have been published showing high success rates for the Draf type III procedure. The factors that cause restenosis or failure of surgery were also studied. There is no consensus in defining the success of frontal sinus drilling approaches. Some authors describe the success as the rate of symptom improvement; others describe the failure of surgery such as the rate of restenosis or the rate of surgical revision. ▶ Table 44.2 displays results of some series.

In their meta-analysis, Anderson and Sindwani described that the improvement of the symptoms was achieved in 82.2% of cases. That was consistent with the rate of needed revision surgery, which stood at 13.9% (85/612).[13] Similar results were reported by Georgalas et al who examined 122 patients after a Draf type III procedure and found an 88% improved symptoms rate. Nevertheless, further 32% of cases required a revision surgery.[5]

Tran et al analyzed 77 consecutive patients with CRS who underwent a Draf type III procedure. They used the reduction of the size of the ostium as a way to define the

Table 44.2 Results in the drilling of frontal sinus

Author	Cohort	Revision surgery rate (%)	Symptoms improvement (%)	Restenosis rate (%)	Follow-up (mo)	Complications rate (%)
Wormald[4]	83	7	75	7	21.9	0
Banhiran et al[7]	72	7	75	5.6	22.0	0
Shirazi et al[17]	97	23	98	-	18.0	1
Tran et al[14]	77	13	–	33%[a]	29.2	–
Georgalas et al[5]	122	32	88	9.7	33.0	0
Eloy et al[16]	120	–	73	12.5	24.6	7.5
Hildenbrand et al[20]	24	4	–	4	25.6	0
Naidoo et al[18]	229	5	100	3	45.0	0
Ting et al[22]	204	29.9	70.1	29.9	122.4	5.8
Illing et al[19]	67	4.4	100	3%[b]	34.0	0

[a]Reduction of the intraoperative frontal ostium area of more than 60%.
[b]Reduction of the intraoperative frontal ostium area of more than 50%.

success of the surgery. All patients presented a reduction in the size of the area, and 33% presented a reduction greater than 60% from the initial size. These were considered the restenosis group. Only 13% ($n = 9$) of the cases required revision surgery, and only one of these was not in the restenosis group.[14]

Osteoneogenesis was believed to lead to surgery failure. There is only one study that has analyzed the relationship between bone formation, mucociliary clearance, and the final size of the frontal sinus. It was an animal model (14 sheep) performed by Rajapaksa et al in 2004. They found histological evidence of neo-osteogenesis in 56% of the biopsies. However, no worsened mucociliary clearance in those with neo-osteogenesis was found. In addition, the average reduction of the neo-ostium was 28%, and they also did not find a relationship with the new bone formation.[8]

Some authors have found other factors that may favor restenosis. In 2007, Shirazi et al published a retrospective analysis of 97 patients with a revision surgery rate of 23%. In 82% of these patients, the ASA triad and allergies were present. The authors found a failure rate significantly higher among patients with sensitivity to aspirin, nasal polyposis, asthma, and multiple environmental allergies.[17] Georgalas et al also reported a trend toward restenosis in the patients with ASA triad and cystic fibrosis.[5] In other series, the size of the neo-ostium and the "eosinophilic mucin CRS" were found to be significant factors in predicting the rate of postoperative restenosis.[14] This is opposite to what was described by DeConde and Smith in their review,[10] as shown later, although in some series no causes associated with an increased risk of closure were found.[16]

There are also surgical factors that may influence the success rate. One of the few reviews on this subject was recently published by DeConde and Smith. Fifteen publications on Draf IIa and 24 articles on Draf III were analyzed. They concluded that there is evidence to affirm that larger openings of the frontal sinus (> 4.5 mm in Draf IIa) in both nondrilling and drilling approaches present lower rates of restenosis. They also reported that development of the instrumentation and a better knowledge of the frontal anatomy seem to have improved results in frontal sinus surgery: the postoperative endoscopic patency rate reported for Draf type III procedures in the last 10 years ranged from 67.6 to 92% in contrast to the first 10 years when the results were found to be between 27.3 and 100%.[10]

44.4 Complications

Performing a Draf type III may lead to certain complications, including dural injury and cerebrospinal fluid (CSF) leak, orbital injury, and injury to the nasal bones and skin.[13] Most series reported a very low risk of major complications (< 1%).[5,18,19] Thus, most of the articles described the Draf type III procedure as a safe and well-tolerated

procedure when performed by experienced surgeons.[13] A reasonable hypothesis would be to think that frontal sinus drilling approaches present a higher complication rate than nondrilling approaches because they are more aggressive, but so far there are no studies comparing both.

44.5 Controversies and Opinions

The definition of success for drilling approaches of the frontal sinus has not been standardized. The complete resection of the tumor is the most common benchmark in the cases where this is the indication for the drilling approach.[5] However, when the surgery addresses CRS, the definition of success is not so clear. Patency of the frontal sinus, complete resolution or improvement of the symptoms, and the revision surgery rate were used in different series as a definition of surgical success. These benchmarks coincide in most patients. However, several series also described patients with complete frontal sinus stenosis after surgery without further symptoms and therefore not needing any rescue surgery.[5]

Several variants of the Draf type III technique have been described in the literature. One of them describes the coverage of the bare bone with mucosal flaps from the nasal septum. It would reduce the time of healing and the osteogenesis, thus improving the final results of the procedure.[20] However, this has not yet been proven.

44.6 Unanswered Questions

Drilling approaches of the frontal sinus were usually compared with external approaches in the literature, both being used as a salvage surgery. Therefore, the characteristics of the patients who underwent nondrilling approaches or drilling approaches of the frontal sinus were usually not comparable. Thus, comparison of the results and safety of both techniques is not feasible.

Further research with randomized clinical trials would be necessary to compare the results and complications of nondrilling and drilling approaches of the frontal sinus. In addition, such studies would support the understanding of which patients would benefit from a Draf type III as a primary surgery.

Although several factors associated with an increased risk of restenosis, as described earlier, have been studied, there is no way to predict when a patient will present restenosis after a Draf type III. This would certainly allow a frequent follow-up or a more aggressive debridement. Also, larger case series with a higher level of evidence would help detect risk factors for restenosis and failure of the surgery allowing performance of more aggressive surgeries or more frequent follow-ups in these risk patients.[10,21]

Finally, one factor cannot be measured, but might be taken into account: the heat generated on the drilled bone potentially promoting a reactive osteoneogenesis and restenosis.

Recommended Readings

One of the fundamentals of frontal sinus surgery is a correct knowledge of the anatomy. Therefore it would be recommendable to read the following:

- Wormald PJ. Endoscopic sinus surgery. 3rd ed. New York, NY: Thieme; 2013.
- Lund VJ, Stammberger H, Fokkens WJ, et al. European position paper on the anatomical terminology of the internal nose and paranasal sinuses. Rhinol Suppl 2014;24:1–14.

In order to maneuver with the best possible surgical technique, it is important to understand the different approaches of the frontal sinus and the classic indications of each one:

- Draf W. Endonasal frontal sinus drainage type I-III according to Draf. In: Kountakis S, Senior B, Draf W, eds. The Frontal Sinus. Berlin: Springer; 2005:219–232.
- Draf W. Endonasal micro-endoscopic frontal sinus surgery: The Fulda concept. Oper Tech Otolaryngol Head Neck Surg 1991;2:234–240.

The most recently published revisions of the drilling frontal sinus approaches are also recommended to understand the indications and results of this surgery:

- Anderson P, Sindwani R. Safety and efficacy of the endoscopic modified Lothrop procedure: a systematic review and meta-analysis. Laryngoscope 2009;119 (9):1828–1833.
- DeConde AS, Smith TL. Outcomes after frontal sinus surgery: an evidence-based review. Otolaryngol Clin North Am 2016;49(4):1019–1033.

Since the endoscopic drilling approaches of frontal sinus have been described, many case series have been published in the literature. According to their impact, follow-up time, and/or cohort size, some of the most important studies are the following:

- Georgalas C, Hansen F, Videler WMJ, Fokkens WJ. Long term results of Draf type III (modified endoscopic Lothrop) frontal sinus drainage procedure in 122 patients: a single centre experience. Rhinology 2011;49:195–201.
- Eloy P, Vlaminck S, Jorissen M, et al. Type III frontal sinusotomy: surgical technique, indications, outcomes, a multi-university retrospective study of 120 cases. B-ENT 2011;7(Suppl 17):3–13.
- Naidoo Y, Bassiouni A, Keen M, Wormald PJ. Long-term outcomes for the endoscopic modified Lothrop/Draf III procedure: a 10-year review. Laryngoscope 2014;3 (5):412–417.

References

[1] Wormald PJ. Endoscopic Sinus Surgery. 3rd ed. New York, NY: Thieme; 2013

[2] Lund VJ, Stammberger H, Fokkens WJ, et al. European position paper on the anatomical terminology of the internal nose and paranasal sinuses. Rhinol Suppl. 2014(24):1–34

[3] Weber RK, Hosemann W. Comprehensive review on endonasal endoscopic sinus surgery. GMS Curr Top Otorhinolaryngol Head Neck Surg. 2015; 14:Doc08

[4] Wormald PJ. Salvage frontal sinus surgery: the endoscopic modified Lothrop procedure. Laryngoscope. 2003; 113(2):276–283

[5] Georgalas C, Hansen F, Videler WMJ, Fokkens WJ. Long term results of Draf type III (modified endoscopic Lothrop) frontal sinus drainage procedure in 122 patients: a single centre experience. Rhinology. 2011; 49:195–201

[6] Draf W. Endonasal frontal sinus drainage type I-III according to Draf. In: Kountakis S, Senior B, Draf W, eds. The Frontal Sinus. Berlin: Springer; 2005:219–232

[7] Banhiran W, Sargi Z, Collins W, Kaza S, Casiano R. Long-term effect of stenting after an endoscopic modified Lothrop procedure. Am J Rhinol. 2006; 20(6):595–599

[8] Rajapaksa SP, Ananda A, Cain TM, et al. Frontal ostium neo-osteogenesis and restenosis after modified endoscopic Lothrop procedure in an animal model. Clin Otolaryngol. 2004; 29:386–388

[9] Valdes CJ, Bogado M, Samaha M. Causes of failure in endoscopic frontal sinus surgery in chronic rhinosinusitis patients. Int Forum Allergy Rhinol. 2014; 4(6):502–506

[10] DeConde AS, Smith TL. Outcomes after frontal sinus surgery: an evidence-based review. Otolaryngol Clin North Am. 2016; 49(4):1019–1033

[11] Draf W. Endonasal micro-endoscopic frontal sinus surgery: the Fulda concept. Oper Tech Otolaryngol Head Neck Surg. 1991; 2:234–240

[12] Gross WE, Gross CW, Becker D, Moore D, Phillips D. Modified transnasal endoscopic Lothrop procedure as an alternative to frontal sinus obliteration. Otolaryngol Head Neck Surg. 1995; 113(4):427–434

[13] Anderson P, Sindwani R. Safety and efficacy of the endoscopic modified Lothrop procedure: a systematic review and meta-analysis. Laryngoscope. 2009; 119(9):1828–1833

[14] Tran KN, Beule AG, Singal D, Wormald PJ. Frontal ostium restenosis after the endoscopic modified Lothrop procedure. Laryngoscope. 2007; 117(8):1457–1462

[15] Naidoo Y, Bassiouni A, Keen M, Wormald PJ. Risk factors and outcomes for primary, revision, and modified Lothrop (Draf III) frontal sinus surgery. Int Forum Allergy Rhinol. 2013; 3(5):412–417

[16] Eloy P, Vlaminck S, Jorissen M, et al. Type III frontal sinusotomy: surgical technique, indications, outcomes, a multi-university retrospective study of 120 cases. B-ENT. 2011; 7 Suppl 17:3–13

[17] Shirazi MA, Silver AL, Stankiewicz JA. Surgical outcomes following the endoscopic modified Lothrop procedure. Laryngoscope. 2007; 117(5):765–769

[18] Naidoo Y, Bassiouni A, Keen M, Wormald PJ. Long-term outcomes for the endoscopic modified Lothrop/Draf III procedure: a 10-year review. Laryngoscope. 2014; 124(1):43–49

[19] Illing EA, Cho do Y, Riley KO, Woodworth BA. Draf III mucosal graft technique: long-term results. Int Forum Allergy Rhinol. 2016; 6 (5):514–517

[20] Hildenbrand T, Wormald PJ, Weber RK. Endoscopic frontal sinus drainage Draf type III with mucosal transplants. Am J Rhinol Allergy. 2012; 26(2):148–151

[21] DeConde AS, Suh JD, Mace JC, Alt JA, Smith TL. Outcomes of complete vs targeted approaches to endoscopic sinus surgery. Int Forum Allergy Rhinol. 2015; 5(8):691–700

[22] Ting JY, Wu A, Metson R. Frontal sinus drillout (modified Lothrop procedure): long-term results in 204 patients. Laryngoscope. 2014; 124(5):1066–1070

45 Indications for Operating the Frontal Sinus: Primary Surgery or Always Second Line?

Nsangou Ghogomu and David B. Conley

Abstract

Should frontal sinus surgery be done primarily or always secondarily for frontal chronic rhinosinusitis (CRS)? Historically, chronic sinus outflow obstruction was considered the etiology of frontal CRS, and thus surgery limited to the osteomeatal complex (OMC) or frontal recess (Draf I/anterior ethmoidectomy) was the logical first surgery following failure of medical management. Our current understanding of the etiology of CRS suggests a multifactorial disease that includes a broad range of inflammatory mediators as well as mucociliary dysfunction that persist even in the presence of sinus ostial and recess patency. With this in mind, the goal of frontal sinus surgery is not only the relief of obstruction but also the provision of access for saline irrigation and topical medications such as steroids. This is much more likely to be accomplished following sinus ostial (at least Draf II) surgery where diseased septations consisting of mucosa and bone as well as part of the frontal beak are removed. With the advent of steroid-eluting frontal ostium implants, the risk of postoperative frontal sinus ostium stenosis has decreased, making surgery of the frontal ostium safer than it was just a few years ago. We thus consider Draf IIa as the first-line surgery in frontal CRS, except in the rare case of reversible inflammatory conditions such as mild unilateral CRS without nasal polyps (CRSsNP) associated with OMC obstruction.

Keywords: chronic rhinosinusitis, frontal sinus, anterior ethmoidectomy, osteomeatal complex, Draf, Lothrop, endoscopic modified Lothrop procedure

45.1 Introduction

In determining the extent of primary frontal sinus surgery for chronic rhinosinusitis (CRS), one must first determine what pathophysiologic change is sought from the planned anatomic modification. If obstruction of the osteomeatal complex (OMC) causes frontal CRS, simple outflow patency achieved by anterior ethmoidectomy would result in good outcomes for most patients. If the majority of frontal CRS is multifactorial mucosal inflammatory disease with associated dysfunction of mucociliary clearance, it stands to reason that the primary goal of frontal sinus surgery is provision of significant topical access to improve mucociliary clearance and decrease underlying inflammation. In this chapter, we break the question about the timing and extent of frontal sinus surgery into five logical and fundamental questions, which,

taken together, build the foundation to support our ultimate conclusion:

- Does OMC/frontal recess obstruction cause frontal CRS?
- Is anterior ethmoidectomy (Draf I) optimal as first-line surgery for frontal CRS?
- What are the clinical characteristics of patients who fail Draf I?
- Why is Draf I not successful in some patients with frontal CRS?
- Is primary Draf IIa effective as an initial surgical intervention for frontal CRS?

45.2 Controversies and Opinions

45.2.1 Does OMC/Frontal Recess Obstruction Cause Frontal CRS?

Evidence

In 1944, A.C. Hilding described the vector of mucociliary clearance in the frontal sinus: from the superior intersinus septum, it traveled laterally, then inferiorly, and finally medially, ultimately being carried out the frontal ostium and down the frontal recess. In 1967, Messerklinger published a landmark article that added a critical additional finding: in the medial aspects of the frontal sinus, ostium, and recess, the vector of mucociliary clearance is superior, effectively directing mucus into the frontal sinus (▶ Fig. 45.1). In the normal frontal sinus ostium, with these opposing vectors so close together, a

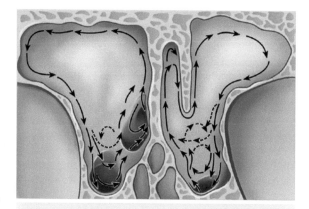

Fig. 45.1 Mucociliary flow through the frontal sinus, ostium, and recess. Note the retrograde flow into the frontal sinus. Source: Reproduced from Philpott C, Tassone P, Clark M. Bullet Points in ENT. Postgraduate and Exit Exam Preparation. 1st Edition. Thieme; 2014.

certain amount of recirculation is inevitable. In the setting of more viscous secretions or obstruction of the frontal recess, an increasing amount of mucus collecting at the ostium gets picked up by the upward mucus current and is recirculated into the frontal sinus.[1]

OMC is the area where the drainage pathways of the maxillary, anterior ethmoid, and frontal sinus converge. The pathogenesis of acute bacterial sinusitis of the frontal, maxillary, and anterior ethmoid sinuses is believed to be due to obstruction of the OMC following viral infection, followed by bacterial superinfection of stagnant sinus secretions.[2] Odontogenic infection may also start in the maxillary sinus, and spread via the OMC to involve adjacent sinuses.[3] The presence of mucociliary flow from the frontal recess into the ostium as well as the significantly increased recirculation in the setting of inflammation makes the frontal sinus particularly susceptible to infections starting in the OMC, and may delay its recovery from these infections.

Logical extension of this theory would support the hypothesis that CRS without nasal polyps (CRSsNP) is simply caused by prolonged obstruction of the sinus drainage pathways, with the OMC or proximal frontal recess being responsible for chronic frontal sinusitis. As recently as 2011, this theory appeared to still have widespread acceptance and was often quoted in the background of articles on CRSsNP.[4]

The concept of OMC or proximal frontal recess obstruction as the principal pathophysiologic mechanism of CRS has been brought into question by the results of several studies. In 1990, Wallace et al looked at CTs of patients with frontal 'sinus disease' and found that of 117 patients, 84 (72%) had OMC disease with normal frontal sinuses, 32 (27%) had frontal sinus disease without OMC involvement, and 17 (15%) had bilateral OMC disease but finding of only 1 diseased frontal sinus.[5] This study has innumerable weaknesses including failure to distinguish "disease" from "patency" and OMC from frontal recess, as well as failure to clearly define symptoms and duration of disease in the patient population. However, it appropriately questions whether obstruction of the frontal sinus drainage pathway causes adjacent sinus disease, or whether an underlying inflammatory process is responsible for simultaneous development of disease in the frontal sinuses and the OMC.

In 2003, Pruna published a case control study comparing the dimensions of the OMC in patients with normal CT scans (40) to those with well-defined untreated CRSsNP (64). Of particular interest, they found no difference in frontal recess and ethmoid infundibulum widths in the cases and controls. They found that when ethmoid mucosal thickening was present, similar finding was present in 97% of maxillary sinuses. However, when maxillary mucosal thickening was present, there was ethmoid thickening in only 29% of cases. They concluded that anterior chronic sinus disease did not necessarily begin in the OMC.[6]

In 2011, Leung et al looked at the CT scans of 144 patients with CRSsNP and 123 with CRS with nasal polyps (CRSwNP). In patients with CRSsNP, they found a significantly higher rate of frontal sinus disease in patients with OMC disease compared to those without (54 vs. 24%). However, they also found that in patients with CRSsNP, 25% of frontal and 50% of anterior ethmoid disease were not associated with obstruction of the OMC. In patients with CRSwNP, there was no difference in frequency of frontal sinus disease in patients with and without associated OMC disease (75 vs. 70%). They concluded that CRSwNP and many cases of CRSsNP may not be postobstructive in nature.[4] A very similar study was performed in 2013, comparing the rate of OMC obstruction in patients with ipsilateral maxillary, ethmoid, or frontal eosinophilic and noneosinophilic CRS. They found no association between OMC obstruction and disease in the ethmoid and frontal sinus for both subtypes. They found that while there was a high rate of maxillary sinusitis associated with an occluded OMC, 50% of maxillary sinusitis was associated with a patent OMC.[7] These findings were both in line with a retrospective study in 2010 looking at the CT of 106 patients with CRS where they found that 35% of patients with CRS of the maxillary, ethmoid, or frontal sinuses had nondiseased OMCs (▶ Table 45.1)[8].

Opinion

- Unilateral frontal (CRSsNP) associated with anterior ethmoid disease may be post-obstructive in origin.
- Bilateral frontal CRSsNP is correlated with, but not caused by, OMC obstruction. OMC obstruction may secondarily contribute to worsening of already-present CRSsNP via a postobstructive mechanism.

Table 45.1 Frequency of patent OMC in the setting of frontal CRS

	Wallace et al 1990	Chandra et al 2010[a]	Leung et al 2011		Snidvongs et al 2013
			CRSsNP	CRSwNP	
Number of patients	117	106	144	123	70
OMC patency rate	27%	35%	25%	30%	36%

Abbreviations: CRS, chronic rhinosinusitis; CRSsNP, CRS without nasal polyps; CRSwNP, CRS with nasal polyps; OMC, osteomeatal complex.
[a]In this study, data were pooled for maxillary, ethmoid, and frontal sinus disease.

- Frontal CRSwNP or eosinophilic mucin CRS (EMCRS) is not associated with or caused by obstruction of the OMC.

45.2.2 Is Anterior Ethmoidectomy (Draf I) Optimal as First-Line Surgery for Frontal CRS?

Evidence

The research into the pathophysiology of frontal CRS suggests that some, but not all, frontal sinus disease is associated with obstruction of the frontal recess or OMC. If this association is in fact a true causal mechanism, anterior ethmoidectomy should be an effective treatment in some cases of frontal CRS.

Becker et al did a retrospective study looking at the impact of Draf I (anterior ethmoidectomy) on chronic frontal sinusitis in 77 patients (33 unilateral, 44 bilateral disease, 121 sinuses) followed for a mean of 27 months. Approximately half of the cohort had polyps. They defined surgical failure as symptomatic disease that failed medical management and had confirmed opacification on CT scan. By that criteria, failure rate was found to be 14/121 (11.5%). Risk factors for failure included polyps with asthma and Samter's triad.[9]

A recent nonrandomized prospective study was performed by Abuzeid et al comparing outcomes of patients with frontal CRS who underwent either anterior ethmoidectomy or Draf IIa surgery. There was a significant selection bias in that patients who were selected for Draf IIa had a significantly higher rate of nasal polyps, prior surgery, asthma, and aspirin-exacerbated respiratory disease (AERD). Their primary outcome, 22-item Sino-Nasal Outcome Test (SNOT-22) score, was found to be similar at 1 year in both groups.[10]

These studies suggest that anterior ethmoidectomy may be a reasonable first step in patients with nonpolypoid disease, and those with polyps without asthma or AERD. Unfortunately, these studies have many methodological flaws, which make it difficult to determine when Draf I is sufficient. First, no published studies do a side-to-side comparison of patients with similar disease randomized to Draf I versus Draf II. Next, Becker et al only evaluated symptomatic patients, thus failing to include patients with asymptomatic frontal recess stenosis in their assessment of failure rate. Finally, Abuzeid et al only looked at SNOT-22 scores and did not report on patency rates at 1-year follow-up following Draf I.

Opinion

- These studies do suggest that in selected patients, surgery limited to the anterior ethmoids could be effective in the long term.

- The quality of the studies looking at Draf I efficacy for frontal CRS has significant weaknesses, making conclusions regarding its long-term efficacy difficult to make.

45.2.3 What Are the Clinical Characteristics of Patients Who Fail Draf I?

Evidence

The study by Becker et al concluded that patients with polyps, asthma, or AERD were likely to fail Draf I. The study by Abuzeid et al appeared to support those findings by demonstrating successful outcomes following Draf I as determined by SNOT-22 scores in carefully selected patients who were significantly less likely to have polyps, asthma, or severe disease.[9,10] Given the weakness of current evidence to support primary Draf I, alternative analysis of a study looking at patients getting revision Draf IIa procedures provides additional insight into the question of who fails primary Draf I procedures.

Naidoo et al published a study that included patients who underwent full FESS with Draf IIa. These patients were classified as "primary" if they had never undergone any sinus surgery and "revision" if they had previously undergone limited surgery not including the frontal ostium (Draf I). If all patients were equally at risk of failing Draf I procedures, you would expect an equal distribution of comorbidities between the primary and secondary Draf IIa populations in this study. However, their data revealed that compared to the population of all patients presenting for their first surgery, those who had previously undergone Draf I and failed were significantly more likely to have asthma, polyps, or EMCRS (► Table 45.2).[11]

Opinion

- Based on our current understanding of the disease pathophysiology combined with results of a few Draf I

Table 45.2 Increased frequency of asthma, polyps, and EMCRS in patients who failed Draf I

Characteristics	Patients presenting for first FESS	Patients who previously failed Draf I
Total patients	118	221
Asthma	4%	10%
Allergy	6%	7%
Polyps	7%	14%
EMCRS	3%	11%

Abbreviations: EMCRS, eosinophilic mucin chronic rhinosinusitis; FESS, functional endoscopic sinus surgery.

outcome studies, we predict that patients with mild unilateral frontal CRSsNP associated with OMC obstruction could get lifelong benefit from Draf I surgery.

- Patients at high risk of failing Draf I surgery during their lifetime include patients with:
  - Severe unilateral CRSsNP.
  - Bilateral or diffuse (anterior and posterior) mild CRSsNP.
  - CRSwNP.
  - EMCRS.
  - Comorbid asthma or AERD.

45.2.4 Why Is Draf I not Successful in Some Patients with Frontal CRS?

Evidence

As our understanding of CRS evolves, it appears that the primary benefit of sinus surgery is the provision of improved access for topical steroids and saline irrigation to the sinuses.[12] Saline irrigation assists with clearance of mucus rendered stagnant by microbe- and inflammation-induced acquired ciliary dysfunction.[13] Topical steroids have well-known broad anti-inflammatory effects and have been consistently found to be beneficial in both types of CRS, with greater benefits seen in polyp patients and following sinus surgery.[14,15] The success of any surgery in patients with frontal CRS depends on its ability to provide adequate access for these topical treatments.

A single study has been performed specifically looking at access of nasal irrigations to the frontal sinus in patients who had undergone endoscopic sinus surgery including Draf I. In this study, they included Technetium 99 m labeled saline douche, spray, and nebulizer and used scans to measure the level of radioactivity in each of the sinuses. Among the nine Draf I patients, only two had evidence of any radioactivity in the frontal sinus, and this was only seen with douching.[16]

Opinion

- Cases of frontal CRS, both obstructive and nonobstructive, require topical steroids and saline irrigations to decrease inflammation and compensate for acquired ciliary dysfunction.
- Draf I does not provide adequate access for saline irrigations or topical steroids.

45.2.5 Is Primary Draf IIa Effective as an Initial Surgical Intervention for Frontal CRS?

Evidence

Naidoo et al retrospectively looked at 210 primary Draf IIa procedures that had been performed as the first surgical intervention following failure of medical therapy. At

16 months, they had a 92% patency rate in a moderate-risk population in which 68% of patients had polyps and 29% had asthma. The only risk factor for failure was intra-op frontal ostium size less than 5 mm.[17] A significant part of the success of primary Draf IIa is likely attributable to the improved access for irrigations relative to Draf I. Studies looking into the effectiveness of topical medication and irrigation delivery to the frontal sinus following Draf IIa demonstrate an 81% rate of access and 25% rate of lavage in the vertex head position.[18]

Recently, an intrapatient randomized controlled trial of frontal sinus steroid-eluting implants following Draf IIa in 89 patients with similar asthma and polyp rates as those in the Naidoo et al study demonstrated significant benefits at 30- and 90-day follow-up including the following: (1) larger size of the frontal sinus ostium (5.9 vs. 4.4 mm) and (2) significantly decreased rate of ostium occlusion or stenosis (21 vs. 46%).[19] The postoperative use of the steroid-eluting frontal sinus implants will only lead to improvements in the already excellent 92% patency rate reported after Draf IIa and, consequently, improved disease control due to improved access for topical steroids and irrigation.

While Draf IIa appears superior to Draf I as the initial surgery for the majority of frontal CRS, recent evidence suggests that Draf III may be even better up front. First, access and lavage rates following Draf III are significantly better than those seen in Draf IIa based on research using cadavers (access 81 vs. 100%; lavage 25 vs. 88%)[18] as well as computational fluid dynamics.[20] This improved topical access correlates with improved outcomes following Draf III compared to Draf IIa procedures. In a study of 339 patients with frontal CRS followed for 2 years after Draf IIa procedure, 14% of the cohort failed and required a Draf III/endoscopic modified Lothrop procedure (EMLP). In this cohort, the rate increased to 17% when polyps were present, 28% when polyps and asthma were present, and 50% when asthma, polyps, and a Lund–Mackay score greater than 16 were present.[11] Bassiouni and Wormald published a head-to-head comparison of patients with polyps who underwent either Draf IIa or III procedures. At 21 months, polyp recurrence rates were lower in all Draf III patients (16 vs. 26%), but the benefit was even more impressive in the presence of asthma (16 vs. 40%), or AERD (11 vs. 55%).[21] These outcomes have ushered in an era where Draf III may be appropriate as a primary surgical intervention in patients with very severe polyp disease, or those associated with asthma or AERD.

Opinion

- Primary Draf IIa is safe and effective and should be used as the initial surgery in the majority of patients with frontal CRS.
- Steroid-eluting frontal sinus implants significantly decrease the risk of postoperative/iatrogenic frontal

sinus stenosis, making primary Draf IIa even safer to perform than it was just a few years ago.

- In some patients with more severe disease, Draf III/EMLP, rather than Draf IIa, may be more appropriate as the first-line surgery.

45.3 Case Studies

45.3.1 Case 1: Mild Diffuse CRSwNP Involving the Frontal Sinus

A 39-year-old man presents with 3 years of progressive nasal congestion and decreased olfaction. He denies history of asthma or AERD. Endoscopy reveals a middle meatus edema bilaterally. CT scan revealed diffuse mild mucosal thickening including the anterior ethmoids and frontal sinus with a total Lund–Mackay score of 9 (▶ Fig. 45.2). The patient failed to have any symptom resolution following a course of topical steroids, oral steroid burst, and oral antibiotics. He was taken to surgery where full functional endoscopic sinus surgery (FESS) including Draf IIa was performed. Intra-op, small polyps were identified. The maximum achievable anteroposterior dimensions of the frontal ostia without drilling of the frontal beak was 5 mm. Given the relatively mild disease present, rather than drill down the frontal beak, steroid-eluting implants were placed in the frontal ostium (▶ Fig. 45.3).

45.3.2 Case 2: Failed Draf I Procedure Requiring at least Draf IIa—Ciliary Dysfunction?

The patient is a 49-year-old man with a history of bilateral CRSsNP who had undergone bilateral FESS with Draf I and unilateral frontal trephination 10 years prior during a severe exacerbation of CRS. Symptoms improved, but slowly recurred over the last 12 months. CT performed after failing appropriate medical therapy during one of his exacerbations revealed very healthy right sinuses, but persistent left frontal and maxillary sinus mucosal disease in spite of a widely patent OMC, suggesting possible ciliary dysfunction (▶ Fig. 45.4a, b). He was taken to the OR for EMLP to maximize access for irrigation and topical steroids. Since surgery, symptoms as well as endoscopic and imaging findings have normalized.

45.3.3 Case 3: Severe CRSwNP Requiring EMLP as Initial Surgical Intervention

A 28-year-old man presents with 6-month history of decreased sense of smell. Changes were progressive and associated with postnasal drip and bilateral nasal congestion. He has a history of asthma. Nasal endoscopy revealed polypoid changes in the bilateral middle meatus. He had a limited response to oral prednisone burst and topical steroids and his symptoms recurred shortly after completion. CT scan following appropriate medical management revealed complete opacification of all sinuses (▶ Fig. 45.5). Full FESS with EMLP were performed and steroid-eluting implants were placed in the ethmoid as well as frontal sinuses.

45.3.4 Case 4: Odontogenic Frontal CRS

A 68-year-old man presents with odontogenic chronic sinusitis refractory to antibiotic therapy. He was scheduled for simultaneous removal of the offending tooth as well as FESS. Given the fact that minimal disease was present in the frontal sinus (▶ Fig. 45.6a) and this had

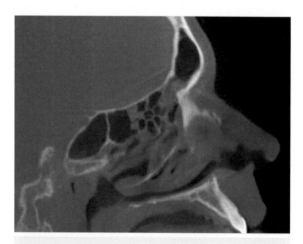

Fig. 45.2 Preoperative CT showing mild diffuse disease and narrow frontal ostium.

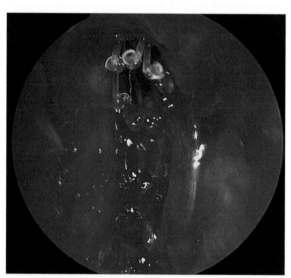

Fig. 45.3 Narrow frontal ostium intra-op requiring placement of steroid-eluting implant.

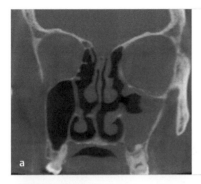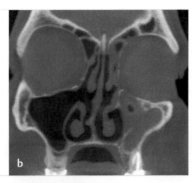

Fig. 45.4 (a,b) Preoperative CT demonstrating chronic rhinosinusitis in spite of patent osteomeatal complex.

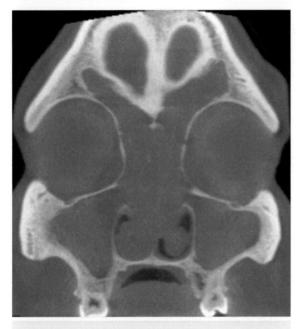

Fig. 45.5 Preoperative CT of a patient who underwent endoscopic modified Lothrop procedure up front for chronic rhinosinusitis with nasal polyposis.

clearly originated in a maxillary molar (▶ Fig. 45.6b), moved to the OMC and anterior ethmoid first, we planned to do a maxillary antrostomy and limited anterior ethmoidectomy. Intra-op, a tremendous amount of purulence and inflamed mucosa was present. After opening the anterior ethmoid and identifying the frontal recess, we realized it was so narrow and the mucosa at that level was so inflamed that the likelihood of stenosis causing secondary frontal sinusitis in the future was too great (▶ Fig. 45.7a). We thus proceeded with a Draf IIa procedure (▶ Fig. 45.7b). The patient did very well.

45.4 Unanswered Questions

- The main controversy is whether simple alleviation of an obstructed frontal recess is adequate in the management of frontal CRS. In this chapter, we argue that Draf IIa should be the starting point for the majority of cases of frontal CRS.
- The recommendations made against Draf I as primary surgery in this chapter are due to the low quality of the research on Draf I and extrapolations made from higher quality, but indirectly related research on Draf IIa outcomes. It would be ideal to have a well-designed, prospective, randomized study comparing Draf I to Draf IIa in similar patient cohorts; however, with the current state of knowledge, this may not be ethical.
- Given the expectation that Draf I would fail in the cases of postobstructive frontal CRS if acquired ciliary dysfunction is present, research better delineating which sinuses are predisposed to this will better guide treatment decisions regarding choice of surgery in obstructive disease.
- We argue that Draf I provides very poor access to the frontal sinus for irrigations. This is based on a very old study that does not use some of the more complex methodology available today. An updated study following Draf I surgery would help shed light on this question.

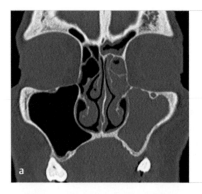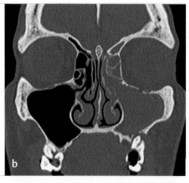

Fig. 45.6 (a,b) Preoperative CT of odontogenic sinusitis.

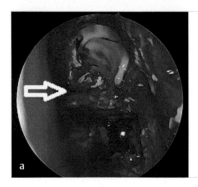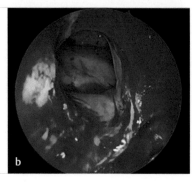

Fig. 45.7 (a) Intra-op picture of purulence in the ethmoids associated with extremely narrow and inflamed frontal recess (*arrow* to slitlike frontal recess). **(b)** Widely patent frontal ostium after Draf IIa.

References

[1] Hilding AC. III The Physiology of Drainage of Nasal Mucus IV. Drainage of the Accessory Sinuses in Man: Rationale of Irrigation of the Infected Maxillary Sinuses. Annals of Otology, Rhinology & Laryngology. 1944;53(1):35–41

[2] Messerklinger W. On the drainage of the normal frontal sinus of man. Acta Otolaryngol. 1967; 63(2):176–181

[3] DeMuri G, Wald ER. Acute bacterial sinusitis in children. Pediatr Rev. 2013; 34(10):429–437, quiz 437

[4] Onişor-Gligor F, Lung T, Pintea B, Mureşan O, Pop PB, Juncar M. Maxillary odontogenic sinusitis, complicated with cerebral abscess: case report. Chirurgia (Bucur). 2012; 107(2):256–259

[5] Leung RM, Kern RC, Conley DB, Tan BK, Chandra RK. Osteomeatal complex obstruction is not associated with adjacent sinus disease in chronic rhinosinusitis with polyps. Am J Rhinol Allergy. 2011; 25 (6):401–403

[6] Wallace R, Salazar JE, Cowles S. The relationship between frontal sinus drainage and osteomeatal complex disease: a CT study in 217 patients. AJNR Am J Neuroradiol. 1990; 11(1):183–186

[7] Pruna X. Morpho-functional evaluation of osteomeatal complex in chronic sinusitis by coronal CT. Eur Radiol. 2003; 13(6):1461–1468

[8] Snidvongs K, Chin D, Sacks R, Earls P, Harvey RJ. Eosinophilic rhinosinusitis is not a disease of ostiomeatal occlusion. Laryngoscope. 2013; 123(5):1070–1074

[9] Chandra RK, Pearlman A, Conley DB, Kern RC, Chang D. Significance of osteomeatal complex obstruction. J Otolaryngol Head Neck Surg. 2010; 39(2):171–174

[10] Becker SS, Han JK, Nguyen TA, Gross CW. Initial surgical treatment for chronic frontal sinusitis: a pilot study. Ann Otol Rhinol Laryngol. 2007; 116(4):286–289

[11] Abuzeid WM, Mace JC, Costa ML, et al. Outcomes of chronic frontal sinusitis treated with ethmoidectomy: a prospective study. Int Forum Allergy Rhinol. 2016; 6(6):597–604

[12] Naidoo Y, Bassiouni A, Keen M, Wormald PJ. Risk factors and outcomes for primary, revision, and modified Lothrop (Draf III) frontal sinus surgery. Int Forum Allergy Rhinol. 2013; 3(5):412–417

[13] Harvey RJ, Psaltis A, Schlosser RJ, Witterick IJ. Current concepts in topical therapy for chronic sinonasal disease. J Otolaryngol Head Neck Surg. 2010; 39(3):217–231

[14] Gudis D, Zhao KQ, Cohen NA. Acquired cilia dysfunction in chronic rhinosinusitis. Am J Rhinol Allergy. 2012; 26(1):1–6

[15] Snidvongs K, Kalish L, Sacks R, Craig JC, Harvey RJ. Topical steroid for chronic rhinosinusitis without polyps. Cochrane Database Syst Rev. 2011(8):CD009274

[16] Kalish L, Snidvongs K, Sivasubramaniam R, Cope D, Harvey RJ. Topical steroids for nasal polyps. Cochrane Database Syst Rev. 2012; 12: CD006549

[17] Wormald PJ, Cain T, Oates L, Hawke L, Wong I. A comparative study of three methods of nasal irrigation. Laryngoscope. 2004; 114 (12):2224–2227

[18] Naidoo Y, Wen D, Bassiouni A, Keen M, Wormald PJ. Long-term results after primary frontal sinus surgery. Int Forum Allergy Rhinol. 2012; 2(3):185–190

[19] Barham HP, Ramakrishnan VR, Knisely A, et al. Frontal sinus surgery and sinus distribution of nasal irrigation. Int Forum Allergy Rhinol. 2016; 6(3):238–242

[20] Smith TL, Singh A, Luong A, et al. Randomized controlled trial of a bioabsorbable steroid-releasing implant in the frontal sinus opening. Laryngoscope. 2016; 126(12):2659–2664

[21] Zhao K, Craig JR, Cohen NA, Adappa ND, Khalili S, Palmer JN. Sinus irrigations before and after surgery-Visualization through computational fluid dynamics simulations. Laryngoscope. 2016; 126(3):E90–E96

[22] Bassiouni A, Wormald PJ. Role of frontal sinus surgery in nasal polyp recurrence. Laryngoscope. 2013; 123(1):36–41

46 Economic and Quality-of-Life Evaluation of Surgery and Medical Treatment for Chronic Rhinosinusitis

Caroline S. Clarke, Carl M. Philpott, and Steve Morris

Abstract

Chronic rhinosinusitis (CRS) is a common disorder in the general population with a number of symptoms that markedly impact on quality of life. There is also a substantial financial burden to the NHS and wider society through health care consultations and through loss of productivity in the workplace. Although there are some established medical and surgical treatment options and guidelines, use of these is variable, partly due to insufficient evidence of effectiveness and cost-effectiveness, especially in regard to direct unbiased comparison between surgical and medical treatments. This chapter explores the tools that are currently available to measure CRS costs including the evidence base to date. It also discusses the differences between the available patient-reported health-related quality-of-life tools such as the condition-specific 22-Item Sinonasal Outcome Test (SNOT-22) and generic tools such as the EuroQoL (EQ-5D). In considering the overall cost-effectiveness of strategies for managing a condition, there is an inherent need to consider evidence to support the use of interventions in clinical practice. This remains a controversial area with a need for more trials for both medical and surgical treatments, and these controversies are discussed further in this chapter. The chapter assists the reader to understand the economic and quality-of-life implications of CRS and to appreciate the cost and cost-effectiveness implications of the medical and surgical treatments that are currently available.

Keywords: chronic rhinosinusitis, endoscopic sinus surgery, cost-effectiveness, quality of life

46.1 Published Evidence

46.1.1 What is Known about the Economic Burden of Chronic Rhinosinusitis?

Chronic rhinosinusitis (CRS) is a common disorder that affects approximately 11% of adults in the United Kingdom, with estimated rates in Europe varying from 6.9 to 27.1%.[1] These prevalence estimates depend in part on the source of sampling, as studies based on symptom profiles alone will overestimate the disease, whereas numbers of patients with CRS diagnosed by a specialist in line with international guidelines such as the European Position Paper on Rhinosinusitis and Nasal Polyps that require confirmation of symptoms with endoscopic and/or radiological changes[2] are likely to be an underestimate.

Studies measuring the economic burden of CRS often use observational datasets.[3,4,5] Using such datasets for retrospective cost analyses requires various assumptions to be made regarding the classification of patients within the dataset as being CRS patients. Nevertheless, in the United Kingdom, for example, one can examine longitudinal data from the Clinical Practice Research Datalink (CPRD)[6] and see the patterns of activity in primary care. A recent look at this data source showed that the average rhinosinusitis patient (including all types of acute and chronic sinusitis) visited their general practitioner (GP) about four times over a 12-month period in 2009 to 2011, and in doing so accrued direct costs to the National Health Service (NHS), including the receipt of multiple prescriptions (91% receiving antibiotics).[7]

Sinus surgery is one treatment option for CRS, and approximately one in three CRS patients referred to secondary care will undergo surgery (Hospital Episode Statistics [HES] data from England and Wales).[8] In the United Kingdom Sinonasal Audit of 2001, which recruited 3,128 patients who underwent surgery for CRS in a prospective observational study, the 5-year follow-up data for patients highlighted the issue of revision surgery, showing that, at 5 years, 19.1% had undergone further sinus surgery or a polypectomy since their original operation,[9] suggesting that their original surgery had perhaps failed in some way. This appeared to be higher in those with polyps (CRSwNPs, 20.6%) than in those without polyps (CRSsNPs, 15.5%). Furthermore, in cases of CRSwNPs where a simple polypectomy was initially performed, there was a significant risk of revision surgery compared to those who had also received additional sinus surgery at the first encounter.[10] To consider the burden of cost for revision surgery within the English NHS, we can combine the figures from the annual HES data for admissions with the NHS Reference Costs of approximately £1,500 per case for each surgical admission,[11,12] and estimate that the total cost to the NHS is likely to be over £30 million per year.[10] The proportion of revision surgeries estimated from the Chronic Rhinosinusitis Epidemiology Study (CRES) was 50%, meaning that an estimated £15 million is spent each year on revision sinus surgery or polypectomies. To date, there remains a lack of randomized controlled trials for sinus surgery[13] and as such it has been included in the National Institute for Health and Care Excellence (NICE) Database of Uncertainties about the Effects of Treatments (UK DUETs).[14]

In the United States, Bhattacharyya[15] estimated the health care burden for CRS using the Medical Expenditure Panel Survey (MEPS) and found that direct costs related to consultations, prescriptions, and emergency visits exceeded $8.6 billion in 2007[15] ($9.8 billion in 2016 prices[16]). He showed that adult CRS patients had three to four outpatient consultations and five repeat prescriptions annually compared to those without CRS, giving a bill of $772 per year per CRS patient. Using outpatient data, another U.S. study found that 12 to 26% of patients had four to eight medications coded for CRS.[17] Further work in Taiwan[18] showed that CRS patients had significantly more outpatient visits (3.9 vs. 1.4, $p < 0.001$) and costs (US$77.70 vs. US$19.40, $p < 0.001$) in 1 year from an initial physician visit in 2010 compared with patients in a control group.

46.1.2 What Are the Wider Costs of CRS?

Direct costs of CRS related to prescriptions, appointments, and surgical and other interventions can be quantified from health care datasets such as CPRD and HES in the United Kingdom or medical insurance databases in North America, as discussed earlier. However, these do not reveal other costs of the disease such as time off work (absenteeism), time spent in lower productivity at work due to illness (presenteeism), costs to patients in purchasing over-the-counter medications or other private health care expenditure, or travel to and from doctors' appointments, which are also important. Data on these wider costs are available from some European and American prospective studies. A key impact is that of CRS on productivity in the workplace. Recently in the United Kingdom, the national CRES collected data from CRS patients seeking treatment in secondary care and found levels of anxiety and depression that were significantly higher than a reference control population, with 25 to 31% reporting anxiety and/or depression compared to 19% of control patients.[19] This was consistent with the results of a Swedish study where anxiety and depression were seen in 28% of CRS patients,[20] and 57% of CRS patients reported absenteeism. Another study suggested that the morbidity of CRS was such that patients' reported quality-of-life (QOL) impairment was greater than that for lower back pain, angina, congestive heart failure, or chronic obstructive pulmonary disease (COPD).[21] CRS, therefore, has the potential to have a significant effect on an individual's functioning and productivity and, since it primarily affects those in middle age with a mean of 52 years,[22] this impacts workforce productivity and as such has been found to be one of the top 10 most costly diseases for U.S. employers.[23] Rudmik et al used annual daily wage rates in an attempt to determine the cost of lost productivity caused by CRS.[24] They found that a mean of 24.6 and 38.8 workdays were lost per CRS patient per year due to absenteeism and presenteeism, respectively, with a total of 21.2 household days lost for daily sinus care requirements; the resulting annual productivity cost was $10,077 per CRS patient and was directly related to worse

disease-specific QOL as measured using the SNOT-22 questionnaire.

46.1.3 What Is the Impact of CRS on QOL?

CRS patients have worse QOL than people without chronic conditions and comparable QOL to those with other chronic conditions. Disease-specific and generic measures have been used in a number of studies to assess this.

Impact on Disease-Specific QOL—SNOT-22

Erskine et al assessed SNOT-22 scores measured as part of the CRES,[25,26] which included those presenting to secondary care outpatient clinics and diagnosed according to the European Position Paper on Rhinosinusitis and Nasal Polyps 2 by an ENT (ear, nose, and throat) surgeon as having CRS. Erskine et al found that healthy controls reported a mean SNOT-22 total score of 12.1 (standard deviation [SD]: 13.9) out of a possible total of 110, whereas those with CRS (without nasal polyps) reported a mean SNOT-22 score of 45.7 (SD: 21.1), indicating that they experienced more and/or stronger negative impacts of the type assessed in the SNOT-22 questionnaire.[19] Those CRS patients with polyps or with allergic fungal rhinosinusitis reported a similar mean SNOT-22 score of 44.4 (SD: 21.6). These figures suggest that CRS patients with or without polyps suffer adverse effects as measurable via the SNOT-22 and experience a lower CRS-related QOL compared to healthy people.

A number of other studies also reported similar results, namely, patients with CRS experienced reduced QOL as expressed through higher SNOT-22 scores.[24,27,28,29]

Impact on Generic QOL—EQ-5D, SF-36, and SF-12

When considering the disease-specific QOL, research by various researchers agrees that generic QOL scores for CRS sufferers are worse for the general population, and comparable to sufferers of other chronic conditions. For example, the mean QOL score found using the 5-level EQ-5D version (EQ-5D-5L) for CRS patients in a recent feasibility study was 0.7553[30] and the trans-European GALEN study also demonstrated a lower health-related QOL in CRS patients compared to those without CRS.[31] This can be compared to the data on COPD patients from the United States, who had an EQ-5D-3 L QOL score of 0.79[32] and to European data on patients who had a stroke 4 months previously, with median EQ-5D-3 L QOL score of 0.77, or mean of 0.69.[33]

Other studies in the United Kingdom and United States have also reported worse EQ-5D-5 L, 12-Item Short Form Survey (SF-12), and SNOT-22 scores for CRS patients compared to patients with no chronic illnesses.[30,34] A comparison of patients' QOL at baseline as assessed using the three different measures concluded that higher SNOT-22 scores (i.e., worse CRS-related QOL) were associated with lower utility scores derived from the EQ-5D-5 L measure and lower mental component score (MCS) and physical component score (PCS) calculated from responses to the SF-12 questionnaire (i.e., worse generic health-related QOL).[28]

If the individual domains within these generic QOL questionnaires are considered, it can be seen that aspects of CRS patients' lives concerned with mobility and self-care are often not strongly affected, whereas levels of loss of QOL due to pain or discomfort, and anxiety or depression, are more pronounced, and the impact on people's performance of their usual activities (e.g., work, study, housework, family, or leisure activities) is also considerable.[19,28,35,36,37]

Qualitative Work Assessing Impact of CRS on Patients

Qualitative work exploring the experiences and opinions of CRS patients regarding their disease and the impact it has on various different aspects of their life, including problems with repeated or unsuccessful medical treatments, duration of symptoms, impact on daily living (e.g., loss of sense of smell), and the perceived need for integrated management of their condition across specialties (allergy and respiratory), has also highlighted the impact that this chronic condition has on patients' overall QOL, in terms of both their physical and mental health.[38,39]

46.1.4 Cost and Cost-Effectiveness of Treatment for CRS

Comparing Costs of Medical and Surgical Treatments

Medical treatment costs for CRS tend to include prescription costs and costs of appointments with primary care physicians and at secondary care outpatient clinics. These tend to be a lot lower than the costs of surgery, although these can continue for many years as CRS is a chronic condition.

A commonly quoted estimate of the overall cost burden of CRS was published by Bhattacharyya, who estimated annual direct costs of CRS to exceed $8.6 billion in 2007 in the United States ($9.8 billion in 2016 prices[16]), which were predominantly attributed to physician office visits, emergency department encounters, and medication use.[15] The same paper reported the mean yearly cost of medically treated CRS to be $772 (US in 2007). Rudmik et al. estimated average annual costs of $965 (US in 2013).[40] These estimates are much lower than estimated costs of ESS, which appear to vary considerably both within and

between countries and may reflect the varying extent of intervention between practitioners and also variations in coding for procedures. In Canada, the cost per outpatient day surgery patient was estimated at CAN$3,510 per case.[41] In the English NHS, costs paid by clinical commissioning groups for ESS vary between £1,771 and £2,299. Some changes may have been seen over the last decade as ESS is now more frequently performed as day surgery.[42] Further examples from the United States and Canada have shown significant reductions in health care utilization levels within 13 weeks postoperatively in patients undergoing surgery.[43] An American study in 2011 estimated the 45-day postoperative costs to be $772,675.

Cost-effectiveness studies in CRS are uncommon[2,9,44,45] but do offer some evidence of the costs of perioperative medical treatment.[46] The combined package of prescriptions, clinic visits, investigations, and the ESS increase to as high as $2,449 in the year before ESS, with the bulk of the cost in the last 6 months before surgery. In the year after surgery, costs dropped to an average of $1,564 per annum and further in the second year after ESS to $1,118 per year.[2,46] Another American study also looked at perioperative costs in 2014 and showed a significant decline in postoperative resource use but noted that all CRS patients require continuous baseline levels of health care utilization.[47] In another North American study considering those who had respiratory comorbidities in addition to their CRS, health care costs also reduced after surgical intervention, and asthma was found to be a main determinant of the associated costs.[48] It is important to note that comparing costs before and after surgery is not equivalent to comparing costs without and with surgery. To perform the latter comparison, random allocation to continued medical management or to surgery would be required.

Comparing Effects and Cost-Effectiveness of Medical and Surgical Treatments

Patients and their doctors are often faced with a choice over whether to have surgery to treat their CRS or to continue with medical management of their symptoms. There is little direct evidence that compares these two strategies, especially in terms of cost-effectiveness, and the published studies that are available are often not based on a randomized protocol.

The current CRS treatment pathway recommends medical management as the primary treatment, moving on to surgery when this is judged by the patient and their clinician to have failed. There is little consensus among national and international guidelines regarding the length and exact nature of maximum medical therapy or when is the best time to offer surgery.[49]

A handful of studies in the United States have evaluated ESS compared to medical therapy in CRS patients.[40,50,51,52] These studies carry significant risks of bias as they have tended to include nonrandomized patients who have failed on medical management and are offered a choice of continued medical management or ESS plus medical management. A U.S. cohort study reported that those patients choosing to undergo surgery had a lower baseline QOL than those who chose to remain on medical management and experienced significantly higher levels of improvement than patients who remained on medical management in several outcomes, including reduced direct and indirect costs.[51] In U.S. patients, Rudmik et al demonstrated that patients suffering from refractory CRS may reach stability after ESS, with 54% of patients achieving long-term postoperative QOL scores higher than the U.S. norm of 0.81.

A Canadian study simulated a risk analysis, using costs to Medicare, QOL, and complication rates reported in the literature. Three perspectives were used: the Medicare patient perspective, societal perspective, and universal health care perspective. The research question was concerned with estimating the threshold at which risks associated with repeated courses of oral corticosteroid (OCS) exceeded the risks associated with surgery. The results suggested that surgery was preferred over medical therapy where patients required OCS more than once every 2 years in CRS with nasal polyps, once per year in CRS without polyps/asthma, or twice per year for patients with Samter's triad.[52]

An attempt was made to estimate the long-term cost-effectiveness of ESS compared to continued medical management for patients with refractory CRS via a decision analytic model that used values for average costs and effects in CRS from various published sources.[40] The simulated patient pathway included three possible health states that were created based on QOL scores from a published clinical trial, and transition probabilities between these states were based on published data from nonrandomized observational studies. The U.S. third-party payer perspective was used to calculate costs and effects over a 30-year time horizon, comparing ESS followed by medical therapy to continued medical therapy alone. The incremental cost-effectiveness ratio (ICER) was calculated and suggested that the surgery strategy was likely to be the more cost-effective, although the results carried significant caveats due to the paucity of direct evidence available for the model and subsequent structural and parameter assumptions that were required to be made.

There is certainly growing evidence of the positive impact of sinus surgery on the lower respiratory tract as seen with analyses of data from both the U.K. primary care data in the Clinical Research Practice Datalink (CPRD)[53] and from the U.K. Sinonasal Audit,[54] including demonstrating that rates of late-onset asthma are influenced by the delay between diagnosis and surgical intervention.

A further study by Hopkins and colleagues examined the timing of offering surgery and the impact that this had on rates of health care resource use. Dates of diagnosis in CRS patients were determined in electronic health care datasets in the United Kingdom and United States, and patients were grouped into those who had ESS early after their diagnosis, that is, within 12 months, and those who had ESS late, that is, more than 5 years after the identified diagnosis date.[55,56] Both the U.K. and U.S. data showed that rates of health care use, including visits to health care professionals and CRS-related prescriptions, were lower after surgery in the group undergoing surgery within the first year after diagnosis than in those undergoing surgery at a later time. This suggests that undergoing surgery earlier in the treatment pathway could offer reductions in cost and therefore possible improvements in cost-effectiveness.

46.2 Controversies Surrounding the Cost-Effectiveness of Treatment for CRS

As with any economic evaluation that aims to compare a surgical and nonsurgical intervention, there is a potential problem with equipoise. In order to have equipoise, both options available must be understood to be similarly effective and carry similar levels of risk. It has historically been common for both patients and physicians to consider that surgery is a last resort and should only be offered when all medical options have failed, due to the inherent risks associated with undergoing a surgical procedure. Therefore, it is often difficult to recruit to randomized controlled clinical trials where participants will be randomized to options that include surgery and those who do not because surgery tends to be seen as an extreme option. This implies that potential participants could have a strong preference for which treatment they would want to be randomized to, and so either they are reluctant to be randomized, or it is possible that they might be more likely to drop out of the trial if they are unhappy with their randomly allocated treatment. As a result, although we present in this chapter a variety of results that broadly agree with each other, there is likely to be bias in the results reported due to the patient populations that were included in the studies. These have tended to be patients who are eligible for surgery, or who have already had surgery, and so are likely to be the more ill of those patients diagnosed with CRS. There have also mostly been small sample sizes in the studies published so far, which also introduces uncertainty into studies' results and into the conclusions and inferences that can be drawn. There is not always a distinction made between patients with and without nasal polyps, but this is potentially an important marker for more severe disease.

A further challenge to the economic evaluation of CRS is that observational studies using preexisting datasets do not yield QOL data from patients and do not give direct evidence of health states. Observational studies can be

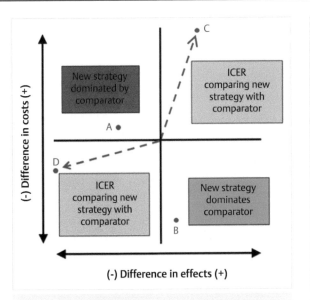

Fig. 46.1 The cost-effectiveness plan comparing the new strategy with the comparator.

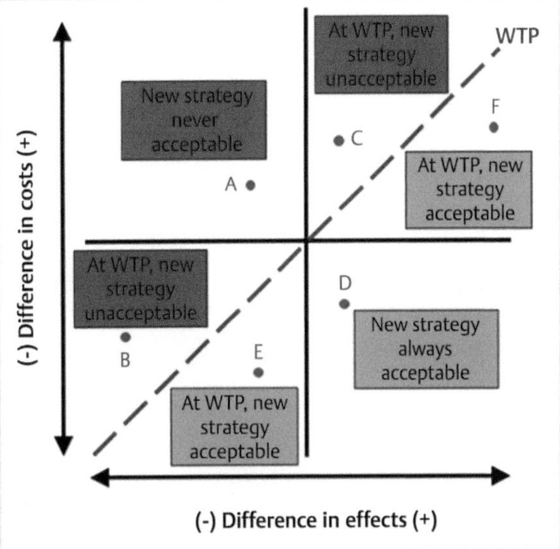

Fig. 46.2 Cost-effectiveness acceptability of the new strategy compared to the old (WTP, willingness-to-pay threshold).

performed using electronic health records as described earlier, and the outcomes available in these datasets tend to relate to rates of revision surgery and other clinical resource-based outcomes, rather than QOL outcomes, as the SNOT-22, EQ-5D, and SF-36/SF-12 are not routinely collected for CRS patients. This means that assumptions must be made both regarding the health states that patients pass through along their treatment journey and regarding QOL scores that are attached to these health states.

As CRS is a chronic disease, the impact of a successful intervention might be expected to last for a number of years. Clinical trials usually only collect data on each patient for 6 or 12 months, and then costs and effects past the end of that time frame must be estimated via a decision analytic model, using various assumptions regarding the evolution of these costs and effects.

Given that treatment failure may significantly affect both costs and outcomes,[57,58] future studies should consider cost and QOL impacts that might include the need for additional investigations, additional treatments for resistant organisms (in relation to antimicrobial use), and additional side effects from more toxic treatments.

46.3 Unanswered Questions and Future Research

To address the gaps in evidence identified earlier, more economic evaluations, especially those using quality-adjusted life years (QALYs) as the effectiveness outcome, are needed, and they should be based as far as possible on data that have bias removed or avoided as far as possible. The gold standard for unbiased data is randomized controlled trials; so, economic evidence from this type of source should be sought where possible.

Suggested Readings

Agborsangaya CB, Lahtinen M, Cooke T, Johnson JA. Comparing the EQ-5D 3 L and 5L: measurement properties and association with chronic conditions and multimorbidity in the general population. Health Qual Life Outcomes. 2014; 12:74

Brazier JE, Roberts J. The estimation of a preference-based measure of health from the SF-12. Med Care. 2004; 42(9):851–859

Dieleman JL, Baral R, Birger M, et al. US spending on personal health care and public health, 1996–2013. JAMA. 2016; 316(24):2627–2646

Dolan P. Modeling valuations for EuroQol health states. Med Care. 1997; 35 (11):1095–1108

Drummond M, Sculpher MJ, Claxton K, Stoddart GL, Torrance GW. Methods for the Economic Evaluation of Health Care Programmes. New York, NY: Oxford University Press; 2015

EQ-5D–3 L User Guide: Basic information on how to use the EQ-5D–3 L instrument. Secondary EQ-5D–3 L User Guide: Basic information on how to use the EQ-5D–3 L instrument 2015. Available at: https://euroqol.org/wp-content/uploads/2016/09/EQ-5D-3L_UserGuide_2015.pdf

EQ-5D–5 L User Guide: Basic information on how to use the EQ-5D–5 L instrument. Secondary EQ-5D–5 L User Guide: Basic information on how to use the EQ-5D–5 L instrument 2015. Available at: https://euroqol.org/wp-content/uploads/2016/09/EQ-5D-5L_UserGuide_2015.pdf

Fenwick E, Claxton K, Sculpher M. Representing uncertainty: the role of cost-effectiveness acceptability curves. Health Econ. 2001; 10(8):779–787

Guide to the Methods of Technology Appraisal. 2013. London, 2013

Hancox RJ, Milne BJ, Taylor DR, et al. Relationship between socioeconomic status and asthma: a longitudinal cohort study. Thorax. 2004; 59(5):376–380

Herdman M, Gudex C, Lloyd A, et al. Development and preliminary testing of the new five-level version of EQ-5D (EQ-5D-5L). Qual Life Res. 2011; 20 (10):1727–1736

Horsman J, Furlong W, Feeny D, Torrance G. The Health Utilities Index (HUI): concepts, measurement properties and applications. Health Qual Life Outcomes. 2003; 1(1):54

Hunter RM, Baio G, Butt T, Morris S, Round J, Freemantle N. An educational review of the statistical issues in analysing utility data for cost-utility analysis. Pharmacoeconomics. 2015; 33(4):355–366

Husereau D, Drummond M, Petrou S, et al. CHEERS Task Force. Consolidated Health Economic Evaluation Reporting Standards (CHEERS) statement. Value Health. 2013; 16(2):e1–e5

Jenkinson C, Layte R. Development and testing of the UK SF-12 (short form health survey). J Health Serv Res Policy. 1997; 2(1):14–18

Kozyrskyj AL, Kendall GE, Jacoby P, Sly PD, Zubrick SR. Association between socioeconomic status and the development of asthma: analyses of income trajectories. Am J Public Health. 2010; 100(3):540–546

McHorney CA, Ware JE, Jr, Lu JF, Sherbourne CD. The MOS 36-item Short-Form Health Survey (SF-36): III. Tests of data quality, scaling assumptions, and reliability across diverse patient groups. Med Care. 1994; 32(1):40–66

Morris S, Devlin N, Parkin D, Spencer A. Economic Analysis in Health Care. 2nd ed. Chichester, UK: John Wiley & Sons; 2012

Mulhern B, Feng Y, Shah K, et al. Comparing the UK EQ-5D-3 L and the English EQ-5D-5 L value sets. Pharmacoeconomics 2017

Office for National Statistics. Health Inequalities. Decennial Supplement No. 15. London: The Stationary Office; 1997

Office for National Statistics. Secondary. https://www.ons.gov.uk/methodology/classificationsandstandards/otherclassifications/thenationalstatisticssocioeconomicclassificationnnssecrebasedonsoc2010

Rudmik L. Economics of chronic rhinosinusitis. Curr Allergy Asthma Rep. 2017; 17(4):20

Rudmik L, Mace J, Soler ZM, Smith TL. Long-term utility outcomes in patients undergoing endoscopic sinus surgery. Laryngoscope. 2014; 124(1):19–23

Shaw M, Dorling D, Davey Smith G. Poverty, social exclusion, and minorities. In: Marmot M, Wilkinson G, eds. Social Determinants of Health. Oxford: Oxford University Press; 2006

Ware J, Jr, Kosinski M, Keller SDA. A 12-Item Short-Form Health Survey: construction of scales and preliminary tests of reliability and validity. Med Care. 1996; 34(3):220–233

Ware JE, Gandek B, Kosinski M, Snow KK, New England Medical Center. Health I. SF-36 health survey: manual and interpretation guide. Boston, MA: The Health Institute, New England Medical Center; 1993

Ware JE. How to Score Version 2 of the SF-12 Health Survey (with a Supplement Documenting Version 1). Lincoln, RI: QualityMetric Inc.; 2002

Ware JE, Jr, Sherbourne CD. The MOS 36-item short-form health survey (SF-36). I. Conceptual framework and item selection. Med Care. 1992; 30(6):473–483

Ware JE. User's manual for the SF-36v2 Health Survey. London: Quality Metric; 2007

References

[1] Hastan D, Fokkens WJ, Bachert C, et al. Chronic rhinosinusitis in Europe: an underestimated disease. A GA2LEN study. Allergy. 2011; 66(9):1216–1223

[2] Fokkens WJ, Lund VJ, Mullol J, et al. European Position Paper on Rhinosinusitis and Nasal Polyps 2012. Rhinol Suppl. 2012; 23(23):3 p preceding table of contents–, 1–298

[3] Blackwell DL, Lucas JW, Clarke TC. Summary health statistics for U.S. adults: national health interview survey, 2012. Vital Health Stat 10. 2014(260):1–161

[4] Halawi AM, Smith SS, Chandra RK. Chronic rhinosinusitis: epidemiology and cost. Allergy Asthma Proc. 2013; 34(4):328–334

[5] Xu Y, Quan H, Faris P, et al. Prevalence and incidence of diagnosed chronic rhinosinusitis in Alberta, Canada. JAMA Otolaryngol Head Neck Surg. 2016; 142(11):1063–1069

[6] Medicines & Healthcare products Regulatory Authority (MHRA). Clinical Practice Research Datalink. Secondary Clinical Practice Research Datalink 2018. Available at: https://www.cprd.com/intro.asp

[7] Gulliford MC, Dregan A, Moore MV, et al. Continued high rates of antibiotic prescribing to adults with respiratory tract infection: survey of 568 UK general practices. BMJ Open. 2014; 4(10):e006245

[8] NHS. Hospital Episode Statistics, 2015

[9] Hopkins C, Slack R, Lund V, Brown P, Copley L, Browne J. Long-term outcomes from the English national comparative audit of surgery for nasal polyposis and chronic rhinosinusitis. Laryngoscope. 2009; 119(12):2459–2465

[10] Philpott C, Hopkins C, Erskine S, et al. The burden of revision sino-nasal surgery in the UK-data from the Chronic Rhinosinusitis Epidemiology Study (CRES): a cross-sectional study. BMJ Open. 2015; 5(4):e006680

[11] Hospital Episode Statistics. Department of Health; 2013

[12] NHS reference costs. Secondary NHS reference costs 2017. https://improvement.nhs.uk/resources/reference-costs/

[13] Sharma R, Lakhani R, Rimmer J, Hopkins C. Surgical interventions for chronic rhinosinusitis with nasal polyps. Cochrane Database Syst Rev. 2014(11):CD006990

[14] NICE. Database of Uncertainties of Treatments

[15] Bhattacharyya N. Incremental health care utilization and expenditures for chronic rhinosinusitis in the United States. Ann Otol Rhinol Laryngol. 2011; 120(7):423–427

[16] Social Science Research Unit, UCL Institute of Education. CCEMG - EPPI-Centre Cost Converter. Secondary CCEMG - EPPI-Centre Cost Converter 2016. https://eppi.ioe.ac.uk/costconversion/default.aspx

[17] Smith WM, Davidson TM, Murphy C. Regional variations in chronic rhinosinusitis, 2003–2006. Otolaryngol Head Neck Surg. 2009; 141(3):347–352

[18] Chung SD, Hung SH, Lin HC, Lin CC. Health care service utilization among patients with chronic rhinosinusitis: a population-based study. Laryngoscope. 2014; 124(6):1285–1289

[19] Erskine SE, Hopkins C, Clark A, et al. Chronic rhinosinusitis and mood disturbance. Rhinology. 2017; 55(2):113–119

[20] Sahlstrand-Johnson P, Ohlsson B, Von Buchwald C, Jannert M, Ahlner-Elmqvist M. A multi-centre study on quality of life and absenteeism in patients with CRS referred for endoscopic surgery. Rhinology. 2011; 49(4):420–428

[21] Gliklich RE, Metson R. The health impact of chronic sinusitis in patients seeking otolaryngologic care. Otolaryngol Head Neck Surg. 1995; 113(1):104–109

[22] Philpott C, Erskine S, Hopkins C, et al. CRES Group. A case-control study of medical, psychological and socio-economic factors influencing the severity of chronic rhinosinusitis. Rhinology. 2016; 54(2):134–140

[23] Goetzel RZ, Hawkins K, Ozminkowski RJ, Wang S. The health and productivity cost burden of the "top 10" physical and mental health conditions affecting six large U.S. employers in 1999. J Occup Environ Med. 2003; 45(1):5–14

[24] Rudmik L, Smith TL, Schlosser RJ, Hwang PH, Mace JC, Soler ZM. Productivity costs in patients with refractory chronic rhinosinusitis. Laryngoscope. 2014; 124(9):2007–2012

[25] Erskine SE, Hopkins C, Clark A, et al. CRES Group. SNOT-22 in a control population. Clin Otolaryngol. 2017; 42(1):81–85

[26] Erskine S, Hopkins C, Kumar N, et al. A cross sectional analysis of a case-control study about quality of life in CRS in the UK; a comparison between CRS subtypes. Rhinology. 2016; 54(4):311–315

[27] Hopkins C, Gillett S, Slack R, Lund VJ, Browne JP. Psychometric validity of the 22-item Sinonasal Outcome Test. Clin Otolaryngol. 2009; 34(5):447–454

[28] Bewick J, Morris S, Hopkins C, Erskine S, Philpott C. Health utility reporting in Chronic Rhinosinusitis patients. Clin Otolaryngol. 2018; 43(1):90–95

[29] Kennedy JL, Hubbard MA, Huyett P, Patrie JT, Borish L, Payne SC. Sinonasal outcome test (SNOT-22): a predictor of postsurgical improvement in patients with chronic sinusitis. Ann Allergy Asthma Immunol. 2013; 111(4):246–251.e2

[30] Bewick J, Ahmed S, Carrie S, et al. The value of a feasibility study into long-term macrolide therapy in chronic rhinosinusitis. Clin Otolaryngol. 2017; 42(1):131–138

[31] Lange B, Holst R, Thilsing T, Baelum J, Kjeldsen A. Quality of life and associated factors in persons with chronic rhinosinusitis in the general population: a prospective questionnaire and clinical cross-sectional study. Clin Otolaryngol. 2013; 38(6):474–480

[32] Lin FJ, Pickard AS, Krishnan JA, et al. CONCERT Consortium. Measuring health-related quality of life in chronic obstructive pulmonary disease: properties of the EQ-5D-5 L and PROMIS-43 short form. BMC Med Res Methodol. 2014; 14:78

[33] Golicki D, Niewada M, Karlińska A, et al. Comparing responsiveness of the EQ-5D-5 L, EQ-5D-3 L and EQ VAS in stroke patients. Qual Life Res. 2015; 24(6):1555–1563

[34] Atlas SJ, Metson RB, Singer DE, Wu YA, Gliklich RE. Validity of a new health-related quality of life instrument for patients with chronic sinusitis. Laryngoscope. 2005; 115(5):846–854

[35] Crump RT, Lai E, Liu G, Janjua A, Sutherland JM. Establishing Utility Values for the 22-Item Sino-Nasal Outcome Test (SNOT-22) Using a Crosswalk to the EuroQol–Five-Dimensional Questionnaire–Three-Level Version (EQ-5D-3L). Hoboken, NJ: Wiley-Blackwell; 2017

[36] Abdalla S, Alreefy H, Hopkins C. Prevalence of sinonasal outcome test (SNOT-22) symptoms in patients undergoing surgery for chronic rhinosinusitis in the England and Wales National prospective audit. Clin Otolaryngol. 2012; 37(4):276–282

[37] Gliklich RE, Metson R. The health impact of chronic sinusitis in patients seeking otolaryngologic care. Otolaryngol Head Neck Surg. 1995; 113(1):104–109

[38] Erskine SE, Verkerk MM, Notley C, Williamson IG, Philpott CM. Chronic rhinosinusitis: patient experiences of primary and secondary care: a qualitative study. Clin Otolaryngol. 2016; 41(1):8–14

[39] Erskine SE, Notley C, Wilson AM, Philpott CM. Managing chronic rhinosinusitis and respiratory disease: a qualitative study of triggers and interactions. J Asthma. 2015; 52(6):600–605

[40] Rudmik L, Soler ZM, Mace JC, Schlosser RJ, Smith TL. Economic evaluation of endoscopic sinus surgery versus continued medical therapy for refractory chronic rhinosinusitis. Laryngoscope. 2015; 125(1):25–32

[41] Au J, Rudmik L. Cost of outpatient endoscopic sinus surgery from the perspective of the Canadian government: a time-driven activity-based costing approach. Int Forum Allergy Rhinol. 2013; 3(9):748–754

[42] Bajaj Y, Sethi N, Carr S, Knight LC. Endoscopic sinus surgery as day-case procedure. J Laryngol Otol. 2009; 123(6):619–622

[43] Department of Health and Social Care. 2009–10 NHS Reference Costs Publication. London: Department of Health and Social Care; 2011

[44] Bhattacharyya N. Clinical outcomes after endoscopic sinus surgery. Curr Opin Allergy Clin Immunol. 2006; 6(3):167–171

[45] Bhattacharyya N. Symptom outcomes after endoscopic sinus surgery for chronic rhinosinusitis. Arch Otolaryngol Head Neck Surg. 2004; 130(3):329–333

[46] Bhattacharyya N, Orlandi RR, Grebner J, Martinson M. Cost burden of chronic rhinosinusitis: a claims-based study. Otolaryngol Head Neck Surg. 2011; 144(3):440–445

[47] Benninger MS, Holy CE. Endoscopic sinus surgery provides effective relief as observed by health care use pre- and postoperatively. Otolaryngol Head Neck Surg. 2014; 150(5):893–900

[48] Benninger MS, Holy CE. The impact of endoscopic sinus surgery on health care use in patients with respiratory comorbidities. Otolaryngol Head Neck Surg. 2014; 151(3):508–515

[49] Hopkins C, Lund V. Does time to endoscopic sinus surgery impact outcomes? Prospective findings from the National Comparative Audit of Surgery for Nasal Polyposis and Chronic Rhinosinusitis. Rhinology. 2015; 53(1):10–17

[50] Smith KA, Smith TL, Mace JC, Rudmik L. Endoscopic sinus surgery compared to continued medical therapy for patients with refractory chronic rhinosinusitis. Int Forum Allergy Rhinol. 2014; 4(10):823–827

[51] Smith TL, Kern RC, Palmer JN, et al. Medical therapy vs surgery for chronic rhinosinusitis: a prospective, multi-institutional study. Int Forum Allergy Rhinol. 2011; 1(4):235–241

[52] Leung RM, Dinnie K, Smith TL. When do the risks of repeated courses of corticosteroids exceed the risks of surgery? Int Forum Allergy Rhinol. 2014; 4(11):871–876

[53] Hopkins C, Andrews P, Holy CE. Does time to endoscopic sinus surgery impact outcomes in chronic rhinosinusitis? Retrospective analysis using the UK clinical practice research data. Rhinology. 2015; 53(1):18–24

[54] Hopkins C, Rimmer J, Lund VJ. Does time to endoscopic sinus surgery impact outcomes in chronic rhinosinusitis? Prospective findings from the National Comparative Audit of Surgery for Nasal Polyposis and Chronic Rhinosinusitis. Rhinology. 2015; 53(1):10–17

[55] Hopkins C, Andrews P, Holy CE. Does time to surgery impact on outcomes from endoscopic sinus surgery? Retrospective analysis using the UK clinical practice research data. Rhinology. 2015; 51(1):18–24

[56] Benninger MSP, Holy C, Hopkins C. Early versus delayed endoscopic sinus surgery in patients with chronic rhinosinusitis: impact on health care utilization. Otolaryngol Head Neck Surg. 2015; 152(3):546–552

[57] Smith RCJ. The Economic Burden of Antimicrobial Resistance: Why It Is More Serious than Current Studies Suggest. Technical Report. London: London School of Hygiene and Tropical Medicine; 2012

[58] React Group. Economic aspects of antibiotic resistance. 2007. Available at: http://www.reactgroup.org/uploads/publications/react-publications/economic-aspects-of-antibiotic-resistance.pdf

47 Training Models and Techniques in Frontal Sinus Surgery

Abdulaziz Al-Rasheed, Philip A. Chen, and Marc A. Tewfik

Abstract

Endoscopic sinus surgery (ESS) and frontal sinus surgery pose unique training challenges owing to the complex and variable anatomy, as well as the risk of major complications. Moreover, ESS requires a certain set of technical abilities differing from that of most surgical procedures. Surgical simulation provides an alternative solution to develop these skills in a safe environment. We describe in this chapter the technologies and training models available for the training of frontal sinus surgery.

Keywords: frontal sinus surgery, training models, surgical simulation

47.1 Introduction

Surgical management of inflammatory disease in the frontal sinus is considered by many to be among the most challenging in the realm of endoscopic sinus surgery. Surgery of the frontal sinus poses unique challenges due to anatomical complexity, risk of complications, and a high failure rate.[1] With regard to anatomy, the cellular patterns in the frontal recess and the anatomy of the outflow tract are highly variable.[2,3] Adding to the complexity, the space is surrounded by critical structures including the orbit and the brain. As a result, the risk of major complication is a constant concern to the operating surgeon,[4] causing many to be very tentative when operating in this area. Unfortunately, the surgeon's uncertainty can result in inadequate surgery with failure to improve or even worsen symptomatology due to frontal recess stenosis.[5,6] Thus, knowledge of the anatomy, precise preoperative planning, and meticulous surgical execution are paramount for a successful surgical outcome in frontal sinus surgery. In order to enhance surgeons' understanding of the anatomy and surgical planning, we describe in this chapter recent advances in surgical education including a three-dimensional (3D) conceptualization module to teach frontal sinus anatomy and surgery, followed by simulation models to practice surgical steps.

47.2 Published Evidence

In order to improve understanding of the frontal sinus anatomy, Wormald elaborated a 3D conceptualization method to establish the pattern of the frontal sinus anatomy and drainage pathway.[7] Following review of the CT scan in triplanar view, he encouraged the use of building blocks representing each cell identified in the frontal recess and frontal sinus. Using this methodology, the agger nasi is the key to understanding the anatomy and

surgical planning. Subsequently, using coronal and para-sagittal scans in tandem, each cell is identified and placed in relation to the other cells. Finally, the frontal sinus drainage pathway is identified primarily using the axial CT images, followed superiorly to inferiorly and plotted around the cells in the frontal recess. More recently, the International Frontal Sinus Anatomy Classification (IFAC)[8] was published in order to simplify and harmonize the nomenclature of the important cells affecting the frontal sinus drainage pathway.

Using this building block method to understand the anatomy, the Scopis Building Blocks computer software has recently been developed. This software allows the user to draw building blocks on the CT scan itself in all three dimensions and resize and place them over the cells within the viewer (▶ Fig. 47.1). Importantly, the frontal sinus drainage pathway can also be drawn directly on the CT scan, creating an accurate 3D anatomical image. This system allows the surgeon to visualize the 3D anatomy of the frontal recess and the surrounding cells in order to formulate a surgical plan. Furthermore, this system can be utilized as a teaching module by affording an opportunity for the trainee to review the CT scan and then use the program to interact with the frontal sinus anatomy, create a 3D building blocks conceptualization, and identify the drainage pathway. This has been shown to improve the residents' ability in recognizing cells of the frontal recess on CT scans.[9]

In regard to task training for surgical skills, virtual reality (VR) surgical simulators have the advantage of providing trainees with an opportunity to practice surgical maneuvers in a low-risk environment. Furthermore, the dynamic nature of the VR software permits programming different clinical variations to improve training content and allow for individualized, proficiency-based training. Many of the VR surgical simulators currently available also have the advantage of providing feedback through analysis of different performance metrics (e.g., time to complete a task, percentage of normal tissue removed, contact with vital structure, and force measurements). This built-in assessment functionality permits self-directed learning and proficiency-based training.

The ES3 was the first VR sinus surgery simulator developed in 1998 by Lockheed Martin.[10] Although the ES3 demonstrated tangible benefits for resident training, it is no longer in production and there are fewer than a handful of devices in North America.[11] After the discontinuation of the ES3, other VR simulator models for ESS have been created; however, many of these devices were not validated.[12] The McGill simulator for ESS is a VR simulator with advanced 3D and tissue characteristic. The simulator is capable of measuring objective performance metrics in

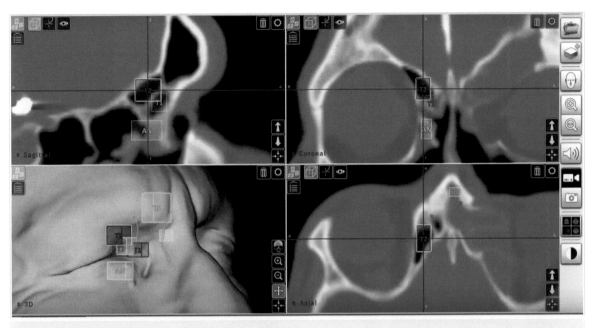

Fig. 47.1 Preoperative surgical planning on the Scopis program.

order to provide the trainee with constructive feedback to improve performance.[13] However, VR simulators are limited in their ability to mimic tool–tissue interactions and few have been able to successfully simulate haptic feedback (▶ Fig. 47.2 and ▶ Fig. 47.3).

In recent years, 3D printing, also known as rapid prototyping, has been utilized to create surgical simulators. Surgical simulation models range from part-task simulators to procedure-specific simulators. As with VR, these synthetic models give trainees the opportunity to practice specific surgical skills in a low-risk environment.

3D printing is a methodology using 3D computer-aided design datasets for producing 3D haptic physical model. Recently, this technology has been used by different surgical specialties in order to create high-fidelity models for surgical training. An example in the field of otolaryngology is the development of a 3D printed temporal bone model using computed tomography data. The model is considered highly realistic and an excellent replica for temporal bone surgical training.[14]

Rapid prototyping models enhance 3D learning especially in challenging anatomical conditions. Furthermore, the possibility of training surgical procedures in general as well as patient-specific procedures in complex cases improves the surgeon's abilities and results.[15] The preoperative simulation of a specific and complex surgery provides a unique opportunity to employ surgical steps in order to determine the best operating strategy.[16]

At our center, we developed a 3D printed simulator of the osteomeatal complex and the frontal sinus by segmenting a CT scan of the paranasal sinuses.[17] The model has both bony and soft-tissue consistencies (▶ Fig. 47.4). After performing a set of tasks on the model by expert

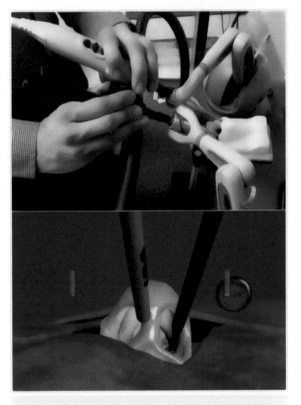

Fig. 47.2 Virtual reality simulator with the user placing the endoscope and the microdebrider within the nasal cavity.

participants, the model rated highly in terms of haptic feedback and surgical experience. Furthermore, the model could significantly differentiate between expert and novice

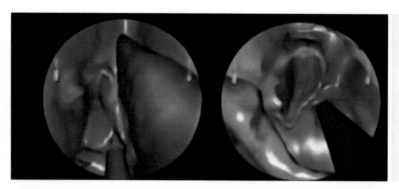

Fig. 47.3 Virtual view of user performing sphenoidotomy.

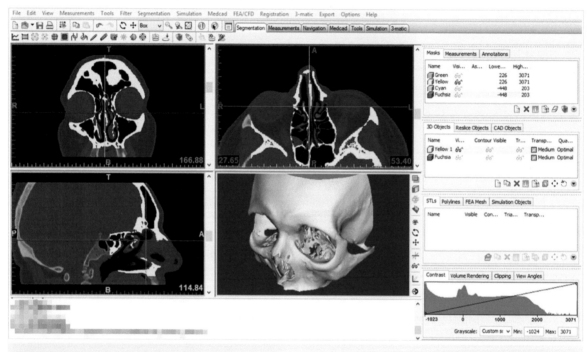

Fig. 47.4 Mimics program used for the segmentation process.

surgeons, which makes it helpful to train the residents and give feedback on the surgical performance (▶ Fig. 47.5 and ▶ Fig. 47.6). Participants also highly rated performing the surgical maneuvers required for the frontal recess dissection. The advantage of 3D printed model is the ability to print the variable frontal recess anatomy and enable the trainee to perform the maneuvers required in a safe environment. Furthermore, it allows the trainee to practice manipulating angled endoscopes and the special instruments necessary to operate in this delicate area.

However, 3D printing technologies do have limitations. To start, the printer and materials are expensive to acquire. Second, for this model in particular, additional labor was required by cleaning off excess support materials (wax) before use. However, with advancements in technology, the direction toward cheaper models with little to no wax materials and a more lifelike feel is the hope

to fully enable the trainee to practice in a safe and realistic environment.

47.3 Controversies and Opinions

Surgery of the frontal sinus poses unique challenges. Not only can surgical intervention of the frontal sinus be difficult to execute well, but teaching the topic also has challenges. The age-old surgical training model of "see one, do one, teach one" is a vast oversimplification, especially in an anatomical region as complex as the frontal sinus. In this traditional intraoperative setting, opportunities to perform specific procedures such as frontal sinus surgery are sporadic, and are regularly combined with a mismatch between resident ability and procedure complexity. This mismatch can frustrate the learner and impede progress and learning.[18,19]

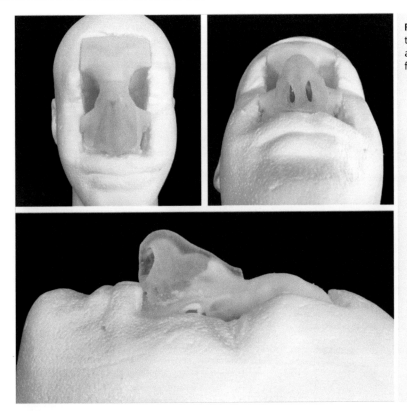

Fig. 47.5 The printed model containing two distinctive materials simulating bone and soft tissue mounted within a Styrofoam head.

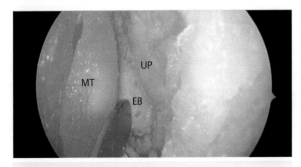

Fig. 47.6 Endoscopic view of the middle meatus (MT, middle turbinate; EB, ethmoid bulla; UP, uncinate process).

In an ideal situation, the complex training of a competent surgeon addresses three main learning objectives relevant to each individual trainee: cognitive, affective, and psychomotor domains.[20] In order to improve the cognitive domain, it is important for the trainee to analyze and formulate a surgical plan; this is followed by practicing the surgical steps in order to improve the psychomotor domain.

The use of simulation models affords deliberate learning and practice of surgical skills in a safe environment. One anticipates that learned skills in a simulation setting translate into confidence and improved performance in live surgery.[21] While simulation in endoscopic sinus surgery remains in early stages, a considerable challenge of existing simulators is an inability to accurately reproduce the complexity and heterogeneous anatomy of the frontal sinuses.

47.4 Unanswered Questions

Frontal sinus surgery remains one of the most challenging aspects of current rhinology practice. Frontal recess anatomy is variable, often confusing, and commonly affected by pathology. Superimpose this fact with the narrow confines of the surgical corridor and the frequent need for angled instruments and endoscopes and the challenges become obvious. In order to advance the teaching of frontal sinus surgery, a broad training curriculum encompassing the 3D conceptualization of preoperative imaging and simulation of the surgical maneuvers needs to be developed and validated. The possible application of validated measures of performance on the simulator could provide critical benchmarking data. These data are relevant to the future application of simulation curricula for endoscopic sinus surgery training.

References

[1] Kennedy DW, Senior BA. Endoscopic sinus surgery. A review. Otolaryngol Clin North Am. 1997; 30(3):313–330

[2] Stammberger H, Hosemann W, Draf W. Anatomic terminology and nomenclature for paranasal sinus surgery. Laryngorhinootologie. 1997; 76(7):435–449

[3] Lee D, Brody R, Har-El G. Frontal sinus outflow anatomy. Am J Rhinol. 1997; 11(4):283–285

[4] Krings JG, Kallogjeri D, Wineland A, Nepple KG, Piccirillo JF, Getz AE. Complications of primary and revision functional endoscopic sinus surgery for chronic rhinosinusitis. Laryngoscope. 2014; 124(4):838–845

[5] Ramadan HH. Surgical causes of failure in endoscopic sinus surgery. Laryngoscope. 1999; 109(1):27–29

[6] Valdes CJ, Bogado M, Samaha M. Causes of failure in endoscopic frontal sinus surgery in chronic rhinosinusitis patients. Int Forum Allergy Rhinol. 2014; 4(6):502–506

[7] Wormald P-J. Three-dimensional building block approach to understanding the anatomy of the frontal recess and frontal sinus. Oper Tech Otolaryngol Head Neck Surg. 2006; 17(1):2–5

[8] Wormald P-J, Hoseman W, Callejas C, et al. The International Frontal Sinus Anatomy Classification (IFAC) and Classification of the Extent of Endoscopic Frontal Sinus Surgery (EFSS). Int Forum Allergy Rhinol. 2016; 6(7):677–696

[9] Chen PG, Bassiouni A, Taylor CB, et al. Teaching residents frontal sinus anatomy using a novel 3-dimensional conceptualization planning software-based module. Am J Rhinol Allergy. 2018; 32(6):526–532

[10] Fried MP, Kaye RJ, Gibber MJ, et al. Criterion-based (proficiency) training to improve surgical performance. Arch Otolaryngol Head Neck Surg. 2012; 138(11):1024–1029

[11] Wiet GJ, Stredney D, Wan D. Training and simulation in otolaryngology. Otolaryngol Clin North Am. 2011; 44(6):1333–1350, viii–ix

[12] Javia L, Deutsch ES. A systematic review of simulators in otolaryngology. Otolaryngol Head Neck Surg. 2012; 147(6):999–1011

[13] Varshney R, Frenkiel S, Nguyen LHP, et al. National Research Council Canada. Development of the McGill simulator for endoscopic sinus surgery: a new high-fidelity virtual reality simulator for endoscopic sinus surgery. Am J Rhinol Allergy. 2014; 28(4):330–334

[14] Hochman JB, Rhodes C, Kraut J, Pisa J, Unger B. End user comparison of anatomically matched 3-dimensional printed and virtual haptic temporal bone simulation: a pilot study. Otolaryngol Head Neck Surg. 2015; 153(2):263–268

[15] Knox K, Kerber CW, Singel SA, Bailey MJ, Imbesi SG. Rapid prototyping to create vascular replicas from CT scan data: making tools to teach, rehearse, and choose treatment strategies. Catheter Cardiovasc Interv. 2005; 65(1):47–53

[16] Mavili ME, Canter HI, Saglam-Aydinatay B, Kamaci S, Kocadereli I. Use of three-dimensional medical modeling methods for precise planning of orthognathic surgery. J Craniofac Surg. 2007; 18(4):740–747

[17] Alrasheed AS, Nguyen LHP, Mongeau L, Funnell WRJ, Tewfik MA. Development and validation of a 3D-printed model of the ostiomeatal complex and frontal sinus for endoscopic sinus surgery training. Int Forum Allergy Rhinol. 2017; 7(8):837–841

[18] Nogueira JF, Stamm AC, Lyra M, Balieiro FO, Leão FS. Building a real endoscopic sinus and skull-base surgery simulator. Otolaryngol Head Neck Surg. 2008; 139(5):727–728

[19] Reznick RK, MacRae H. Teaching surgical skills: changes in the wind. N Engl J Med. 2006; 355(25):2664–2669

[20] Wiggins JS. Book Reviews: Taxonomy of Educational Objectives, The Classification of Educational Goals, Handbook II: Affective Domain by David R. Krathwohl, Benjamin S. Bloom, and Bertram B. Masia. New York: David McKay Company, 1964. Pp. vii + 196. Educ Psychol Meas. 1965; 25(3):895–897

[21] Bhatti NI, Ahmed A. Improving skills development in residency using a deliberate-practice and learner-centered model. Laryngoscope. 2015; 125 Suppl 8:S1–S14

48 Augmented Reality in Frontal Sinus Surgery

Pavol Šurda and Martyn Barnes

Abstract

Navigation in endoscopic sinus surgery has emerged as a critical tool in the last decades. The rhinologist in the operating room is limited by transformation of the information from the three-dimensional (3D) surgical field to two-dimensional (2D) sections on the navigation screen. Therefore, the surgeon is confronted with the mental task of integrating these two image datasets. Augmented reality might be a way to overcome this problem. The virtual data may be used for preoperative planning (3D reconstruction from slices of CT scan) or intraoperative navigation. Intraoperative navigation can be simply informative (such as textual or numerical values relevant to what is under observation) or consisting of 3D virtual objects inserted within the real environment in spatially defined positions.

Keywords: augmented reality, scopis, Navigation, Telemedicine, frontal sinus surgery, building blocks, preoperative planning

48.1 Role of Augmented Reality in Preoperative Planning

There is still some confusion about the difference between augmented reality (AR) and virtual reality (VR) and the different uses. **AR** uses technology to *superimpose information* (such as images and sounds) on the world we see—it *adds to normal reality*, while **VR** *creates a computer-generated environment* for the user to interact with and be fully immersed in—it *replaces normal reality*. The newest AR software uses the features of both technologies to provide a better understanding of sinus anatomy, which is probably the most important prerequisite for endoscopic sinus surgery (ESS).

The most basic example of preoperative AR is the fusion of MRI scan and the picture of patient's sagittal photograph using the Android/iPhone overlay application. Precise alignment of virtual datasets is critical. This technique was used to depict the lesion's surface projection onto the skin of the head.[1]

Advanced AR planning software allows the transformation of the sinus anatomy into 3D models from slices of patient's CT scan. This 3D model can be later annotated in order to highlight the area of interest (tumor, frontal sinus outflow, neurovascular structures). For example, in case of tumor removal, the surgeon can examine the anatomy from different angles and better understand the position of critical structures in relation to the tumor and learn how to avoid them.[2] The experience can be maximized with 3D glasses, which enhance the perception of

depth, or the construct can be 3D printed into a real model.

48.2 Role of Augmented Reality during Surgery

Preoperative planning is only a small fraction of what AR can offer. The keystone of AR is to bring that plan into the operating room and fuse the annotated preoperative images with intraoperative endoscopic view on the surgical navigation platform. This enables the surgeon to see "behind the corner" and also to avoid the critical neurovascular structures (orbital wall, ethmoid roof, optic nerve, internal carotid artery).

There are several systems with this unique feature. Scopis Hybrid Navigation (Scopis GmbH, Berlin, Germany) offers a novel preoperative planning phase, known as Building Blocks for frontal recess anatomy (as proposed by Wormald; ▶ Fig. 48.1).[3] Furthermore, this navigation system incorporates technology for the calibration of standard endoscopic image with CT scan-derived models, a variation of an approach originally proposed as image-enhanced endoscopy. Intraoperatively, the AR views provided useful information before starting the dissection, as the AR permitted the surgeon to "see" the relevant structures without formally removing the uncinated process or any other tissue. This may have important implications for balloon catheter dilatation of sinus ostia. Image-guided surgery (IGS) with AR may also function as a "target avoidance" mechanism. AR may mark structures so that their location is clear, before they are exposed during surgery. ▶ Fig. 48.2 shows this concept of "antitargeting" by illustrating the presence of the optic nerve without direct exposure of the optic nerve. The internal carotid artery could be highlighted in a similar fashion.[4,5] Recently, Scopis merged the capabilities of Microsoft HoloLens and AR. By donning a pair of the HoloLens glasses, the surgeon can see a holographic visualization of the overlay and preplanned image, which allows a better spatial orientation within the complex anatomy of sinonasal cavity. Additionally, surgeons can keep their eye on the operative field, and use gestures to place virtual monitors onto their visual field. Other companies also expanded their portfolio of AR navigation systems. Solution from Karl Storz (Tüttlingen, Germany) is an adapter (NAV1 Endoscope Tracker), which is attached to the endoscope. The result is an enhanced image with information obtained from the preoperative virtual planning.[6]

There is evidence from published studies that the use of surgical navigation (also known as IGS) for ESS is associated with a lower risk of major and total complications

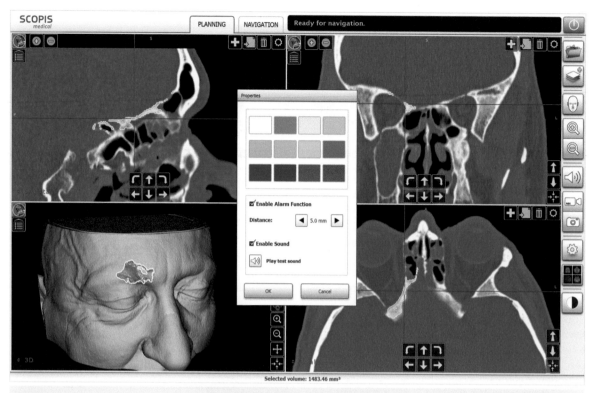

Fig. 48.1 Scopis Hybrid Navigation Planning software (Scopis GmbH) includes tools to annotate the critical areas such as skull base with a yellow color. (This image is provided courtesy of Scopis GmbH, Berlin, Germany.)

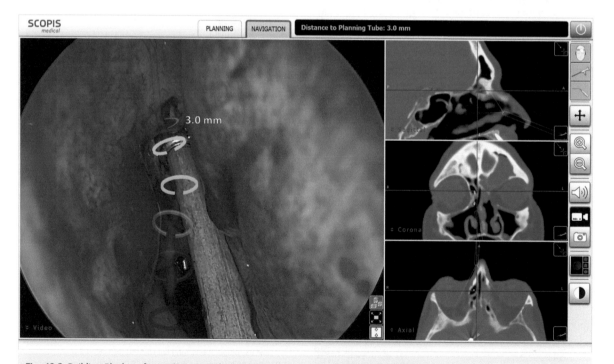

Fig. 48.2 Building Blocks software (Scopis GmbH) permits the user to annotate the preoperative CT scan. In this instance, navigation shows the frontal sinus outflow pathway with an *orange line*. (This image is provided courtesy of Scopis GmbH, Berlin, Germany.)

compared with non-IGS sinus surgery.[7] Both the American Academy of Otolaryngology–Head and Neck Surgery[8] and a working group in Australian rhinology[9] endorse the use of IGS during ESS in select cases based on expert consensus and literature evidence.

However, AR in sinus surgery is still novel; therefore, the literature describing the efficacy is limited.[2,4,5] Dixon et al focus on a role of AR in training. Due to close proximity to dangerous structures, ESS in early years of training can be associated with increased mental demand, effort, and frustration. ARS seems to reduce the task workload for trainees performing ESS and may be a valuable intraoperative teaching aid.[10] In skull base surgery, annotated AR overlays of planned trajectory and neurovascular anatomy were highly valuable in reaching the sellar floor safely in redo procedures, with no additional operative time or hardware setup required.[11,12] One of the limitations may be a single head-up display, which can distract the user and cause an inattentional blindness. This can be corrected by a submonitor.[13]

Another type of AR is the Google Glass (GG), which offers quite a different experience. GG is essentially a smartphone in the form of a pair of conventional spectacles with built-in small screen that allows hands-free access to electronic information through voice command.[14,15] Its connectivity via Wi-Fi makes GG potentially useful for the needs of telemedicine.[16] The main advantages of the intraoperative use are as follows: the access to electronic medical literature including instructional videos or patient records for a quick reference, connection to the operating theater's information system to monitor a patient's vital signs, and speech-to-text dictation (e.g., of major intraoperative findings) for more detailed and accurate documentation. Moreover, GG can be used as a tool for telemedicine where the members of the surgical team or other specialties could communicate; hence, GG may facilitate intraoperative decision-making.[17]

GG represents a novel breakthrough technology in the field of surgery, but we feel a need to mention several limitations. Literature review showed that authors struggled with a short battery life[18] and poor image quality (screen resolution is 640 × 360 pixels).[19,20] In telemedicine, the use of GG was limited by network delay and also line of sight where the operating surgeon had to tilt the head unnaturally to keep the image on the display so the surgeon B could see the surgical field.[17]

We believe that AR-assisted navigation may be superior to the traditional navigation in the field of sinus surgery as it reduces the task workload and mental stress of the surgeon by merging the surgical field 3D real-world environment to 2D sections on the navigation screen into one comprehensive view.[10] However, further studies must be performed to provide their utility.

References

[1] Hou Y, Ma L, Zhu R, Chen X, Zhang J. A low-cost iPhone-assisted augmented reality solution for the localization of intracranial lesions. PLoS One. 2016; 11(7):e0159185

[2] Agbetoba A, Luong A, Siow JK, et al. Educational utility of advanced three-dimensional virtual imaging in evaluating the anatomical configuration of the frontal recess. Int Forum Allergy Rhinol. 2017; 7 (2):143–148

[3] Wormald P-J. Three-dimensional building block approach to understanding the anatomy of the frontal recess and frontal sinus. Oper Tech Otolaryngol Head Neck Surg. 2006; 17(1):2–5

[4] Citardi MJ, Agbetoba A, Bigcas JL, Luong A. Augmented reality for endoscopic sinus surgery with surgical navigation: a cadaver study. Int Forum Allergy Rhinol. 2016; 6(5):523–528

[5] Li L, Yang J, Chu Y, et al. A novel augmented reality navigation system for endoscopic sinus and skull base surgery: a feasibility study. PLoS One. 2016; 11(1):e0146996

[6] The KARL STORZ navigation family. 2017. Available from: https://www.karlstorz.com/gb/en/navigation.htm

[7] Dalgorf DM, Sacks R, Wormald PJ, et al. Image-guided surgery influences perioperative morbidity from endoscopic sinus surgery: a systematic review and meta-analysis. Otolaryngol Head Neck Surg. 2013; 149(1):17–29

[8] American Academy of Otolaryngology – Head and Neck Surgery. Position Statement: intra-operative use of computer aided surgery. 2012. Available from: http://www.entnet.org/Practice/policyIntraOperativeSurgery.cfm

[9] Stelter K, Ertl-Wagner B, Luz M, et al. Evaluation of an image-guided navigation system in the training of functional endoscopic sinus surgeons. A prospective, randomised clinical study. Rhinology. 2011; 49 (4):429–437

[10] Dixon BJ, Chan H, Daly MJ, Vescan AD, Witterick IJ, Irish JC. The effect of augmented real-time image guidance on task workload during endoscopic sinus surgery. Int Forum Allergy Rhinol. 2012; 2(5):405–410

[11] Yoshino M, Saito T, Kin T, et al. A microscopic optically tracking navigation system that uses high-resolution 3D computer graphics. Neurol Med Chir (Tokyo). 2015; 55(8):674–679

[12] Kawamata T, Iseki H, Shibasaki T, Hori T. Endoscopic augmented reality navigation system for endonasal transsphenoidal surgery to treat pituitary tumors: technical note. Neurosurgery. 2002; 50(6):1393–1397

[13] Dixon BJ, Daly MJ, Chan HH, Vescan A, Witterick IJ, Irish JC. Inattentional blindness increased with augmented reality surgical navigation. Am J Rhinol Allergy. 2014; 28(5):433–437

[14] Glauser W. Doctors among early adopters of Google Glass. CMAJ. 2013; 185(16):1385

[15] Aldaz G, Shluzas LA, Pickham D, et al. Hands-free image capture, data tagging and transfer using Google Glass: a pilot study for improved wound care management. PLoS One. 2015; 10(4):e0121179

[16] Ye J, Zuo Y, Xie T, et al. A telemedicine wound care model using 4G with smart phones or smart glasses: A pilot study. Medicine (Baltimore). 2016; 95(31):e4198

[17] Chang JY, Tsui LY, Yeung KS, Yip SW, Leung GK. Surgical vision: Google Glass and surgery. Surg Innov. 2016; 23(4):422–426

[18] Paro JA, Nazareli R, Gurjala A, Berger A, Lee GK. Video-based self-review: comparing Google Glass and GoPro technologies. Ann Plast Surg. 2015; 74 Suppl 1:S71–S74

[19] Rahimy E, Garg SJ. Google Glass for recording scleral buckling surgery. JAMA Ophthalmol. 2015; 133(6):710–711

[20] Hashimoto DA, Phitayakorn R, Fernandez-del Castillo C, Meireles O. A blinded assessment of video quality in wearable technology for telementoring in open surgery: the Google Glass experience. Surg Endosc. 2016; 30(1):372–378

49 Robotic Surgery: Beyond DaVinci

Paul Breedveld

Abstract

During frontal sinus surgery and endoscopic endonasal surgery, faraway locations in the skull have to be reached with minimal damage to healthy tissues. Starting at DaVinci, this chapter describes the newest developments in the field of steerable and maneuverable surgical instrumentation allowing the surgeon to move along complex 3D pathways in the skull with entrance via narrow anatomic corridors. The chapter will end with the future perspective of multibranched, snakelike instrumentation suited for complex 3D motion along the dense and delicate anatomy in the skull.

Keywords: endoscopic endonasal surgery, robotic surgery, master–slave system, steerable instrument, shape memory system, follow-the-leader propagation, 3D printing

49.1 Published Evidence

49.1.1 Shortcomings of DaVinci

During endoscopic endonasal surgery (EES), surgical instruments are inserted through a narrow anatomic corridor starting at the nostrils, passing the nasal cavity, and running through openings in the sphenoid sinus to enter the sella turcica that cradles the pituitary gland. During resection of, for example, pituitary gland adenoma, this anatomic corridor confines the reachable surgical area to a relatively small, narrow space behind the sphenoid sinus. Complete removal of pituitary gland adenoma, especially those that extend behind delicate neural or vascular structures, cannot always be achieved, requiring the need for surgical access from other locations or transfer to conventional open craniotomy.

The restricted workspace behind the narrow anatomic corridor is due to a lack of instrument maneuverability, as current skull base procedures are carried out with rigid instrumentation. The maneuverability can be expanded by using instruments with a steerable tip, that is, instruments that contain a mechanism at the end of the shaft that functions like a wrist and allows the tip to be bent in all directions. Although hardly used in skull base surgery, steerable instruments are quite common in other surgical fields such as laparoscopic surgery, the most successful one being the EndoWrist developed by the U.S. company Intuitive Surgical. Controlled by DaVinci, instruments equipped with the EndoWrist mechanism can be steered in all directions, intuitively controlled by the surgeon using dedicated moveable handles and looking at the image of a 3D endoscope on a monitor in a console. Seen from a technical perspective, DaVinci belongs to the robotic class of "master–slave systems," in which the steerable instruments are considered "slaves" that precisely follow the motion of the "masters," that is, the moveable handles controlled by the surgeon.

Even though DaVinci is an ingenious device applied with success in surgical procedures such as prostatectomy, the system suffers from a number of drawbacks that limit its application to other surgical fields. First of all, the system is huge, with a set of large robotic arms requiring a lot of space above the patient—too large for EES. Besides, DaVinci is very expensive and the EndoWrist instruments are highly complex. Composed out of tiny custom-made parts such as miniature pulleys and complex frame elements, the instruments are expensive and limited to a lifespan of only 10 surgical procedures. One of the main lifespan-limiting factors is material fatigue of the steel cables that are wound over pulleys with a too small diameter as compared to the thickness of the cables, causing damage to the cables after frequent use.[1] EndoWrist was developed as a strongly miniaturized version of conventional pulley mechanisms such as those found in large-scale technical applications. For the required 5-mm surgical instrument diameter, however, squeezing down such conventional mechanisms leads to large mechanical complexity and limited lifespan as the mechanism is not well suited for the required miniature size.

49.2 Steering at Greater Simplicity

At the Bio-Inspired Technology (BITE) group at Delft University of Technology (TU Delft), an explorative study was carried out on the application of 3D printing technology for steerable surgical instrumentation. 3D printing is an emerging manufacturing technique enabling easy, low-cost manufacture of complex 3D shapes without a need for elaborate conventional machining such as milling or lathing. In a search for a better alternative for the EndoWrist, we invented a novel grasping forceps with a steerable tip composed out of only five 3D-printed parts controlled by two steering cables. The miniature pulleys of the EndoWrist were replaced by specially shaped convex surfaces with a large radius so that cable fatigue will not occur. Being a strongly simplified version of the EndoWrist with similar size and steering characteristics, a series of steerable instrument prototypes with the name "DragonFlex" was developed.[1,2] ▶ Fig. 49.1 shows the latest version, 3D-printed from resin in an Envisiontec printer. Being world's first 3D-printed steerable surgical grasping forceps, DragonFlex offers very good steering properties at high stiffness and without cable fatigue, showing great potential for disposable use thanks to the ease of the 3D printing process. A drawback, however, is that the used resin is not

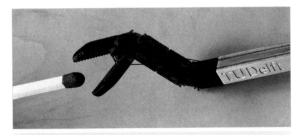

Fig. 49.1 Prototype of DragonFlex: world's first 3D-printed steerable grasping forceps, 5-mm thick, with match as size reference. The steerable tip, printed from resin and steerable in all directions over an angle of 90 degrees, contains only five individual parts controlled by two steering cables. The shaft was milled from metal in this prototype due to restrictions in the maximum printable length of the shaft in the used 3D printing machine. The DragonFlex was developed in the BITE group at TU Delft in a close collaboration with the Netherlands Organization for Applied Scientific Research (TNO) and the Austrian Center for Medical Innovation and Technology (ACMIT).[1,2]

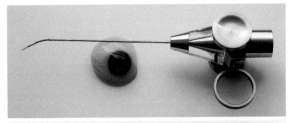

Fig. 49.2 Prototype of the I-Flex steerable grasping forceps with artificial glass eye at the background as size reference. The squid-inspired tip of the I-Flex contains six cables for steering and a seventh cable that controls the gripper. Having an ultrathin diameter of only 0.9 mm, the tip is steerable in all directions over an angle of 90 degrees. The I-Flex was developed in the BITE group at TU Delft in collaboration with the Rotterdam Eye Hospital.

biocompatible and still too fragile for use in clinical practice. Combining steering with bipolar electrosurgery,[3] we are currently experimenting with precise 3D printing of stainless steel to obtain a more robust, biocompatible device.

49.3 Steering at Reduced Dimensions

Although by simplifying the conventional pulley mechanism, DragonFlex reaches the size limitations of current 3D printing technology, making it nearly impossible to downsize the mechanism to diameters less than 5 mm.[2] In an attempt to find an even simpler solution, a creative exploration of biological methods for steering and maneuvering in nature was carried out. Biology follows alternative design pathways often leading to amazingly clever solutions potentially applicable to the medical technology domain. Lacking hard skeletal support, squid tentacles are, for example, composed out of ingenious compositions of interacting muscles arranged in layers and bundles, with muscle fibers oriented in multiple directions. By selectively tensioning and relaxing muscles, tentacles can be maneuvered in a remarkable variety of poses.[4] Transferring this structure to the medical technology domain led to the invention of our patented "cable-ring" mechanism, in its simplest embodiment consisting of two standard coil springs, an outer spring, and an inner spring with a smaller diameter, with in between a ring of cables that are all fixed to the tip. Pulling at some cables while releasing the others causes the mechanism to bend. A great advantage of the cable-ring mechanism is that it can be constructed entirely out of commercially available low-cost parts.[5] The cable-ring mechanism was used to

develop the world's thinnest prototype steerable grasping forces, called the "I-Flex" (▶ Fig. 49.2), with a diameter of only 0.9 mm, combining omnidirectional steering with precise control using a pincer grip. Although initially developed as a handheld steerable instrument for surgery within the eye, the steering mechanism of the I-Flex is suited for a great many surgical applications, including EES.

49.4 Controversies and Opinions

49.4.1 Maneuvering beyond DaVinci

Although the above-mentioned steerable instruments can all be used to "grasp around a corner," their motion is still limited to a steering angle of maximally 90 degrees. In order to increase the steering range, Hong et al[6] developed a novel robotic system for maxillary sinus surgery using instruments with a 4-mm steerable tip composed out of 17 stainless steel ball-and-socket joints. The joints are interconnected by two hollow nitinol tubes and two stainless steel cables, allowing an overall steering angle of 270 degrees along a circular arc. A gripper is located at the end of the tip and the instrument was tested in phantom skulls showing promising results. No clinical studies have yet been reported.

Maneuvering beyond a circular arc, Coemert et al[7] developed a "multisteerable" instrument for skull base surgery, containing two individually steerable tip segments with a diameter of 3.3 mm, allowing S-shaped curves in one single plane. A more advanced instrument for maxillary sinus surgery was developed by Yoon et al.[8] The multisteerable tip consists of two 5-mm segments that can both be steered in all directions, allowing motion along spatial S-shaped curves. Each segment consists of a series of ball-and-socket joints containing rings with holes to guide steering cables. Two versions of the system were built: one with a CMOS (complementary metal oxide semiconductor) camera and one with a gripper.

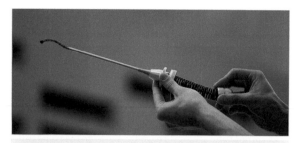

Fig. 49.3 Prototype of the HelixFlex: a multi-steerable instrument suited for complex 3D-maneuvering through narrow anatomic corridors. The tip, inspired by a squid-tentacle, diameter 5 mm, uses a novel combination of parallel cables and helically oriented cables to enable rotation and translation of the tip in all directions with a fixed position of the instrument shaft. The construction of the instrument is entirely mechanical and the tip can be intuitively controlled by a joystick on the handle. The HelixFlex was developed in the BITE group at TU Delft.[9]

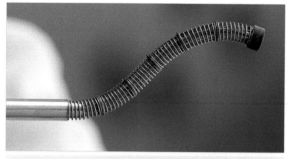

Fig. 49.4 Close-up of tip of HelixFlex, diameter 5 mm, showing the combination of 6 parallel and 12 helically oriented cables used to control the tip.[9]

Using robotic master–slave control, the system was tested in the maxillary sinus area of a human phantom, with promising results.

In a desire to avoid complex robotic technology by developing handheld multisteerable instruments for EES, we developed a new steering mechanism inspired by helically oriented muscle layers in a squid tentacle. In the resulting "HelixFlex" prototype,[9] we combined parallel with helical steering cables, the parallel cables enabling steering over circular arcs and the helical cables enabling spatial **S**-shaped curves (▶ Fig. 49.3 and ▶ Fig. 49.4). HelixFlex functions like a mechanical handheld master–slave system in the sense that the end of the handle contains a joystick, the "master," which can be translated and rotated in all directions relative to the shaft. The joystick movements are precisely copied to a motion of the tip, the "slave," enabling intuitive control in a wide 3D motion range without the use of a robot.

49.5 Maneuvering Like a Snake

The instruments described till now in this chapter all have straight and rigid instrument shafts with steerable tips that can be bent and twisted. Due to the rigidity of the shaft, their application is still limited to a confined workspace at the end of a straight anatomic corridor. Maneuvering a steerable instrument tip further along the delicate anatomy at the skull base would require the shaft to be entirely flexible, which is not possible with these instruments. Looking again at nature, a solution would be a miniature biological snakelike device that can manoeuver its body along any arbitrary 3D path. Maneuvering such a snakelike instrument is referred to as follow-the-leader (FTL) propagation, in which the head of the "snake" is regarded as the leader that is actively steered by the surgeon. As the snakelike instrument moves

forward, the curved track initiated by the head is transferred backward along the body of the snake that automatically follows the created path. This enables maneuvering along dense anatomic environments while reducing the surgical access to a minimum.

In the research group led by Webster at Vanderbilt University, novel "concentric tube robots" consisting of a series of concentric prebent tubes of superelastic nitinol have been developed for EES.[10,11] Telescopically moving the concentric tubes relative to one another results in a snakelike motion with a restricted motion range limited to the prebent shape of the interacting tubes. A way to realize unrestricted FTL propagation is to use a long, flexible shaft with a large number of segments that can be controlled individually, similar to the skeleton of a biological snake. Following our squid-inspired cable ring approach, we devised a prototype snakelike instrument, called "MemoFlex," containing 14 steering segments controlled by 56 steering cables at a diameter of 5 mm (▶ Fig. 49.5). We are currently investigating methods to control this device by using FTL propagation, which can in principle be realized by connecting the cables individually to miniature electric motors that are located either in the flexible shaft itself [12] or in a control unit at the base of the device[13] (▶ Fig. 49.6). The shape of the snakelike instrument is then driven by the motors and controlled by a computer in which the 3D trajectory is stored. This trajectory can either be determined beforehand from CT or MRI images, or be created during the procedure by the surgeon using a dedicated joystick to control the instrument head, for example, by observing the image of a miniature camera that is located in the head. It may be clear that this way of controlling will lead to a complex snakelike robotic device. Systems enabling FTL propagation have already been developed for a number of other surgical fields, such as natural orifice transluminal endoscopic surgery (NOTES),[12] robotic colonoscopy,[14] and robotic thoracic surgery,[15] all current solutions leading to devices that are either too complex, too thick for EES, or deploying FTL propagation with insufficient precision. We are currently exploring alternative ways to control snakelike

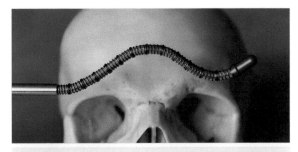

Fig. 49.5 Prototype of the MemoFlex: a multisteerable instrument suited for snakelike motion along with delicate anatomy, with an artificial skull in the background. The tip, 5-mm thick and 12-cm long, is composed out of 14 individually controllable segments, driven by 56 steering cables, allowing snakelike motion along complex 3D paths.

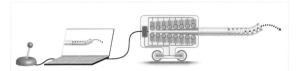

Fig. 49.6 Schematic picture of a method to control MemoFlex. The steering cables (*red*) are fixed to individual segments in the tip and guided to a control unit where they are controlled by electric motors (*yellow*). A computer is used to memorize the shape of the instrument and to control the electric motors in such a way that the shape is transmitted backward along the tip when the instrument is moved forward. In this way, maneuvering along curved 3D trajectories can be facilitated, however, at the expense of considerable electromechanical complexity.

instruments for EES, using advanced 3D-printing technology and a mechanical shape memory system that fits in a compact, handheld system without a need for electric actuation.[16]

49.6 Future Steps toward Clinical Practice

From the overview above, it is clear that the research on snakelike instrumentation is still in a very early phase with many technical challenges ahead, such as reducing control complexity and simplifying the construction of the snakelike shafts as to make them suitable for low-cost disposable use. Before testing these systems in a clinical setting, first well-working technical prototypes have to be created to solve these challenges. Using relatively simple handheld steerable instruments for EES and frontal sinus surgery will clearly be a great step forward as it gives the surgeon a better access to difficult-to-reach locations in the skull. Several companies are currently working on such instruments, among which is the Dutch company DEAM. The impact of advanced snakelike devices suited for reaching locations far beyond the current frontiers is still unclear as surgical procedures for such instruments do not yet exist. Yet, the general idea of being able to reach a great number of locations in the skull by using ultrathin, snakelike instruments with the lowest possible risk of damage to healthy tissues is very appealing. It is the author's expectation that systematic researches on intuitive controls[17] and worldwide research on snakelike multibranched instruments[18,19] will be a great drive for the future of surgery, eventually leading to surgical devices such as the one in ▶ Fig. 49.7 that go far beyond the possibilities of the existing instrumentation.

49.7 Unanswered Questions

The area of 3D printing is rapidly evolving, offering great future possibilities for patient-specific instrumentation

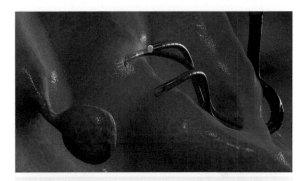

Fig. 49.7 An artist's impression of a surgical instrument consisting of three individual branches and moving along a complex 3D path to reach an atomic location of concern.

and advanced robotic surgical tools. The question is, however, whether high-tech robotic technology will counterbalance the relative simplicity and reliability of handheld instrumentation. Are we heading for a high-tech future in which the surgeon will be part of an advanced robotic system in which surgery is assisted by high-tech devices that do part of the surgeon's work? Or will there be a counterdevelopment in which all this technical complexity will be reduced so that the surgeon's craftsmanship will play a more dominant role? Whatever we are heading for, the surgeon should be in the center of the technical developments and not the technology itself. Robotic or handheld, the future will lie in the advancement of clever, yet affordable surgical devices optimally adapted to the surgeon's experience and skills, leading to new possibilities that reach beyond DaVinci.

Acknowledgments

Among the many students, PhDs, and technicians that have worked on the research described in this chapter, the author would especially like to thank MSc student Iris van Leeuwen for reviewing the state-of-the-art in novel devices for skull base surgery, and PhDs Costanza Culmone, Paul Henselmans, Ewout Arkenbout, Giada

Gerboni, and Filip Jelinek, as well as instrument makers David Jager, Menno Lageweg, and Remi van Starkenburg, for their valuable contribution to the developed instrument prototypes. The design of the DragonFlex steerable grasping forceps has been supported by the Center for Translational Molecular Medicine (CTMM) and our research on the development of snakelike instrumentation for skull base surgery is supported by the Netherlands Organization for Scientific Research (NWO), domain Applied and Engineering Sciences (TTW), which is partly funded by the Ministry of Economic Affairs.

References

[1] Jelinek F, Pessers R, Breedveld P. DragonFlex smart steerable laparoscopic instrument. J Med Device. 2014; 8(1)::1–9

[2] Jelinek F, Breedveld P. Design for additive manufacture of fine medical instrumentation: DragonFlex case study. J Mechan Design. 2015; 137 (11)::1–7

[3] Sakes A, Hovland K, Smit G, Geraedts J, Breedveld P. Design of a novel 3D-printed 2-DOF steerable electrosurgical grasper for minimally invasive surgery. J Med Device. 2017; 12(1)::1–15

[4] van Leeuwen JL, Kier WM. Functional design of tentacles in squid: linking sarcomere ultrastructure to gross morphological dynamics. Philos Trans R Soc Lond B Biol Sci. 1997; 352(1353):551–571

[5] Breedveld P, Scheltes JS, Blom EM, Verheij JEI. A new, easily miniaturized steerable endoscope. Squid tentacles provide inspiration for the Endo-Periscope. IEEE Eng Med Biol Mag. 2005; 24(6):40–47

[6] Hong W, Xie L, Liu J, Sun Y, Li K, Wang H. Development of a novel continuum robotic system for maxillary sinus surgery. IEEE/ASME Trans Mechatron. 2018; 23(3):1226–1237

[7] Coemert S, Gao A, Carev JP, et al. Development of a snake-like dexterous manipulator for skull base surgery. 38th Annual International Conference of the IEEE Engineering in Medicine and Biology Society, EMBS; 2016:5087–5090

[8] Yoon H-S, Jeong JH, Yi B-J. Image-guided dual master-slave robotic system for maxillary sinus surgery. IEEE Trans Robot. 2018; 34 (4):1098–1111

[9] Gerboni G, Henselmans PWJ, Arkenbout EA, van Furth WR, Breedveld P. HelixFlex: bioinspired maneuverable instrument for skull base surgery. Bioinspir Biomim. 2015; 10(6):066013

[10] Gilbert HB, Neimat J, Webster RJ, III. Concentric tube robots as steerable needles: achieving follow-the-leader deployment. IEEE Trans Robot. 2015; 31(2):246–258

[11] Swaney PJ, Gilbert HB, Webster RJ, III, Russell PT, III, Weaver KD. Endonasal skull base tumor removal using concentric tube continuum robots: a phantom study. J Neurol Surg B Skull Base. 2015; 76 (2):145–149

[12] Son J, Cho CN, Kim KG, et al. A novel semi-automatic snake robot for natural orifice transluminal endoscopic surgery: preclinical tests in animal and human cadaver models (with video). Surg Endosc. 2015; 29(6):1643–1647

[13] Palmer D, Cobos-Guzman S, Axinte D. Real-time method for tip following navigation of continuum snake arm robots. Robot Auton Syst. 2014; 62(10):1478–1485

[14] Loeve A, Breedveld P, Dankelman J. Scopes too flexible...and too stiff. IEEE Pulse. 2010; 1(3):26–41

[15] Ota T, Degani A, Schwartzman D, et al. A highly articulated robotic surgical system for minimally invasive surgery. Ann Thorac Surg. 2009; 87(4):1253–1256

[16] Henselmans PWJ, Gottenbos S, Smit G, Breedveld P. The Memo Slide: an explorative study into a novel mechanical follow-the-leader mechanism. Proc Inst Mech Eng H. 2017; 231(12):1213–1223

[17] Fan C, Jelínek F, Dodou D, Breedveld P. Control devices and steering strategies in pathway surgery. J Surg Res. 2015; 193(2):543–553

[18] Arkenbout EA, Henselmans PWJ, Jelínek F, Breedveld P. A state of the art review and categorization of multi-branched instruments for NOTES and SILS. Surg Endosc. 2015; 29(6):1281–1296

[19] https://journals.sagepub.com/doi/10.1177/0954411919876466

50 Pathophysiology of the Failed Frontal Sinus and Its Implications for Medical Management

Li-Xing Man, Zeina Korban, and Samer Fakhri

Abstract

Recalcitrant or recurrent frontal sinus disease after sinus surgery may be due to improper patient selection as well as local and systemic causes. Surgery should be avoided when the chief complaint is sinus headache or sinus pain. Common local sources of failure include incomplete surgical dissection, the lateralized middle turbinate, neo-osteogenesis, and poor postoperative care. When there is continued frontal sinus disease despite optimal surgery and meticulous postoperative care, systemic factors must be assessed and considered in order to devise a comprehensive and effective management plan.

Keywords: aspirin-exacerbated respiratory disease, middle turbinate lateralization, neo-osteogenesis, non-steroidal anti-inflammatory drug (NSAID)-exacerbated respiratory disease, patient selection, postoperative care

50.1 Introduction

The frontal sinus poses a technical challenge with regard to surgical treatment due to its complex three-dimensional anatomy, narrow drainage pathways, proximity to critical structures, and difficult access requiring specialized angled telescopes and instrumentation. Stepwise surgical approaches have been advocated with the goal of obtaining wide frontal sinusotomies to optimize ventilation and drainage and to allow access to topical medications and nasal saline irrigation. Patient selection plays a key role in determining surgical success. Persistent or recurrent frontal sinus disease following sinus surgery is higher than in other sinuses due to multiple factors. Subsets of patients continue to suffer from mucosal edema and inflammation despite appropriate sinus surgery and optimal postoperative medical therapy. Most causes of failure of frontal sinus surgery are attributed to the surgical technique and local factors. Systemic causes may also contribute, especially in cases of suboptimal outcome despite proper surgical technique and postoperative care. In this chapter, we review patient selection, local and systemic factors that may lead to a failed frontal sinus, and the subsequent recommended medical management.

50.2 Failure due to Errors in Patient Selection

A primary principle of medicine and surgery is that a proposed therapy is most successful when the treatment goals are defined in the context of a clear diagnosis. The corollary of this axiom is that a wrong diagnosis often leads to erroneous or unnecessary interventions and thus persistence or even worsening of the condition. This is most true when we consider the indications for sinus surgery in the patient with the chief complaint of **headache and facial pain**. Unfortunately, there is a general belief among patients and many physicians, including otolaryngologists, that chronic headache and facial pain are often rhinogenic in origin. The terms "sinus headache" and "sinus pain" are ingrained in our societal and medical cultures despite a large body of evidence indicating that isolated chronic headache and facial pain are overwhelmingly primary in nature. A majority of "sinus headache" patients without significant inflammatory sinonasal findings meet diagnostic criteria for migraine.[55,2] These patients will often have rhinologic complaints that are high in symptom severity or affect them psychosocially.[3] Even when rhinosinusitis is confirmed with nasal endoscopy or computed tomography (CT), a primary headache disorder may serve as a comorbid condition. These patients may be most benefited by interdisciplinary otolaryngologic-neurologic therapy.[4]

One should recognize, however, that select sinonasal conditions that are CT and endoscopy negative may be associated with symptoms in the pain domain, such as the controversial entity of sinonasal contact points. In these instances, careful evaluation of the patient should be undertaken including referral to a neurology headache specialist. Surgery is considered an option in exceptional circumstances and is only offered when pharmacotherapy fails to relieve the symptoms. The clinical evidence supporting surgery as an effective treatment for contact point headache or facial pain is weak.[5] Unfortunately, many are too quick to perform sinus surgery on headache patients who do not have sinus disease. This has created a pool of patients with iatrogenic frontal sinus disease and persistence or worsening of their primary headache syndrome. These are the most devastated, dissatisfied, and outright angry patients encountered in our practice. Therefore, it is imperative to accurately diagnose and properly select patients for sinus surgery to prevent such failures.

50.3 Local Causes of Recalcitrant Frontal Sinus Disease

Recalcitrant isolated frontal sinus disease is most often due to a local etiology, which includes intrinsic patient factors as well as intraoperative or postoperative issues. **Frontal recess inflammatory mucosal disease** is a primary cause of failure of frontal sinus surgery.[6] Significant mucosal disease of the frontal sinus outflow tract due to microbial infections or eosinophilic inflammation at the time of surgery may lead to suboptimal mucosal healing and more vigorous scarring and neo-osteogenesis postoperatively. There is strong evidence in the literature that the use of preoperative anti-inflammatory medical therapy in this patient group leads to better perioperative mucosal healing.[7]

Patient anatomy also plays a key role. The anteroposterior dimension of the frontal recess from the nasofrontal beak to the skull base insertion of the ethmoid bulla is approximately 1 cm and correlates to the anteroposterior dimension of the agger nasi.[8] If there is a prominent nasofrontal beak or if the slope of the anterior ethmoid skull base is unfavorable, the maximum anterior-to-posterior dimensions of the frontal sinusotomy may be limited (▶ Fig. 50.1). Similarly, if the intercanthal distance is small—even if there is no clinical hypotelorism—the lateral-to-medial width of the ethmoid cavity may limit the planned sinusotomy. Short-term (1-year) frontal sinus patency after endoscopic frontal sinusotomy has been reported to range from 81 to 92%.[9,10,11,12] Fewer studies have examined long-term (>3 years) results, with reported frontal recess patency rates ranging from 68 to 88%.[13,14] Both Hosemann et al and Naidoo et al found that creating a frontal sinus ostium of at least 5 mm at the time of surgery is positively correlated with long-term patency.[9,12] In addition, restricted width of the ethmoid cavity may limit access of postoperative topical therapy and may place the middle turbinate in closer proximity to the lateral nasal wall, therefore potentially facilitating scarring.

Incomplete surgical dissection at the time of frontal sinusotomy is a common cause of recurrent or persistent disease.[49] Clearly, the extent of dissection at the time of the initial surgery should be dictated by the nature and extent of the disease. There are cases in which a complete frontal recess dissection is not warranted based on disease extent and configuration and hence a more limited frontal recess surgery would be appropriate. However, in many patients with frontal sinus/frontal recess disease, the initial dissection often falls short of accomplishing its goals of proper ventilation and drainage due to suboptimal dissection of the frontal recess. Valdes et al reviewed 109 frontal sinuses in 66 patients undergoing revision frontal sinusotomy for causes of failure. They found that retained ethmoid and frontal recess partitions contributed to the need for revision frontal sinusotomy.[6] Localized patterns of failure included retained agger nasi cell (73%), residual non–agger nasi ethmoid cells (32%; ▶ Fig. 50.2), residual frontal cells (25%), or most often a combination thereof (▶ Fig. 50.3). They classified the

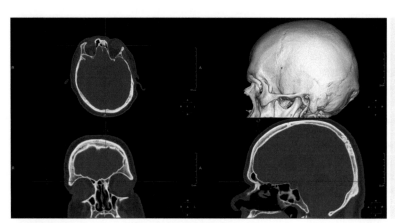

Fig. 50.1 Unfavorable frontal sinus anatomy. A prominent nasofrontal beak and unfavorable slope of the frontal sinus posterior table narrow the anterior-to-posterior dimensions of the frontal recess.

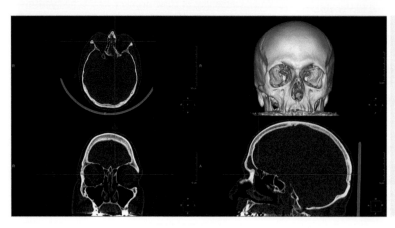

Fig. 50.2 Frontal sinus disease secondary to residual partition of a posteriorly based frontoethmoid cell.

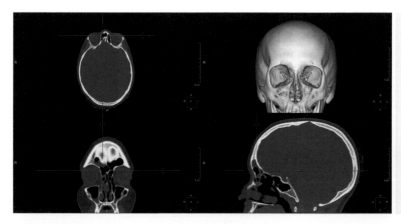

Fig. 50.3 Frontal sinus disease secondary to retained agger nasi as well as residual anterior and posterior frontoethmoid cells.

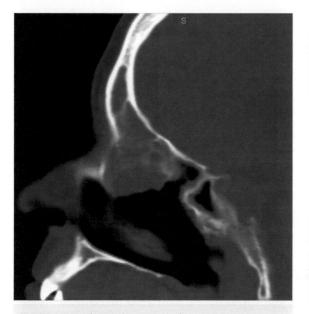

Fig. 50.4 Frontal sinus disease secondary to neo-osteogenesis in the frontal recess.

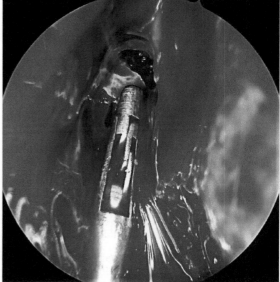

Fig. 50.5 Meticulous removal of bone fragments from the frontal recess reduces the risk of postoperative scarring and neo-osteogenesis.

residual ethmoid and frontal cells to be secondary to suboptimal surgical technique and concluded that meticulous and complete dissection is paramount to successful primary frontal sinusotomy. Similarly, Otto et al found that retained anteriorly based ethmoid cells (53%) and retained agger nasi (13%) were common findings in 298 frontal recesses undergoing revision frontal sinusotomy, with obstruction of the frontal recess directly related to prior surgery up to 75% of the time.[15]

Valdes et al found that **neo-osteogenesis** within the frontal recess (46%) was also a common cause of failure (▶ Fig. 50.4).[6] There is a paucity of data on the association between inadequate removal of debris and bone fragments from the frontal recess at the end of surgery and neo-osteogenesis after routine frontal sinusotomy. Nevertheless, residual bone dust as well as inflammatory fibrin and blood clots in the frontal recess have been proposed

as a cause of restenosis after Draf III frontal sinusotomy.[16] Bone fragments should be carefully removed during frontal sinusotomy to reduce the nidus for postoperative inflammation and neo-osteogenesis (▶ Fig. 50.5).[17] Frontal sinus punches should be cleaned regularly during the procedure to prevent spillage of free bony and mucosal fragments in the surgical field. Gentle atraumatic technique and avoidance of mucosal stripping are paramount to minimize scarring, stenosis, and neo-osteogenesis.

Scarring of a **lateralized middle turbinate** (30–48%) is another frequent finding in revision frontal sinusotomy (▶ Fig. 50.6).[6,15] One review found that middle turbinate lateralization was not associated with patient-reported symptoms but possibly led to earlier need for revision surgery.[18] A lateralized middle turbinate scarred to the lamina papyracea or lateral nasal wall may compromise

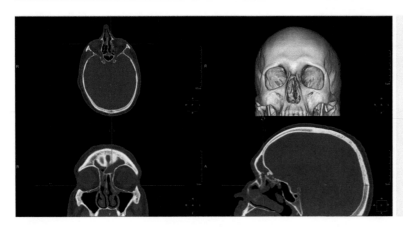

Fig. 50.6 Middle turbinate lateralization. A lateralized middle turbinate (coronal view) and neo-osteogenesis and residual frontoethmoid cell partitions (sagittal view) result in continued frontal sinus disease.

the frontal sinus outflow tract and lead to secondary frontal sinusitis. Indeed, myriad techniques for keeping the middle turbinate medialized after surgery have been described, including inducing scarring of the middle turbinate to the septum as well as the use of sutures, middle meatal spacers, and basal lamella relaxing incisions among other methods.[19,20,21,22] Nevertheless, middle turbinate lateralization continues to be cited as a leading cause for endoscopic sinus surgery failure.[22] Frontal sinus rescue, as described by Kuhn et al, is an effective method of dealing with the lateralized middle turbinate in revision frontal sinus surgery.[23,24] This technique involves removing the synechiae between the middle turbinate and the lateral structures, dissecting the mucosa off the medial and lateral aspects of the bony middle turbinate, resecting the middle turbinate bone at the skull base, and rotating the flap of frontal sinus mucosa superiorly and medially to cover the roof of the nasal vault and create a fully mucosalized frontal sinus outflow tract.[17,23,24]

Meticulous **postoperative care** may also play a role in preventing failure of frontal sinus surgery. The evidence, however, is based on endoscopic sinus surgery generally rather than specifically for postfrontal sinusotomy. A 2011 systematic review of postoperative care after endoscopic sinus surgery found that sinonasal saline irrigations started 24 to 48 hours after surgery improved short-term postoperative symptoms and endoscopic appearance.[25] Likewise, postoperative debridement is recommended for reducing the risk of synechiae formation and middle turbinate lateralization.[17,25,26] Postoperative antibiotics may reduce crusting and improve short-term symptoms, but may precipitate side effects such as gastrointestinal upset and bacterial resistance. The routine practice of prescribing postoperative antibiotics was initially adopted to prevent packing-associated toxic shock syndrome. The authors of the above-mentioned 2011 systematic review recommended the use of postoperative antibiotics,[25] but a more recent systematic review and meta-analysis did not demonstrate any statistically significant reduction in infection, symptoms, or endoscopic appearance with such practice.[27] Indeed, the

use of perioperative antibiotics is no longer recommended.[51] The use of perioperative corticosteroids reduces intraoperative blood loss and improves the quality of the surgical field, potentially shortening operative time.[52,53,54] The use of corticosteroids in the immediate postoperative period, however, has not been shown to affect long-term patient quality of life or surgical outcomes. Therefore, current practice guidelines do not advise the use of perioperative corticosteroids.[51] The use of steroid-impregnated nasal dressings may improve the early postoperative healing after surgery[28] and obviate the benefits of short-term early postoperative systemic corticosteroids.[29] More recently, the placement of a commercially available bioabsorbable steroid-releasing implant in the frontal sinus opening at the end of surgery has been shown to decrease the rate of restenosis, the need for surgical interventions, and the need for systemic steroid interventions compared to the use of no implant after surgery.[30] There has not been a comparison between the commercially available steroid-eluting implant versus other methods to deliver topical steroid locally via bioabsorbable or nonabsorbable spacers.[31] A recent study found no improvement in postoperative outcomes with the use of commercially available steroid-releasing implants versus traditional, non-resorbable middle meatal spacers.[50]

50.4 Systemic Causes of Recalcitrant Frontal Sinus Disease

A systematic diagnostic approach should be employed when refractory frontal sinusitis is encountered despite optimal surgery and appropriate postoperative care. Nasal endoscopy with assessment of the previously achieved frontal sinusotomy should be performed, noting the presence of scarring, mucosal or polypoid edema, purulence, and/or neo-osteogenesis. CT imaging is complementary to evaluate areas not visualized on endoscopy, such as the frontal sinus in a completely stenotic frontal recess. It is also used to characterize local causes of failure, including presence of middle turbinate lateralization, residual frontoethmoid cells, and neo-osteogenesis. Finally, CT evaluation helps in assessing the burden of persistent or recurrent disease. When there is continued frontal sinus disease despite the mitigation of local factors, one must consider systemic causes of recalcitrant disease. In reality, the spectrum of recurrent postoperative frontal sinus disease often encompasses both systemic and local factors. Accurate assessment of the differential contribution of each is imperative to devise a comprehensive and effective management plan.

Recalcitrant postoperative frontal sinus disease due to systemic factors may be associated with any of the clinical subtype of CRS. It is beyond the scope of this chapter to list and discuss each of the phenotypes, clinical subtypes, and endotypes, and their impact on success or failure of frontal sinus surgery.[32] However, it is important to recognize that certain clinical entities within CRS, such as **eosinophilic mucin CRS** (EMCRS) and **allergic fungal rhinosinusitis** (AFRS) portend a poorer overall prognosis and are associated with a higher refractory sinus disease and increased rate of revision surgery.[33]

A particular condition that requires special attention is **aspirin-exacerbated respiratory disease** (AERD), a subset of EMCRS with severe eosinophilic features. AERD refers to patients with asthma, CRS with nasal polyposis, and respiratory reactions to cyclooxygenase-1 (COX-1) inhibitors. Multiple studies confirm that AERD patients will have recurrent sinonasal disease following sinus surgery, often with poorer outcomes compared to patients without AERD.[34,35] Those who fail surgery and a diagnosis of AERD is suspected should undergo an aspirin challenge test. If the diagnosis of AERD is confirmed, aspirin desensitization should be considered as part of the postoperative management plan.

There is level I evidence demonstrating **aspirin desensitization** followed by high-dose aspirin therapy improves sinonasal and pulmonary symptoms while decreasing corticosteroid use.[36,37,38] Although the optimum dosage of aspirin after desensitization is unknown, aspirin 650 mg twice daily has been shown to control symptoms better than 325 mg twice daily.[39] Nevertheless, not all AERD patients will benefit from aspirin desensitization. A long-term retrospective review of 172 AERD patients undergoing desensitization found that 14% discontinued aspirin therapy due to side effects and an additional 19% did not experience any clinical improvement.[40]

Medications targeting the leukotriene pathway with **leukotriene receptor antagonists** such as montelukast or 5-lipoxygenase inhibitors such as zileuton also may be helpful. Uncontrolled studies suggest that montelukast may reduce nasal symptom scores in patients with nasal polyposis, but these studies were not limited to AERD patients.[41,42] Approximately twice as many AERD patients report that zileuton is very effective for their symptoms compared to montelukast.[43] Zileuton is less frequently prescribed, however, due to cost, concern for liver toxicity, and the need for hepatic transaminase monitoring.

The advent of humanized monoclonal antibodies targeting type 2 inflammation has altered the treatment landscape for NERD and other forms of eosinophilic CRS and nasal polyposis. Dupilumab, a monoclonal antibody targeting the Interleukin 4 (IL-4) alpha-subunit receptor, is approved for the treatment of inadequately controlled CRS with nasal polyposis, moderate-to-severe asthma, and moderate-to-severe atopic dermatitis in the United States and the European Union among other countries.[56,57] By modulating both IL-4 and IL-13, it improved endoscopic grading, Sinonasal Outcome Test (SNOT)-22, and CT imaging scores in patients with nasal polyposis.[58] Dupilumab also improved sense of smell as well as reduced the need for systemic oral corticosteroid use and sinus surgery. Patients with NERD demonstrated the greatest benefit, with significant and dramatic improvement in treatment and disease outcomes along with control of their lung function and concomitant asthma.[56,59]

Omalizumab is a humanized monoclonal antibody that inhibits free immunoglobulin E (IgE) from binding to its high-affinity receptor. In clinical trials, it reduced nasal polyp, nasal congestion, SNOT-22 scores compared with controls, resulting in omalizumab becoming the second biologic approved for the management of nasal polyposis in the United States and European Union.[60]

Monoclonal antibodies targeting IL-5 (mepolizumab, reslizumab) and IL-5-alpha receptor (benralizumab) have also shown promise in eosinophilic CRS with nasal polyposis. Multiple double-blind, placebo-controlled studies investigating mepolizumab showed statistically significant reductions in endoscopic nasal polyp scores, polyp size and improvement in sense of smell, congestion, and the need for surgery in patients with corticosteroid refractory nasal polyposis.[61,62] Post-hoc analysis of reslizumab trials for asthma indicates that reslizumab improves pulmonary function and reduces asthma exacerbations in subjects with concomitant asthma and CRS with nasal polyposis, with or without NSAID sensitivity.[63] Phase III trials are ongoing for benralizumab in the treatment of CRS with nasal polyposis.[64,65]

These new biologics potentially provide powerful new options to treat inflammatory disease to control exacerbations and reduce the need for oral corticosteroids, antibiotics, and surgery. The high cost of monoclonal antibodies, however, may limit their utility and implementation.[66,67] Indeed, cost-benefit and cost-utility analyses indicate that at current prices biologics are not cost effective for the treatment of asthma and nasal polyposis.[68,69] Moreover, one must remember that treatment of systemic inflammatory disease is not a substitute for proper surgical patient selection and fastidious surgical technique in frontal sinus surgery.

Clearly, there are many other clinical subtypes and etiologies within CRS that may be associated with recalcitrant postoperative frontal sinus disease. These include but are not limited to patients with CRS with nasal polyps, AFRS, eosinophilic granulomatosis with polyangiitis, ciliary dysmotility, common variable immunodeficiency, biofilm with pus, and others. Accurate diagnosis is critical to effective treatment implementation and often requires a high index of suspicion for unusual etiologies. Tailored and sustained medical treatment is often necessary to reverse disease recurrence and reestablish health and function to the diseased frontal sinus.

50.5 Conclusion

Surgical management of the frontal sinus is particularly challenging due to the complex and narrow confines of its anatomical drainage pathways. Proper diagnosis and patient selection before surgery is key to optimize success. The spectrum of persistent and recurrent frontal sinus disease encompasses both local factors and systemic causes. In general, failure of frontal sinus surgery due to local factors often requires revision corrective surgery. On the other hand, failure due to systemic factors calls for an appropriate medical management strategy tailored to the underlying pathophysiology.

References

[1] Schreiber CP, Hutchinson S, Webster CJ, Ames M, Richardson MS, Powers C. Prevalence of migraine in patients with a history of self-reported or physician-diagnosed "sinus" headache. Arch Intern Med. 2004; 164(16):1769–1772

[2] Patel ZM, Kennedy DW, Setzen M, Poetker DM, DelGaudio JM. "Sinus headache": rhinogenic headache or migraine? An evidence-based guide to diagnosis and treatment. Int Forum Allergy Rhinol. 2013; 3 (3):221–230

[3] Lal D, Rounds AB, Rank MA, Divekar R. Clinical and 22-item Sino-Nasal Outcome Test symptom patterns in primary headache disorder patients presenting to otolaryngologists with "sinus" headaches, pain or pressure. Int Forum Allergy Rhinol. 2015; 5(5):408–416

[4] Lal D, Rounds A, Dodick DW. Comprehensive management of patients presenting to the otolaryngologist for sinus pressure, pain, or headache. Laryngoscope. 2015; 125(2):303–310

[5] Harrison L, Jones NS. Intranasal contact points as a cause of facial pain or headache: a systematic review. Clin Otolaryngol. 2013; 38(1):8–22

[6] Valdes CJ, Bogado M, Samaha M. Causes of failure in endoscopic frontal sinus surgery in chronic rhinosinusitis patients. Int Forum Allergy Rhinol. 2014; 4(6):502–506

[7] Wright ED, Agrawal S. Impact of perioperative systemic steroids on surgical outcomes in patients with chronic rhinosinusitis with polyposis: evaluation with the novel Perioperative Sinus Endoscopy (POSE) scoring system. Laryngoscope. 2007; 117(11, Pt 2) Suppl 115:1–28

[8] Jacobs JB, Lebowitz RA, Sorin A, Hariri S, Holliday R. Preoperative sagittal CT evaluation of the frontal recess. Am J Rhinol. 2000; 14(1):33–37

[9] Hosemann W, Kühnel T, Held P, Wagner W, Felderhoff A. Endonasal frontal sinusotomy in surgical management of chronic sinusitis: a critical evaluation. Am J Rhinol. 1997; 11(1):1–9

[10] Friedman M, Landsberg R, Schults RA, Tanyeri H, Caldarelli DD. Frontal sinus surgery: endoscopic technique and preliminary results. Am J Rhinol. 2000; 14(6):393–403

[11] Chandra RK, Palmer JN, Tangsujarittham T, Kennedy DW. Factors associated with failure of frontal sinusotomy in the early follow-up period. Otolaryngol Head Neck Surg. 2004; 131(4):514–518

[12] Naidoo Y, Wen D, Bassiouni A, Keen M, Wormald PJ. Long-term results after primary frontal sinus surgery. Int Forum Allergy Rhinol. 2012; 2(3):185–190

[13] Friedman M, Bliznikas D, Vidyasagar R, Joseph NJ, Landsberg R. Long-term results after endoscopic sinus surgery involving frontal recess dissection. Laryngoscope. 2006; 116(4):573–579

[14] Chan Y, Melroy CT, Kuhn CA, Kuhn FL, Daniel WT, Kuhn FA. Long-term frontal sinus patency after endoscopic frontal sinusotomy. Laryngoscope. 2009; 119(6):1229–1232

[15] Otto KJ, DelGaudio JM. Operative findings in the frontal recess at time of revision surgery. Am J Otolaryngol. 2010; 31(3):175–180

[16] Rotenberg BW, Ioanidis KE, Sowerby LJ. Development of a novel T-tube frontal sinus irrigation catheter. Am J Rhinol Allergy. 2016; 30 (5):356–359

[17] Schaitkin BM, Man L-X. Endoscopic approach to the frontal sinus. In: Myers EN, Snyderman CH, eds. Operative Otolaryngology: Head and Neck Surgery. 3rd ed. Philadelphia, PA: Elsevier; 2017

[18] Bassiouni A, Chen PG, Naidoo Y, Wormald PJ. Clinical significance of middle turbinate lateralization after endoscopic sinus surgery. Laryngoscope. 2015; 125(1):36–41

[19] Bolger WE, Kuhn FA, Kennedy DW. Middle turbinate stabilization after functional endoscopic sinus surgery: the controlled synechiae technique. Laryngoscope. 1999; 109(11):1852–1853

[20] Chen W, Wang Y, Bi Y, Chen W. Turbinate-septal suture for middle turbinate medialization: a prospective randomized trial. Laryngoscope. 2015; 125(1):33–35

[21] Lee JM, Grewal A. Middle meatal spacers for the prevention of synechiae following endoscopic sinus surgery: a systematic review and meta-analysis of randomized controlled trials. Int Forum Allergy Rhinol. 2012; 2(6):477–486

[22] Getz AE, Hwang PH. Basal lamella relaxing incision improves endoscopic middle meatal access. Int Forum Allergy Rhinol. 2013; 3 (3):231–235

[23] Kuhn FA, Javer AR, Nagpal K, Citardi MJ. The frontal sinus rescue procedure: early experience and three-year follow-up. Am J Rhinol. 2000; 14(4):211–216

[24] Citardi MJ, Javer AR, Kuhn FA. Revision endoscopic frontal sinusotomy with mucoperiosteal flap advancement: the frontal sinus rescue procedure. Otolaryngol Clin North Am. 2001; 34(1):123–132

[25] Rudmik L, Soler ZM, Orlandi RR, et al. Early postoperative care following endoscopic sinus surgery: an evidence-based review with recommendations. Int Forum Allergy Rhinol. 2011; 1(6):417–430

[26] Orlandi RR, Kingdom TT, Hwang PH, et al. International Consensus Statement on Allergy and Rhinology: Rhinosinusitis. Int Forum Allergy Rhinol. 2016; 6 Suppl 1:S22–S209

[27] Saleh AM, Torres KM, Murad MH, Erwin PJ, Driscoll CL. Prophylactic perioperative antibiotic use in endoscopic sinus surgery: a systematic review and meta-analysis. Otolaryngol Head Neck Surg. 2012; 146 (4):533–538

[28] Côté DW, Wright ED. Triamcinolone-impregnated nasal dressing following endoscopic sinus surgery: a randomized, double-blind, placebo-controlled study. Laryngoscope. 2010; 120(6):1269–1273

[29] Dautremont JF, Mechor B, Rudmik L. The role of immediate postoperative systemic corticosteroids when utilizing a steroid-eluting spacer following sinus surgery. Otolaryngol Head Neck Surg. 2014; 150(4):689–695

[30] Smith TL, Singh A, Luong A, et al. Randomized controlled trial of a bioabsorbable steroid-releasing implant in the frontal sinus opening. Laryngoscope. 2016; 126(12):2659–2664

[31] ClinicalTrials.gov. Steroid Delivery to the Frontal Sinus Opening with a Bioabsorbable Implant vs. a Bioabsorbable Nasal Dressing. 2017. Available at: https://clinicaltrials.gov/ct2/show/results/NCT03188822. Accessed February 19, 2021

[32] Dennis SK, Lam K, Luong A. A review of classification schemes for chronic rhinosinusitis with nasal polyposis endotypes. Laryngoscope Investig Otolaryngol. 2016; 1(5):130–134

[33] Younis RT, Ahmed J. Predicting revision sinus surgery in allergic fungal and eosinophilic mucin chronic rhinosinusitis. Laryngoscope. 2017; 127(1):59–63

[34] Adelman J, McLean C, Shaigany K, Krouse JH. The role of surgery in management of Samter's triad: a systematic review. Otolaryngol Head Neck Surg. 2016; 155(2):220–237

[35] Stevens WW, Peters AT, Hirsch AG, et al. Clinical characteristics of patients with chronic rhinosinusitis with nasal polyps, asthma, and aspirin-exacerbated respiratory disease. J Allergy Clin Immunol Pract. 2017; 5(4):1061–1070.e3

[36] Stevenson DD, Pleskow WW, Simon RA, et al. Aspirin-sensitive rhinosinusitis asthma: a double-blind crossover study of treatment with aspirin. J Allergy Clin Immunol. 1984; 73(4):500–507

[37] Świerczyńska-Krępa M, Sanak M, Bochenek G, et al. Aspirin desensitization in patients with aspirin-induced and aspirin-tolerant asthma: a double-blind study. J Allergy Clin Immunol. 2014; 134(4):883–890

[38] Esmaeilzadeh H, Nabavi M, Aryan Z, et al. Aspirin desensitization for patients with aspirin-exacerbated respiratory disease: a randomized double-blind placebo-controlled trial. Clin Immunol. 2015; 160 (2):349–357

[39] Lee JY, Simon RA, Stevenson DD. Selection of aspirin dosages for aspirin desensitization treatment in patients with aspirin-exacerbated respiratory disease. J Allergy Clin Immunol. 2007; 119(1):157–164

[40] Berges-Gimeno MP, Simon RA, Stevenson DD. Long-term treatment with aspirin desensitization in asthmatic patients with aspirin-exacerbated respiratory disease. J Allergy Clin Immunol. 2003; 111 (1):180–186

[41] Kieff DA, Busaba NY. Efficacy of montelukast in the treatment of nasal polyposis. Ann Otol Rhinol Laryngol. 2005; 114(12):941–945

[42] Yelverton JC, Holmes TW, Johnson CM, Gelves CR, Kountakis SE. Effectiveness of leukotriene receptor antagonism in the postoperative management of chronic rhinosinusitis. Int Forum Allergy Rhinol. 2016; 6 (3):243–247

[43] Ta V, White AA. Survey-Defined Patient Experiences With Aspirin-Exacerbated Respiratory Disease. J Allergy Clin Immunol Pract. 2015; 3(5):711–718

[44] Bobolea I, Barranco P, Fiandor A, Cabañas R, Quirce S. Omalizumab: a potential new therapeutic approach for aspirin-exacerbated respiratory disease. J Investig Allergol Clin Immunol. 2010; 20(5):448–449

[45] Bergmann KC, Zuberbier T, Church MK. Omalizumab in the treatment of aspirin-exacerbated respiratory disease. J Allergy Clin Immunol Pract. 2015; 3(3):459–460

[46] Porcaro F, Di Marco A, Cutrera R. Omalizumab in patient with aspirin exacerbated respiratory disease and chronic idiopathic urticaria. Pediatr Pulmonol. 2017; 52(5):E26–E28

[47] Phillips-Angles E, Barranco P, Lluch-Bernal M, Dominguez-Ortega J, López-Carrasco V, Quirce S. Aspirin tolerance in patients with non-steroidal anti-inflammatory drug-exacerbated respiratory disease following treatment with omalizumab. J Allergy Clin Immunol Pract. 2017; 5(3):842–845

[48] Buchheit KM, Laidlaw TM. Update on the management of aspirin-exacerbated respiratory disease. Allergy Asthma Immunol Res. 2016; 8(4):298–304

[49] Nakayama T, Asaka D, Kuboki A, Okushi T, Kojima H. Impact of residual frontal recess cells on frontal sinusitis after endoscopic sinus surgery. Eur Arch Otorhinolaryngol. 2018 Jul;275(7):1795–1801

[50] Rawl JW, McQuaitty RA, Khan MH, et al. Comparison of steroid-releasing stents vs nonabsorbable packing as middle meatal spacers. Int Forum Allergy Rhinol. 2020 Mar;10(3):328–333

[51] Fokkens WJ, Lund VJ, Hopkins C, et al. European Position Paper on Rhinosinusitis and Nasal Polyps 2020. Rhinology. 2020 Feb 20;58 (Suppl S29):1–464

[52] Wright ED, Agrawal S. Impact of perioperative systemic steroids on surgical outcomes in patients with chronic rhinosinusitis with polyposis: evaluation with the novel Perioperative Sinus Endoscopy (POSE) scoring system. Laryngoscope. 2007;117:1–28

[53] Ecevit MC, Erdag TK, Dogan E, Sutay S. Effect of steroids for nasal polyposis surgery: a placebo controlled, randomized, double-blind study. Laryngoscope. 2015;125:2041–5

[54] Gunel C, Basak HS, Bleier BS. Oral steroids and intraoperative bleeding during endoscopic sinus surgery. B-ENT 2015;11:123–8

[55] Schreiber CP, Hutchinson S, Webster CJ, Ames M, Richardson MS, Powers C. Prevalence of migraine in patients with a history of self-reported or physician-diagnosed "sinus" headache. Arch Intern Med. 2004; 164(16):1769–1772

[56] Laidlaw TM, Mullol J, Fan C, Zhang D, Amin N, Khan A, Chao J, Mannent L; Dupilumab improves nasal polyp burden and asthma control in patients with CRSwNP and AERD. J Allergy Clin Immunol Pract. Sep-Oct 2019;7(7):2462–2465

[57] Castro M, Corren J, Pavord ID, Maspero J, Wenzel S, Rabe KF, et al. Dupilumab efficacy and safety in moderate-to-severe uncontrolled asthma. N Engl J Med 2018;378:2486–96

[58] Bachert C, Han JK, Desrosiers M, et al. Efficacy and safety of dupilumab in patients with severe chronic rhinosinusitis with nasal polyps (LIBERTY NP SINUS-24 and LIBERTY NP SINUS-52): results from two multicentre, randomised, double-blind, placebo-controlled, parallel-group phase 3 trials. Lancet. 2019;394(10209):1638–1650

[59] Laidlaw TM, Bachert C, Amin N, et al. Dupilumab improves upper and lower airway disease control in chronic rhinosinusitis with nasal polyps and asthma. Ann Allergy Asthma Immunol. 2021 Jan 16:S1081-1206(21)00020-X

[60] Gevaert P, Omachi TA, Corren J, et al. Efficacy and safety of omalizumab in nasal polyposis: 2 randomized phase 3 trials. J Allergy Clin Immunol. 2020 Sep;146(3):595–605

[61] Effect of mepolizumab in severe bilateral nasal polyps. Available at: https:// clinicaltrials.gov/ct2/show/NCT03085797. Accessed September 5, 2019

[62] Gevaert P, Van Bruaene N, Cattaert T, et al. Mepolizumab, a humanized anti-IL-5 mAb, as a treatment option for severe nasal polyposis. J Allergy Clin Immunol 2011

[63] Weinstein SF, Katial RK, Bardin P, et al. Effects of reslizumab on asthma outcomes in a subgroup of eosinophilic asthma patients with self-reported chronic rhinosinusitis with nasal polyps. J Allergy Clin Immunol Pract. 2019 Feb;7(2):589–596

[64] Efficacy and Safety Study of Benralizumab for Patients With Severe Nasal Polyposis (OSTRO). Available at: https://clinicaltrials.gov/ct2/show/NCT03401229. Accessed March 14, 2021

[65] Efficacy and Safety Study of Benralizumab in Patient With Eosinophilic Chronic Rhinosinusitis With Nasal Polyps (ORCHID). Available at: https://clinicaltrials.gov/ct2/show/NCT04157335. Accessed March 14, 2021

[66] Fokkens WJ, Lund V, Bachert C, et al. EUFOREA consensus on biologics for CRSwNP with or without asthma. Allergy. 2019 Dec;74 (12):2312–2319

[67] Roland LT, Smith TL, Schlosser RJ, et al. Guidance for contemporary use of biologics in management of chronic rhinosinusitis with nasal polyps: discussion from a National Institutes of Health-sponsored workshop. Int Forum Allergy Rhinol. 2020 Sep;10(9):1037–1042

[68] Anderson WC, Szefler SJ. Cost-effectiveness and comparative effectiveness of biologic therapy for asthma: To biologic or not to biologic? Ann Allergy Asthma Immunol . 2019 Apr;122(4):367–372

[69] Scangas GA, Wu AW, Ting JY, et al. Cost utility analysis of dupilumab versus endoscopic sinus surgery for chronic rhinosinusitis with nasal polyps. Laryngoscope. 2021 Jan;131(1):E26–E33

Index

Note: Page numbers set **bold** or *italic* indicate headings or figures, respectively.

A

accessory air cells 9, 11, **14**, 15
acute bacterial rhinosinusitis (ABRS) 325
acute viral rhinosinusitis (AVRS) 325
adenocarcinoma 226
- intestinal-type 226
aerosinusitis 156
agger nasi air cells 12, **13**, 15, 19, 26, 28, 33, 133, 333
- anterior wall 33
- anterior ethmoid 33, 43
- anterior wall removal 39
- elevating medial posterior 41
- incised uncinate process *33*
- middle meatus *38*
- posterior ethmoid *43*
agger-bullar classification (ABC) 336
allergic fungal disease **107**, 309
allergic fungal rhinosinusitis (AFRS) 70, 71, 182, **182, 183,** 375
American Academy of Otolaryngology-Head and Neck Surgery (AAOHNS) 325
American Joint Committee on Cancer staging system 230
anterior ethmoidal arteries (AEAs) 14, **14**, 20, 26, 28, 95, 111, 115, 285
- septal branch of 21
- injury 58, 65, 66, 69, 73, 74, 87, **111**, 113, 230
anterior skull base surgery
- complications 91
- overview of 87–88
- tips/tricks 91
anteroposterior (AP) distance, narrow 104
anterosuperior cells 20
antibiotics, oral 158, 163, 164, 240, 315, 348
appropriate medical therapy (AMT) 178
arterial blood oxygenation 2, 5
arterial blood supply, of frontal sinus 22
aspirin desensitization 375
aspirin exacerbated respiratory disease (AERD) 182, **182-183,** 184, 185, 272, 273, 317, 321, 346, 375
augmented reality (AR), in frontal sinus surgery 363
- Building Blocks software *364*
- Google Glass (GG) 365
- image-guided surgery (IGS) **363**
- preoperative planning **363**
- Scopis Hybrid Navigation Planning software *364*
axillary flap
- approach 38–39,104
- incision line *38*
- mucosal flap *39*

B

balloon sinus procedures (BSP) 156, 239, 304, 308, 309, 314, 321, 326, 328–330
- catheter, insertion of *311*
- complications **310**
- contraindications **309**
- controversies/opinions **307**
- diffuse vs. localized CRS **308**
- endoscopic view *317*
- illumination, external visualization of 311
- level 1 evidence **304**
- meta-analyses of standalone dilation studies 306
- miscellaneous uses **309**
- nonrandomized studies **307**
- polyp disease **309**
- preoperative preparation **309**
- published evidence **304**
- Randomized controlled trial (RCT) 305
- Randomized Evaluation of Maxillary Antrostomy versus Ostial Dilation Efficacy through Long- Term Follow-Up (REMODEL) 305
- right frontal ostium 311
- training requirements **310**
- unanswered questions
-- cost-effectiveness **311**
-- extrapolation, to wider patient cohort **312**
barosinusitis **156**, 314, 326, 328–330
- atmospheric pressure 159
- cabin maximum compression 157
- case studies, frontal headaches **159**
- clinical presentation/ investigations **156**
- epidemiology/etiology **156**
- left frontal sinusotomy, intraoperative photograph 160
- management **157**
- Weissman/Garges barotrauma classification 158
basal lamella, anterior/posterior ethmoid 41
beta-2 transferrin ((β2T) 118, 251
bilateral computer-assisted sinus surgery (BiCASS) 247
bimanual instrumentation 56, 94
Bio-Inspired Technology (BITE) 366
bipedalism 2
bleeding diathesis 114, 257
bone hyperplasia 275
bone marrow, fatty conversion 3
bone pneumatization 3
bony expansion 2, 137, 186, 246
bulla ethmoidalis (BE) 9, **15**,19
bulla intact approach **28**

C

Caicedo reverse septal flap (CRSF) 94
carboxymethylcellulose (CMC) surface 126
Castelnuovo frontal sinus probe 30
- medial wall and drainage pathway *42*
cerebrospinal fluid (CSF) 82
- anterior skull defect, transnasal endoscopic views *262*
- case studies **260**
- clinical presentation/ investigations **257**
- complications **185**, **260**
- diagnostic tools 257
- endoscopic management **256**
- endoscopic vs open repair **259**
- epidemiology/etiology **256**
-- congenital **256**
-- neoplasia **256**
-- spontaneous **257**
-- trauma **256**
- etiologies **256**
- fistulas 52, 118
- intraoperative transnasal endoscopic views *261*
- leak 13, 59, 64, 106, 229, 256
- management **258**
- meningioma, dural repair post resection of *260*
- outcomes **260**
- postprocedural adjuvants **259**
- postprocedural care **259**
- rhinorrhea 256
- surgical management
-- endoscopic **258**
-- extracranial **259**
-- intracranial **259**
cerebrovascular accident (CVA) 241
chronic invasive fungal rhinosinusitis (CIFRS) **244**, **245**
chronic obstructive pulmonary disease (COPD) 352
chronic rhinosinusitis (CRS) 26, 64, 102, 122, 161, 176, **182**, 219, 244, 275, 314, 325, 340, 351, **351**
- complications **186**
- controversies, treatment cost-effectiveness **354**
- cost and cost-effectiveness **353**
- disease-specific QOL-SNOT-22 **352**
- economic burden **351**
- economic/quality-of-life evaluation **351**
- generic QOL-EQ-5D **352**
- goals of surgery **183**
- impact of **352**
- maxillary/ethmoid sinuses **184**
- qualitative work assessing impact **353**
- quality-of-life (QOL) 161
- wider costs **352**
Chronic Rhinosinusitis Epidemiology Study (CRES) 351

chronic rhinosinusitis with nasal polyps (CRSwNP) 29, 47, 48, 50, 65, 72, 102, 109, 111, 113, 124, **134**, 135, 136, 138, 162, 176, 177,**182–186**,189, 201, 241, 245, 275, 307, 309, 316, 317, 320, 321, 325, 345, 351, 352, 354, 375
- in frontal ostium 185
- middle meatus 48
- persistent/recurrent 102
- with proptosis 186
chronic rhinosinusitis without nasal polyposis (CRSsNP) 159, 176, 241, 345
- appropriate medical therapy **178**
- epidemiology **176**
- frontal recess size **178**
- healed Draf IIb procedure/ unilateral frontal floor resection, right endoscopic view of *180*
- management **178**
- osteomeatal complex **177**
- pathophysiology **177**
- persistent frontal sinusitis, radiological images of *177*
- physiological factors **178**
- specific medical therapy **179**
- surgical management **179**
- topical medications, delivery of **178**
Chronic Sinusitis Survey (CSS) 278
Clinical Practice Research Datalink (CPRD) 351, 354
complications, frontal sinus surgery
- anterior skull base injury/ cerebrospinal fluid leak 118
- bleeding **115**
- cases navigation systems 113
- endoscopic approaches 113, **113**
- epidemiology/etiology **113**
- failure to accomplish **113**
- infection **116**
- mucocele formation **117**
- orbital injury **119**
- overview of **113**
- pain **115**
- prevention of **119**
-- perioperative technique **120**
-- postoperative care **120**
- scar/stenosis **117**
computer-assisted surgery 28 *34, 37, 43, 47, 49*
concha bullosa, middle meatus 46
continuous positive airway pressure (CPAP) 259
coronal approach 21, 22
corticosteroid 103, 114, 115, 120, 126, 129, 130, 131, 138, 144, 163, 178, 179, 240, 244, 308, 354, 374, 375
- intranasal 120, 126, 130, 178

– oral 103, 144, 354, 375
cranialization 151,**152**, 153, 190, 233, 239, 251–253, 259, 283
craniomaxillofacial (CMF) fractures 250
cribriform plate, lateral lamella 13, 84
crista olfactoria 23
cyclooxygenase-1 (COX-1) inhibitors 182, 321, 375
cyclooxygenase-2 (COX-2) inhibitors 115
cystic fibrosis (CF) 161, 182
– clinical presentation/ investigations **161**
– complications **169**
– corticosteroids **163**
– dornase alfa **164**
– Draf IIb, hand instrument *167*
– endoscopic approaches **165**
– epidemiology/etiology **161**
– medical therapy **163**
– nasal saline irrigations **163**
– oral antibiotics **164**
– radiographic abnormalities **162**
– surgical therapy **164**
– transnasal endoscopic view *169*
cystic fibrosis transmembrane conductance regulator (CFTR) modulators **164**

D

Draf frontal sinusotomy
– case examples **28**
– complications management **47**
– surgical steps **26**
Draf I 107, **315**
– classification **27**
Draf IIa 47, 52, 65, 71, 87, *88*, 105, 113, 114, 117, 123, 125, 174, 179, 182, 184, **185**, 192, 219, 223, 238, 239, 253, 269, 285, 300, 314, **315**, 317, 342, 344, 346, **347**, 348, 349, *350*
– anatomy **52**
– bone resection *52*
– complications **53**
– lateral approach **52**
– median approach **52**
– olfactory filament *53*
– Samter's triad 185
Draf IIb 82
– anterior ethmoid artery injury **58**
– approach 220
– case studies **57**
– cerebrospinal fluid (CSF) leak **57**
– complications **57**
– difficulties, tips 57, **57**
– illustration of *54*
– indications **54**
– modifications of **55**
– modified central-lothrop procedure (Eloy IIF) **56**
– modified hemi-lothrop procedure (Eloy IIC) **55**
– modified mini-lothrop procedure (Eloy IID) **55**
– modified subtotal-lothrop procedure (Eloy IIE) **55**
– orbital injury **58**
– overview of **54**
– recurrence/chronic scarring **57**

Draf III (endoscopic modified lothrop) **64**
– anterior ethmoidal nerve *68*
– anterior frontal sinus wall, visualization of *67*
– anterior septectomy *66*
– approach 220
– in allergic fungal sinusitis 185
– case studies
–– chronic frontal sinusitis, with a high posterior frontal cell **71**
–– chronic frontal sinusitis-Riedel's procedure reversal **72**
– complications **73**, *74*
–– hemorrhage *73*
–– orbital injury *74*
–– skin injury *74*
–– skull base injury, cerebrospinal fluid leak *74*
– contraindications **64**
– ethmoidal slit/cribroethmoidal foramen *68*
– frontal sinus neo-ostium, stenosis of *74*
– indications **64**
– landmarks *67*
– lateral-to-medial/inside-out technique **64**
–– bilateral Draf IIa 65
–– flaps, harvesting of 65
–– middle turbinate, axilla of 66
–– nasal beak, bone of 66
–– partial anterior septectomy 65
– laterally based flap, anterior incisions of *65*
– lothrop procedure, modifications of 54, 55, 56, 82, 87, 114, 117, 118, 209, 219, 233, 239, 283, 299, 321, 340, 343, 347, 349
– medially based middle turbinate flap *65*
– nasal beak, drillout of *67*
– outside-in/medial-to-lateral technique **66**
–– anterior skull base 69
–– harvesting mucosal flaps 69
–– natural ostium, joining up 70
–– neo-ostium, maximize 70
–– septal window 69
– patient's nasal symptoms 71
– posterior wall, drillout of *67*
– postoperative management *72*
– preoperative/postoperative computational fluid dynamic models *124*
– Samter's triad 184
– silastic sheet, placement of *69*
– surgical steps **64**
drilling, frontal sinus
– approaches of **340–341**
– classic indications of 340
– complications **342**
– controversies/opinions **342**
– published evidence **340**
– results 341

E

endonasal approaches, anatomy **18**
endonasal endoscopic surgery (EES) **283**
– cerebrospinal fluid leaks **285**
– far lateral frontal sinus surgery, evolution of **285**

endoscopic endonasal orbital transposition 81, 83
– contraindications 81
– ethmoidal roof, with anterior ethmoidal artery *85*
– lateral frontal sinus lesions 81
– posterior wall, erosion of 82
– sinonasal lesion, MRI in T1 sequence *84*
– technical solutions 84
endoscopic endonasal technique
– cadaveric dissection performing *83*
– case studies **83**
– complications
–– CSF leak *84*
–– damage of trochlea *86*
–– retrobulbar hemorrhage *86*
– ethmoidal roof, intraoperative endoscopic view *102*
– indications **81**
– intraoperative endoscopic view *84*
– nasal fossa, MRI in T1 sequence **101**
– surgical steps **82**
– tips/tricks **83**
endoscopic frontal sinus surgery (EFSS) 6, 59, 107, **107**
– grades 1–3 **107**
– *See also* Lothrop procedure
eosinophilic mucin CRS (EMCRS) 375
eosinophilic mucinous fungal rhinosinusitis (EFRS) 244
epidural abscesses 235
ethmoid sinus 2
– formation mechanisms 9
– lamina papyracea 12
– olfactory cartilaginous capsule 2
ethmoidal bulla (EB) 26
– anterior and posterior ethmoid *41*
– frontal recess, upper boundary of *333*
ethmoidectomy, gas bolus *4*
ethmoturbinals 9
European Position Paper on Rhinosinusitis (EPOS) 18, 157
European Position Paper on Rhinosinusitis and Nasal Polyps (EPOS2012) 162
evo-devo theory 12, 15
expanded endoscopic endonasal approaches (EEAs)
– anterior skull base approaches **93**
– case studies, esthesioneuroblastoma (transcribriform approach) **96**, *97*
– complications/management **96**, *99*
–– cerebrospinal fluid fistulas *99*
–– cranial nerves injury *99*
–– postoperative infection *99*
–– vascular complications *96*
– indications **93**
– inverted U *95*
– operative setup *94*
– postoperative considerations **95**
– principles **93**
– reconstruction **95**
– surgical technique **94**
– tips/tricks *96*

– transcribriform approach **94**
– transplanum/transtuberculum approach **95**
– tuberculum sellae meningioma, endoscopic transtuberculum/ transplanum approach **96**
eyelid
– schematic drawings of *23*
– superior eyelid approach 23

F

facial pain 161, 162, 173, *189*, 207, 221, 245, 246, 325, 328, 329, 371
facial trauma 78, 119, 309
failure, frontal sinus
– errors, in patient selection **371**
– medical management, implications **371**
– overview of **371**
– pathophysiology of **371**
– recalcitrant frontal sinus disease
–– local causes of **371**
–– systemic causes of **374**
fibro-osseous lesions 217–218, **284**
– approaches **222**
– characteristics of 218
– clinical presentation/ investigations **221**
–– histology **222**
–– radiological features **221**
– consent **222**
– fibrous dysplasia 217
–– anatomical locations **218**
–– clinical presentation/ investigations **218**
–– epidemiology/etiology **217**
–– malignancy **219**
–– pathology **218**
–– radiological features **218**
– management **219**, **222**
–– conservative **219**
–– surgical indications **219**
– ossifying fibroma **220**
–– anatomical locations **220**
–– characteristics/growth/variants **220**
–– epidemiology/etiology **220**
–– post-operative care **224**
– surgical steps **222**
fibroma, cemento-ossifying 220
fibrous dysplasia (FD) 6, 81, 142, 153, 173, 174, 217, **217**, 219, 277
flaps, frontal sinus surgery
– case studies
– difficult flap elevation **272**
–– Draf IIb, single flap **271**
–– Draf IIc, double flaps **271**
–– Draf III, double flaps **272**
– controversies/opinions
–– flaps feasibility **271**
–– future studies **270**
–– promising outcome, for flaps **270**
– local mucoperiosteal flaps 271
– posterior-based nasoseptal flap 269
– published evidence
–– background **268**
–– literature review/surgical techniques **269**

-- rationale for flaps 268
- septoturbinal flap elevation 270
- surgical tips **273**
Flexner-Wintersteiner rosettes 228
follow-the-leader (FTL)
    propagation 368
forced expiratory volume in 1
    second (FEV1) 164
frontal bullar cells (FBC) 76, 157,
    333
frontal nasal sinus drainage
    pathway (FSDP) 11, 26, 32
frontal recesses (FR) 18, 26, 28, 38
- anterior ethmoid 32
- computer-assisted surgery *34*
- endoscopic view of 91
- ethmoidal bulla 34
- frontal sinus opening *36*
- incomplete dissection *115*
- inflammatory mucosal disease
    371
frontal sinus drainage pathway
    (FSDP) 165
- intact supra bulla cell *32*
- with intact supra bulla cell *31*
frontal sinus rescue (FSR)
    procedure 59, 222
- complications **60**
- healed frontal sinus *62*
- overview of **59**
- reverse procedure **60**
- revision FSR procedure 59
- right paranasal sinuses, coronal
    views of *61*
- right/left postoperative frontal
    sinus 62
- surgical steps **59**
- tips/tricks **62**
frontal sinus surgery
- asthma/polyps/EMCRS,
    frequency of 346
- augmented reality 363
- case studies
-- anterior ethmoidectomy **346**
-- Draf IIa-ciliary dysfunction **348**
-- failed Draf I procedure **348**
-- evidence **344, 346–347**
-- odontogenic frontal CRS **348**
-- opinion **345–347**
-- mild diffuse CRSwNP **348**
-- patent frequency 345
-- surgical intervention **347**
-- clinical characteristics **346**
-- evidence **346**
-- opinion **346**
- controversies/opinions **344**
- cost-effectiveness acceptability
    355
- indications for operating **344**
- mucociliary flow *344*
- OMC/frontal recess obstruction
    344
- overview of **344**
frontoethmoidal cells 20, 28, *32,
    33, 45–47,* 65, 165, **177,** 191,
    309, 310, **333,** 335, *336, 337*
- agger-bullar classification 336
- anatomy/classification of **333**
- frontal cell types I to IV 333
- frontal pneumatization 334
- Kuhn's classification 338
functional endoscopic sinus
    surgery (FESS) 26, 109, 158,
    183, *186,* 238, 256, 304, 320,
    348
fungal frontal sinusitis

- allergic and nonallergic **244**
- bony expansion *246*
- case studies **247**
- clinical presentation/
    investigations
-- acute invasive fungal
    rhinosinusitis **245**
-- chronic invasive fungal
    rhinosinusitis **245**
-- eosinophilic mucinous
    rhinosinusitis **245**
-- granulomatous invasive fungal
    sinusitis **245**
-- sinus mycelia **246**
- complications **247**
- epidemiology/etiology **244**
-- acute invasive fungal
    rhinosinusitis **244**
-- chronic invasive fungal
    rhinosinusitis **244**
-- eosinophilic fungal sinus
    disease **244**
-- sinus mycelia **244**
- medical management **247**
- Philpott-Javer endoscopic
    staging system 247, 248
- surgical and postoperative
    management **247**

G

Gasket seal procedure 213
Glasgow Benefit Inventory
    (GBI) 320
Global Osteitis Scoring Scale
    (GOSS) 275, 277

H

Hadad-Bassagaisteguy flap
    (HBF) 94
Haemophilus influenzae 233
Hajek-Koffler punch 105
Haller's air cells 12
Hospital Episode Statistics
    (HES) 351

I

image-guided surgery (IGS) 283,
    299, 363
- anterior ethmoid osteoma
    obstructing *302*
- applications **300**
- clinical/quality-of-life outcomes
    301
- complications **300**
- controversies/opinions **301**
- cost **301**
- Draf III sinusotomy *302*
- future use **301**
- indications **299, 301**
- medicolegal concerns **301**
- position statement 299
- published evidence **300**
- revision rate **300**
- surgical training **301**
immunoglobulin E (IgE) 375
In-Office Sinus dilation (ORIOS II)
    study 307
incremental cost-effectiveness
    ratio (ICER) 354
inflammation-induced osteoblastic
    activity 103

infundibulum 4, 10, 13, 15, 18, 19,
    22, 26, 50, 52, 177, 250, 309,
    340, 345
inter-frontal sinus septal cell (ISSC)
    14, 28, 333
International Civil Aviation
    Organization (ICAO) Standard
    158
International Classification of
    Complexity(ICC) 101
International Frontal Sinus
    Anatomy Classification (IFAC)
    27, 59, 335, 358
inverted papilloma (IP) 64, 76, 81,
    83, 84, 134, 142, 144, **205, *206,
    208, 209,* 211,** 212-214, 270,
    282–284, *289, 290, 297*
- case studies 211
-- IP, excisional biopsy of 211
-- left respiratory nasal
    obstruction and epistaxis 211
-- recurrent left frontoethmoidal
    IP 211
- clinical presentation/
    investigations 207
- complications 212, 214
- Draf type III frontal sinusotomy,
    endoscopic intraoperative
    view 210
- epidemiology/etiology 205
-- endoscopic endonasal
    approaches 214
-- inverted papilloma of 206
-- surgical treatment 206
- gadolinium enhancement,
    preoperative and postoperative
    MR imaging 213
- inverted papilloma vegetating,
    endoscopic view of 212
- management 208
- preoperative MR imaging
    213–214

K

Kuhn-Bolger frontal sinus curette
    36

L

lamina papyracea (LP) 9, **12,** 26
lateral lesions, extreme
- complications 283
- controversies/opinions **287**
-- cerebrospinal fluid leaks **285**
-- far lateral frontal sinus surgery,
    evolution of **285**
-- fibro-osseous lesions **284**
-- inverted papillomas **284**
-- mucoceles **283**
- endoscopic approaches, lateral
    limits of 294
- inverted papilloma patient
    289–290
- isolated lateral supraorbital
    mucocele *291*
- lateral frontal sinus lesions 288
- published evidence **282**
- suspicious left-sided far lateral
    frontal sinus lesion *292*
- traditional external approaches
    282
Lund-Mackay score (LMS) 325,
    341

Lund-MacKay(LM) classification
    307
Lynch-Howarth approach 239

M

malignant disease
- case studies **231**
- clinical presentation/
    investigation **229**
- complications **231**
- epidemiology/etiology
    226
- esthesioneuroblastoma *229*
- fascia lata graft, defect closed
    231
- Hyams' grading scale 229
- lateral rhinotomy, operative
    exposure *230*
- management **230**
- staging **230**
Manufacturer and User
    Facility Device Experience
    (MAUDE) 311
maxillary sinus mucosa biopsy 4
mean arterial pressure (MAP) 97
median drainage 27, 82, 153, 197,
    283, 287
Medical Expenditure Panel Survey
    (MEPS) 351
middle meatus 13, 19, 34, *37-39,
    48,* 107, 126, 131, 162, 177, 208,
    212, 236, 250, 309, 348, *361*
middle turbinate (MT) 9, *10,* **15,**
    26, 28, 59
middle turbinate lateralization
    102, 114, 115, 126, 133,
    373–375
mucoceles, frontal sinus
- classification **189**
- clinical presentation **188**
- epidemiology **188**
- extra-frontal mucocele
    extension 189
- frontal drainage pathway,
    narrow AP dimension of *191*
- investigations **189**
- management algorithm **190,**
    192
- medial presentation, in
    parasagittal plane *190*
- outcomes **193**
- pathology **188**
- radiological classification of
    190
- terminology **187**
multilayer technique 85, 214
multiplanar reconstruction (MPR)
    336, *337*

N

National Institute for Health and
    Care Excellence (NICE) 351
natural orifice transluminal
    endoscopic surgery (NOTES)
    368
NO synthetase (NOS)
- calcium-independent isoform
    of 4
- nasal administration 4
neuroendocrine small cell
    carcinoma *227*

O

office-based frontal sinus procedures **133**
- anatomic considerations **133**
- balloon catheter dilation **138**
- case studies
-- frontal mucoceles **136**
-- nasal polyps **138**
- controversies **138**
- emerging technologies **139**
- frontal mucocele-intact bulla approach **134**, *137*
- nasal irrigations/topical therapies **136**
- nasal polyps **134**
- outpatient endoscopic frontal polypectomy *138*
- patient selection **133**
- postoperative management/ procedures **135**
- surgical steps **135** **136**
optimization and refinement of technique in in-Office sinus dilation (ORIOS) 138
orbital abscess 233–237, **241**
orbital cellulitis 12, 70, 200, 233, 235, 240, 241, 272
orbital, medial and superior decompression 286
ossifying fibroma (OF) 64, 81, 217, 218, **220**, *221*
- consent
- epidemiology and etiology **220**
- juvenile psammomatoid OF 220
- juvenile trabecular OF 220
- management **222**
- surgical steps **222**
osteitis/frontal sinus
- case studies **279**
- clinical implications **278**
- clinical presentation/ investigations **277**
-- radiological features, in CT **277**
-- radiological features, on SPECT **278**
- epidemiology/etiology **275**
-- allergy **276**
-- bacteriology **276**
-- biofilms **277**
-- definitions **275**
-- incidence **277**
-- pathophysiology **275**
- management **278**
- prognostic factor **278**
osteomas, frontoethmoidal **195**
- case studies **200**
-- acute frontal sinusitis **202**
-- giant frontal osteoma **202**, **202**
-- left frontal headaches **200**, **202**
- clinical presentation/ investigations **196**
- contraindications to endoscopic approach 200
- endoscopic approach, limits of **197**
- epidemiology/etiology **195**
- external approaches **197**
- frontal osteoma, through anterior frontal plate *196*
- frontal sinus osteoma grading system 198
- histology **196**
- management **196**
- osteoma, drilling of *201*
- pneumocephalus *197*

- surgery, in osteomas *198*
- typical osteoma removal *196*
osteomyelitis, acute
- anatomical and pathological causes of 234
- ARS complications
-- classification of 233
-- surgical intervention 240
- case studies
-- cerebral abscess **241**
-- epidural abscess **241**
-- external drainage 242
-- orbital abscess **241**
-- subdural abscess **241**
-- subperiosteal abscess **241**
- cerebral abscess CT *237*
- clinical presentation/ investigations **234**
- epidemiology/etiology **233**
- epidural abscess *238*
- etiology **234**
- frontal sinus drainage techniques **238**
- intracranial complications **235**, 236
-- management of **240**
-- orbital **233-234**, **240**
- investigations **236**
- orbital abscess 237
- osseous complications **236**, **241**
osteoplastic flap (OPF) 64, 76, 82, 83, **147**, 148, 150, 153, 154, 188, 190, 197, 198, 202, 209, 230, 233, 239, 247, 252, 259, 284, 300, 340
- bicoronal incision *148*
- Caldwell X-ray *149*
- complications **150**
- indications **147**
- sinusoidal bicoronal incision *148*
- surgical approaches/ advantages/ disadvantages 147, 284
- tips/tricks **150**
- with obliteration **147**, **149**
- without obliteration **147**
-- anterior table, removal of **148**
-- exposure **148**
-- preparation **147**

P

paranasal sinuses
- blood oxygenation **3**
- function of **5**
- nitric oxide **3**
patient-reported outcome measures (PROMS) 307, **320**
- acute rhinosinusitis, nasal endoscopy 328
- controversies/opinions **321**
- in frontal sinus treatment **321**
- in rhinology **320**
- left trigeminal nerve, MRI demonstrating vascular compression *331*
- middle turbinate/ethmoid cell *327*
- nasal endoscopy *327, 329*
- studies summary **322**
pneumosinus dilatans (PD) 5, 169, **173**

- clinical presentation/ investigations 173
- complications **174**
- diagnosis 173
- epidemiology/etiology 173
- management **174**
- overview of **173**
postoperative management 130
- absorbable packings 127
- dressings and toilet 126
- drug-eluting stents **129**
- endoscopic debridement 130
- frontal drillout cavity, intraoperative image of *127*
- inert stents **129**
- intranasal packing **126**
- nonabsorbable packs **126**
- office-based frontal sinus procedures **135**
- pack/not to pack **128**
- packing materials, selection *128*
- saline irrigations **130**
- sinus ostia, natural history of **126**
- topical treatments 130-131
Pott's puffy tumor 142, 234, 276, *239*, **241**

Q

quality-adjusted life years (QALYs) 355
quality-of-life (QOL) 161, 300, **301**, 307, 315, **351**, 352

R

randomized controlled trial (RCT) 304, 305, 321, 347, 351, 355
Randomized Evaluation of Maxillary Antrostomy versus Ostial Dilation Efficacy through Long-Term Follow-Up (REMODEL) trial 304, 305, 306, 312
recessus terminalis (TR) 13, 15, 19, 309, 333, 335
revision endoscopic frontal sinus surgery **101**
- axillary flap technique **105**
- case studies **109**
- choice of procedure **104**
- complications
-- anterior ethmoid artery **111**
-- cerebrospinal fluid leak **112**
-- frontal sinus surgery 101, 104, 111, 182, 184
-- orbital injury **112**
-- scarring/restenosis **111**
- computer-assisted navigation, during surgery **104**
- endoscopes/equipment **104**
- frontal sinus mini-trephine **106**
-- International classification of complexity 102
- incomplete dissection **102**
- indications **101**
- middle turbinate, lateralization of **102**
- narrow frontal ostium/ extensive supra agger/bulla frontal cells **107**
- neo-osteogenesis **103**
- ongoing mucosal disease **102**

- overview of **101**
- patient selection **103**
- pedicled flap/initial rolled flap *108*
- preoperative planning **104**
- retained cells, in frontal recess/ extending **107**
- scarring/synechiae **103**
- tips/tricks **109**
rhinorrhea 83, 103, 158, 161, *197*, 207, 211, 229, 231, 251, 256, 257, 271, 326
Rhinosinusitis Disability Index (RSDI) 278, 321
rhinosinusitis outcome measure (RSOM) scores 162, 278, 301
Riedel's procedure
- and cranialization of 151
- frontal sinus, cranialization of **151**
- historic perspective/literature review/main indications **151**
-- indications **152**
-- technique **152**
- patient post cranialization *153*
- surgical steps *152*
robotic surgery
- bone fragments, meticulous removal of *373*
- clinical practice **369**
- controversies/opinions **367**
- DaVinci **366-367**
- DragonFlex, prototype *367*
- future steps **369**
- HelixFlex
-- close-up of *368*
-- functions 368
-- prototype of *368*
- I-Flex, prototype of *367*
- maneuvering **367**
- MemoFlex
-- prototype of *369*
- snake **368**
- steering
-- at greater simplicity **366**
-- at reduced dimensions **367**

S

Sinus Allergy and Migraine Headache Study (SAMS) 326
squamous cell carcinoma (SCC) 82, 83, 205, 226, *227*
suction-powered microdebrider (PolypVac) 138
superficial muscular aponeurotic system (SMAS) 21
supra agger cell 19
- bulla frontal cell 19
- frontal cell 19
supra agger frontal cell
-- access **46**
-- medial posterior *48*
- identification of *46, 48*
- posterior wall
-- identifying **36**
-- removing of **36**
- Stammberger circular cutting punch *49*
supra bulla cell (SBC) 19, 28, 133, 333
- frontal cell
-- computer-assisted surgery *43*
-- exposure of *42*
-- removal 43

surgical sinusotomy, minimum vs. maximal
- balloon dilation **314**
- case studies **316**
-- aspirin-exacerbated respiratory disease (AERD) 317
-- headache and frontal sinusitis 317
-- left forehead and periorbital pain 316
- controversies/opinions 316
- published evidence 314
symptoms, frontal sinus disease **325**
- case studies
-- coronary artery disease 327
-- frontal headache, complaints of **330**
-- post-OP nasal endoscopy **328**
-- recurrent sinus infections 328
-- trigeminal nerve, compression of **330**
- controversies/opinions 326
- diagnoses causing symptoms **326**
- published evidence **325**

T

terminal recess (TR) 18, 19, 26, 52, 309, 335
topical antibiotics **131**, **163**, 164, 179
topical therapy
- distribution 122
- to frontal sinus 122
- tips/tricks 125
training models/techniques, in frontal sinus surgery
- controversies/opinions **360**
- mimics program *360*
- overview of **358**
- published evidence **358**

- scopis program, preoperative surgical planning *359*
- Styrofoam head, printed model *361*
- user performing sphenoidotomy, virtual view of *360*
- virtual reality simulator *359*
transseptal approach
- advantages **77**
- background **76**
- disadvantages **77**
- indications/contraindications **76**
- surgical steps **77**
transseptal frontal sinusotomy (TSFS)
- advantages **77**
- background **76**
- case studies **78**
- complications **78**
- disadvantages **77**
- indications/contraindications **76**
- point of difficulty 79
- surgical steps 78
- tips/tricks **78**
trephines, mini/maxi **142**
- case studies **144**
- closure 143
- complications **144**
- frontal sinus trephination 143
- incision/soft tissue 142
- indications **142**
- left frontal sinus, lumen of *143*
- skin hooks *143*
- surgical planning 142
- tips/tricks **144**
- modified central-lothrop procedure (Eloy IIF) **56**
- modified endoscopic Lothrop procedure (MELP) 87

- modified hemi-Lothrop procedure (Eloy IIC) 55, **55**, 82
- modified mini-Lothrop procedure (Eloy IID) **55**, *56*
- modified subtotal-Lothrop procedure (Eloy IIE) **55**, *56*, 82
trauma, frontal sinus
- case studies **253**
- clinical presentation **251**
- complications **253**
- epidemiology/etiology **250**
-- anatomy **250**
-- trauma mechanism **250**
- frontal sinus fractures, guideline for primary treatment *253*
- imaging/paraclinical investigations **251**
- management **251**
- surgical decision-making **252**
- surgical techniques **251**

U

uncinate process (UP) 9, **12**, 18, 26, *29–30*, 35
- anterior and posterior ethmoid *34, 37, 41*
- anterior wall *40*
- Blakesley forceps *30*
- bony lamellas, removing *31*
- dissecting remnants *31*
- medial posterior wall, dissecting/elevating *33*
- postsurgery middle meatus/anterior ethmoid *34*
- removing remnants *31*
- specimen of *30*
- swinging door technique *30*
undifferentiated sinonasal carcinoma 227

V

virtual reality (VR)
- in frontal sinus surgery, preoperative planning **363**
- surgical simulators 358
Visual Analog Score (VAS) 306, 321

W

Wormald frontal sinus malleable instruments 104

1

12-Item Short Form Survey (SF-12) 352

2

20-Item Sinonasal Outcome Test (SNOT-20) 320
22-item Sino-Nasal Outcome Test (SNOT-22) score 138, 346

3

31-item rhinosinusitis outcome measure (RSOM-31) 320
36-Item Short Form Survey (SF-36) 320

5

5-level EQ-5D version (EQ-5D-5L) 352